BASIC AND CLINICAL NUTRITION

Editors

W. P. T. JAMES

Director
Dunn Clinical Nutrition Centre
Addenbrookes Hospital
Cambridge, England

ROBERT H. HERMAN

Chief, Endocrine - Metabolic Service
Department of the Army
Letterman Army Medical Center
San Francisco, California

GEORGE A. BRAY

Professor of Medicine
Harbor/UCLA Medical Center
Torrance, California

Vol. 1   Vitamin E   A Comprehensive Treatise, *edited by Lawrence J. Machlin*

Vol. 2   Vitamin D   Molecular Biology and Clinical Nutrition, *edited by Anthony W. Norman   (In Preparation)*

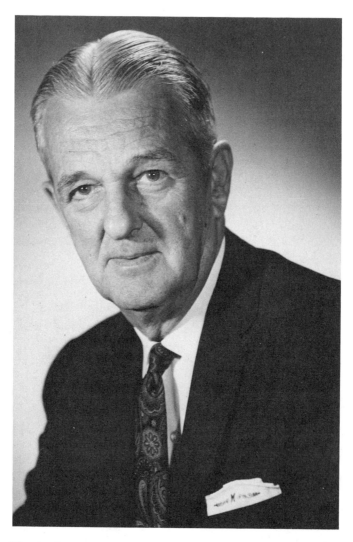

This book is dedicated to Dr. Karl E. Mason, who devoted most of his professional life to the investigation of the effects of vitamin E deficiencies in animals. His studies, spanning five decades, were classic examples of careful, well-controlled, and well-written experiments; and they have served as the foundation for much of the work presented here.

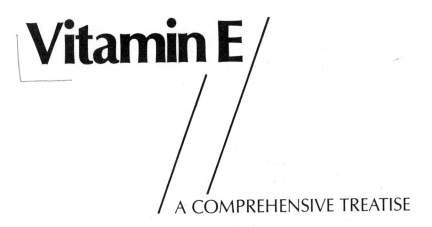

Vitamin E

A COMPREHENSIVE TREATISE

Edited by

Lawrence J. Machlin

Department of Clinical Nutrition
Hoffmann-La Roche Inc.
Nutley, New Jersey

MARCEL DEKKER, INC.   New York and Basel

Library of Congress Cataloging in Publication Data
Main entry under title:

Vitamin E : A Comprehensive Treatise.

(Basic and clinical nutrition ; v. 1)
Includes index.
1. Vitamin E. I. Machlin, Lawrence J. , [date]
II. Series. [DNLM: 1. Vitamin E. W1 CL741 / QU179
V837]
QP772. T6V57   612'. 399   80-12467
ISBN 0-8247-6842-6

MARCEL DEKKER, INC.

270 Madison Avenue, New York, New York 10016

Current printing (last digit):
10 9 8 7 6 5 4 3 2 1

PRINTED IN THE UNITED STATES OF AMERICA

PREFACE

There is more myth and controversy concerning vitamin E than any other single nutrient. This confusion reflects the many gaps in our knowledge of this vitamin. In addition, communication between the various authorities is poor. Clinicians are often unaware of the many studies describing the biochemical and pathological consequences of feeding vitamin E-deficient diets to laboratory animals, or of the many observations [1, 2] of the symptoms of vitamin E deficiency in farm animals fed natural rations. On the other hand, nutritionists and biochemists are not acquainted with the many clinical observations in which vitamin E status has been found to be important.

There is still some disagreement on how the vitamin functions at the cellular and molecular level, on its nutritional role, and on the therapeutic usefulness of the vitamin. However, scientific efforts are continuing at a sufficient rate to justify five conferences concerning this vitamin since 1971 [2-6]. Indeed, recent experimentation has clarified many of the issues and problems concerning this vitamin. For example, the relationship of polyunsaturated acids and selenium to vitamin E has been elucidated. Increasingly sophisticated studies on the structure and function of subcellular particles and cell membranes are advancing our understanding of the cellular role of vitamin E. Recent studies on the role of vitamin E in the immune process, in platelet physiology, in hemolytic anemias, and in protection against environmental pollutants has further added to the interest in this vitamin. Moreover, the role of vitamin E in anemia in premature infants, in malabsorption, and in intermittent claudication is increasingly being recognized.

Although several good reviews of many aspects of vitamin E are available [7-11], there is no single comprehensive source of current information concerning this vitamin. In the following monograph, we hope to provide such a source which will be useful to nutritionists, biochemists, students, clinicians and others who seek an objective, comprehensive, and authoritative reference on vitamin E.

I would like to thank Dr. Jack C. Bauernfeind and Dr. Myron Brin for much useful advice and encouragement in the preparation of this book. In addition, the excellent editorial assistance of Ms. Lynda Horn is gratefully acknowledged, as well as the help of Dr. H. Ronald Kaback, Dr. Nathan Brot, Dr. George Cardinale, Dr. Lester Packer, Dr. Herbert Sheppard, and Dr. Stanley Shapiro, who also reviewed several of the manuscripts.

Lawrence J. Machlin

1. N. Lannek, Wissenshaft. Veroff. Deutsch. Gesell. Ernahr. 16:145-160 (1967).
2. J. Moustagaard and J. Hyldgaard-Jensen (eds.), Acta Agric. Scand. (Suppl. 19:11-128) (1973).
3. P. P. Nair and H. J. Kayden, Ann. N.Y. Acad. Sci. 203:1-247 (1972).
4. M. K. Horwitt (ed.), Amer. J. Clin. Nutr. 27:939-1194 (1974).
5. N. Shimazono and Y. Takagi (eds.), International Symposium on Vitamin E. Tokyo, Kyoritsu Shuppan Co., 1972.
6. C. de Duve and O. Hayaishi (eds.), International Symposium on Tocopherol, Oxygen, and Biomembranes, Sept. 2-3, 1977, Lake Yamanaka, Japan, Elsevier, Amsterdam, 1977.
7. The Vitamins, Vol. 5. Edited by W. H. Sebrell and R. S. Harris. New York, Academic, 1972, pp. 165-317.
8. H. H. Draper, in Fat-Soluble Vitamins. Edited by R. A. Morton. New York, Pergamon, 1970, pp. 333-393.
9. J. G. Bieri, Nutr. Rev. 33:161-167 (1975).
10. M. L. Scott, in Fat-Soluble Vitamins. Edited by H. F. De Luca. New York, Plenum, 1978, pp. 133-210.
11. J. G. Bieri and P. Farrell, Vit. Horm. 34:31-75 (1976).

CONTRIBUTORS

JACK BAUERNFEIND, M.S., Ph.D.[1] Nutrition Research Coordinator, Biochemical Nutrition Department, Roche Research Center, Hoffmann-La Roche Inc., Nutley, New Jersey

GEORGE L. CATIGNANI, Ph.D.[2] Staff Fellow, Laboratory of Nutrition and Endocrinology, National Institute of Arthritis, Metabolism, and Digestive Diseases, National Institutes of Health, Bethesda, Maryland

LAURENCE M. CORWIN, Ph.D. Professor of Microbiology and Nutritional Sciences, Department of Microbiology, Boston University School of Medicine, Boston, Massachusetts

INDRAJIT D. DESAI, M.Sc., Ph.D. Professor of Nutrition, Division of Human Nutrition, The University of British Columbia, Vancouver, British Columbia, Canada

HAROLD H. DRAPER, Ph.D. Professor and Chairman, Department of Nutrition, College of Biological Science, University of Guelph, Guelph, Ontario, Canada

PHILIP M. FARRELL, M.D., Ph.D. Associate Professor, Department of Pediatrics, University of Wisconsin, Madison, Wisconsin

HUGO E. GALLO-TORRES, M.D., M.Sc., Ph.D. Research Group Chief, Department of Biochemical Nutrition, Hoffmann-La Roche Inc., Nutley, New Jersey

MACHIEL J. HARDONK, Ph.D. Professor of Histochemistry, Department of Pathology, Faculty of Medicine, University of Groningen, Groningen, The Netherlands

MAX K. HORWITT, Ph.D. Professor Emeritus, Department of Biochemistry, St. Louis University School of Medicine, St. Louis, Missouri

---

[1] Retired

[2] Present affiliation: Assistant Professor, Department of Food Science, North Carolina State University, Raleigh, North Carolina

CAESAR E. HULSTAERT, Ph.D. Senior Lecturer, Center for Medical
Electron Microscopy, Faculty of Medicine, University of Groningen,
Groningen, The Netherlands

S. KASPAREK.[3] Research Division, Hoffmann-La Roche Inc., Nutley,
New Jersey

M. MARGARET KING, Ph.D.[4] Biomembrane Research Laboratory,
Oklahoma Medical Research Foundation, Oklahoma City, Oklahoma

ABBAS E. KITABCHI, M.D., Ph.D. Professor of Medicine and Biochemistry, Departments of Medicine and Biochemistry, and Program
Director, Clinical Research Center, University of Tennessee Center
for the Health Sciences; Chief, Division of Endocrinology and
Metabolism, Veterans Administration Hospital, Memphis, Tennessee

LAWRENCE J. MACHLIN, Ph.D. Senior Research Group Chief,
Department of Clinical Nutrition, Hoffmann-La Roche Inc., Nutley,
New Jersey

WILBUR L. MARUSICH, M.S. Assistant Research Group Chief,
Animal Health Research Department, Research Division, Hoffmann-
La Roche Inc., Nutley, New Jersey

KARL E. MASON, Ph.D.[5] Consultant, National Institute of Arthritis,
Metabolism, and Digestive Diseases, National Institutes of Health,
Bethesda, Maryland

PAUL B. McCAY, Ph.D.[6] Head, Biomembrane Research Laboratory,
Oklahoma Medical Research Foundation, Oklahoma City, Oklahoma

DANIEL B. MENZEL. Ph.D. Professor of Pharmacology and Medicine and
Director, Laboratory of Environmental Pharmacology and Toxicology,
Duke University Medical Center, Durham, North Carolina

IZAÄK MOLENAAR, M.D., Ph.D. Professor of Submicroscopic Cytology,
Center for Medical Electron Microscopy, Faculty of Medicine, University
of Groningen, Groningen, The Netherlands

JAMES S. NELSON, M.D.[7] Professor of Pathology and Professor of
Pathology in Pediatrics, Washington University School of Medicine,
St. Louis, Missouri

---

[3] Present affiliation: Department of Process Systems Development and
Improvement, Hoffmann-La Roche Inc., Nutley, New Jersey

[4] Additional present affiliation: Associate in Research Biochemistry and
Molecular Biology, University of Oklahoma Health Sciences Center,
Oklahoma City, Oklahoma

[5] Deceased

[6] Additional present affiliation: Professor of Biochemistry and
Molecular Biology, University of Oklahoma Health Sciences Center,
Oklahoma City, Oklahoma

[7] Additional present affiliation: U.S. Senior Scientist Awardee, Humboldt
Foundation, Institut für Neuropathologie, Freie Universitat Berlin, Berlin,
West Germany

LESTER PACKER, Ph.D.   Professor of Physiology, Department of
    Physiology-Anatomy, University of California, Berkeley, California
ROBERT P. TENGERDY, Ph.D.   Professor of Microbiology, Department
    of Microbiology, Colorado State University, Fort Collins, Colorado
JUDIE R. WALTON, Ph.D. [8]   Physiologist, Department of Physiology-
    Anatomy, University of California, Berkeley, California

---

8   Present affiliation: Biomedical Scientist, Department of Biomedical
    Sciences, Lawrence Livermore Laboratory, Livermore, California

CONTENTS

Preface   iii

Contributors   v

1/   THE FIRST TWO DECADES OF VITAMIN E HISTORY   1
Karl E. Mason

2/   CHEMISTRY OF TOCOPHEROLS AND TOCOTRIENOLS   7
S. Kasparek

3/   ASSAY METHODS   67
Indrajit D. Desai

4/   TOCOPHEROLS IN FOODS   99
Jack Bauernfeind

5/   BIOCHEMISTRY   169

Part 5A   ABSORPTION   170
Hugo E. Gallo-Torres

Part 5B   TRANSPORT AND METABOLISM   193
Hugo E. Gallo-Torres

Part 5C   BIOGENESIS   268
Harold H. Draper

Part 5D   NUTRIENT INTERRELATIONSHIPS   272
Harold H. Draper

5/   Part 5E   BIOCHEMICAL FUNCTION   289

     Section 1   Vitamin E: Its role as a biological free radical
         scavenger and its relationship to the microsomal mixed-
         function oxidase system   289
     Paul B. McCay and M. Margaret King

     Section 2   Role in nucleic acid and protein metabolism   318
     George L. Catignani

     Section 3   The role of Vitamin E in mitochondrial metabolism   332
     Laurence M. Corwin

     Part 5F   HORMONAL STATUS IN VITAMIN E DEFICIENCY   348
     Abbas E. Kitabchi

     Part 5G   ROLE IN FUNCTION AND ULTRASTRUCTURE
         OF CELLULAR MEMBRANES   372
     Izaäk Molenaar, Caesar E. Hulstaert, and Machiel J. Hardonk

6/   ROLE OF VITAMIN E IN PLANTS, MICROBES, INVERTE-
         BRATES, AND FISH   391
     Harold H. Draper

7/   PATHOLOGY OF VITAMIN E DEFICIENCY   397
     James S. Nelson

8/   DISEASE RESISTANCE: IMMUNE RESPONSE   429
     Robert P. Tengerdy

9/   VITAMIN E AS AN IN VIVO LIPID STABILIZER AND ITS
         EFFECT ON FLAVOR AND STORAGE PROPERTIES
         OF MILK AND MEAT   445
     Wilber L. Marusich

10/ COUNTERACTION OF ENVIRONMENTAL EFFECTS   473

     Part 10A   PROTECTION AGAINST ENVIRONMENTAL
         TOXICANTS   474
     Daniel B. Menzel

     Part 10B   FREE RADICAL DAMAGE AND PROTECTION:
         RELATIONSHIP TO CELLULAR AGING AND CANCER   495
     Judie R. Walton and Lester Packer

Contents

11/ HUMAN HEALTH AND DISEASE   519

   Part 11A   DEFICIENCY STATES, PHARMACOLOGICAL
       EFFECTS, AND NUTRIENT REQUIREMENTS   520
   Phillip M. Farrell

   Part 11B   INTERPRETATION OF HUMAN REQUIREMENTS
       FOR VITAMIN E   621
   Max K. Horwitt

12/ EPILOGUE   637
   Lawrence J. Machlin

INDEX   647

1 THE FIRST TWO DECADES OF VITAMIN E HISTORY*

KARL E. MASON[†]
National Institute of Arthritis,
Metabolism, and Digestive Diseases
National Institutes of Health
Bethesda, Maryland

I have selected the period 1922-1942 as the first two decades of vitamin E history. By 1922, the existence of vitamins A, B (now B_1), and C had been established and that of vitamin D was essentially assured. It had also been recognized by Osborne and Mendel [1] and by Mattill and Conklin [2] that semipurified diets providing an adequacy of these vitamins, although producing good growth and vigor of the laboratory rat, often failed to support reproduction. The monograph of Long and Evans on the estrous cycle of the rat had appeared in 1922, and the effects of dietary changes on its duration were recorded the following year by Evans and Bishop [3]. It was against this backdrop that Evans and Bishop [4] demonstrated the existence of an unknown dietary factor, first called factor X, the inadequacy of which resulted in fetal death and resorption in the laboratory rat. They also recognized wheat germ and lettuce as sources of this fat-soluble factor. Three years later (1925), Evans [5] stated: "We have adopted the letter E as the next serial alphabetical designation, the antirachitic vitamin now being known as vitamin D." Meanwhile, Sure [6] had jumped the gun, proposing the same designation for comparable reasons in 1924.

The basal semipurified diet employed by Evans and Bishop, composed of casein, starch, lard, butter fat, salts, and brewer's yeast, was one developed by Osborne and Mendel as a diet providing superior growth and vigor in the rat. Recognizing the inadequacy of this diet for reproduction unless supplemented with fresh lettuce, Dr. Mendel suggested that a graduate student explore this sterility problem. I was the fortunate graduate student who was selected to pursue the problem in the spring of 1922.

---

*Adopted from K. E. Mason, Fed. Proc., 36:235 (1977).
[†]Deceased.

My studies concerned a description of the process of degeneration in the germinal epithelium of the male rat which was preventable, but not reparable, by supplements of fresh lettuce [7]. These findings were corroborated by Evans. In 1925, when we simultaneously presented preliminary reports on our observations [5, 8], we were not aware of a brief description of testicular atrophy in rats fed diets with milk as the primary source of protein, as reported by Mattill and Stone [9] in 1923, or of the more contemporary report by Mattill et al. [10] describing the histological changes involved and relating them to dietary inadequacy of "factor X." These pioneer studies of Mattill and his colleagues deserved more recognition than they received.

This first five-year history of vitamin E, recognized solely as a dietary factor necessary for fertility in the male and female rat, may be considered complete with the appearance of the classic monograph of Evans and Burr [11] in 1927. Over the next decade, or two, one witnessed endless, but futile efforts to obtain evidence of practical applications of this new discovery in terms of prevention and treatment of reproductive failures in veterinary and clinical medicine. For the most part, revelations of the next five years became meaningful only at later periods. Adamstone [12] described the formation of a lethal ring in the blastoderm of vitamin E-deficient chick embryos, followed early in the second decade by his description of testis degeneration in the E-deficient chick [13]. Olcott and Mattill [14] recorded their initial observations on the associations of antioxidants or inhibitols and vitamin E in lettuce oil, an early forecast of what was to come in terms of the antioxidant function of the tocopherols [15]. There were also inklings that vitamin E might be more than just an antisterility vitamin. In 1928, Evans and Burr [16] reported a paralysis in suckling young of low-E mother rats, sometimes associated with spontaneous recovery—yet, the related lesions of skeletal muscles went unrecognized for ten years [17]. Meanwhile, in 1931, Pappenheimer and Goettsch [18], employing semipurified diets such as used by Evans and Burr, described "nutritional encephalomalacia" in the chick. Undoubtedly influenced by current opinion that vitamin E was required only for reproduction, they looked in vain for other causative factors. In that same year Goettsch and Pappenheimer [19] described what they properly termed "nutritional muscular dystrophy" in guinea pigs and rabbits fed a natural food diet treated with ferric chloride in ether, a procedure that Waddell and Steenbock [20] had shown to cause destruction of vitamin E. Unfortunately, under the experimental conditions employed, supplements of wheat germ oil failed to prevent the muscle lesions. As will be noted later, the satisfactory resolution of this dilemma required two advances in knowledge of cod-liver oil-vitamin E interrelationships extending over a nine-year period.

Early in the second decade of vitamin E history, another facet of this confusing picture was the report of Pappenheimer and Goettsch [21] that, in ducklings fed diets producing only encephalomalacia in chicks, there occurred only widespread lesions of skeletal muscles and that such lesions did not appear in ducklings fed diets producing nutritional muscular dystrophy in guinea pigs and rabbits. Vitamin E deficiency was not specifically implicated until six years later when Pappenheimer [22] reported prevention of the duckling myopathy by oral administration of α-tocopherol. Adding further confusion were reports of Morgulis and associates [23,24] that, in rabbits fed ferric chloride-treated diets, nutritional muscular dystrophy was due to lack of two dietary factors: vitamin E and a water-soluble factor. It remained for Mackenzie and associated [25] to disprove the need for a water-soluble factor. In this same period came a description of paralysis in adult, E-deficient rats by Ringsted [26] and the first description of a brown pigment, since referred to as a ceroid or ceroid-like pigment, observed by Martin and Moore [27] in the uterus of E-deficient rats. There also appeared the observations of Madsen et al. [28] that the addition of cod-liver oil to synthetic or natural food diets induced muscular dystrophy in guinea pigs, rabbits, and goats. Although destruction of vitamin E was not specifically indicated, these studies provided one step toward establishing deficiency of vitamin E as the sole cause of nutritional muscular dystrophy. The second step will be referred to later.

For fifteen years, vitamin E research had been severely hampered by lack of a source more potent than wheat germ oil and by dependence upon a time-consuming and not completely reliable bioassay procedure for determining the vitamin E content of plant and animal tissues. Long-cherished hopes were fulfilled when, in 1936, Evans et al. [29] reported the isolation from wheat germ oil of an alcohol having marked biological activity, for which they proposed the name α-tocopherol and provided the correct chemical formula ($C_{29}H_{50}O_2$). The following year they reported isolation from vegetable oils of two other tocopherols, for which they proposed the names β- and γ-tocopherol, and made note of their lesser biological activity [30]. Almost simultaneously, Olcott and Emerson [15] presented evidence that these tocopherols were effective antioxidants but not in proportion to their biological activity. In 1938, the structural formula for α-tocopherol was provided by Fernholz [31].

During the last half of the second decade, there were several important developments relative to manifestations of vitamin E deficiency states. First, Olcott's revelation [17] that paralysis of suckling young of low-E mother rats, described in 1928 by Evans and Burr [11] and later explored by others for neurological lesions, was a counterpart of the nutritional muscular dystrophy observed but not explained by Goettsch and Pappenheimer [19] in the guinea pig and rabbit some seven years earlier. Second, came the description of "exudative diathesis" in vitamin E-deficient chicks by Dam and Glavind [32], the genesis of which is now recognized as also related to a deficiency of selenium. There followed, from Dam's laboratory, evidence of the antiencephalomalacia property of α-tocopherol [33], a virtue later recognized as being possessed by certain nonbiological antioxidants. And, finally, came the observations of Mackenzie et al. [25] that lack of α-tocopherol alone, uncomplicated by lack of any water-soluble factor, was responsible for the myopathic changes previously described in the rabbit, and those of Mackenzie et al. [34] and Shimotori et al. [35] demonstrating that, if cod-liver oil and α-tocopherol were fed on alternate days, muscle lesions did not occur. This clear-cut evidence that cod-liver oil and other lipids high in unsaturated fatty acids can inactivate vitamin E in the diet (especially in the presence of ferric salts and also within the digestive tract) did much to clarify the important role of this vitamin in protecting against nutritional muscular dystrophy.

During this period, there were also pleasant surprises in the chemical arena. In Holland, Emmerie and Engel [36] described their ferric chloride-dipyridyl method for determining the vitamin E content of foods, later widely applied to blood and other tissues. A long-felt need was filled. A special surprise was the announcement of the chemical synthesis of α-tocopherol by Karrer et al. [37] at the Hoffmann-La Roche laboratories in Basel. Two similar syntheses were reported later that year by Lee Smith et al. at the University of Minnesota [38], while vigorous efforts toward the same goal were being made by Walter John in Goettingen and by Alexander Tood and Jack Drummond in England. The latter two were later knighted, but for other accomplishments. The early history of vitamin E chemistry has been carefully documented by Smith [39].

This international popularity of vitamin E was also reflected in the first symposium on vitamin E, organized by Jack Drummond and Alfred Bacharach and held in London on April 22, 1939. Invited speakers were Emmerie and Engel, Karrer and Bergel, Martin and Moore, Alexander Todd, Evan Shute, Vogt-Moller, and myself. Before an audience of about 100, 15 papers were presented in a one-day session. It was a lively meeting at an exciting period in vitamin E history.

It is noteworthy that, during the years 1936-1938, when attention was focused on the chemistry and synthesis of vitamin E, Kenneth Hickman was applying "molecular distillation" to the physical separation of natural tocopherols from plant oils. Distillation Products, Inc., at Rochester, New York, with Hickman as director of research (1938-1948), became an ever-expanding source of natural tocopherols and an important center for research on their chemical and biological properties. Other persons who were active in this research deserve mention: Stanley Ames, Mei Dju, Norris Embree, Philip Harris, David Herting, Edwin Hove, and Mary Quaife. Concurrently, at the Hoffmann-La Roche laboratories in Basel, Switzerland, important advances were being made concerning the chemical and biological properties of the synthetic tocopherols under the direction of Doctors Paul Karrer and Saul Rubin, respectively.

It is evident that during the first two decades of vitamin E history essentially all manifestations of its experimentally induced deficiency became apparent, and the chemical nature and biological activity of at least three members of the tocopherol family were well established. The major question then was, and still is, whether the tocopherols have functions other than those of biological antioxidants. And, it may be added, despite innumerable reports of the efficacy of α-tocopherol in preventing or curing an endless number of human maladies, we are still awaiting a clear definition of the role of this vitamin in human health.

REFERENCES *

1. T. B. Osborne and L. B. Mendel, J. Biol. Chem. 38:223 (1919).
2. H. A. Mattill and R. E. Conklin, J. Biol. Chem. 44:137 (1920).
3. H. M. Evans and K. S. Bishop, J. Metab. Res. 3:233 (1923).
4. H. M. Evans and K. S. Bishop, Science 56:650 (1922).
5. H. M. Evans, Proc. Natl. Acad. Sci. USA 11:373 (1925).
6. B. Sure, J. Biol. Chem. 58:693 (1924).
7. K. E. Mason, J. Exp. Zool. 45:159 (1926).
8. K. E. Mason, Proc. Natl. Acad. Sci. USA 11:377 (1925).
9. H. A. Mattill and N. C. Stone, J. Biol. Chem. 55:443 (1923).
10. H. A. Mattill, J. S. Carman, and M. M. Clayton, J. Biol. Chem. 61:729 (1924).
11. H. M. Evans and G. O. Burr, Memoir Univ. Calif., 1927, p. 8.
12. F. B. Adamstone, J. Morphol. 52:47 (1931).
13. F. B. Adamstone and L. E. Card, J. Morphol. 56:339 (1934).
14. H. S. Olcott and H. A. Mattill, J. Biol. Chem. 93:59 (1931).
15. H. S. Olcott and O. H. Emerson, J. Amer. Chem. Soc. 59:1008 (1937).
16. H. M. Evans and G. O. Burr, J. Biol. Chem. 76:273 (1928).
17. H. S. Olcott, J. Nutr. 15:221 (1938).
18. A. M. Pappenheimer and M. Goettsch, J. Exp. Med. 53:11 (1931).
19. M. Goettsch and A. M. Pappenheimer, J. Exp. Med. 54:145 (1931).

---

*An excellent account of historical developments of this same period and photographs of most of the investigators to whom reference has been made may be found in "The Pioneer History of Vitamin E," by H. M. Evans, Vit. Horm. 20:379 (1962).

20. J. Waddell and H. Steenbock, J. Biol. Chem. 80:431 (1928).
21. A. M. Pappenheimer and M. Goettsch, J. Exp. Med. 59:35 (1934).
22. A. M. Pappenheimer, Proc. Soc. Exp. Biol. Med. 45:457 (1940).
23. S. Morgulis and H. C. Spencer, J. Nutr. 11:573 (1936).
24. S. Morgulis, V. M. Wilder, and S. H. Epstein, J. Nutr. 16:219 (1938).
25. C. G. Mackenzie, M. D. Levine, and E. V. McCollum, J. Nutr. 20:399 (1940).
26. A. Ringsted, Biochem. J. 29:788 (1935).
27. A. J. P. Martin and T. Moore, J. Chem. Ind. 55:236 (1936); 57:973 (1938); J. Hyg. 39:643 (1939).
28. L. L. Madsen, C. M. McCay, and L. A. Maynard, Proc. Soc. Exp. Biol. Med. 30:1434 (1933).
29. H. M. Evans, O. H. Emerson, G. A. Emerson, J. Biol. Chem. 113:319 (1936).
30. O. H. Emerson, G. A. Emerson, A. Mohammad, and H. M. Evans, J. Biol. Chem. 122:99 (1937).
31. E. J. Fernholz, Amer. Chem. Soc. 60:700 (1938).
32. H. Dam and J. Glavind, Skand. Arch. Physiol. 89:299 (1939).
33. H. Dam, J. Glavind, O. Bernth, and E. Hagens, Nature (Lond.) 142:1157 (1938).
34. C. G. Mackenzie, J. B. Mackenzie, and E. V. McCollum, J. Nutr. 21:225 (1941).
35. N. G. Shimotori, G. A. Emerson, and H. M. Evans, J. Nutr. 19:547 (1940).
36. A. Emmerie and C. Engel, Rec. Trav. Chim. 57:1351 (1938); 58:283 (1939).
37. P. Karrer, H. Fritzche, B. H. Ringier, and H. Salomon, Helv. Chim. Acta 21:520 (1938); Nature (Lond.) 141:1057 (1938).
38. L. I. Smith, H. E. Ungnada, and W. W. Pritchard, Science 88:37 (1938).
39. L. I. Smith, Chem. Rev. 27:287 (1940).

2 CHEMISTRY OF TOCOPHEROLS AND TOCOTRIENOLS

S. KASPAREK
Hoffmann-La Roche Inc.
Nutley, New Jersey

I.	Introduction	8
II.	Discovery of Tocopherols and Tocotrienols	8
III.	Structure and Stereochemistry	9
IV.	Nomenclature	14
V.	Reactions	15
	A. Oxidation	15
	B. Thermolysis	24
	C. Miscellaneous Reactions	24
	D. Conversions of α-Tocopherylquinone	25
VI.	Physicochemical Properties	26
	A. Melting Point	26
	B. Optical Activity	26
	C. Ultraviolet (UV) Spectra	26
	D. Infrared (IR) Spectra	28
	E. Nuclear Magnetic Resonance (NMR) Spectra	28
	F. Mass Spectra	28
	G. X-ray Diffraction	28
	H. Chromatography	28
VII.	Synthesis	29
	A. Introduction	29
	B. Total Synthesis	30
	C. Partial Synthesis	39
	D. Synthesis of Synthetic Components of Tocopherols and Tocotrienols	40
VIII.	Biosynthesis	48

IX. Structure-Biological Activity   49
    A. Introduction   49
    B. Effect of Functional Groups   49
    C. Effect of Stereoisomerism   51
X. Metabolites of Tocopherols   51
    References   53

I. INTRODUCTION

Since the first report on substances that exhibit vitamin E activity appeared in literature in the 1920s, extensive research on the chemistry of these compounds has been conducted. This chapter will give a brief account of the most important aspects of the chemistry of tocopherols and tocotrienols; the major papers describing the elucidation of structures of these compounds, their properties, and efficient methods of synthesis are reviewed. Attention has been focused on the stereochemistry of tocopherols and tocotrienols which bears an effect on their biological activities. A section dealing with trivial and systematic nomenclature of tocopherols and tocotrienols has been included to indicate the need for an unambiguous system to correctly identify compounds in biological assays.

    A number of comprehensive reviews on the chemistry of tocopherols and tocotrienols previously appeared [1-16]. This review covers the literature up to June, 1975.

II. DISCOVERY OF TOCOPHEROLS AND TOCOTRIENOLS

"Substance X" contained in natural foodstuffs prevented sterility in rats reared on a special dietary regime. This finding reported by Evans and Bishop [17] gave impetus to the investigation of compounds whose biological potency is referred to today as the activity of vitamin E. The vitamin-like nature of "substance X" was recognized and given the letter E to include it in the family of other already known vitamins [17, 18]. The results of Evans and Bishop [17, 19] were confirmed by independent work of Sure [18, 20, 21] and Mattill and coworkers [22-24]. Further research carried out by Evans and co-workers led to the isolation of a homogeneous substance which was named α-tocopherol. Subsequently, two additional substances exhibiting the biological activity of α-tocopherol, albeit in lower degree, were isolated and designated as β-tocopherol and γ-tocopherol, respectively [25-28]. The richest source of α- and β-tocopherol was found in wheat germ oil [26]. However, the investigation of other vegetable oils, i.e., cottonseed [29], lettuce, rice germ, and other seed-germ oils, showed that they contained considerable amounts of substances exhibiting the activity of α-tocopherol [25,30]. A substance named δ-tocopherol was added to the trio of tocopherols when it was isolated from soybean oil [31].

The multiple nature of these vegetable oil components having α-tocopherol activity was further augmented by the isolation of other active substances initially named ξ₁-tocopherol and ξ₂-tocopherol from palm oil and wheat bran and from rice, respectively [32], ε-tocopherol from wheat bran [32-35], and η-tocopherol from rice [36]. However, these substances were shown to be chemically distinctly different from the tocopherols in that they possessed a high degree of unsaturation. It was suggested that they be named α-, β-, and γ-tocotrienol, respectively [37,38]. The fourth member of this group, δ-tocotrienol, was later isolated from palm oil [37] and Hevea latex [38].

III. STRUCTURE AND STEREOCHEMISTRY

The assignment of a structure for α-tocopherol was the subject of various studies [39-47]. Karrer and co-workers [48,49] proposed that α-tocopherol was a coumaran derivative of the structure I. However, the correct structure was established by Fernholz [50] by degradation studies of α-tocopherol using pyrolysis and chromic acid oxidation. The hydroquinone II, lactone III (R = $C_{16}H_{33}$), dimethylmaleic anhydride IV, ketone V (R = $C_{15}H_{31}$), acid VI, diacetyl VII, olefin VIII [57], and acetone were obtained by the degradation. It was postulated that α-tocopherol was a cyclic ether represented by the structure IX (R^1-R^3 = Me), with the indicated numbering of the system. Since the tocopherols differ only in the number of methyl

MeCOCH₂R

V.

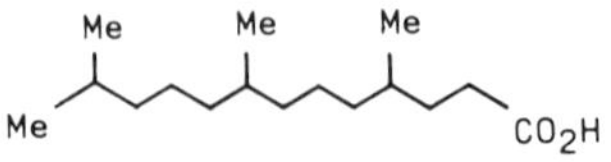

VI

VII

MeCOCOMe

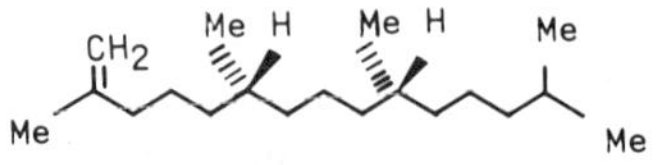

VIII

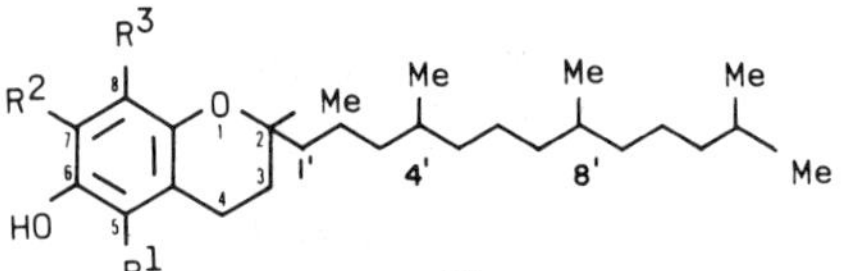

IX

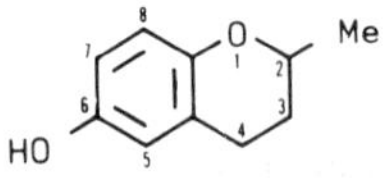

X

groups in the aromatic ring in IX they can be regarded as derivatives of
2-methyl-6-chromanol (X) onto which a saturated 16-carbon isoprenoid
chain is attached at C-2 and which is methylated at C-5, C-7, and C-8,
respectively. The proposed structures of natural tocopherols are shown in
Table 1.

The establishment of the structures of tocopherols was an important
step for structure elucidation of tocotrienols. It has been shown [37,54]
that α-tocotrienol and hydrogenation yielded α-tocopherol, which implied
structure XI (R = Me) for α-tocotrienol with the indicated numbering of
the system. Similarly, the structures of other tocotrienols were established. They are shown in Table 2.

The structure of tocopherols indicate three centers of asymmetry at
C-2, C-4', and C-8', respectively. The tocotrienols possess one center
of asymmetry at C-2 in addition to the sites of geometrical isomerism at

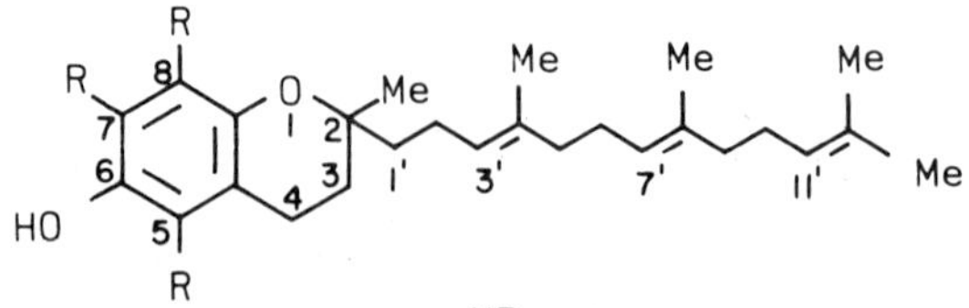

XI

TABLE 1   Structure of Natural Tocopherols

Compound	R^1	R^2	R^3	Reference
α-Tocopherol	Me	Me	Me	39–50
β-Tocopherol	Me	H	Me	40–42, 44, 51, 52
γ-Tocopherol	H	Me	Me	51, 53
δ-Tocopherol	H	H	Me	31

C-3' and at C-7'. Thus, a number of stereoisomers of tocopherols and tocotrienols can exist. It has been shown by Isler and co-workers [57] that natural α-tocopherol has 2R, 4'R, 8'R [58] configuration by relating natural α-tocopherol to phytol XII (R = OH) of established R configuration at C-7 and C-11 [59a, b] and with (–)linalool XIII of established R configuration [60]. Oxidative degradation products of α-tocopherol (e.g., structures XIV, XV,

TABLE 2   Structure of Natural Tocotrienols

Compound	R^1	R^2	R^3	Reference
α-Tocotrienol	Me	Me	Me	32, 33, 54, 55
β-Tocotrienol	Me	H	Me	32, 54, 55
γ-Tocotrienol	H	Me	Me	37, 56
δ-Tocotrienol	H	H	Me	37

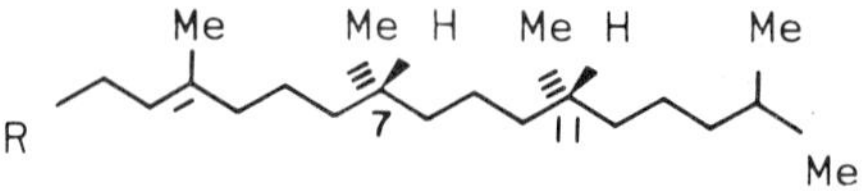

Me   Me H   Me H   Me

R

7   11

Me

Me

XII

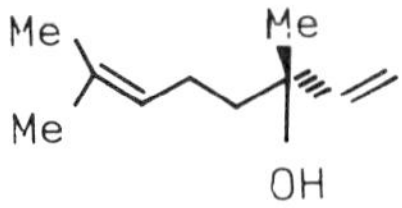

Me   Me
\ |
Me   Me
         OH

XIII

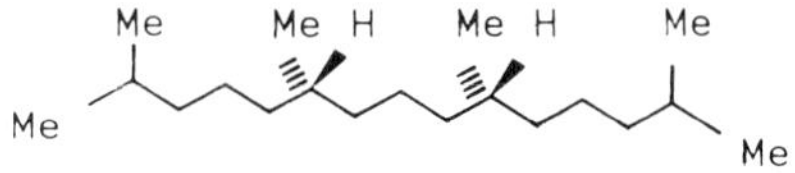

Me   Me H   Me H   Me

Me   Me

XVII

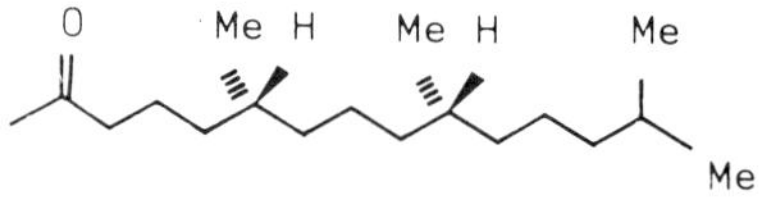

O   Me H   Me H   Me

XIV   Me

Me Me H   Me H   Me

O   O   Me

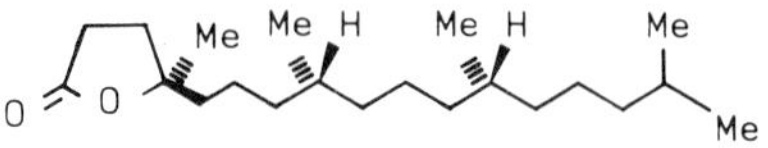

XVIII

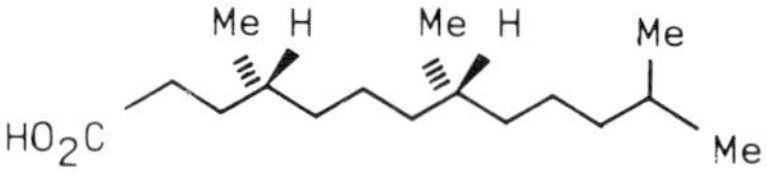

Me H   Me H   Me

HO_2C Me

XV

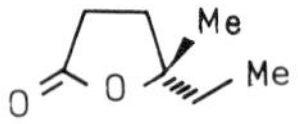

Me
O   Me
O   Me

XIX

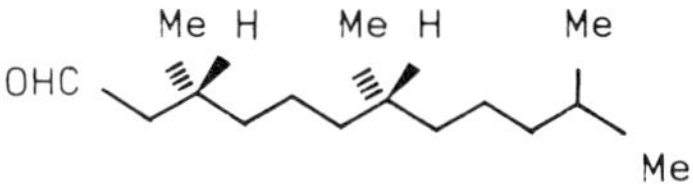

Me H   Me H   Me

OHC

Me

XVI

Me
Me   O   Me
                 ////CHO
HO
        Me

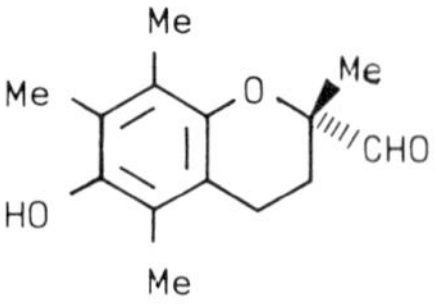

XX

XVI, and XVII) were shown to be identical with those prepared synthetically from (7R, 11R)-phytol XII (R = OH). The 2R configuration of α-tocopherol was assigned by comparing molecular rotation of the lactone XVIII obtained from α-tocopherol and of XIX obtained synthetically from XIII. Additional proof was provided [61] by total synthesis of (2R, 4'R, 8'R)-α-tocopherol from the aldehyde XX. Based on these conclusions, natural β- and γ-tocopherol [54] have been assigned 2R, 4'R, 8'R configuration.

Natural α-, β-, and γ-tocotrienol each have been shown to have (2R̲),3'-trans̲,7'-trans̲ configuration [54-56]. All natural tocopherols and tocotrienols, have R̲ configuration at C-2. The epimer of α-tocopherol, i.e., (2S̲,4'R̲,8'R̲)-α-tocopherol, was prepared by Isler and co-workers, [61,62].

The stereochemical structures of the tocopherols XXI-XXIII (R^1-R^3 = H, Me) and tocotrienols XXIV and XXV (R^1-R^3 = H, Me) are shown herein.

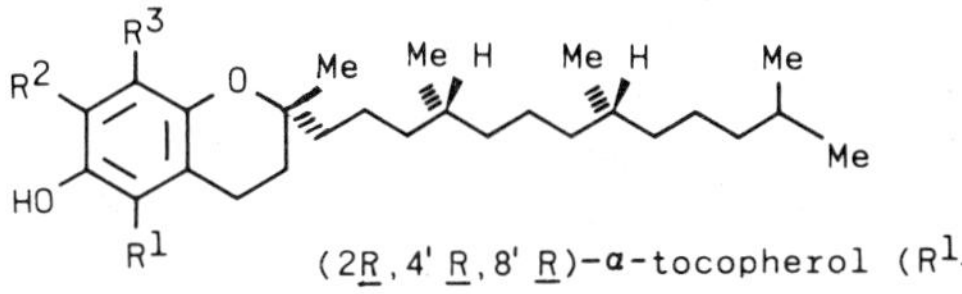

(2R̲,4'R̲,8'R̲)-α-tocopherol (R^1-R^3 = Me)

XXI

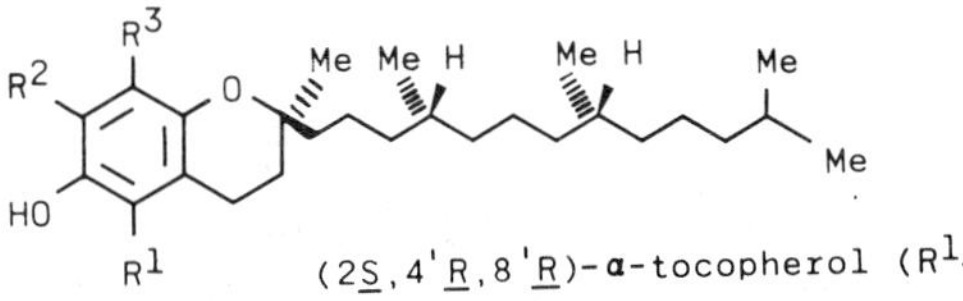

(2S̲,4'R̲,8'R̲)-α-tocopherol (R^1-R^3 = Me)

XXII

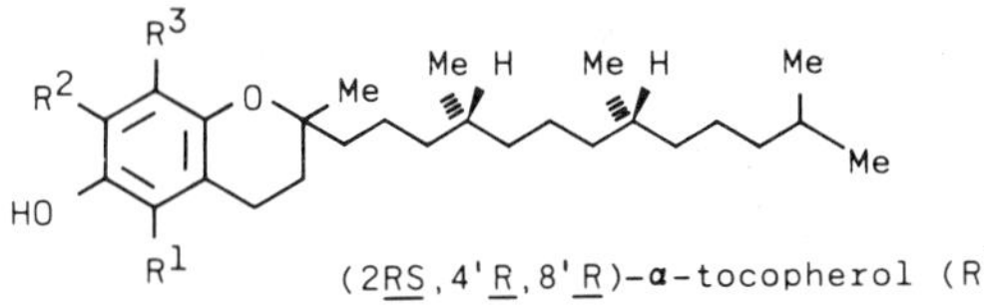

(2RS̲,4'R̲,8'R̲)-α-tocopherol (R^1-R^3 = Me)

XXIII

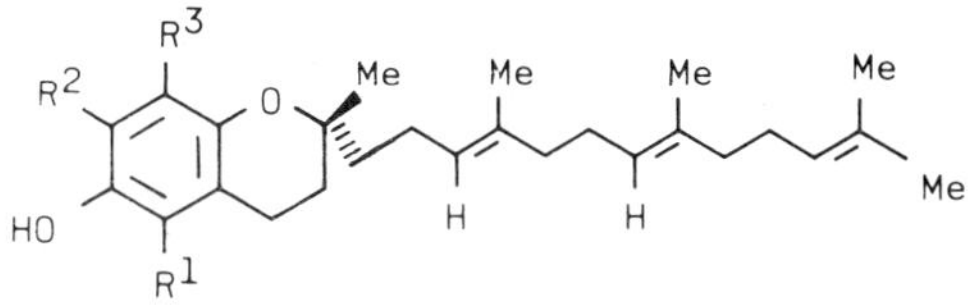

(2R̲),3'E̲,7'E̲-α-tocotrienol (R^1-R^3 = Me)

XXIV

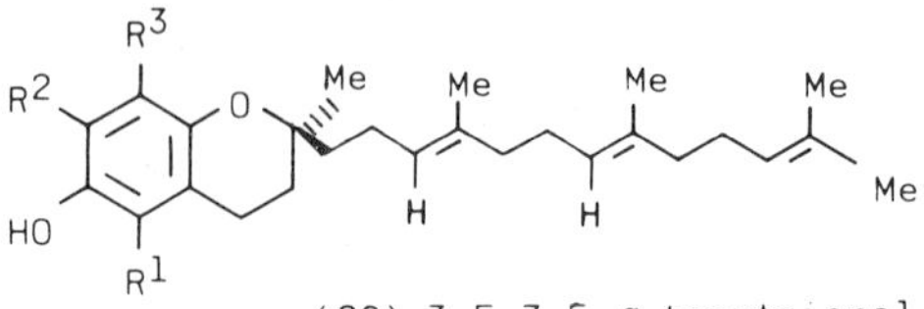

(2$\underline{S}$),3 $\underline{E}$,7 $\underline{E}$-α-tocotrienol (R^1-R^3 = Me)   **XXV**

IV. NOMENCLATURE

There has been considerable inconsistency in the literature concerning the nomenclature of tocopherols and tocotrienols. Natural α-tocopherol has been referred to as $\underline{d}$-α-tocopherol on the basis of the positive sign of rotation of plane-polarized light in ethanol solution [63]. However, the direction of optical rotation of α-tocopherol is solvent dependent; for example, in benzene solution the sign of rotation is opposite, i.e., $\underline{l}$ [63]. Synthetic α-tocopherol obtained from natural, optically active, or synthetic, racemic phytol has been specified as $\underline{dl}$-α-tocopherol [46, 48, 64]. However, the synthesis of α-tocopherol using natural, optically active phytol gives a mixture of epimers differing only in the configuration at C-2 while the synthesis using synthetic racemic phytol affords a mixture of eight dia-stereomers of α-tocopherol. The epimer of natural $\underline{d}$-α-tocopherol, pre-pared synthetically, has been designated $\underline{l}$-α-tocopherol; however, it showed a positive rotation in ethanol solution [65]. There has been no sys-tem of nomenclature to specify the diastereomeric mixture of α-tocopherol.

Some authors designated the asymmetric carbon in question as [C*2-$\underline{d}$,$\underline{l}$; C*4', 8'-$\underline{d}$]-α-tocopherol [66] or [(-)-at C-2-α-tocopherol] [67]. The letters $\underline{D}$ and $\underline{L}$ [68] have been used to specify the configuration at C-4' and C-8', respectively [65], because natural phytol has been found to have 7-$\underline{D}$, 11-$\underline{D}$ configuration [59a, b].

According to the recommendations of the IUPAC-IUB Commission on Biochemical Nomenclature* [69] all the above specifications should be abandoned. It has been recommended that:

1. 2-Methyl-2-(4', 8', 12'-trimethyltridecyl)-6-chromanol IX (R^1-R^3 = H) be named tocol and all tocopherols should be regarded as its derivatives.

2. The term tocopherol should be used as the generic descriptor for all mono-, di-, and trimethyltocols.

3. 2-Methyl-2-(4', 8', 12'-trimethyltrideca-3', 7', 11'-trienyl)-6-chromanol XI (R = H) be named tocotrienol and all tocotrienols should be regarded as its derivatives.

---

*International Union of Pure and Applied Chemistry—International Union of Biochemistry Commission on Biochemical Nomenclature.

4. The term vitamin E should be used as the generic descriptor for all tocol and tocotrienol derivatives qualitatively exhibiting the biologic activity of α-tocopherol. Statements such as vitamin E deficiency and vitamin E activity illustrate the use of this term.

5. The natural stereoisomer of α-tocopherol is to be named (2R, 4'R, 8'R)-α-tocopherol; the name α-tocopherol should not be used without specifying the configuration. All other stereoisomers of tocopherols should be named accordingly.

6. Trivial names are allowed to briefly describe the configuration of a tocol or a tocotrienol. Unless otherwise stated, it is understood that the configuration of natural α-tocopherol is 2R, 4'R, 8'R. Thus, RRR- α-tocopherol can be used for the natural α-tocopherol isomer. The epimer of natural α-tocopherol, i.e., (2S, 4'R, 8'R)-α-tocopherol, can be briefly named 2-epi-α-tocopherol. A mixture of RRR- and SRR-α-tocopherol obtained synthetically can be named 2-ambo-α-tocopherol (ambo = Latin for both). The reduction product of natural α-tocotrienol is a mixture of four diastereomeric α-tocopherols and can be called 4'-ambo, 8'-ambo- α -tocopherol. Synthetic α-tocopherol from synthetic phytol or isophytol is a mixture of four racemates and should be named all-rac-α-tocopherol.

7. Italicized prefixes d-, l-, and d,l, if still used for RRR-α-tocopherol and all-rac-α-tocopherol, should be replaced by lowercase letters in brackets, i.e., [d] and [dl].

Table 3 lists the recommended trivial names for tocopherols and tocotrienols. Table 4 lists the Chemical Abstracts' systematic names.

V. REACTIONS

A. Oxidation

RRR-α-Tocopherol treated with chromic acid gives the degradation products IV, VII, XIV, XV, XVIII, XXVI, and XXVII [50, 57]. The lactone XVIII was also obtained by oxidation of 5, 7, 8-trimethyltocol with potassium permanganate [43]. 5, 8- and 7, 8-Dimethyltocol were oxidized similarly [51, 53].

α-Tocopherylquinone XXVIII was obtained on oxidizing 5, 7, 8-trimethyltocol with nitric acid [70, 71, 74], silver nitrate [41, 70, 72, 73, 76], ferric chloride [41, 72, 75], auric chloride [76], ceric sulfate [77], benzoyl peroxide [78], lead tetraacetate [79, 80], carbon tetrachloride in ethanol [80a], and nitrogen dioxide [80b]. It has been suggested that RRR-α-tocopherol protects lung tissue from the effects of nitrogen dioxide in polluted air by reacting with nitrogen dioxide to form XXVIII [80b].

TABLE 3   IUPAC-IUB Commission on Biochemical Nomenclature
Recommended (1973) Trivial Names of α-Tocopherol and α-Tocotrienol

Name used in the literature	Structure
α-Tocopherol d-α-Tocopherol (+)-α-Tocopherol	IX (R^1 - R^3 = Me)
d-α-Tocopherol [C*-2-d; C*4', 8'-d]-α-Tocopherol (+)-at C-2-α-Tocopherol 2D, 4'D, 8'D-α-Tocopherol	XXI (R^1 - R^3 = Me)
l-α-Tocopherol (-)-α-Tocopherol L-α-Tocopherol [C*-2-l; C*4', 8'd]-α-Tocopherol 2L, 4'D, 8'D-α-Tocopherol	XXII (R^1 - R^3 = Me)
dl-α-Tocopherol [C*-2-dl; C*4', 8'-d]-α-Tocopherol (±)-at C-2-α-Tocopherol DL-α-Tocopherol 2DL, 4'D, 8'D-α-Tocopherol	XXIII (R^1 - R^3 = Me) IX (R^1 - R^3 = Me)
ζ_1-Tocopherol ζ_2-Tocopherol α-Tocotrienol Tocochromanol-3 rac-all-trans-α-Tocotrienol	XI (R = Me)
(2R)-all-trans-α-Tocotrienol	XXIV (R^1 - R^3 = Me)
(2S)-all-trans-α-Tocotrienol	XXV (R^1 - R^3 = Me)

Description of compounds	Recommended trivial names
α-Tocopherol of unspecified configuration	5, 7, 8-Trimethyltocol
Natural or synthetic α-tocopherol of specified configuration	(2R, 4'R, 8'R)-α-Tocopherol RRR-α-Tocopherol [d]-α-Tocopherol
Epimer of natural α-tocopherol prepared synthetically	(2S, 4'R, 8'R)-α-Tocopherol SRR-α-Tocopherol 2-epi-α-Tocopherol
A mixture of synthetic 2R, 4'R, 8'R-α-tocopherol with 2S, 4'R, 8'R-α-tocopherol	2-ambo-α-Tocopherol
A mixture of four pairs of enantiomers of synthetic α-tocopherol	all-rac-α-Tocopherol [dl]-α-Tocopherol
A mixture of four isomers of α-tocopherol, i.e., (2R, 4'R, 8'R) + (2R, 4'S, 8'R) + (2R, 4'R, 8'S) + (2R, 4'S, 8'S)-α-tocopherol	4'ambo-8'-ambo-α-Tocopherol
	5, 7, 8-Trimethyl-all-trans-tocotrienol (2RS)-2'-trans, 7'-trans-tocotrienol
	(2R), 3'-trans, 7'-trans-α-Tocotrienol
	(2S), 3'-trans, 7'-trans-α-Tocotrienol 2-epi-α-Tocotrienol

TABLE 4   Chemical Abstracts' Systematic Nomenclature of Tocopherols
and Tocotrienols

Substance	Chemical Abstracts' name	Registry no.
α-Tocopherol	6-Chromanol, 2,5,7,8-tetramethyl-2-(4,8,12-trimethyltridecyl)-	10191-41-0
	2H-1-Benzopyran-6-ol, 3,4-dihydro-, 2,5,7,8-tetramethyl-2-(4,8,12-trimethyltridecyl)-	
β-Tocopherol	6-Chromanol, 2,5,8-trimethyl-2-(4,8,12-trimethyltridecyl)-	148-03-8
	2H-1-Benzopyran-6-ol, 3,4-dihydro-, 2,5,8-trimethyl-2-(4,8,12-trimethyltridecyl)-	
γ-Tocopherol	6-Chromanol, 2,7,8-trimethyl-2-(4,8,12-trimethyltridecyl)-	7616-22-0
	2H-1-Benzopyran-6-ol, 3,4-dihydro-2,7,8-trimethyl-2-(4,8,12-trimethyltridecyl)-	
δ-Tocopherol	6-Chromanol, 2,8-dimethyl-2-(4,8,12-trimethyltridecyl)-	119-13-1
	2H-1-Benzopyran-6-ol, 3,4-dihydro-, 2,8-dimethyl-2-(4,8,12-trimethyltridecyl)-	
α-Tocotrienol	6-Chromanol, 2,5,7,8-tetramethyl-2-(4,8,12-trimethyl-3,7,11-tridecatrienyl)-	22625-13-4
	2H-1-Benzopyran-6-ol, 3,4-dihydro-2,5,7,8-tetramethyl-2-(4,8,12-trimethyl-3,7,11-tridecatrienyl)-	
β-Tocotrienol	6-Chromanol, 2,5,8-trimethyl-2-(4,8,12-trimethyl-3,7,11-tridecatrienyl)-	49-23-3
	2H-1-Benzopyran-6-ol, 3,4-dihydro-2,5,8-trimethyl-2-(4,8,12-trimethyl-3,7,11-tridecatrienyl)-	

TABLE 4   (continued)

Substance	Chemical Abstracts' name	Registry no.
γ-Tocotrienol	6-Chromanol, 2,7,8-trimethyl-2-(4,8,12-trimethyl-3,7,11-tridecatrienyl)-	14101-61-2
	2H-1-Benzopyran-6-ol, 3,4-dihydro-2,7,8-trimethyl-2-(4,8,12-trimethyl-3,7,11-tridecatrienyl)-	
δ-Tocotrienol	6-Chromanol, 2,8-dimethyl-2-(4,8,12-trimethyl-3,7,11-tridecatrienyl)-	25612-59-3
	2H-1-Benzopyran-6-ol, 3,4-dihydro-2,8-dimethyl-2-(4,8,12-trimethyl-3,7,11-tridecatrienyl)-	

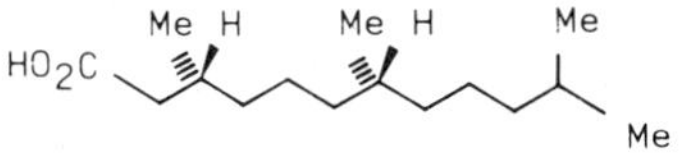

XXVI

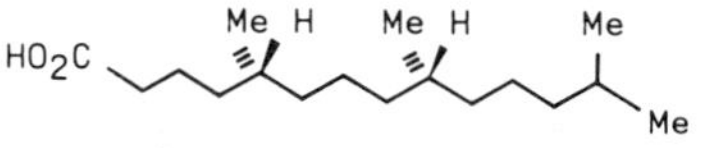

XXVII

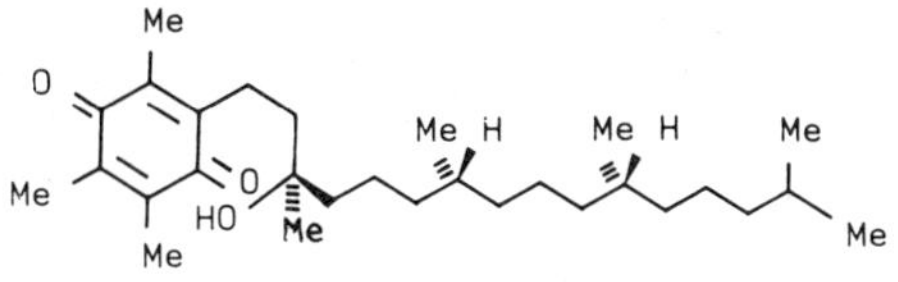

XXVIII

α-Tocored XXIX, the quinone XXX, and tocopurple XXXI were the oxidation products of 5,7,8-trimethyltocol with nitric acid [70,73,74] or ferric chloride [74,81]. 5,8- [63,70] and 7,8-Dimethyltycol [63] were oxidized similarly.

α-Tocopheroxide XXXII (R = Et) was obtained when RRR-α-tocopherol was oxidized with ferric chloride in ethanol in the presence of 2,2'-bipyridyl [82-84]. The ethers are also formed in the reaction of RRR-α-tocopherol with benzoyl peroxide in an alcohol [85]. Ethers XXXII in which R equals Me, Et, iso-Pr, tert-Bu, and octyl were thus prepared [85]. It was assumed that these ethers were formed via the quinone hemiacetal XXXII (R = H) which can be prepared by the oxidation of RRR-α-tocopherol with tetrachloro-o-quinone or N-bromosuccinimide [86,87].

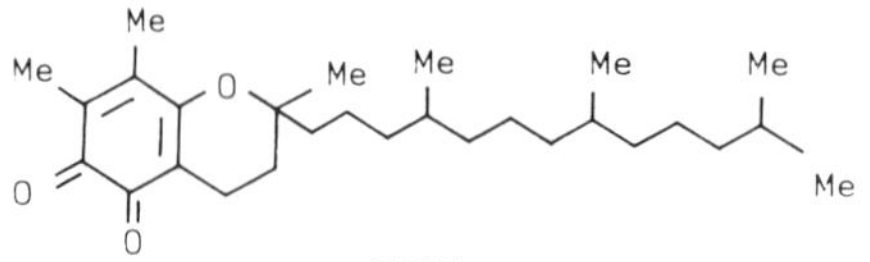

XXIX

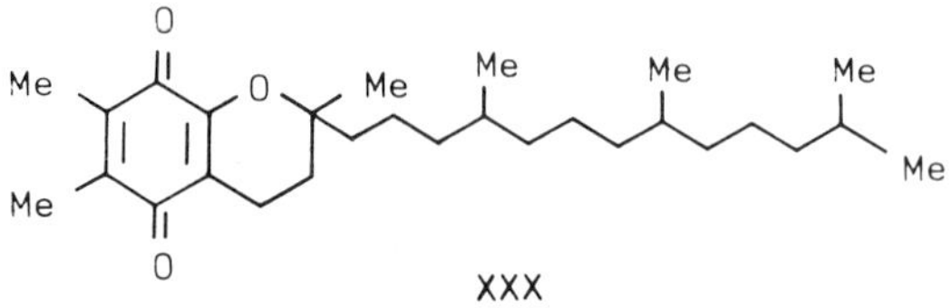

XXX

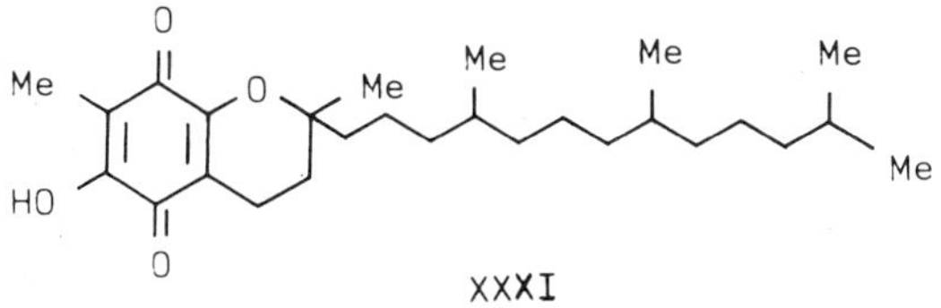

XXXI

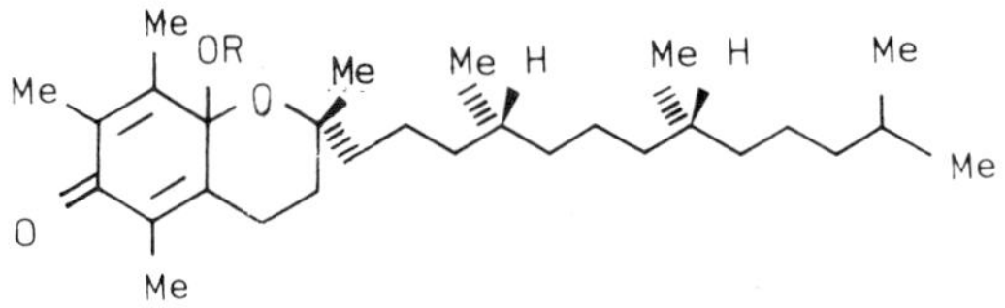

XXXII

The oxidation of 5, 7, 8-trimethyltocol with alkaline ferricyanide [88-93] or with tri-tert-butylphenoxy radical [86] gives products of complex structures, e.g., XXXIII, XXXIV and XXXV. The optical rotation of these oxidation products is frequently utilized for analytic determinations of RRR-α-tocopherol or its stereoisomer 2-epi-α-tocopherol [90]. Similar products were obtained by oxidizing the tocopherols with p-benzoquinone [93-95] or azodiisobutyronitrile [96]. 5, 8-Dimethyltocol, on treatment with p-benzoquinone, afforded XXXVI and XXXVII, while 7, 8-dimethyltocol yielded XXXVIII and XXXIX. 8-Methyltocol reacted similarly [94, 95]. It has been claimed that a metabolite of 5, 7, 8-trimethyltocol having the structure XXXIII is formed in the liver [97]. 2, 3-Dichloro-5, 6-dicyano-p-benzoquinone oxidizes 5, 7, 8-trimethyltocol acetate to give the 3, 4-dehydro compound XL (R = Ac) [92, 98].

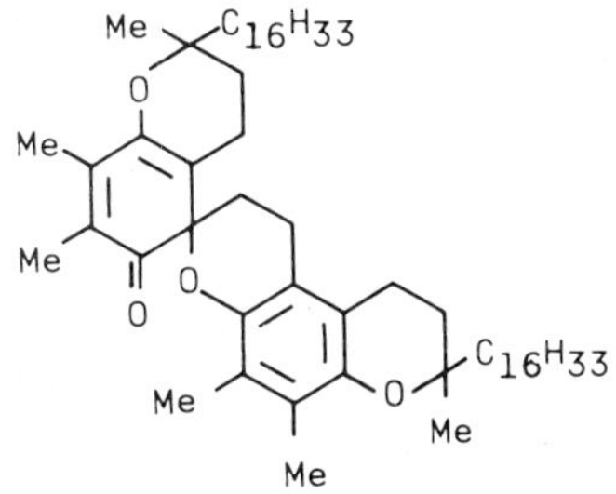

XXXIII

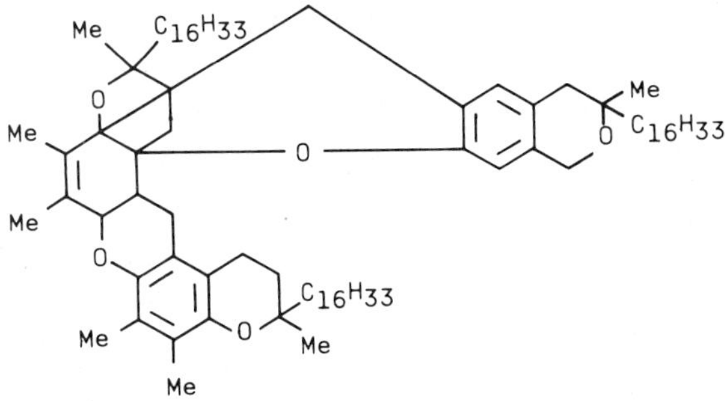

XXXIV

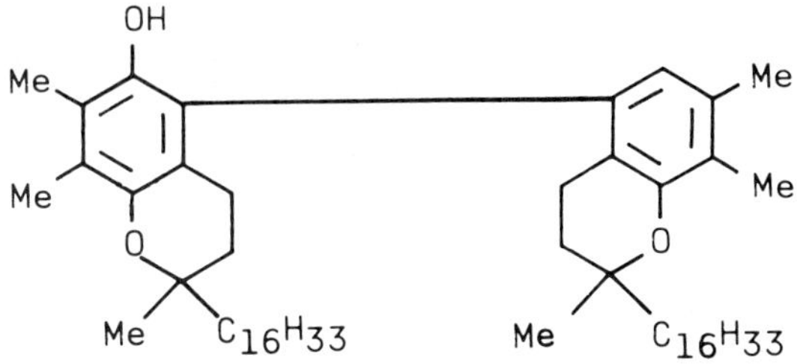

XXXV

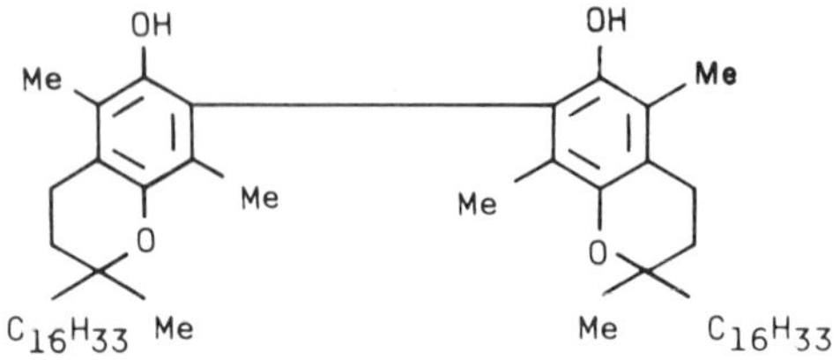

XXXVI

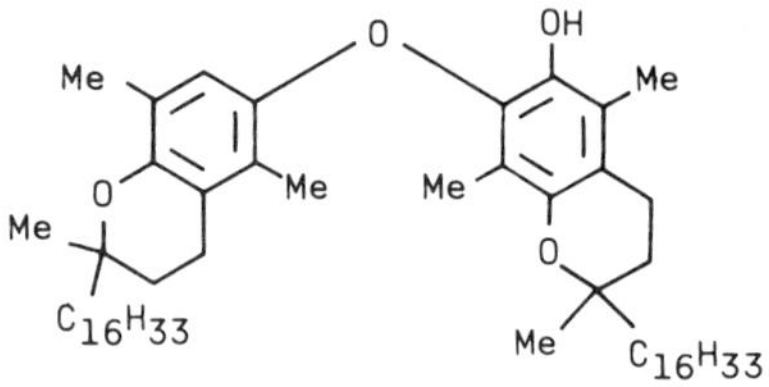

XXXVII

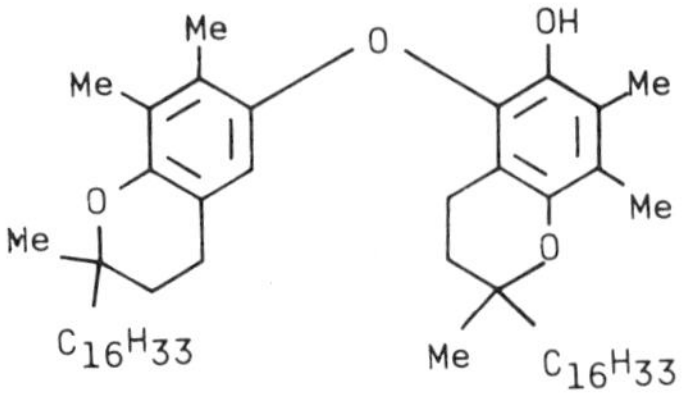

XXXVIII

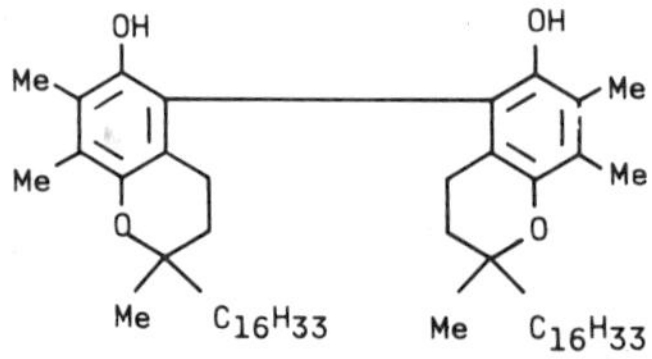

XXXIX

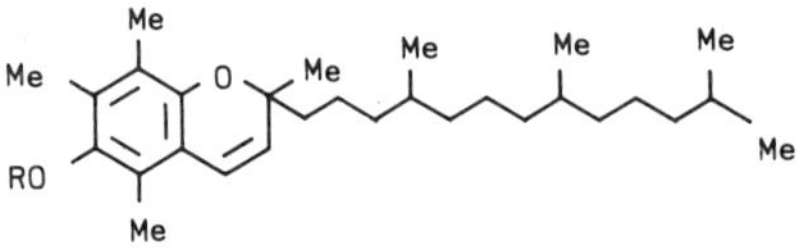

XL

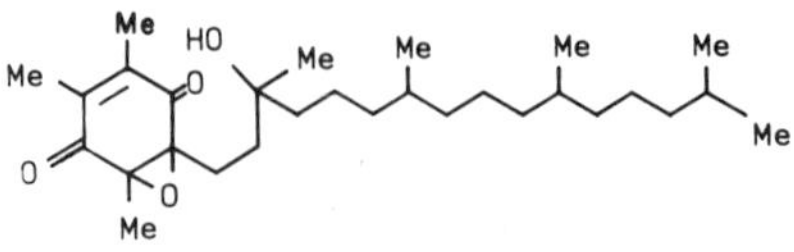

XLI

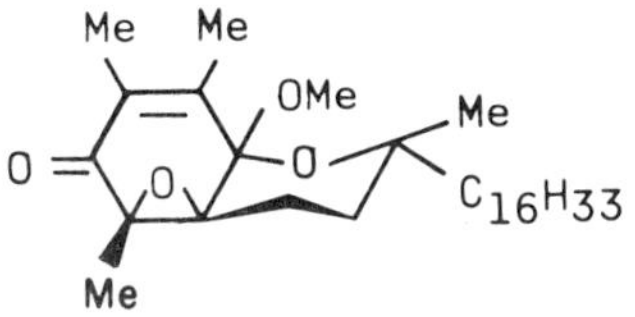

XLII

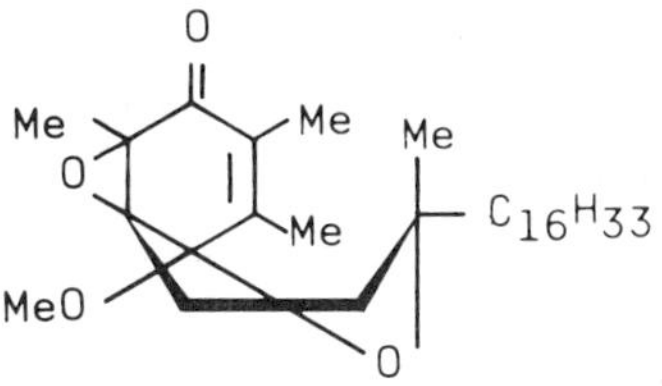

XLIII

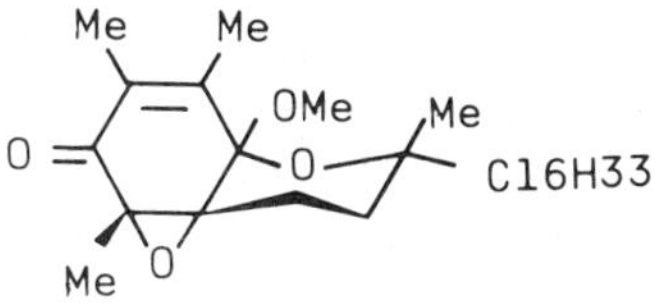

XLIV

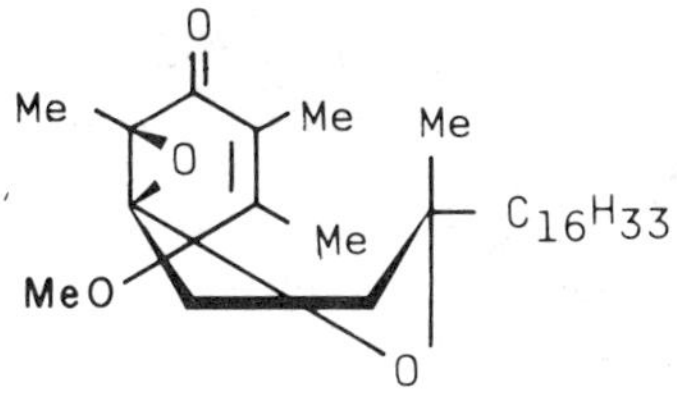

XLV

　　　Recently, a number of studies have been published concerning the oxidation of tocopherols with singlet oxygen. This oxidation is of interest because of a plausible analogous mechanism by which tocopherols function as antioxidants in vivo or in vitro. Grams et al. [99, 100] irradiated [dl]-α-tocopherol in methanol in a Pyrex vessel with a G.E. 300-W tungsten lamp in the presence of proflavin and oxygen and established the structures of the oxidation products as XXXII (R = Me), XXVIII, and the epoxides XLI, XLII, XLIII, XLIV, and XLV. An investigation of the reactivity of tocopherols toward singlet oxygen showed that 5, 7, 8-trimethyltocol had reactivity 1 followed by 5, 8-dimethyltocol (0.50), 7, 8-dimethyltocol (0.26), and 8-methyltocol (0.10). It has been suggested that the reactivity of tocopherols with singlet oxygen is in correlation with their vitamin E activity and that the quenching of singlet oxygen by tocopherols is the mechanism by which tocopherols inhibit lipid peroxidation [101]. Subsequently, other studies were published determining the activity of tocopherols in quenching singlet oxygen [102-104]. Nishikimi and Machlin [105] studied a model compound of tocopherols—6-hydroxy-2, 5, 7, 8-tetramethyl-2-chroman-carboxylic acid XLVI—and found it to be oxidized by the xanthine-xanthine oxidase system. The oxidation was inhibited by superoxide dismutase. It has been suggested that the oxidation is caused by superoxide anion and that the oxidation product is XLVII. It is possible that vitamin E scavenges the superoxide anion generated by membrane-bound enzymes in biological oxidations [105]. The acid XLVI proved to be an excellent antioxidant [105a].

XLVI   XLVII

B. Thermolysis

Thermal degradation of <u>RRR</u>-α-tocopherol, used in structure determination, produced the hydroquinone II and an unsaturated hydrocarbon
that was later identified as being VIII [40, 50, 57]. Trimethylhydroquinone
XLVIII was similarly obtained from 5, 8- and 7, 8-dimethyltocol [44, 51, 52],
while 8-methyltocol yielded 2, 6-dimethylhydroquinone XLIX [31]. Heating
5, 7, 8-trimethyl- or 5, 8-dimethyltocol under pressure with hydrogen
iodide in the presence of acetic acid yielded L and LI, respectively [42].

XLVIII   XLIX

L   LI

C. Miscellaneous Reactions

The phenolic hydroxyl of the tocopherols can be acylated [63, 106],
etherified [30], and phosphorylated [107]. The aromatic ring of tocopherols undergoes nitrosation [34, 108, 109]. Chloromethylation [110] and
hydroxymethylation [111] of the aromatic ring of tocopherols have been

frequently used as the first step to convert 5, 8-dimethyltocol, 7, 8-dimethyltocol, or 8-methyltocol into the higher methylated derivative (see Sec. VII.C).

D. Conversions of α-Tocopherylquinone

α-Tocopherylquinone XXVIII has been implicated as a metabolite of RRR-α-tocopherol in oxidation reactions [80b, 99, 100]. Therefore, a short description of the chemical behavior of α-tocopherylquinone is given.

The opening of the heterocyclic ring of RRR-α-tocopherol to give XXVIII proceeds with the retention of configuration at C-2, C-4', and C-8'. The reduction of XXVIII with ascorbic acid [84] or catalytically [62, 72] yielded hydroquinone LII of unchanged configuration. Subsequent ring reclosure with zinc chloride afforded a mixture of (2RS, 4'R, 8'R)-α-tocopherol [62]. Using concentrated sulfuric acid [112], or 1-butanethiol in acetic acid [113] as the catalyst, it was possible to obtain RRR-α-tocopherol with complete retention of configuration. Acetylation of XXVIII with acetic anhydride in the presence of zinc [114] yielded LIII while treatment with acetyl chloride [112] yielded LIV.

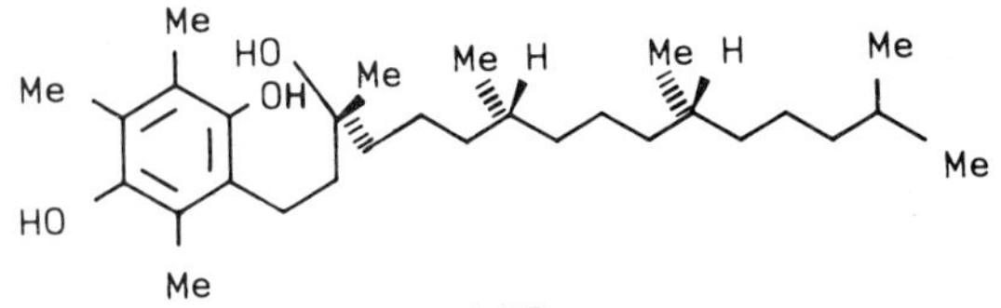

LII

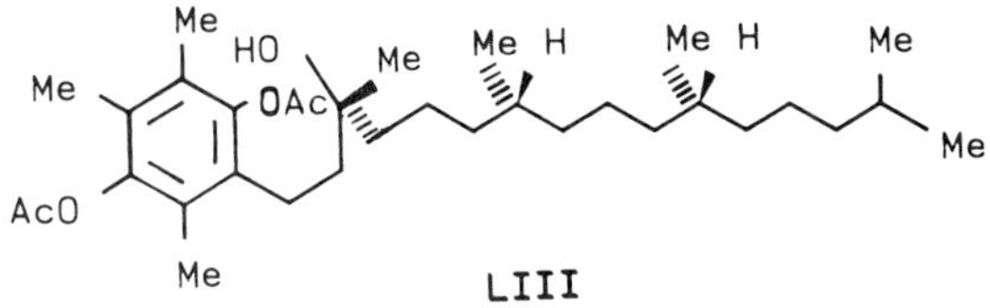

LIII

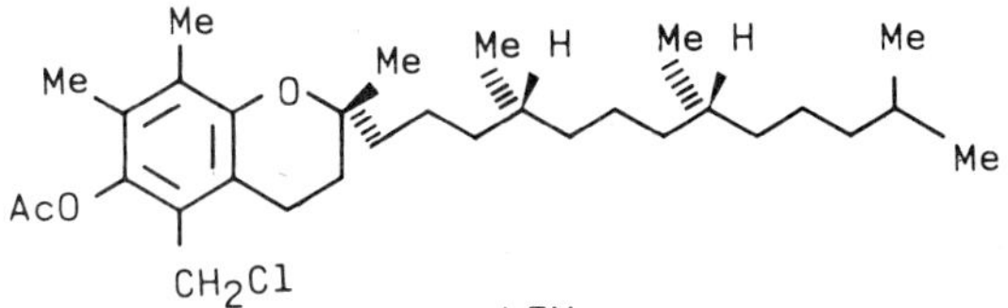

LIV

VI. PHYSICOCHEMICAL PROPERTIES

A. Melting Point

The tocopherols are viscous oils at room temperature, insoluble in water but soluble in aprotic solvents. The melting point of RRR-α-tocopherol was determined to be 2.5-3.5°C [115]. Frequently, esters [63] of tocopherols are used to define purity, e.g., acetate [116], allophanate [63], p-phenylazobenzoate [62], p-nitrophenylurethane [28], and 2,4-dinitrobenzoate [46].

B. Optical Activity

Optical rotation of natural tocopherols is of very small magnitude and is dependent on the nature of the solvent. Thus, α-tocopherol shows

$$\alpha_{546.1}^{25°} + 0.32°$$

in ethanol, while in benzene the rotation is opposite, i.e., -3.0° [31, 63]. Tables 5 and 6 show specific rotations for natural tocopherols and some of their derivatives.

C. Ultraviolet (UV) Spectra

UV spectra of tocopherols and tocotrienols show an absorption at 292-298 mμ in ethanol. Acylation of the phenolic hydroxyl shifts the absorption to 276-285 mμ [34,38,55,56,63,117].

TABLE 5   Specific Rotations of Natural Tocopherols[a]

Compound	Solvent	$\alpha_{546.1}^{25°}$
α-Tocopherol	Ethanol	+0.32°
	Benzene	-3.0°
β-Tocopherol	Ethanol	+2.9°
	Benzene	+0.9°
γ-Tocopherol	Ethanol	+3.2°
	Benzene	-2.4°
δ-Tocopherol	Ethanol	+3.4°
	Benzene	+1.1°

[a] From Ref. 63.

TABLE 6 Specific Rotations of Stereoisomeric α-Tocopherols

Stereoisomer	Reference	α-Tocopherol $[\alpha]_{}^{25°}$ (EtOH)	α-Tocopheryl p-phenylazobenzoate $[\alpha]_{600}^{25°}$ (CHCl$_3$)	K$_3$Fe(CN)$_6$ Oxidation product $[\alpha]_{}^{25°}$ (isooctane)
2R, 4'R, 8'R	62	+0.75°	+7.07°	+26.0°
2S, 4'R, 8'R	62	+0.19°	-7.64°	-25.8°
2RS, 4'R, 8'R	1, 62	+0.38°	0°	0°
2R, 4'RS, 8'RS	61	-	-6.96°	+25.8°
2S, 4'RS, 8'RS	1, 61	-0.14°	-7.47°	-23.6°

D. Infrared (IR) Spectra

The IR spectra of tocopherols and tocotrienols show the usual OH (2.8-3 μm) and CH (3.4-3.5 μm) stretching vibrations [33,118], and a characteristic band at 8.6 μm [33].

E. Nuclear Magnetic Resonance (NMR) Spectra

NMR spectroscopy has been used to differentiate between mono-, di-, and trimethylsubstituted tocols due to the presence or absence of characteristic bands for aromatic hydrogens and/or methyl groups [1]. A novel method has been described for the structural differentiation of tocopherols by means of NMR based on anisotropy indices that allow the assignment of chemical shifts to specific substituents in the aromatic ring of tocopherols [119]. The use of tris(dipivalyloxymethanato)europium as the shift reagent has resulted in a simplification of the spectrum. Thus, it is possible to analyze the spin-spin coupling of hydrogens at C-8, C-7, and C-9 [120]. NMR spectra of 7,8-dimethyl- and 8-methyltocotrienol and of 5,7-dimethyl- and 7-methyltocol have been recorded and discussed [38,56].

F. Mass Spectra

Mass spectra of tocopherols have been used to determine molecular weight and character of the side chain. The mechanism of opening and reclosing the heterocyclic ring of RRR-α-tocopherol was studied using $^{18}O_2$ and mass spectra determination of the reaction products [112]. The fragmentation pattern of tocopherols has been established as being the cleavage of the heterocyclic ring followed by loss of the isoprenoid side chain [121].

G. X-ray Diffraction

X-ray diffraction of tocopherol derivatives was used to differentiate between the stereoisomers of α-tocopherol [61,62].

H. Chromatography

1. Column Chromatography

The tocopherols were separated using a column of Kieselguhr coated with liquid paraffin [117], alumina [32], activated secondary magnesium phosphate [122], alumina, zinc carbonate, and Celite [123], zinc carbonate [31,124], or Floridin Earth [125]. 5,7,8-Trimethyltocol was separated from 5,7,8-trimethyltocotrienol on a polyethylene-Celite column [125a]. Hydroxyalkoxypropyl Sephadex was used to separate tocopherols [125b].

2. Paper Chromatography

Paper coated with Vaseline [126], liquid paraffin [35], silicone [127], or zinc carbonate [34] was used in one-dimensional paper chromatography to determine the tocopherols. A two-dimensional technique using paper impregnated with paraffin was described [34]. Nitrosated tocopherols were separated on paper treated with zinc carbonate or zinc carbonate and liquid paraffin [128].

3. Thin-Layer Chromatography

Silica gel or aluminum oxide with chloroform or benzene as the solvents were used to separate a mixture of all four tocopherols [129-131]. Similar methods have been published [131a,b]. A mixture of tocopherols and tocotrienols was separated by using a two-dimensional technique [132].

4. Gas Chromatography

5,7,8-Trimethyltocol was separated from 7,8-dimethyltocol on columns coated with silicone-rubber gums [133], silicone polymers SE-30, QF-1, poly(ethyleneglycoladipate) [134], SE-52, and a nitrile polysiloxane rubber [135]. Trimethylsilyl ethers of tocopherols were separated on columns of silanized glass with Apiezon L or SE-30 on Anakrom [136a]. Gas chromatography-mass spectrometry method for identification of tocopherols and tocotrienols in vegetable oils was reported [136b].

5. High-Pressure Liquid Chromatography

All natural tocopherols and tocotrienols were readily separated by high-pressure liquid chromatography on a Corasil II column [136c].

VII. SYNTHESIS

A. Introduction

The synthetic methods for tocopherols and tocotrienols that have been described in the literature can be classified as total and partial syntheses.

The total syntheses, in one approach, employ construction of the heterocyclic ring of tocopherols and tocotrienols along with the isoprenoid side chain at C-2 using methylated hydroquinones and an aliphatic reactant as the starting materials. In another approach, the isoprenoid side chain is introduced into the preformed, methylated 1-benzopyran system by the formation of a carbon-carbon bond. Figures 1 and 2 illustrate these approaches.

In partial synthesis, methyl groups are introduced into the aromatic ring of the lower methyl homolog of 5,7,8-trimethyltocol. This method makes it possible to use 5,8-dimethyl-, 7,8-dimethyl, and 8-methyltocol,

which are always present in natural sources, and convert them into the
biologically most active RRR-α-tocopherol.

B. Total Synthesis

1. Synthesis of Tocopherols by Construction of the Substituted
   Heterocyclic Ring

a. 5,7,8-Trimethyltocol: Isler and co-workers [4,137] described the
first attempts to synthesize (2RS,4'R,8'R)-α-tocopherol from trimethylhydroquinone XLVIII and 1,3-dibromophythane LV. Subsequently, Karrer
and co-workers [46,48] published a method for condensing phytyl bromide
XII (R = Br), prepared from natural phytol XII (R = OH), with trimethylhydroquinone LXVIII in petroleum ether with zinc chloride as the catalyst
to obtain a quantitative yield of (2RS,4'R,8'R)-α-tocopherol. The reaction

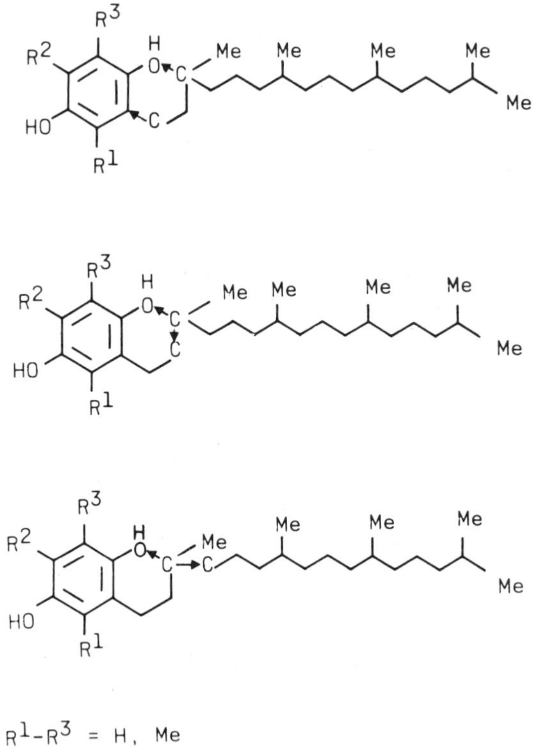

R^1-R^3 = H, Me

FIG. 1   Total synthesis of tocopherols by construction of the substituted
heterocyclic ring.

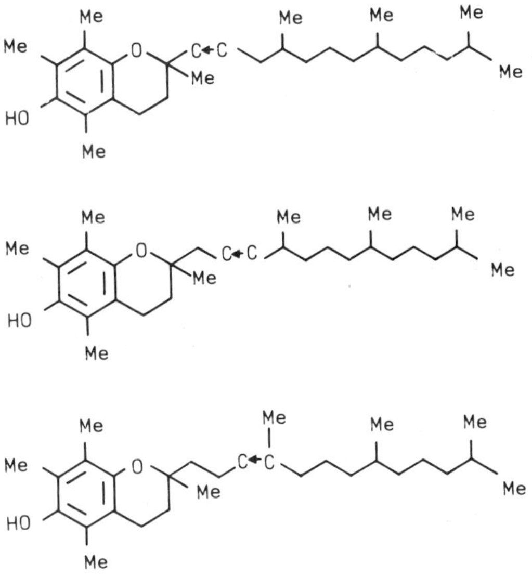

FIG. 2   Total synthesis of tocopherols by construction of the isoprenoid side chain.

presumably proceeds via LVII with ensuing ring closure. This method was later modified by Smith and Ungnade who carried out the reaction in the absence of solvent to obtain high yields of the product [138]. Karrer and Ringier [64] later postulated that the use of phytyl bromide prepared from synthetic phytol would give a mixture of diastereomers of α-tocopherol. However, no attempt had been made to isolate the isomers. The separation of 2R and 2S isomers of α-tocopherol obtained from natural phytol and trimethylhydroquinone was investigated [48, 61, 139], and recently, Robeson and Nelan [65] succeeded in separating the mixture of the epimers via a piperazine complex.

The synthesis of 5, 7, 8-trimethyltocol was also achieved by directly condensing phytol LVI (R = OH) with trimethylhydroquinone XLVIII [140–148]. Recent, mostly patented modifications of these original approaches employ various catalysts and solvents to achieve condensation in high yields. Zinc chloride and trichloroacetic acid in a carboxylic acid ester [149]; powdered aluminum, iron, or tin and boron trifluoride [150]; zinc chloride with sulfuric or p-toluenesulfonic acid and sodium hydrogen sulfate [151]; boron trifluoride and formic acid [152]; zinc dust [153]; zinc chloride and hydrochloric acid [154]; and tin dichloride [155] were used. It was shown [156, 156a] that the addition of boron trifluoride or aluminum chloride to trimethylhydroquinone resulted in the formation of the complex

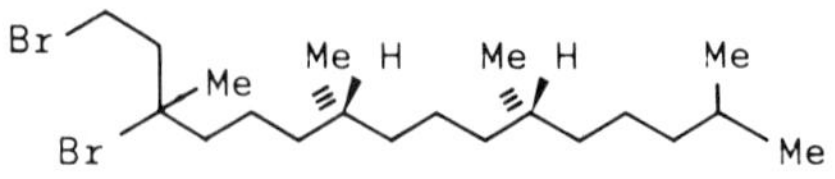

LV

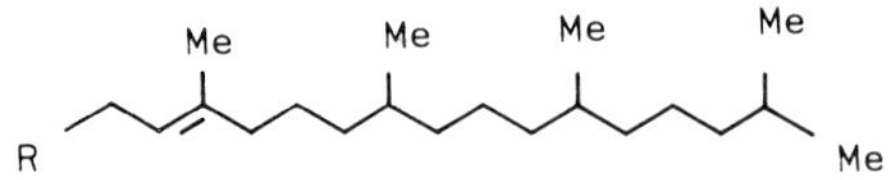

LVI

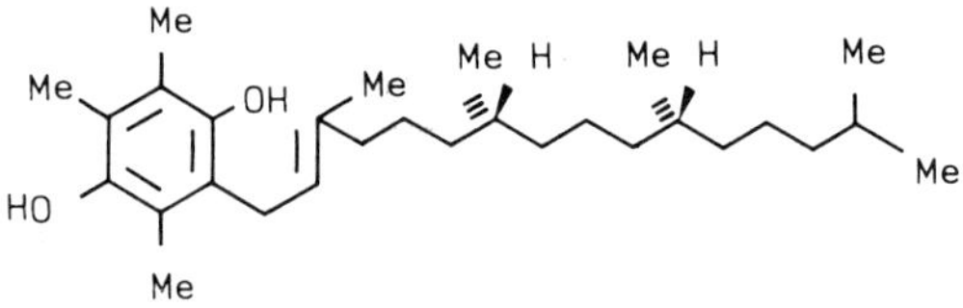

LVII

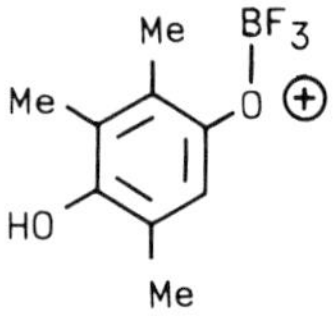

LVIII

LVIII and of protonated phytol or isophytol LIX whose interaction gave all-rac-α-tocopherol in high purity and good yields. Other phytane derivatives were also used in the condensation with trimethylhydroquinone. Smith et al. [157] employed the Claisen method to condense phytadiene LX with trimethylhydroquinone XLVIII in formic acid-acetic acid to obtain 5,7,8-trimethyltocol. In another approach, the halohydrin LXI reacted with trimethylhydroquinone XLVIII in the presence of zinc chloride in acetic acid to give 5,7,8-trimethyltocol [158].

The synthesis has been described based on the respective reactions of isophytol [146,159-162], phytyl acetate [163], phytane-1,3-diol [164,165], phytenic acid [165], and phytyldiphenylphosphate [166] with trimethylhydroquinone. The tertiary alcohol LXII, prepared from the Grignard reagent LXIII and ketone LXIV, was cyclized into 5,7,8-trimethyltocol with hydrogen bromide in acetic acid [167]. A reverse route was described by John and

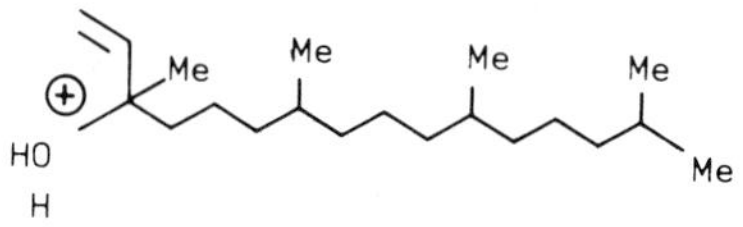

LIX

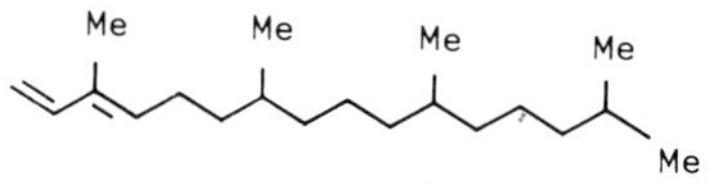

LX

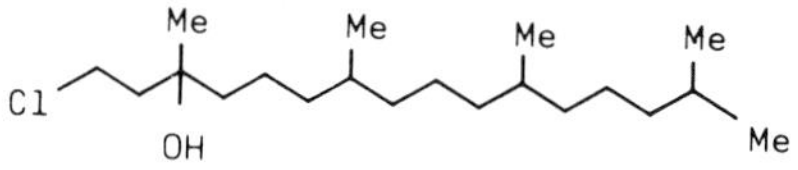

LXI

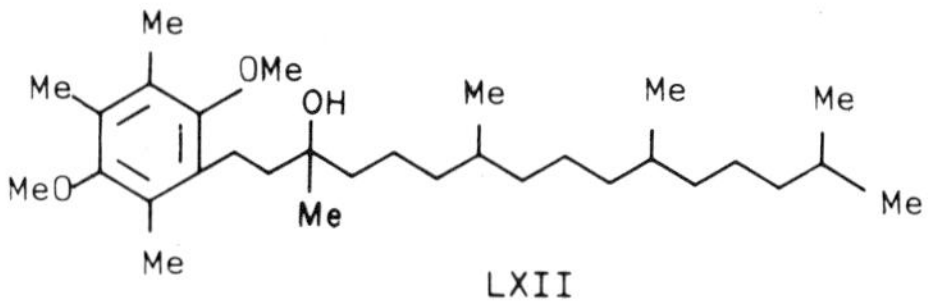

LXII

and Pini [168] who reacted the ketone LXV with the Grignard reagent LXVI followed by ferric chloride oxidation to give the quinone XXVIII which was reduced to the corresponding hydroquinone and cyclized into 5,7,8-trimethyltocol.

b. 5,8-Dimethyltocol: A direct condensation of 2,5-dimethylhydroquinone LXVII (R = H) with phytol LVI (R = OH) or phytyl bromide LVI (R = Br) afforded a mixture of products due to reactivity of LXVII (R = H) at both positions adjacent to the hydroxyl group as compared with trimethylhydroquinone XLVIII. Products of structures like LXVIII were

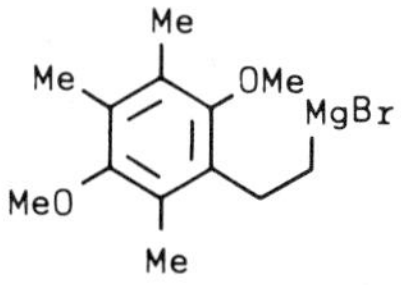

LXIII

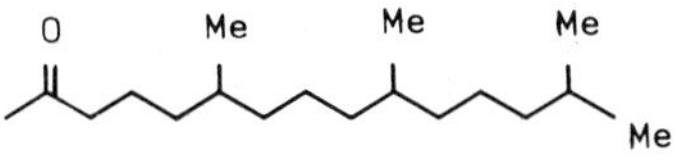

LXIV

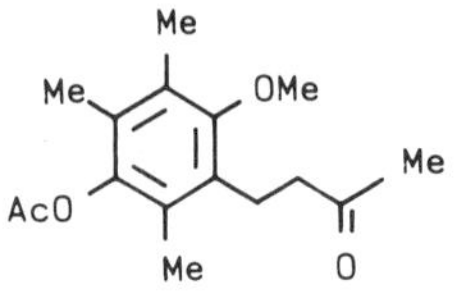

Me
Me   OMe
                    Me
AcO
Me   O

LXV

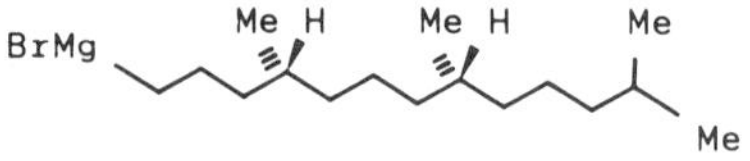

Me H   Me H   Me
BrMg
                        Me

LXVI

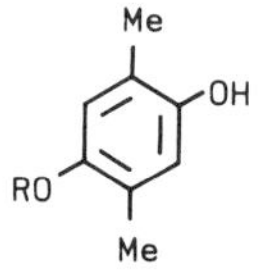

Me
        OH
RO
Me

LXVII

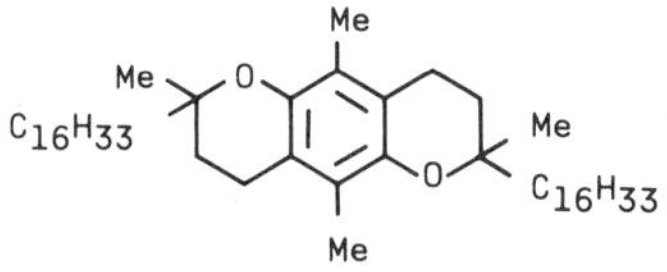

Me
Me   O
C$_{16}$H$_{33}$ Me
                O
                  C$_{16}$H$_{33}$
Me

LXVIII

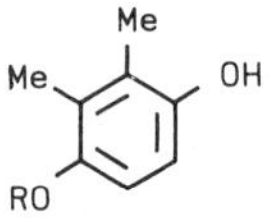

Me
Me   OH
RO

LXIX

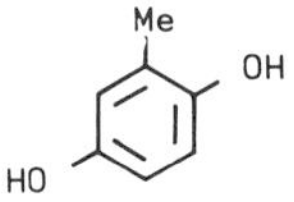

Me
        OH
HO

LXX

Me   O   O
HO   S

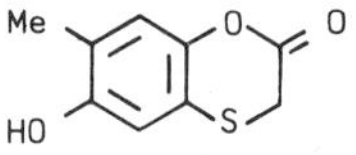

LXXI

formed beside 5,8-dimethyltocol, and the mixture was difficult to separate [48,169,170]. This problem was circumvented by using LXVII (R =
PhCH$_2$, PhCO) where the ortho position to the protected hydroxyl group
was deactivated. The protecting group was removed after the condensation with phytol or phytyl bromide, and the ring closure was achieved as
usual [171]. However, using formic acid as the catalyst, it was possible
to carry out the condensation of phytol LVI (R = OH) with 2,5-dimethyl-
hydroquinone LXVII (R = H) [169] with no undesirable side products.

c. 7,8-Dimethyltocol: The method used for the synthesis of 5,8-dimethyltocol was applied to prepare the isomeric tocol. 2,3-Dimethylhydroquinone LXIX (R = $PhCH_2$, Ac) treated with phytol or phytyl bromide and zinc chloride followed by removal of the protecting group yielded 7,8-dimethyltocol [171].

d. 8-Methyltocol: The synthesis of 8-methyltocol by the reaction of 2-methylhydroquinone LXX and phytol gave a mixture of 5-methyltocol IX (R^1 = Me, R^2 = R^3 = H), 7-methyltocol IX (R^1 = R^3 = H, R^2 = Me), and 8-methyltocol IX (R^1 = R^2 = H, R^3 = Me) [172,173]. The reaction of phytol LVI (R = OH) with 2-methylhydroquinone ethers and esters was studied by Green and coworkers [174] to obtain pure monomethyltocols. It was shown that thio derivatives of hydroquinone were suitable starting material [175]. This method was applied to the preparation of 8-methyltocol. The benzoxathionone LXXI was condensed with phytol followed by Raney nickel desulfurization and hydrolysis to give pure 8-methyltocol albeit in a low yield [176]. High yields of 8-methyltocol acetate were obtained when the acetophenone LXXII was reacted with phytol or isophytol followed by treatment with organic peracids, e.g., peracetic acid [177]. Recently, a general method for the synthesis of monomethyltocols has been reported. Phytyl bromide and tetracarbonylnickel form a π-allylnickel complex LXXIII which reacts with 2-bromo-6-methylhydroquinone diacetate LXXIV. Subsequent treatment with tin dichloride and hydrochloric acid gave 8-methyltocol [177a].

LXXII

LXXIII   LXXIV

e. 5-Methyltocol: Pure 5-methyltocol IX (R^1 = Me, R^2 = R^3 = H) was prepared in low yield by condensation of the thiophenol LXXV with phytol followed by desulfuration [174]. Other methods, i.e., reacting toluquinol ethers with phytol afforded only a mixture of all three monomethyltocols [173, 174]. A good yield of pure 5-methyltocol was obtained by reacting the Grignard reagent LXXVI with the ketone LXIV followed by treatment with acid [175]. A recently reported new method for the synthesis of mono-methyltocols [177a] was applied to the preparation of 5-methyltocol by the reaction of a π-allynickel complex LXXIII with 2-bromo-3-methylhydro-quinone diacetate LXXVII.

LXXV

LXXVI   LXXVII

f. 7-Methyltocol: 7-Methyltocol IX ($R^1 = R^3 = H$, $R^2 = Me$) was prepared analogously to the 5-methyl isomer [177a, 178].

g. 5,7-Dimethyltocol: 5,7-Dimethyltocol IX ($R^1 = R^2 = Me$, $R^3 = H$) was prepared by the reaction of phytol or isophytol and 2,6-dimethylhydro-quinone in the presence of formic acid [178].

h. Tocol: Tocol IX (R^1-R^3 = H) and its alkyl ethers were obtained by condensing phytol with hydroquinone using formic acid as the catalyst [179].

2. Synthesis of Tocopherols by Construction of the Isoprenoid Side Chain

Isler and co-workers [61] described a synthesis of epimeric α-tocopherols starting with the propiolic acid LXXVIII, which was converted into the aldehydes XX and LXXIX. The aldehydes were reacted with the phospho-nium salt LXXX (n = 1) to obtain LXXXI and LXXXII followed by catalytic hydrogenation to yield (2R,4'R,8'R)-α-tocopherol XXI (R^1-R^3 = Me) and (2S,4'R,8'R)-α-tocopherol XXII (R^1-R^3 = Me). In a similar manner, the aldehyde LXXXIII was treated with phosphonium salt LXXXIV to give LXXXV, which was hydrogenated to yield all-rac-α-tocopherol acetate

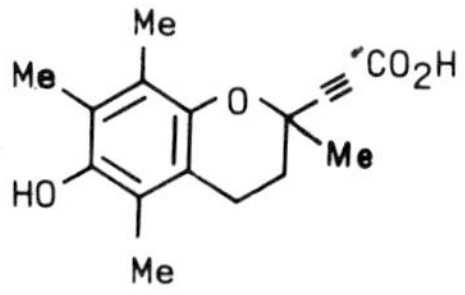

LXXVIII Fig. 1

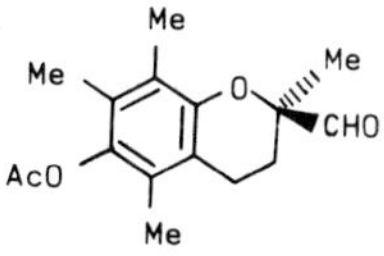

LXXIX Fig 2

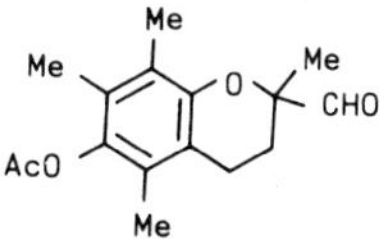

LXXIXa 3

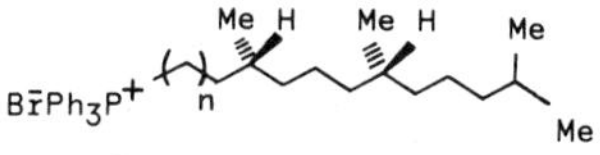

LXXX 4

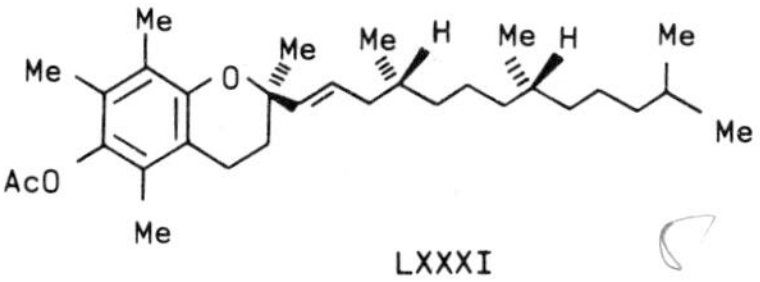

LXXXI 5

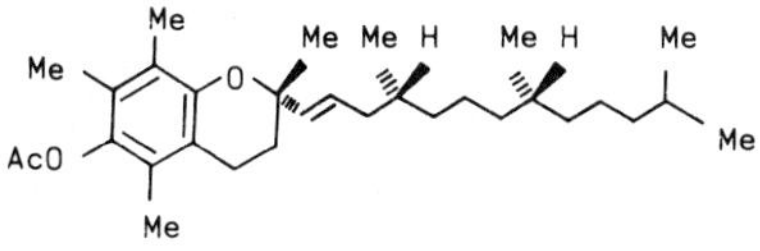

LXXXII 6

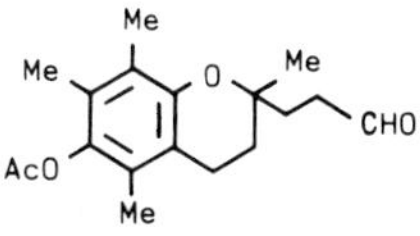

LXXXIII

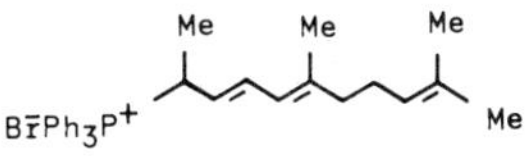

LXXXIV

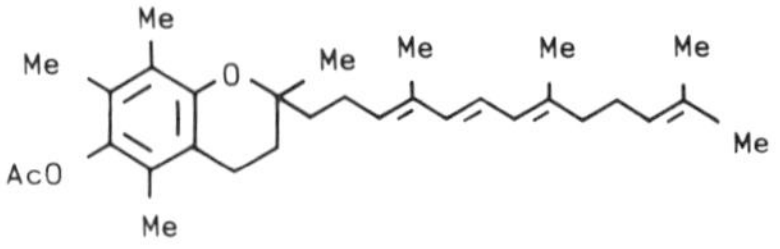

LXXXV 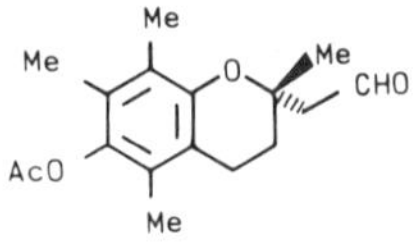   LXXXVI

[180]. The Scott and Saucy group employed the Wittig reaction for coupling
the aldehyde LXXXVI, prepared by a novel method (see Sec. D.3), with
the phosphonium salt LXXX (n = 0) followed by hydrogenation and reductive
saponification to synthesize (2R, 4'R, 8'R)-α-tocopherol [180a].

3. Synthesis of Tocotrienols by Formation of the Substituted
   Heterocyclic Ring

Attempts to prepare 5, 7, 8-trimethyltocotrienol by analogous synthesis that
yielded 5, 7, 8-trimethyltocol failed due to cyclization of the unsaturated
isoprenoid chain under the acidic experimental conditions [181] or yielded
only impure products [182]. The synthesis was achieved, however, by
Isler and co-workers under neutral reaction conditions with the use of boron
trifluoride etherate as the catalyst. Thus, trimethylhydroquinone XLVIII
was condensed with d, l-all-trans-geranyllinalool LXXXVII followed by
oxidation with silver oxide to give the quinone LXXXVIII, which was
refluxed in pyridine to obtain XL (R = H). The latter was reduced with
sodium in alcohol to give 2RS-α-tocotrienol [55]. Similarly, β- [55],
γ-, and δ-tocotrienol [56] were synthesized.

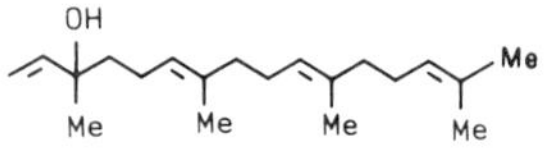

LXXXVII

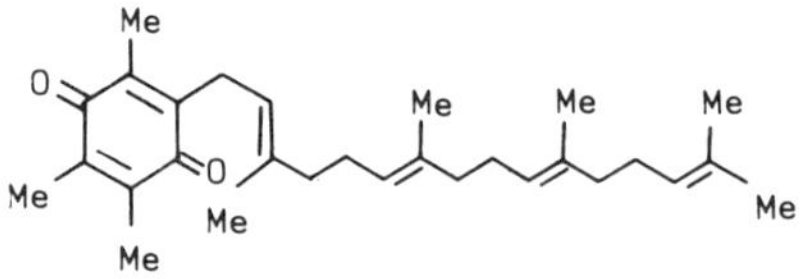

LXXXVIII

4. Synthesis of Tocotrienols by Construction of the Isoprenoid Side Chain

The first total synthesis of (2R), 3'E, 7'E-α-tocotrienol has been recently
achieved by Scott, Saucy, and coworkers. The methods, which are outlined

in Figs. 3 and 4, used the same starting material as for the synthesis of (2R, 4'R, 8'R)-α-tocopherol (see Secs. B.2 and D.3). However, the method in Fig. 3 yielded a mixture of isomeric compounds, i.e., (2R), 3'E, 7'E-α-tocotrienol and the isomer A, which was not possible to separate. The second approach, shown in Fig. 4, resulted in pure (2R), 3'E, 7'E-α-tocotrienol [180a].

C. Partial Synthesis

1. Synthesis of Tocopherols

The methylation of 5,8-dimethyl-, 7,8-dimethyl-, or 8-methyltocol was achieved by chloromethylation with formaldehyde and hydrochloric acid followed by the Clemmensen or catalytic reduction to give 5,7,8-trimethyltocol [110,183-185]. Similarly, 5,7,8-trimethyltocol from the lower methyl homologs was the result of aminomethylation with formaldehyde, ammonia, or a primary amine followed by reduction [186]; formylation with hexamethylenetetramine [187], zinc(II) cyanide [188], or methane trihalides [189]; and hydroxymethylation with formaldehyde [111,190, 191] followed by reduction. Other methods involved first oxidation of

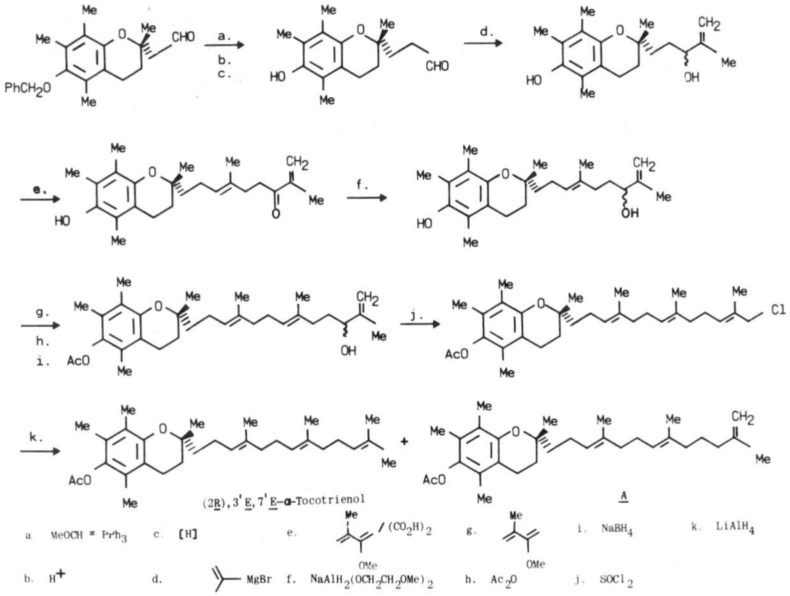

FIG. 3 Total synthesis of (2R), 3'E, 7'E-α-tocotrienol.

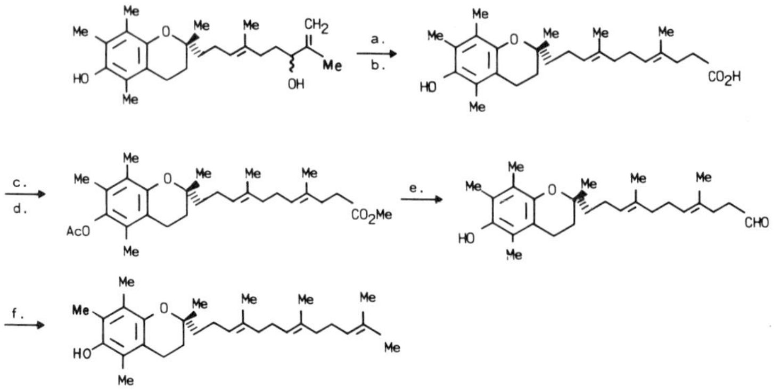

a. MeC(OEt)₃/EtCO₂H   c. MeI/NaHCO₃/DMF   e. DIBAL

b. saponification   d. Ac₂O   f. Ph₃P = CHMe₂

FIG. 4   Total synthesis of (2R̲),3'E̲,7'E̲-α-tocotrienol.

the tocopherol with ferric chloride to the corresponding tocopherylquinone
followed by chloromethylation, reduction, and recyclization [192,193].
These approaches have the disadvantage of yielding a mixture of stereoisomers of α-tocopherol. The reactions have been studied in detail, and
the reaction intermediates have been isolated and identified [33,194].

Hydrogenation of tocotrienols was used to obtain tocopherols and thus
to assign the configuration of the tocotrienols [54,56].

2. Synthesis of Tocotrienols

8-Methyltocotrienol was converted into 5,8-dimethyltocotrienol by
hydroxymethylation followed by reduction [38]. Similar reactions were
carried out with 5,8-dimethyltocotrienol [34,36] and 7,8-dimethyltocotri-
enol [36,56].

D. Synthesis of Synthetic Components of Tocopherols and Tocotrienols

1. Synthesis of Methylated Hydroquinones

a. 2,3,5-Trimethylhydroquinone: 2,3,5-Trimethylphenol LXXXIX,
prepared from 3,5-dimethylphenol XC by the Mannich reaction via XCI,
was coupled with p̲-diazoniumbenzenesulfonic acid. The azo dye was
reduced with sodium hydrosulfite followed by oxidation with ferric chloride
to obtain the quinone XCII, which was reduced to give 2,3,5-trimethyl-
hydroquinone XLVIII [195]. Alternatively, nitrosation of LXXXIX followed

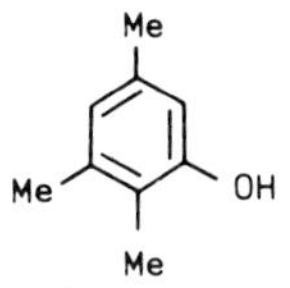

Me
Me   OH
Me

LXXXIX

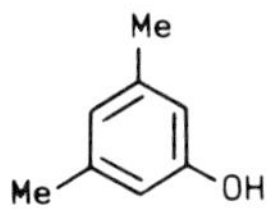

Me
Me   OH

XC

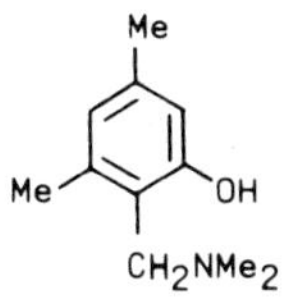

Me
Me   OH
CH₂NMe₂

XCI

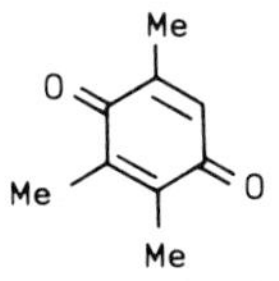

Me
O   Me
Me   O
Me

XCII

by treatment with sodium nitrite in sulfuric acid gave XCII, which was reduced with sodium hydrosulfite to give XLVII [196-199]. A general method for the preparation of polymethylhydroquinones via azo dyes was reported [200]. Oxidation of polymethylphenols with a free para or ortho position with potassium nitrosodisulfonate gave the corresponding quinones, which could be reduced into corresponding hydroquinones in high yields [201]. In another method, 1, 2, 4-trimethyl benzene XCIII was sulfonated and nitrated, the product XCIV reduced into XCV which was oxidized to

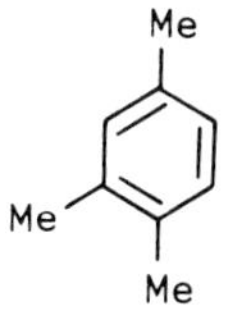

Me
Me
Me

XCIII

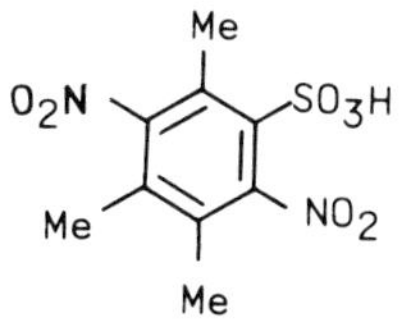

Me
O₂N   SO₃H
Me   NO₂
Me

XCIV

XCVI, and the latter was reduced to give trimethylhydroquinone XLVIII [202-205]. The preparation of trimethylhydroquinone XLVIII from 4-benzyloxyphenol [206], mesitylene [207], isophorone [208], diethyl ketone and benzeneazomalonaldehyde [209] was reported. A new method for the synthesis of trimethylhydroquinone XLVIII was reported by Wehrli and co-workers [210]. The condensation of crotonaldehyde XCVII and the ketone XCVIII gave the cyclohexenone XCIX, which was aromatized over palladium on charcoal to obtain the phenol C. Electrolytic oxidation of compound C in the presence of sodium hydroxylamine disulfonate gave the quinone CI, reduction of which, with sodium hydrosulfite, yielded

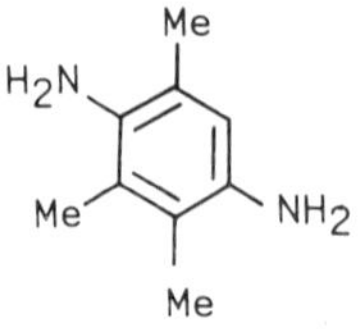

Me
H₂N — (ring, Me, Me, NH₂) — structures...

XCV 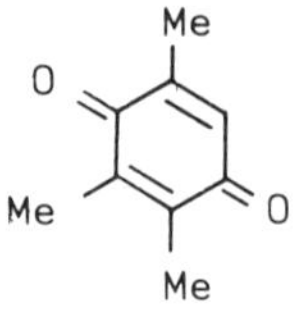   XCVI

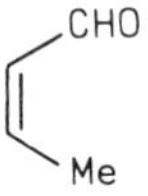

XCVII 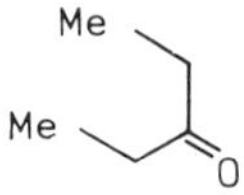   XCVIII

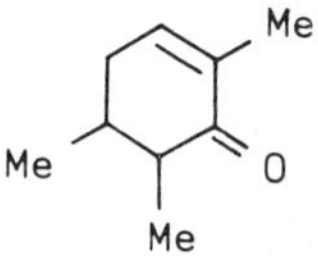

XCIX 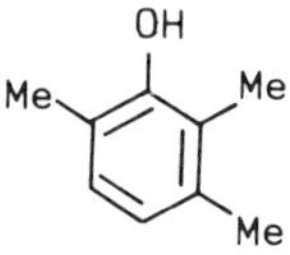   C 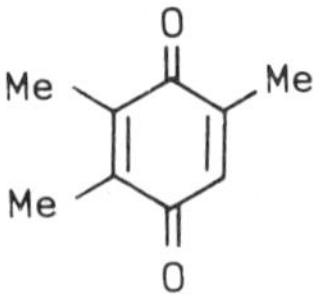   CI

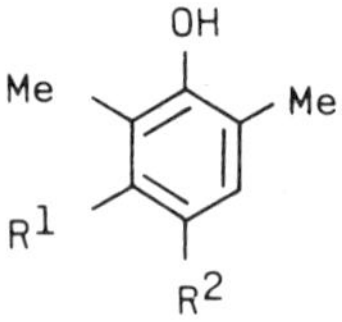

CII 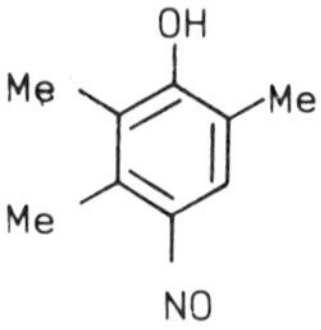   CIII 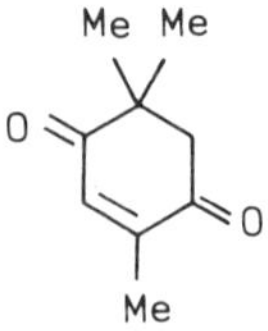   CIV

trimethylhydroquinone XLVIII. Sulfonation of a mixture of 2,4,6-trimethylphenol CII (R^1 = H, R^2 = Me) and 2,3,6-trimethylphenol CII (R^1 = Me, R^2 = H) followed by oxidation with manganese dioxide and hydrogenation yielded XLVIII [211,212]. Alternatively, nitrosation of CII (R^1 = Me, R^2 = H) and hydrogenation of the nitroso derivative CIII in sulfuric acid [213] or oxidation of CII (R^1 = Me, R^2 = H) with thallium sulfate [214] gave XLVIII. Acylation of the quinone CIV followed by hydrolysis yielded XLVIII [215].

b. 2,5-Dimethylhydroquinone: Oxidation of 2,5-dimethylphenol CV
with potassium nitrosodisulfonate [201] or lead tetraacetate [216], coupling
of CV with p-diazoniumbenzenesulfonic acid followed by reduction, oxidation, and reduction [200] were the methods used to prepare 2,5-dimethyl-
hydroquinone CVI. Hydroquinone subjected to the Mannich reaction with
formaldehyde and primary amines RNH_2 afforded CVII which was treated
with acetic anhydride and sodium acetate to give CVIII. The latter was
reduced with Raney nickel to CVI [217,218].

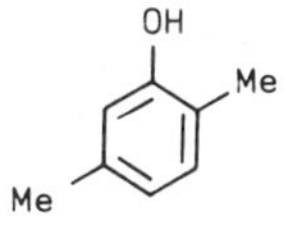

CV

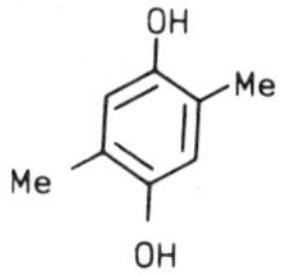

CVI

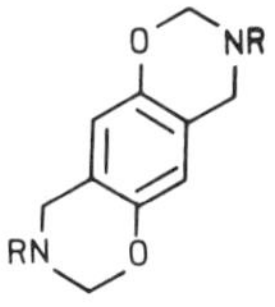

CVII 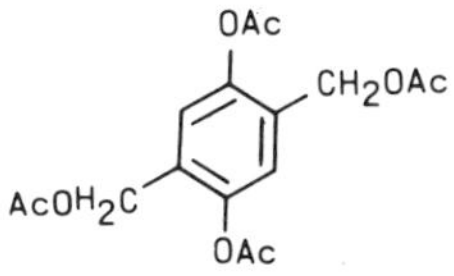   CVIII

c. 2,3-Dimethylhydroquinone: o-Xylene CIX was nitrated, the nitro
derivative reduced to 2,3-dimethylaniline CX and the latter oxidized to
2,3-dimethyl-p-benzoquinone CXI, which on reduction yielded 2,3-dimethyl-
hydroquinone CXII [219]. In another method, 2,3-dimethylphenol CXIII
was coupled with p-diazoniumbenzenesulfonic acid, the obtained azo compound was reduced, and the aminophenol CXIV was oxidized to the corresponding benzoquinone, which then was reduced to give CXII [220-222].
Another route to CXII was described using hydroquinone as the starting
material, which by Mannich reaction gave CXV. Treatment of the latter
with acetic anhydride and sodium acetate followed by Raney nickel hydrogenation yielded CXII [217].

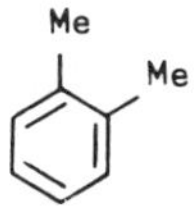

CIX 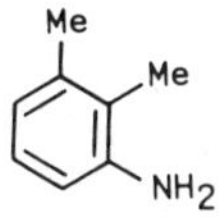   CX 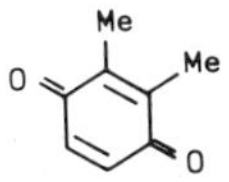   CXI 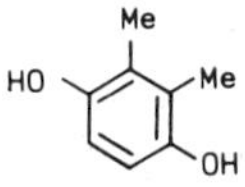   CXII

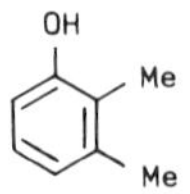

CXIII

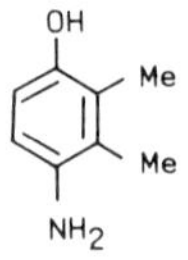

CXIV

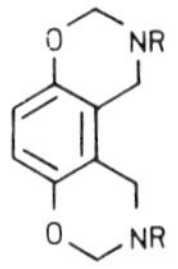

CXV

d. 2-Methylhydroquinone: Oxidation of 2-methylphenol CXVI with potassium nitrosodisulfonate [201] followed by reduction of the resulting benzoquinone was used to prepare 2-methylhydroquinone CXVII.

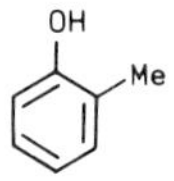

CXVI

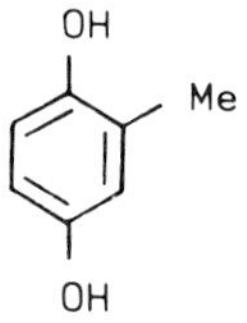

CXVII

2. Synthesis of the Isoprenoid Component of Tocopherols and Tocotrienols

Multistep synthesis of phytol LVI (R = OH) from pseudoionone CXVIII, citral CXIX, or linalool CXX was reported [64, 158, 223, 223a-c]. However, methods using acetone CXXI as the starting material are presently used to produce phytol LVI (R = OH) or isophytol CXXII. Thus, acetone CXXI is

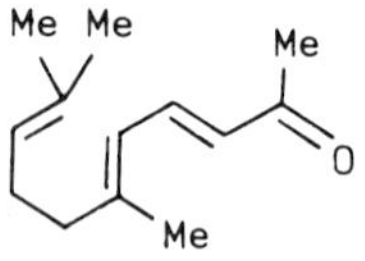

CXVIII

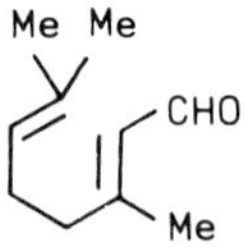

CXIX

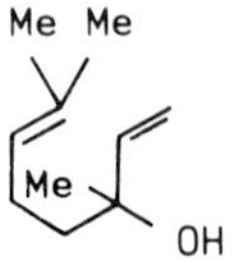

CXX

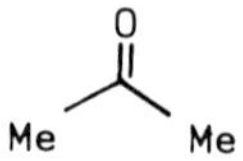

CXXI

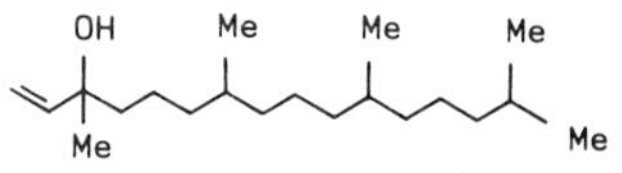

CXXII

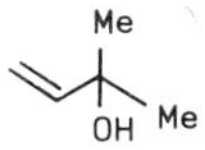

CXXIII

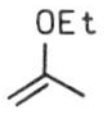

CXXIV

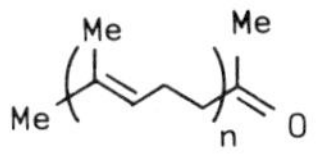

CXXV

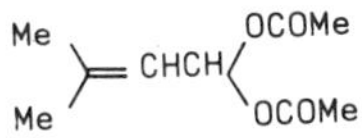

CXXVI

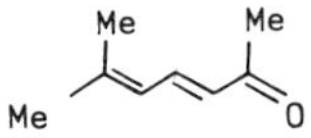

CXXVII

converted by ethynylation and hydrogenation to the tertiary alcohol CXXXIII, which is condensed with 2-ethoxypropene CXXIV by the method of Saucy and Marbet [224] to give the ketone CXXV (n = 1). By repeating this chain extension, the ketone CXXV (n = 3) is obtained and hydrogenated, ethynylated, and, in turn, again hydrogenated to give isophytol CXXII. Rearrangement of the latter gives phytol LVI (R = OH). Analogous chain extension of acetone is performed using acetoacetic ester synthesis [225-228] or a reaction with diketene [229, 230]. In another method, acetone was ethynylated, the acetylenic alcohol was treated with acetic anhydride in the presence of phosphoric acid, and the resulting acetate was isomerized to obtain CXXVI, which was condensed with acetone to give the homologous ketone CXXVII. Repetition of these reactions followed by hydrogenation afforded isophytol CXXII [231]. Phytone XIV was prepared from XXVII by treating the latter with sodium hydride in dimethyl sulfoxide followed by reflux in the presence of aluminum amalgam, and was ethynylated and reduced to give isophytol CXXII [232].

3. Synthesis of 2H-1-Benzopyran System

2,3,5-Trimethylhydroquinone XLVIII was formylated with hexamethylene-
tetramide to give CXXVIII, which was acetylated and subjected to the
Wittig reaction with CXXIX to obtain CXXX. This unsaturated ketone was
hydrogenated, reacted with ethynylmagnesium bromide to yield CXXXI,
which was cyclized to the benzopyran CXXXII. Hydrogenation of the latter
followed by ozonization gave the racemic LXXIXa which was resolved into
XX and LXXIX. Alternatively, CXXXII was reacted with ethylmagnesium
bromide followed by treatment with carbon dioxide to give LXXVIII,
which was hydrogenated, and the olefinic acid ester CXXXIII was
ozonized to give LXXIXa. Yet another approach utilized the acid CXXXIV
as the starting material to prepare LXXIXa [61]. The aldehyde LXXXIII
was prepared by the reaction of 2,3,5-trimethylhydroquinone XLVIII and

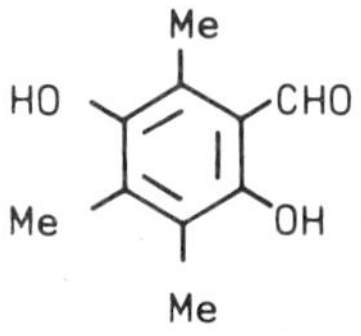

CXXVIII

$Ph_3P = CHCOMe$

CXXIX

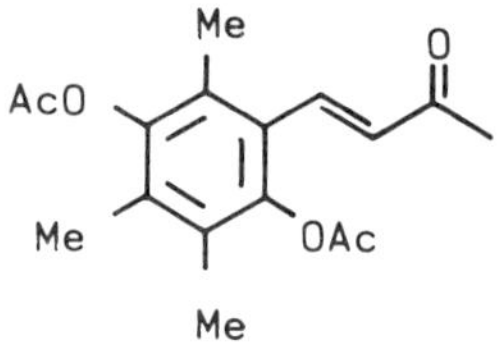

CXXX

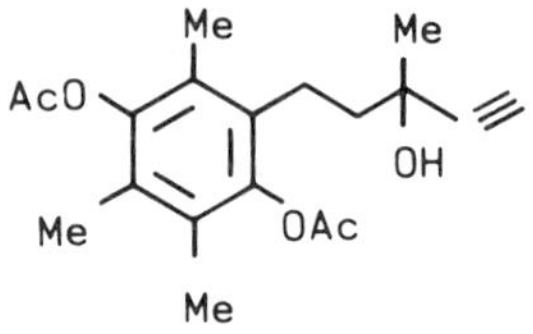

CXXXI

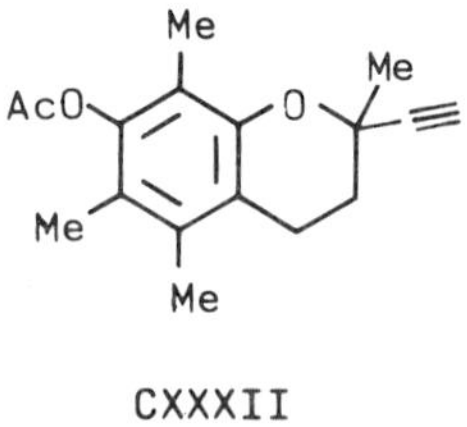

CXXXII

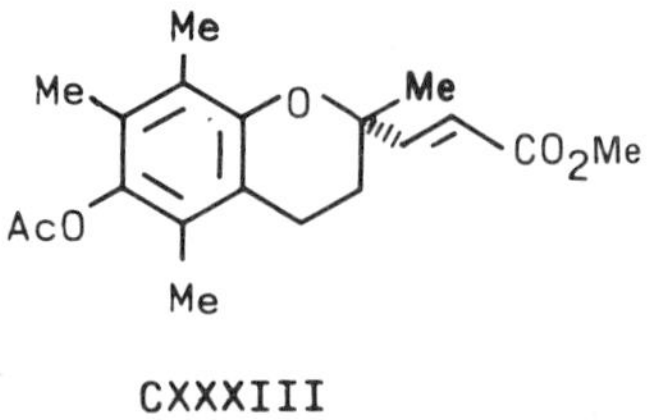

CXXXIII

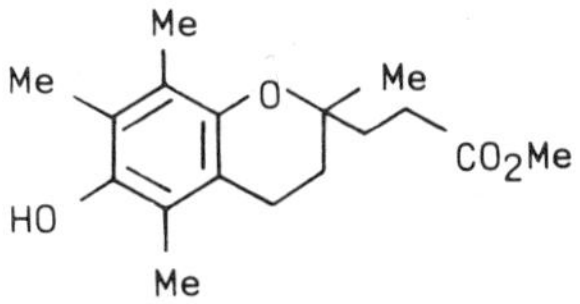

CXXXIV

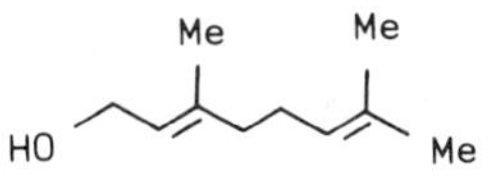

CXXXV

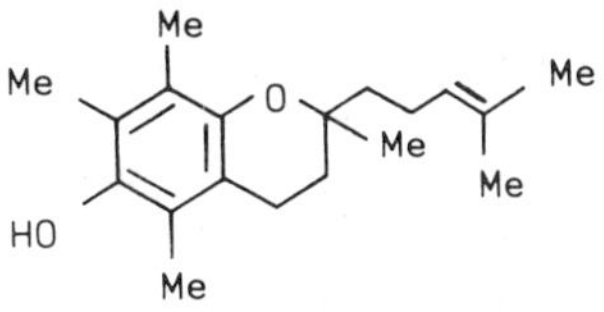

CXXXVI

geraniol CXXXV to give CXXXVI. Subsequent ozonization of the obtained olefin afforded LXXXIII [180]. Recently, a novel method for the preparation of the aldehyde LXXXVI was reported by Scott and Saucy group [180a] and is shown in Fig. 5.

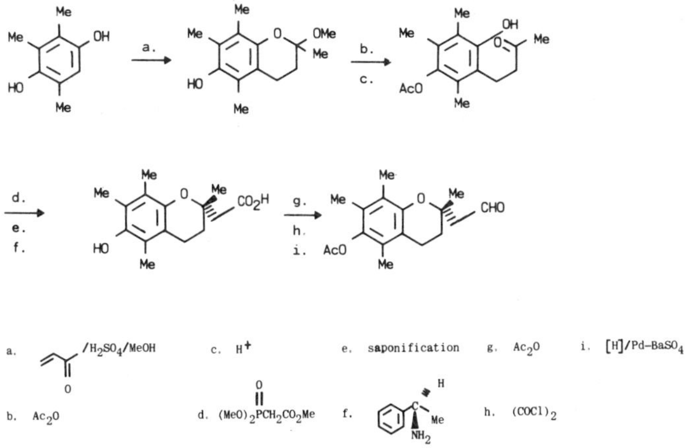

FIG. 5   Synthesis of 2H-1-benzopyran system.

VIII. BIOSYNTHESIS

Experiments with radioactive material administered to higher plants
showed that the aromatic part of the tocopherol molecule might be formed
from tyrosine CXXXVII (R = OH) and that the β-carbon of CXXXVII (R =
OH) or phenylalanine CXXXVII (R = H) could be utilized to form the aromatic methyl groups of the tocopherols [233]. It has been suggested that
one of the biosynthetic steps involves an intramolecular rearrangement of
4-hydroxyphenylpyruvic acid CXXXVIII [234] and that the biosynthetic pathway is as follows [233,234]: shikimic acid CXXXIX → prephenic acid
CXL → CXXXVIII → homogentisic acid CXLI → homoarbutin CXLII → tocopherols. The aromatic methyl groups might also be formed by methyl transfer from l-methionine [233,235,236]. The isoprenoid side chain might be
formed from mevalonic acid CXLIII [237-239] and it was shown that the
isoprenoid units were formed in trans configuration [240]. A detailed
account on the experimental procedures in studying the biogenesis has been
published [241]. There is evidence that tocotrienols are formed first,
followed by methylation and reduction of the side chain. The presence of
RRR-α-tocopherol beside all of the tocotrienols in palm oil [37] and the
fact that 5,8-dimethyl- and 5,7,8-trimethyltocotrienol were found in the
germinating seeds of wheat, in addition to RRR-α- and RRR-β-tocopherol,

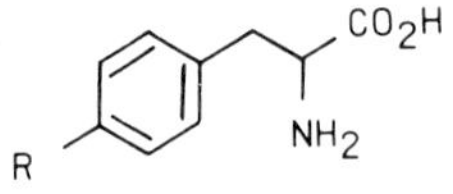

CXXXVII

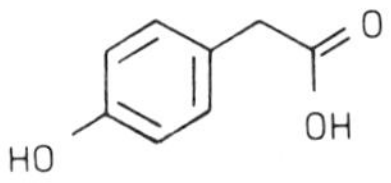

CXXXVIII

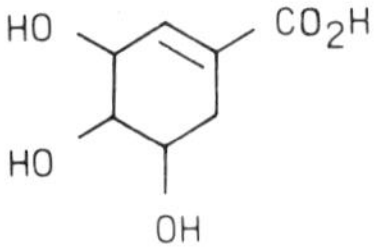

CXXXIX

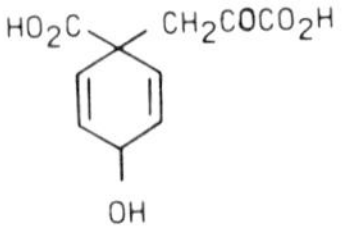

CXL

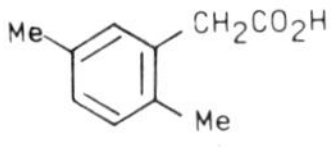

CXLI

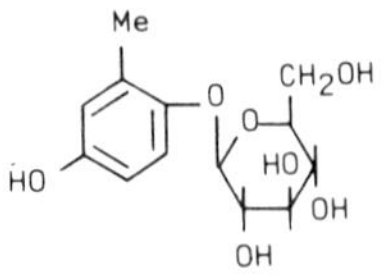

CXLII

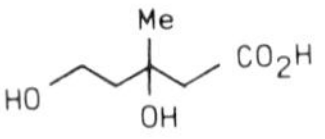

CXLIII

but were absent in the plant after 2 months of growth [242] would support these postulations. Similar contents of tocotrienols and tocopherols are found in pea seeds [242, 243].

IX. STRUCTURE-BIOLOGICAL ACTIVITY

A. Introduction

To define the relation between structure and biological activity of tocopherols and tocotrienols, two structural features of these compounds have to be considered: the presence of hydroxyl and methyl groups in the aromatic part of the molecule and the character of the aliphatic side chain at C-2 of the hetero-ring. In addition, the configuration at C-2, C-4', and C-8' of tocopherols and at C-2, C-3', and C-7' of tocotrienols will have a decisive effect on the activity. It should be pointed out that care has to be taken in comparing the reported values of activity of the assayed material due to the inconsistent nomenclature of these compounds as discussed in Sec. IV. The future synthesis of all stereoisomers of tocopherols and tocotrienols will be a desired undertaking to ascertain the effect of stereoisomerism on the activity.

B. Effect of Functional Groups

The presence of the phenolic hydroxyl in tocopherols is apparently of importance for the activity, although there has been no agreement in the literature as to what role the hydroxyl plays. It has been claimed that the position para to the heterocyclic oxygen is necessary for the activity [106]. However, a number of chromans X with various alkyl groups at C-2 were inactive [2440. When the hydroxyl group was masked as ether or allophanate, a complete inactivity resulted [245]. On the other hand, esterification of the hydroxyl did not alter or only somewhat altered the activity [106, 246]. The replacement of the hydroxyl by amino group does not affect the activity; the α-tocopheramine CXLIV was as active as RRR-α-tocopherol [247]. The fact that it is possible to convert CXLIV by mild oxidation into XXVIII, which is also formed from RRR-α-tocopherol, could support the postulation that the quinone XXVIII is the active compound in the antioxidant activity of RRR-α-tocopherol. However, the quinone XXVIII itself is biologically inactive [76]. Recent

CXLIV

studies [99-104] on oxidation of tocopherols with singlet oxygen showed that formation of the epoxides XLI-XLV might be the major pathway of the antioxidant process involving tocopherols.

The presence of methyl groups in the benzene ring is of primary importance. RRR-α-Tocopherol which is fully methylated in the benzene ring is the most active of all tocopherols in the standard bioassays, i.e., resorption gestation [248-252], muscular dystrophy [253-255], erythrocyte hemolysis [256-259], and encephalomalacia [260, 261]. The loss of methyl groups sharply reduces the activity. RRR-β-Tocopherol shows 25-40% and RRR-γ-tocopherol about 20% of the activity of RRR-α-tocopherol [248-258]. The position of the methyl group influences the activity since the synthetic 5, 7-dimethyltocol with the hydroxyl group flanked at both ortho positions by methyl groups shows about 60% of the α-tocopherol activity [257] as compared with the low activity of 5, 8- or 7, 8-dimethyltocol in which the ortho position to the hydroxyl is not substituted. 5-Methyltocol and 7-methyltocol and tocol do not show any appreciable activity [257]. Homologous alkyl groups in the benzene ring reduce or eliminate the bio-potency [48, 262, 263]. 5-Ethyl-7, 8-dimethyltocol IX (R^1 = Et, R^2 = R^3 = Me), 7-ethyl-5, 8-dimethyltocol IX (R^1 = R^3 = Me, R^2 = Et), and 8-ethyl-5, 7-dimethyltocol IX (R^1 = R^2 = Me, R^3 = Et) had similar chemical and physiochemical properties but differed in biological activity. The 7-ethyl isomer was the most active, and it was suggested that the position of alkyl groups at C-5, C-7, and C-8 affected the activity [262]. Homologous alkyl groups introduced in the benzene ring of tocopherols lowered the activity by a factor of 2 to 5 [263, 263a]. Shortening or elimination of the isoprenoid side chain of 5, 7, 8-trimethyltocol resulted in sharp decrease in activity (by a factor of 10 to 40) [264] or no activity. Thus, CXLV showed 3-5% of [dl]-α-tocopherol activity. No activity was observed with CXLVI and CXLVII [265].

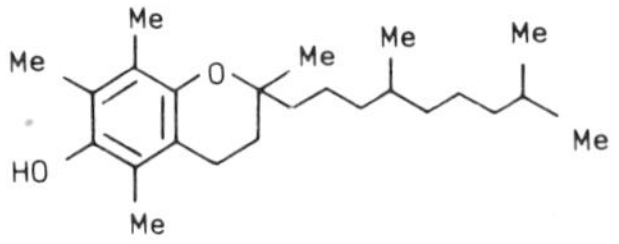

CXLV

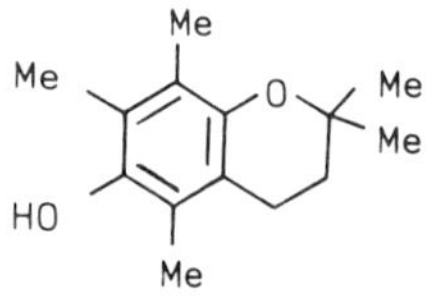

CXLVI

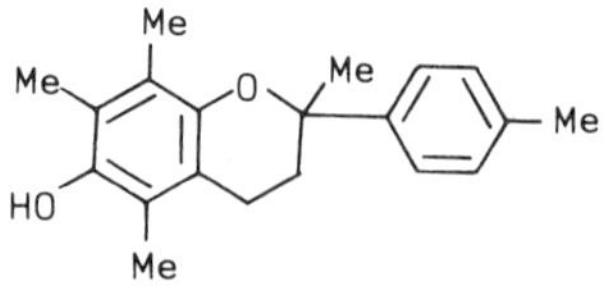

CXLVII

The dependence of activity of tocotrienols on the presence of methyl groups in the benzene ring is apparently the same as for tocopherols. 5, 8-Dimethyltocotrienol shows a negligible activity as compared with 5, 7, 8-trimethyltocotrienol and RRR-α-tocopherol [248-250]. Unsaturation of the side chain causes the decrease in activity of tocotrienols [259].

C. Effect of Stereoisomerism

The differences in biopotency of stereoisomers of α-tocopherol can be seen from the definition of International Unit (IU) for [dl]-α-tocopherol according to the National Formulary [266]:

1 mg [dl]-α-Tocopherol acetate = 1.0 IU

1 mg [dl]-α-Tocopherol   = 1.1 IU

1 mg [d]-α-Tocopherol acetate = 1.36 IU

1 mg [d]-α-Tocopherol   = 1.49 IU

(2R, 4'R, 8'R)-α-Tocopherol has been shown to be about 40% more active than the mixture of epimers, i.e., (2RS, 4'R, 8'R)-α-tocopherol [267]. (2S, 4'R, 8'R)-α-Tocopherol showed about 42% activity of the 2R-epimer [268]. The reported values of activity of (2S, 4'R, 8'R)-α-tocopherol differ, depending on the character of the bioassay, and are in the range of 40% [268] and 20% [255, 260, 269-271]. It has been suggested that the stereoisomerism at C-4' and C-8' affects the biopotency of tocopherols [271] which has been, however, disputed [268, 269]. A recent review on the biological activity of α-tocopherol stereoisomers concluded that (2R, 4'R, 8'R)-α-tocopherol acetate had a biopotency of 1.66 IU/mg while 2-epi-α-tocopherol acetate had a potency of 0.35 IU/mg based on biologic function assays. Hemolysis assays indicated relative activity of 1.53 and 0.56 for (2R, 4'R, 8'R)-α-tocopherol and 2-epi-α-tocopherol acetate, respectively, as compared with the activity of 2-ambo-α-tocopherol and all-rac-α-tocopherol acetate. A redefinition of the International Unit in terms of 1 IU = 0.60 mg of (2R, 4'R, 8'R)-α-tocopherol acetate has been suggested [272]. It has been postulated that the configuration at C-2 is the most important for potency; however, the effect of the configuration at C-4' and C-8' cannot be dismissed [272-274]. From this point of view it becomes obvious how important the task is to synthesize all possible stereoisomers of tocopherols and tocotrienols and assay their activity.

X. METABOLITES OF TOCOPHEROLS

Tocopheronic acid CXLVIII, tocopheronolactone CXLIX and the acid CL were isolated from human and rabbit urine as metabolites of vitamin E.

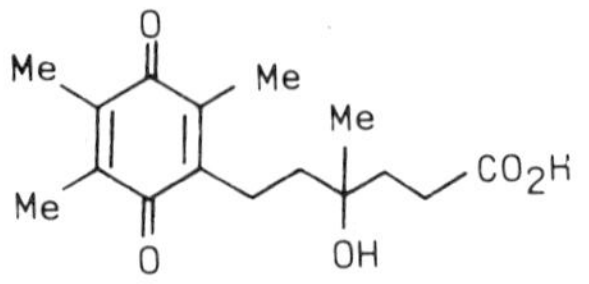

CXLVIII

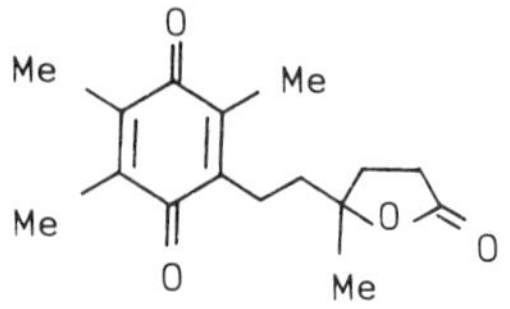

CXLIX

Since these compounds did not exhibit any vitamin E activity, they can be regarded as the products of a detoxification process that involved the formation of their conjugates with glucuronic acid [275, 275a-c]. The tocopherylquinone XXVIII was proved to be formed in liver and muscle [276] and fat deposits [277] of rats. The quinone XXVIII is reduced to the corresponding hydroquinone C LI in rat liver. No reconversion of the hydroquinone C LI to RRR-α-tocopherol occurred [278-280]. The ketoether XXXIII, which is also the oxidation product of 5, 7, 8-trimethyltocol with

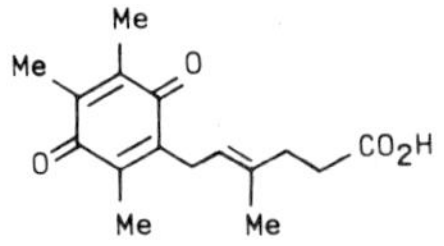

CL

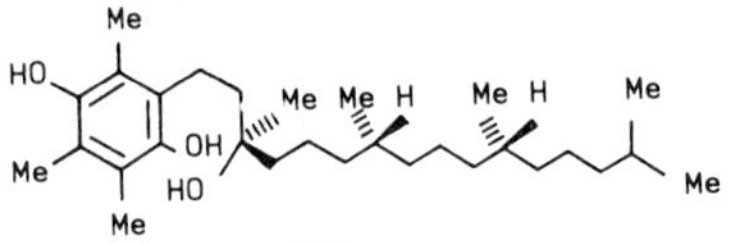

CLI

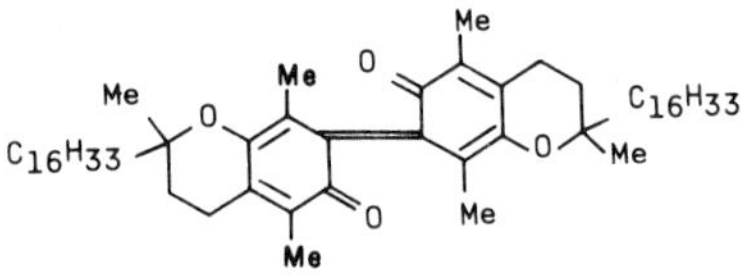

CLII

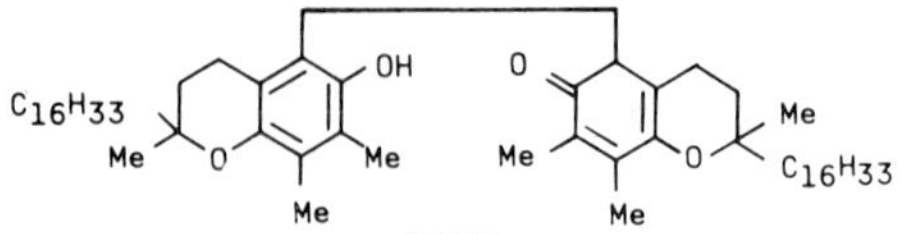

CLIII

potassium ferricyanide (see Sec. V.A), was detected in liver of rats fed with ^{14}C-labeled α-tocopherol [88,89,97,281-283]. The dimer CLII was claimed to be formed in rat and rabbit liver and to be obtained by the oxidation of 5,7,8-trimethyltocol with potassium ferricyanide [284,285]; however, a reappraisal of the structure showed that the compound was CLIII [286].

ACKNOWLEDGMENTS

I wish to thank Dr. G. Saucy for his encouragement during the preparation of this chapter, Drs. J. W. Scott and M. Nishikimi and L. J. Machlin for giving me access to their papers prior to publication, and Drs. G. Saucy J. W. Scott for critically reading the manuscript and for their valuable comments. Thanks are also due to Mrs. M. Loibissio for her skillful secretarial work.

REFERENCES

1. P. Schudel, H. Mayer, and O. Isler, in The Vitamins, Vol. 5. Edited by W. H. Sebrell, Jr. and R. S. Harris, New York, Academic, 1972.
2. H. Mayer and O. Isler, in Methods in Enzymology, Vol. 18. Edited by D. B. McCormic and L. D. Wright, New York, Academic, 1971.
3. D. C. Herting, in Kirk-Othmer Encyclopedia of Chemical Technology, 2nd ed., Vol. 21, Chicago, Interscience Publishers, 1970.
4. O. Isler, P. Schudel, H. Mayer, J. Würsch, and R. Rüegg, in Vitamins and Hormones, Vol. 20. Edited by R. S. Harris and I. G. Wool, New York, Academic, 1962.
5. H. Gutmann and O. Isler, in Ullman's Encyklopädie der Technischen Chemie, 3rd ed. Edited by W. Foerst, Munich, Urban and Schwarzenberg, 1967.
6. L. I. Smith, Chem. Rev. 27:287 (1940).
7. N. Campbell, in Chemistry of Carbon Compounds, Vol. 4. Edited by E. H. Rodd, New York, Elseiver, 1959, p. 929.
8. H. H. Draper, in Fat-Soluble Vitamins, International Encyclopedia of Food and Nutrition, Vol. 9. Edited by R. A. Morton, Elmsford, N.Y., Pergamon, 1970.
9. A. F. Wagner and K. Folkers, in Vitamins and Coenzymes. New York, John Wiley, 1964, p. 363.
10. J. Weichet and E. Knobloch, in Vitamine, Vol. 2. Edited by J. Fragner, Jena, Fischer Verlag, 1965.

11. P. Karrer, Helv. Chim. Acta 22:334 (1939).
12. W. John, Angew. Chem. 52:413 (1939).
13. H. A. Mattill, in The Vitamins, Vol. 3. Edited by W. H. Sebrell and R. S. Harris, New York, Academic, 1954, p. 481.
14. W. Hjarde, E. Leerbeck, and T. Leth, Acta Agric. Scand. Suppl. 1971, p. 87.
15. B. Stalla-Bourdillon, Ind. Chim. Belge 35:13 (1970).
16. T. Rubel, Chemical Process Review, No. 39, Park Ridge, N.J., Noyes Development Corp., 1969.
17. M. Evans and K. S. Bishop, Science 56:650 (1922).
18. B. Sure, J. Biol. Chem. 58:693 (1924).
19. M. Evans and K. S. Bishop, JAMA 99:469 (1932); Amer. J. Physiol. 63:396 (1922); JAMA 81:889 (1922).
20. B. Sure, Science 59:19 (1924).
21. B. Sure, J. Biol. Chem. 62:371 (1925).
22. H. A. Mattill, R. E. Carmen, and M. M. Clayton, J. Biol. Chem. 61:729 (1924).
23. H. A. Mattill and R. E. Conklin, J. Biol. Chem. 44:137 (1920).
24. H. A. Mattill and N. C. Stone, J. Biol. Chem. 55:443 (1923).
25. M. Evans and G. O. Gurr, Proc. Natl. Acad. Sci. USA 11:334 (1925).
26. M. Evans and G. O. Burr, J. Biol. Chem. 76:273 (1928).
27. M. Evans, O. H. Emerson, and G. A. Emerson, J. Biol. Chem. 113:319 (1936).
28. O. H. Emerson, G. A. Emerson, A. Mohammad, and H. M. Evans, J. Biol. Chem. 122:99 (1937).
29. H. S. Olcott, J. Biol. Chem. 107:471 (1934).
30. H. S. Olcott and H. A. Mattill, J. Biol. Chem. 104:423 (1934).
31. J. Green, P. Mamalis, S. Marcinkiewicz, and D. McHale, Chem. Ind. (Lond.) 1960, p. 73.
32. M. H. Stern, C. D. Robeson, L. Weisler, and J. G. Baxter, J. Amer. Chem. Soc. 69:869 (1947).
33. J. Green, D. McHale, S. Marcinkiewicz, P. Mamalis, and P. R. Watt, J. Chem. Soc. 7:3362 (1959).
34. J. Green, S. Marcinkiewicz, and P. R. Watt, J. Sci. Food Agric. 6:274 (1955).
35. P. W. R. Eggitt and L. D. Ward, J. Sci. Food Agric. 4:469 (1953).
36. J. Green and S. Marcinkiewicz, Nature (Lond.) 177:86 (1956).
37. J. F. Pennock, F. W. Hemming, and J. D. Kerr, Biochem. Biophys. Res. Commun. 17:542 (1964).
38. K. J. Whittle, P. J. Dunphy, and J. F. Pennock, Biochem. J. 100:138 (1966).
39. C. S. McArthur and E. M. Watson, Science 86:35 (1937).
40. E. Fernholtz, J. Amer. Chem. Soc. 59:1154 (1937).
41. W. John, Z. Physiol. Chem. 252:222 (1938).

42. W. John, E. Dietzel, and P. Günther, Z. Physiol. Chem. 252:208 (1938).

43. O. H. Emerson, Science 88:40 (1938).

44. F. Bergel, A. R. Todd, and T. S. Work, J. Chem. Soc. 1938:253.

45. L. I. Smith, H. E. Ungnade, and W. W. Prichard, Science 88:37 (1938).

46. P. Karrer, H. Fritzsche, B. H. Ringier, and H. Salomon, Helv. Chim. Acta 21:520 (1938).

47. P. Karrer, H. Salmon, and H. Fritzsche, Helv. Chim. Acta 21:309 (1938).

48. P. Karrer, H. Fritzsche, B. H. Ringier, and H. Salomon, Helv. Chim. Acta 21:820 (1938).

49. P. Karrer, R. Escher, H. Fritzsche, H. Keller, B. H. Ringier, and H. Salomon, Helv. Chim. Acta 21:939 (1938).

50. E. Fernholz, J. Amer. Chem. Soc. 60:700 (1938).

51. O. H. Emerson, J. Amer. Chem. Soc. 60:1741 (1938).

52. W. John, Z. Physiol. Chem. 250:11 (1937).

53. O. H. Emerson and L. I. Smith, J. Amer. Chem. Soc. 62:1869 (1940).

54. O. Isler, H. Mayer, J. Metzger, R. Rüegg, and P. Schudel, Angew. Chem. 75:1030 (1963).

55. P. Schudel, H. Mayer, J. Metzger, R. Rüegg, and O. Isler, Helv. Chim. Acta 46:2517 (1963).

56. H. Mayer, J. Metzger, and O. Isler, Helv. Chim. Acta 50:1376 (1967).

57. H. Mayer, P. Schudel, R. Rüegg, and O. Isler, Helv. Chim. Acta 46:963 (1963).

58. R. S. Cahn, C. K. Ingold, and V. Prelog, Experientia 12:81 (1956).

59a. J. W. K. Burrell, L. M. Jackman, and B. C. L. Weedon, Proc. Chem. Soc. 1959:263.

59b. P. Crabbe, C. Djerassi, E. J. Eisenbraun, and S. Liu, Proc. Chem. Soc. 1959:264.

60. R. H. Conforth, J. W. Cornforth, and V. Prelog, Ann. Chem. 634:197 (1960).

61. H. Mayer, P. Schudel, R. Rüegg, and O. Isler, Helv. Chim. Acta 46:650 (1963).

62. P. Schudel, H. Mayer, J. Metzger, R. Rüegg, and O. Isler, Helv. Chim. Acta 46:333 (1963).

63. J. G. Baxter, C. D. Robeson, J. D. Taylor, and R. W. Lehman, J. Amer. Chem. Soc. 65:918 (1943).

64. P. Karrer and B. H. Ringier, Helv. Chim. Acta 22:610 (1939).

65. C. D. Robeson and D. R. Nelan, J. Amer. Chem. Soc. 84:3196 (1962).

66. P. Karrer and H. Rentschler, Helv. Chim. Acta 26:1750 (1943).

67. P. Schudel, H. Mayer, R. Rüegg, and O. Isler, Chimia 16:368
     (1962).

68. R. P. Linstead, J. C. Lunt, and B. C. L. Weedon, J. Chem. Soc.
     1950:3333.

69. IUPAC-IUB Commission on Biochemical Nomenclature. Nomencla-
     ture of tocopherols and related compounds, recommendations
     (1973). Eur. J. Biochem. 46:217 (1974).

70. W. John and W. Emte, Z. Physiol. Chem. 268:85 (1940); 261:24
     (1939).

71. M. Further and R. E. Meyer, Helv. Chim. Acta 22:240 (1939).

72. W. John, E. Dietzel, and W. Emte, Z. Physiol. Chem. 257:173
     (1939).

73. L. I. Smith, W. B. Irwin, and H. E. Ungnade, J. Amer. Chem. Soc.
     61:2424 (1939).

74. V. L. Frampton, W. A. Skinner, P. Cambour, and P. S. Bailey,
     J. Amer. Chem. Soc. 82:4632 (1960).

75. V. L. Frampton, W. A. Skinner, and P. S. Bailey, Science 116:34
     (1954).

76. P. Karrer and A. Geiger, Helv. Chim. Acta 23:455 (1940).

77. M. Kofler, P. F. Sommer, H. R. Bolliger, B. Schmidli, and
     M. Vecchi, in Vitamins and Hormones, Vol. 20. Edited by R. S.
     Harris and I. G. Wool, New York, Academic, 1962, p. 407.

78. G. E. Inglett and H. A. Mattill, J. Amer. Chem. Soc. 77:6552
     (1965).

79. A. Issidorides, J. Amer. Chem. Soc. 73:5146 (1951).

80. W. H. Harrison, J. E. Gander, E. R. Blakley, and P. D. Boyer,
     Biochim. Biophys. Acta 21:150 (1956).

80a. C. R. Seward, G. V. Mitchell, L. C. Argrett, and E. L. Hove,
     Lipids 4:629 (1969).

80b. H. Selander and J. L. G. Nilsson, Acta Pharm. Suec. 9:125 (1972).

81. V. L. Frampton, W. A. Skinner, Jr., and P. S. Bailey, J. Amer.
     Chem. Soc. 76:282 (1954).

82. C. Martius and H. Eilingsfeld, Ann. Chem. 607:159 (1957).

83. P. D. Boyer, J. Amer. Chem. Soc. 73:733 (1951).

84. W. H. Harrison, J. E. Gander, E. R. Blakley, and P. D. Boyer,
     Biochim. Biophys. Acta 21:150 (1956).

85. C. T. Goodhue and H. A. Risley, Biochemistry 4:854 (1965).

86. W. Dürckheimer and L. A. Cohen, Biochem. Biophys. Res.
     Commun. 9:262 (1962).

87. W. Dürckheimer and L. A. Cohen, J. Amer. Chem. Soc. 86:4388
     (1964).

88. H. H. Draper, A. S. Csallany, and S. N. Shah, Biochim. Biophys.
     Acta 59:527 (1962).

89.　D. R. Nelan and C. D. Robeson, Nature (Lond.) 193:477 (1962); J. Amer. Chem. Soc. 84:2963 (1962).

90.　P. Schudel, H. Mayer, R. Rüegg, and O. Isler, Chimia 16:367 (1962).

91.　W. A. Skinner and P. Alaupovic, J. Org. Chem. 28:2854 (1963).

92.　P. Schudel, H. Mayer, J. Metzger, R. Rüegg, and O. Isler, Helv. Chim. Acta 46:636 (1963).

93.　W. A. Skinner and R. M. Parkhurst, J. Org. Chem. 29:3601 (1964); J. Org. Chem. 31:1248 (1966).

94.　J. L. G. Nilsson, G. D. Daves, Jr., and K. Folkers, Acta Chem. Scand. 22:207 (1968).

95.　D. McHale and J. Green, Chem. Ind. 1963:982; Chem. Ind. 1964:366.

96.　W. A. Skinner, Biochem. Biophys. Res. Commun. 15:469 (1964).

97.　A. S. Csallany and H. H. Draper, J. Biol. Chem. 238:2912 (1963); J. Biol. Chem. 239:574 (1963).

98.　Belg. Patent 635,999 (1962) to Hoffmann-La Roche; Chem. Abstr. 61:13285 (1964).

99.　G. W. Grams, K. Eskins, and G. E. Inglett, J. Amer. Chem. Soc. 94:866 (1972).

100.　G. W. Grams, Tetrahedron Lett. 1971:4823.

101.　G. W. Grams and K. Eskins, Biochemistry 11:606 (1972).

102.　S. R. Fahrenholtz, F. H. Doleiden, A. M. Trozzolo, and A. A. Lamola, Photochem. Photobiol. 20:505 (1974).

103.　B. Stevens, R. D. Small, Jr., and S. R. Perez, Photochem. Photobiol. 20:515 (1974).

104.　C. F. Foote, Ta-Yen Ching, and G. G. Geller, Photochem. Photobiol. 20:511 (1974).

105.　M. Nishikimi and L. J. Machlin, Arch. Biochem. Biophys. 170:684 (1975).

105a.　J. W. Scott, W. M. Cort, H. Harley, D. R. Parrish, and G. Saucy, J. Amer. Oil. Chem. Soc. 51:200 (1974).

106.　V. Demole, O. Isler, B. H. Ringier, H. Salomon, and P. Karrer, Helv. Chim. Acta 22:65 (1939).

107.　P. Karrer and G. Bussmann, Helv. Chim. Acta 23:1137 (1940).

108.　J. Green and S. Marcinkiewicz, Analyst (London) 84:297, 304 (1959).

109.　M. L. Quaife, J. Amer. Chem. Soc. 66:308 (1944).

110.　L. Weisler and A. J. Chechak, U.S. Patent 2,486,542 (1949); Chem. Abstr. 44:2037.

111.　L. Weisler, U.S. Patent 2,640,058 (1953); Chem. Abstr. 48:7643 (1954).

112.　H. Mayer, W. Vetter, J. Metzger, R. Rüegg, and O. Isler, Helv. Chim. Acta 50:1168 (1967).

113. M. A. Oxman and L. A. Cohen, Biochim. Biophys. Acta 113:412 (1966).

114. M. Tishler and N. L. Wendler, J. Amer. Chem. Soc. 63:1532 (1941).

115. C. D. Robeson, J. Amer. Chem. Soc. 65:1660 (1943).

116. C. D. Robeson, J. Amer. Chem. Soc. 64:1487 (1942).

117. P. W. R. Eggit and F. W. Norris, J. Sci. Food Agric. 6:689 (1955).

118. H. Rosenkrantz, J. Biol. Chem. 173:439 (1948).

119. H. Finegold and H. T. Slover, J. Org. Chem. 32:2557 (1967).

120. K. Tsukida, M. Ito, and F. Ikeda, J. Vitaminol. 18:24 (1972).

121. S. E. Scheppele, R. K. Mitchum, C. J. Charles, Jr., K. F. Kinneberg, and G. V. Odell, Lipids 7:297 (1972).

122. F. Bro-Rasmussen and W. Hjarde, Acta Chem. Scand. 11:34; 44 (1957).

123. J. G. Bieri, C. J. Pollard, I. Prange, and H. Dam, Acta Chem. Scand. 15:783 (1961).

124. M. L. Quaife, J. Biol. Chem. 175:605 (1948).

125. A. Emmerie, Ann. N.Y. Acad. Sci. 52:309 (1949).

125a. C. K. Pearson, D. R. Davies, and M. McC. Barnes, Chem. Ind. 1970:275.

125b. J. N. Thompson, P. Erdody, and W. B. Maxwell, Anal. Biochem. 50:267 (1972).

126. F. Brown, Biochem. J. 51:237 (1952); 52:523 (1952).

127. J. A. Brown, Analyt. Chem. 25:774 (1953).

128. S. Marcinkiewicz and J. Green, Analyst 84:304 (1959).

129. A. Seher, Microchim. Acta 1961:308.

130. H. D. Stowe, Arch. Biochem. Biophys. 103:42 (1963).

131. M. K. Govind Rao, S. Venkob Rao, and K. T. Achaya, J. Sci. Food Agric. 16:1 (1965).

131a. H. G. Lovelady, J. Chromatogr. 85:81 (1973); 78:449 (1973).

131b. T. Arantani, K. Mita, and F. Mizui, J. Chromatogr. 79:179 (1973).

132. K. J. Whittle and J. F. Pennock, Analyst 92:423 (1967).

133. N. Nicolaides, J. Chromatogr. 4:496 (1960).

134. P. W. Wilson, E. Kodicek, and V. H. Booth, Biochem. J. 84:524 (1962).

135. P. P. Nair and D. A. Turner, J. Amer. Oil Chem. Soc. 40:353 (1963).

136. H. T. Slover, L. M. Shelley, T. L. Burks, J. Amer. Oil Chem. Soc. 44:161 (1967).

136a. B. C. Rudy, F. P. Mahn, B. Z. Senkowski, A. J. Sheppard, and W. D. Hubbard, J. Assoc. Off. Anal. Chem. 55:1211 (1972).

136b. K. G. M. Rao and E. G. Perkins, J. Agr. Food Chem. 20:240 (1972).

136c. J. F. Cavins and G. E. Inglett, Cereal Chemistry 51:605 (1974).
137.   O. Isler, Mitt. Naturforsch. Ges. Schaffhausen 18:321 (1942-43).
138.   L. I. Smith and H. E. Ungnade, J. Org. Chem. 4:298 (1939).
139.   P. Karrer, A. Kugler, and H. Simon, Helv. Chim. Acta 27:1006
       (1944).
140.   P. Karrer and O. Isler, U.S. Patent 2,411,967 (1938); Chem.
       Abstr. 41:1713 (1947).
141.   F. Bergel, A. Jacob, A. R. Todd, and T. S. Work, Nature
       (London) 142:36 (1938).
142.   F. Bergel, A. M. Copping, A. Jacob, A. R. Todd, and T. S. Work,
       J. Chem. Soc. 1938:1382.
143.   L. I. Smith, H. E. Ungnade, J. R. Stevens, and C. C. Christman,
       J. Amer. Chem. Soc. 61:2615 (1939).
144.   L. F. Fieser, M. Tishler, and N. L. Wendler, J. Amer. Chem.
       Soc. 62:2861 (1940).
145.   F. von Werder, U.S. Patent 2,230,659 (1941); Chem. Abstr.
       35:3270 (1941).
146.   J. Weichet and J. Hodrova, Collect. Czech. Chem. Commun.
       22:595 (1957).
147.   O. Ehrmann, Ger. Patent 1,015,446 (1957); Chem. Abstr. 54:578
       (1960).
148.   K. Nakagawa and S. Muraki, Jap. Patent 11993 (1963); Chem.
       Abstr. 59:13953 (1963); Jap. Patent 18338 (1966); Chem. Abstr.
       67:90966 (1967).
149.   Japan Kokai 73 72,168 (1973); Chem. Abstr. 80:3385 (1974); Japan
       Kokai 73 72,167 (1973); Chem. Abstr. 80:3386 (1974).
150.   Japan Kokai 73 48,472 (1973); Chem. Abstr. 79:105067 (1973).
151.   Ger. Offen. 2,208,795 (1972); Chem. Abstr. 77:164485 (1972).
152.   Japanese Pat. 72 08,821 (1970); Chem. Abstr. 77:34735 (1972).
153.   Japanese Pat. 70 31,662 (1970); Chem. Abstr. 74:53535 (1971).
154.   Japanese Pat. 70 21,835 (1970); Chem. Abstr. 73:77438 (1970).
155.   Japanese Pat. 70 21,712 (1970); Chem. Abstr. 73:76848 (1970).
156.   P. A. Wehrli, R. I. Fryer, and W. Metlesics, J. Org. Chem.
       36:2910 (1971).
156a. O. Ehrmann, Ger. Patent 1,015,446 (1957); Chem. Abstr. 54:578
       (1960).
157.   L. I. Smith, H. E. Ungnade, H. H. Hoehn, and S. Wawzonek,
       J. Org. Chem. 4:311 (1939).
158.   L. I. Smith and J. A. Sprung, J. Amer. Chem. Soc. 65:1276
       (1943).
159.   P. Karrer and O. Isler, U.S. Patent 2,411,969 (1941); Chem.
       Abstr. 41:1713 (1947).
160.   M. E. Maurit, G. V. Smirnova, E. A. Parefnov, I. K. Sarycheva,
       and N. A. Preobrazhenskii, Dokl. Akad. Nauk SSSR 140:1330
       (1961); Chem. Abstr. 56:8672 (1962).

161. J. D. Surmatis and J. Weber, U.S. Patent 2,723,278 (1955);
      Chem. Abstr. 50:10794 (1956).

162. K. Nakajima and S. Kitmura, Jap. Patent 5334 (1967); Chem.
      Abstr. 67:90673 (1967).

163. J. A. Aeschlimann, U.S. Patent 2,307,010 (1943); Chem. Abstr.
      37:3567 (1943).

164. L. Blaha, J. Hodrova, and J. Weichet, Collect. Czech, Chem.
      Commun. 24:2023 (1959).

165. M. Matsui, S. Kitamura, H. Fukawa, and H. Kurihara, Jap.
      Patent 2621-2624 (1962); Chem. Abstr. 58:7911 (1963).

166. I. A. Miller and H. C. S. Wood, Chem. Commun. 1965:40.

167. L. I. Smith and H. C. Miller, J. Amer. Chem. Soc. 64:440 (1942).

168. W. John and H. Pini, Z. Physiol. Chem. 273:225 (1942).

168a. W. John, P. Gunther, and F. H. Rathmann, Z. fur Chemie,
      268:104 (1941).

169. P. Karrer and H. Fritzsche, Helv. Chim. Acta 21:1234 (1938).

170. P. Karrer, H. Koenig, B. H. Ringier, and H. Salomon, Helv.
      Chim. Acta 22:1139 (1939).

171. A. Jacob, M. Steiger, A. R. Todd, and T. S. Work, J. Chem.
      Soc. 1939:542.

172. P. Karrer and H. Fritzsche, Helv. Chim. Acta 22:260 (1939).

173. S. Marcinkiewicz, D. McHale, P. Mamalis, and J. Green,
      J. Chem. Soc. 1959:3377.

174. P. Mamalis, J. Green, S. Marcinkiewicz, and D. McHale,
      J. Chem. Soc. 1959:3350.

175. D. McHale, P. Mamalis, S. Marcinkiewicz, and J. Green,
      J. Chem. Soc. 1959:3358.

176. J. Green, D. McHale, P. Mamalis, and S. Marcinkiewicz,
      J. Chem. Soc. 1959:3374.

177. T. Nakamura, S. Kijima, Japan Kokai 73 91,076 (1973); Chem.
      Abstr. 80:146019 (1974).

177a. S. Inoue, K. Saito, K. Kato, S. Nozaki, and K. Sato, J. Chem.
      Soc. Perkin Trans. 1 1974:2097.

178. D. McHale, P. Mamalis, J. Green, and S. Marcinkiewicz,
      J. Chem. Soc. 1958:1600.

179. P. Mamalis, D. McHale, J. Green, and S. Marcinkiewicz,
      J. Chem. Soc. 1958:1850.

180. T. Ichakawa and T. Kato, Jap. Patent 11064 (1967); Chem. Abstr.
      67:10003 (1967); Jap. Patent 11065 (1967); Chem. Abstr. 67:10001
      (1967).

180a. J. W. Scott, F. T. Bizzarro, D. R. Parrish, and G. Saucy, Helv.
      Chim. Acta 59:290 (1976).

181. P. Karrer and H. Rentschler, Helv. Chim. Acta 27:1279 (1944).

182. D. McHale, J. Green, S. Marcinkiewicz, J. Feeney, and L. H. Sutcliffe, J. Chem. Soc. 1963:784.
183. L. Weisler, U.S. Patent 2,486,539 (1949); Chem. Abstr. 44:2037 (1950).
184. K. C. D. Hickman and L. Weisler, U.S. Patent 2,486,540 (1949); Chem. Abstr. 44:1234 (1950).
185. L. Weisler and A. J. Chechak, U.S. Patent 2,486,542 (1949); Chem. Abstr. 44:2037 (1950).
186. L. Weisler, U.S. Patent 2,519,863 (1950); Chem. Abstr. 45:669 (1951).
187. J. G. Baxter, U.S. Patent 2,592,531 (1952); Chem. Abstr. 47:833 (1953).
188. L. Weisler, U.S. Patent 2,592,628 (1952); Chem. Abstr. 47:1192 (1953).
189. L. Weisler, U.S. Patent 2,592,630 (1952); Chem. Abstr. 47:1192 (1953).
190. L. Weisler, U.S. Patent 2,640,058 (1953); Chem. Abstr. 48:7643 (1954).
191. L. Weisler, U.S. Patent 2,673,858 (1954); Chem. Abstr 49:5533 (1955).
192. F. J. Sevigne, U.S. Patent 2,998,430 (1961); Chem. Abstr. 56:3462 (1962).
193. F. J. Sevigne, U.S. Patent 3,187,011 (1965); Chem. Abstr. 63:8322 (1965).
194. T. Nakamura and S. Kijima, Chem. Pharm. Bull. 19:2318 (1971); 20:1681 (1972); U.S. Patent 3,631,068 (1971); Chem Abstr. 76:85700 (1972).
195. W. T. Caldwell and T. R. Thompson, J. Amer. Chem. Soc. 61:765 (1939).
196. P. Karrer and O. Hoffmann, Helv. Chim. Acta 22:654 (1939); 23:1126 (1940).
197. H. A. Offe and W. Barkow, Chem. Ber. 80:464 (1947).
198. R. J. Boscott, Chem. Ind. 1955:201.
199. E. Daiwa and S. Oshiro, Jap. Patent 4617/65 (1963); Derwent No. 16169 (1965).
200. L. I. Smith, J. W. Opie, S. Wawzonek, and W. W. Prichard, J. Org. Chem. 4:318 (1939).
201. H. J. Teuber and W. Rau, Chem. Ber. 85:1036 (1953).
202. A. Pongratz and K. L. Zirm, Monatsh. Chem. 83:13 (1952).
203. G. Leuschner and K. Pfordte, J. Prakt. Chem. 10:340 (1960).
204. R. Nietzki and J. Schneider, Ber. Deutsch. Chem. Gesellschaft 27:1430 (1894).
205. L. I. Smith, J. Amer. Chem. Soc. 56:472 (1934).

206. W. J. Burke, J. A. Warburton, J. L. Bishop, and J. L. Bills,
     J. Org. Chem. 26:4669 (1961); K. Sato and S. Abe, J. Org. Chem.
     28:1928 (1963).
207. M. Y. Kraft and A. M. Tsyganova, Med. Prom. SSSR 14:27 (1960);
     Chem. Abstr. 55:6426 (1961).
208. I. K. Sarycheva, G. Serebrennikova, L. I. Mitrushkina, and
     N. A. Preobrazhenskii, J. Gen. Chem. USSR 31:2046 (1961).
209. D. Leuchs, Chem. Ber. 98:1335 (1965).
210. P. A. Wehrli, R. I. Fryer, F. Pigott, and G. Silverman, J. Org.
     Chem. 37:2340 (1972); W. Metlesics and P. A. Wehrli, Ger. Offen.
     1,909,164 (1969); Chem. Abstr. 72:12569 (1970).
211. H. Hoever, E. Biller, Ger. Offen. 2,225,543 (1973); Chem.
     Abstr. 80:70533 (1974).
212. L. Rappen, W. Fickert, W. Orth, M. Maurer, and H. Miele, Ger.
     Patent 1,932,362 (1972); Chem. Abstr. 78:110880 (1973).
213. W. E. von Doering, W. J. Farrissey, Jr., F. F. Frulla, and
     D. V. Rao, U.S. Patent 3,683,034 (1972); Chem. Abstr. 77:114031
     (1972).
214. L. LeBris, D. Michelet, and M. Rakoutz, Brit. Patent 1,244,470
     (1971); Chem. Abstr. 75:129533 (1971).
215. J. G. Thweatt and F. H. Rash, Ger. Offen. 2,149,159 (1972);
     Chem. Abstr. 77:19359 (1972).
216. W. Mehlesics, E. Schinzel, H. Vilcsek, and F. Wessely,
     Monatsh. Chem. 88:1069 (1957).
217. D. L. Fields, J. B. Miller, and D. D. Reynolds, J. Org. Chem.
     27:2749 (1962).
218. V. Rericha and M. Protiva, Chem. Listy 45:157 (1951); Chem.
     Abstr. 46:1497 (1952).
219. O. H. Emerson and L. I. Smith, J. Amer. Chem. Soc. 62:141
     (1940).
220. R. T. Arnold and H. E. Zangg, J. Amer. Chem. Soc. 63:1317
     (1941).
221. L. I. Smith and F. L. Austin, J. Amer. Chem. Soc. 64:528 (1942).
222. L. I. Smith and W. H. Tess, J. Amer. Chem. Soc. 66:1523 (1944).
223. F. G. Fischer and K. Löwenberg, Ann. Chem. 475:183 (1929);
     J. Weichet, J. Hodrova, and V. Kvita, Chem. Listy 51:568 (1957).
223a. I. K. Sarycheva, G. A. Vorobeva, N. A. Kuznetsova, and N. A.
     Preobrazhenskii, Zh. Obshch. Khim. 28:647 (1958).
223b. I. K. Sarycheva, Yu. G. Molotkovskii, G. A. Vorobeva, and
     N. A. Preobrazhenskii, Zh. Obshch. Khim. 29:1123 (1959).
223c. J. Redel and J. Boch, French Patent 1,460,512 (1966); Chem.
     Abstr. 67:100279 (1967).
224. G. Saucy and R. Marbet, Helv. Chim. Acta 50:2091 (1967).

225. O. Isler, R. Rüegg, L. H. Chopard-dit-Jean, A. Winterstein, and O. Wiss, Helv. Chim. Acta 41:786 (1958).

226. O. Isler, R. Rüegg, L. H. Chopard-dit-Jean, H. Wagner, and K. Bernard, Helv. Chim. Acta 39:897 (1956).

227. R. Rüegg, U. Gloor, A. Langemann, M. Kofler, C. von Planta, G. Ryser, and O. Isler, Helv. Chim. Acta 43:1745 (1960).

228. R. Rüegg, U. Gloor, R. N. Goel, G. Ryser, O. Wiss, and O. Isler, Helv. Chim. Acta 42:2616 (1959).

229. W. Kimel, J. D. Surmatis, J. Weber, G. O. Chase, N. W. Sax, and A. Ofner, J. Org. Chem. 22:1611 (1957).

230. W. Kimel, N. W. Sax, S. Kaiser, G. G. Eichmann, G. O. Chase, and A. Ofner, J. Org. Chem. 23:153 (1958).

231. M. E. Maurit, G. V. Smirnova, E. A. Parfenov, T. M. Vinkovskaya, and N. A. Preobrazhenskii, J. Gen. Chem. USSR 32:2449 (1963).

232. A. Shigehiro, M. Shiomichi, and S. Kikumasa, Japanese Pat. 11,044 (1967); Chem. Abstr. 67:90965 (1967).

233. G. R. Whistance and D. R. Threlfall, Biochem. J. 109:577 (1968).

234. G. R. Whistance and D. R. Threlfall, Biochem. Biophys. Res. Commun. 28:295 (1967).

235. D. R. Threlfall, G. R. Whistance, and T. W. Goodwin, Biochem. J. 106:107 (1968).

236. K. J. Whittle, B. G. Audley, and J. F. Pennock, Biochem. J. 103:21C (1967).

237. D. R. Threlfall, W. T. Griffiths, and T. W. Goodwin, Biochem. J. 103:831 (1967).

238. K. J. Whittle, P. J. Dunphy, and J. F. Pennock, Biochem. J. 100:138 (1966).

239. W. T. Griffiths, D. R. Threlfall, and T. W. Goodwin, Eur. J. Biochem. 5:124 (1968).

240. O. A. Dada, D. R. Threlfall, and G. R. Whistance, Eur. J. Biochem. 4:329 (1968).

241. D. R. Threlfall and G. R. Whistance, in Methods in Enzymology. Edited by D. B. McCormic and L. D. Wright, Vol. 1, New York, Academic, 1971, p. 369

242. J. Green, J. Sci. Food Agric. 9:801 (1958).

243. T. Baszynski, Acta Soc. Bot. Polon. 30:307 (1961).

244. H. M. Evans, O. H. Emerson, G. A. Emerson, L. I. Smith, H. E. Ungnade, W. W. Prichard, F. L. Austin, H. H. Hoehn, J. W. Opie, and S. Wawzonek, J. Org. Chem. 4:376 (1939).

245. F. v. Werder, T. Moll, and F. Jung, Z. Physiol. Chem. 257:129 (1939).

246. T. Tatsuta, Vitamins 45:247 (1972).

247. L. I. Smith, W. B. Renfrew, and J. W. Opie, J. Amer. Chem.
      Soc. 64:1082 (1942).
248. M. Joffe and P. L. Harris, J. Amer. Chem. Soc. 65:925 (1943).
249. M. H. Stern, C. D. Robeson, L. Weisler, and J. G. Baxter,
      J. Amer. Chem. Soc. 69:869 (1947).
250. R. J. Ward, Br. J. Nutr. 12:226 (1958).
251. H. Gottlieb, F. W. Quackenbush, and H. Steenbock, J. Nutr.
      25:433 (1943).
252. S. R. Ames, M. I. Ludwig, D. R. Nelan, and C. D. Robeson,
      Biochemistry 2:188 (1963).
253. E. L. Hove and P. L. Harris, J. Nutr. 33:95 (1947).
254. M. L. Scott and I. D. Desai, J. Nutr. 83:39 (1964).
255. C. D. Fitch and J. F. Diehl, Proc. Soc. Exp. Biol. Med. 119:553
      (1965).
256. C. S. Rose and P. György, Amer. J. Physiol. 168:414 (1952).
257. J. Bunyan, J. Green, E. E. Edwin, and A. T. Diplock, Biochem. J.
      75:460 (1960).
258. L. Friedman, W. Weiss, F. Wherry, and O. L. Kline, J. Nutr.
      65:143 (1958).
259. T. Tatsuta, Vitamins 1971:185.
260. H. Dam and E. Sondergaard, Z. Ernahrungswiss. 5:73 (1964).
261. W. L. Marusich, G. Ackerman, and J. C. Bauernfeind, Poultry
      Sci. 46:541 (1967).
262. L. I. Smith and W. B. Renfrow, Jr., J. Amer. Chem. Soc. 64:445
      (1942).
263. P. Karrer and O. Hoffmann, Helv. Chim. Acta 22:654 (1939);
      23:1126 (1940).
263a. P. Karrer and R. Schaepfer, Helv. Chim. Acta 24:298 (1941).
264. P. Karrer and K. S. Yap, Helv. Chim. Acta 24:640 (1941).
265. T. Tatsuta, Vitamins 1974:63.
266. The National Formulary, 12th ed., Easton, Pa., Mack Printing Co.,
      1965.
267. P. L. Harris and M. I. Ludwig, J. Biol. Chem. 179:1111 (1949).
268. H. Weiser, G. Brubacher, and O. Wiss, Science 140:80 (1963).
269. S. R. Ames, M. I. Ludwig, D. R. Nelan, and C. D. Robeson,
      Biochemistry, 2:188 (1963).
270. L. A. Witting and M. K. Horwitt, Proc. Soc. Exp. Biol. Med.
      116:655 (1964); J. Nutr. 82:19 (1964).
271. J. Brüggeman, K. H. Niesar, and C. Zentz, Intern. Zeit. für
      Vitaminforsch. 33:180 (1963).
272. S. R. Ames, Lipids 6:281 (1971).
273. B. Century and M. K. Horwitt, Fed. Proc. 24:906 (1965).
274. M. L. Scott, Fed. Proc. 24:901 (1965).
275. E. J. Simon, A. Eisengart, L. Sundheim, and A. T. Milhorat,
      J. Biol. Chem. 221:807 (1956).

275a. M. Watanabe, M. Toyoda, I. Imada, and H. Morimoto, Chem. Pharm. Bull. 22:176 (1974).

275b. M. Watanabe, R. Negishi, I. Imada, M. Nishikawa, and H. Morimoto, Chem. Pharm. Bull. 22:183 (1974).

275c. M. Watanabe, M. Kawada, M. Nishikawa, I. Imada, and H. Morimoto, Chem. Pharm. Bull. 22:566 (1974).

276. A. S. Csallany, H. H. Draper, and S. N. Shah, Arch. Biochem. Biophys. 98:142 (1962).

277. F. Weber and O. Wiss, Helv. Physiol. Pharmacol. Acta 21:131 (1963).

278. C. K. Chow, H. H. Draper, A. S. Csallany, and M. Chiu, Lipids 2:390 (1967).

279. J. Bunyan, J. Green, A. T. Diplock, and E. E. Edwin, Biochim. Biophys Acta 49:420 (1961).

280. J. B. Mackenzie and C. G. Mackenzie, J. Nutr. 72:322 (1960).

281. P. Alaupovic, B. C. Johnson, Q. Crider, H. N. Bhagavan, and B. J. Johnson, Amer. J. Clin. Nutr. (No. 4, Part 2), 9:76 (1961).

282. A. S. Csallany and H. H. Draper, Proc. Soc. Exp. Biol. Med. 104:739 (1960); Arch. Biochem. Biophys. 100:335 (1963).

283. P. Schudel, H. Mayer, J. Metzger, R. Rüegg, and O. Isler, Helv. Chim. Acta 46:636 (1963).

284. H. H. Draper, A. S. Csallany, and M. Chiu, Lipids 2:47 (1967).

285. W. A. Skinner and P. Alaupuvic, Science 140:803 (1963).

286. A. S. Csallany, Int. J. Vit. Nutr. Res. 41:376 (1971).

3 ASSAY METHODS

INDRAJIT D. DESAI
The University of British Columbia
Vancouver, British Columbia, Canada

I.	Introduction	68
II.	Basic Preparatory Procedures	69
	A. General Precautions	69
	B. Sample Preparation	70
	C. Extraction	70
	D. Saponification	70
	E. Molecular Distillation or Microsublimation	71
	F. Preparatory Column Chromatography	72
III.	Chemical and Physical Methods of Analysis	72
	A. Colorimetry	72
	B. Spectrophotometry	73
	C. Spectrofluorometry	74
	D. Column Chromatography	75
	E. Paper Chromatography	76
	F. Thin-Layer Chromatography	77
	G. Gas-Liquid Chromatography	80
	H. Electrochemical Method	81
IV.	Applications of Chemical and Physical Methods	81
	A. Blood	81
	B. Cerebrospinal Fluid	84
	C. Animal Tissues	84
	D. Foods and Feeds	86
	E. Pharmaceuticals	87
V.	Biological Methods	88
	A. Fetal-Resorption Test	89
	B. Erythrocyte-Hemolysis Test	90
	C. Muscular Dystrophy Test	91
	D. Liver-Storage Test	91

    E. Other Methods   92
    F. Standards and Biologic Activities   92
VI. Recent Developments   92
    References   93

I. INTRODUCTION

Vitamin E is now recognized as an important nutrient not only for higher animals but also for humans. The recent editions of the recommended dietary standards for the United States [1, 2] and Canada [3] included, for the first time, specific dietary recommendations and allowances for vitamin E. The increasing interest in the use of vitamin E calls for specific and simple quantitative analytical techniques for determining vitamin E activity in natural and enriched foods, biological materials, and pharmaceutical products. Vitamin E consists of eight naturally occurring chromanols made up of four tocols and four tocotrienols having different stereochemistry and biological activity. The nomenclature suggested by IUPAC-IUB Commission on Biochemical Nomenclature* [4] and used throughout this chapter is presented in Table 1.

Vitamin E activity in food of plant origin derives from α-, β-, γ-, and ζ- tocopherols and corresponding tocotrientols. In animal tissues, α-tocopherol is predominant and is mainly considered for biological activity and dietary calculations. The β-, γ-, and ζ-tocopherols and tocotrienols have lower biological activities, estimated to be 1-50% that of α-tocopherol. Some of these less-active tocopherols, particularly γ-tocopherol, are present in mixed diets and the γ or ζ form occur mainly in vegetable oils, but their relative contribution to the total vitamin E activity in diets has yet to be assessed. In addition, commercial foods and pharmaceutical preparations contain synthetic stable forms of tocopherols such as d- and dl-α-tocopheryl acetates and succinates which require a slightly different approach for their estimation.

There are two major classes of methods available to the analyst for the assay of tocopherols: chemical methods and biological methods. The chemical methods are useful in quantitative and qualitative analysis of tocopherols, whereas biological methods are helpful in estimating the biological effectiveness of the test compounds and samples containing vitamin E activity. A large number of methods exist for the chemical and biological assay of tocopherols, and several elegant reviews covering literature in print up to 1970 have appeared [5-13]. In writing this chapter,

---

*International Union of Pure and Applied Chemistry—International Union of Biochemistry Commission on Biochemical Nomenclature.

TABLE 1   Nomenclature of Naturally Occurring Vitamin E Compounds and Their Abbreviations

Common name	Stereochemical designation	Abbreviation
Tocol		T
α-Tocopherol	5, 7, 8-Trimethyltocol	α-T
β-Tocopherol	5, 8-Dimethyltocol	β-T
γ-Tocopherol	7, 8-Dimethyltocol	γ-T
ζ-Tocopherol	8-Methyltocol	ζ-T
Tocotrienol		T3
α-Tocotrienol	5, 7, 8-Trimethyltocotrienol	α-T3
β-Tocotrienol	5, 8-Dimethyltocotrienol	β-T3
γ-Tocotrienol	7, 8-Dimethyltocotrienol	γ-T3
ζ-Tocotrienol	8-Methyltocotrienol	ζ-T3

I have attempted to present a general outline of various assay methods and to review recent literature on the development of new and improved procedures for suitable application to biological research in the field of vitamin E.

II. BASIC PREPARATORY PROCEDURES

A. General Precautions

The success of vitamin E assay greatly depends on the following factors which should be carefully controlled: (1) cleanliness of the glassware, (2) purity of solvents and chemicals, (3) interference from nonspecific reducing substances, and (4) destruction of tocopherols by light, heat, alkaline conditions, and metal-ion contamination. All glassware should be soaked in chromic acid solutions, washed thoroughly with inorganic detergent, and rinsed repeatedly first with tap water and then with glass-distilled water. Subsequent rinsing of the glassware should be carried out with redistilled ethanol followed by drying by heat or with redistilled acetone. All reagents should be of certified analytical grade. The organic solvents should be spectrograde quality and should be routinely distilled over potassium hydroxide after refluxing with potassium permanganate in all glass apparatus. The first and last fractions of the distillates should be carefully discarded. The solvents should be kept dried over Drierite or anhydrous sodium sulfate and stored in dark bottles. All efforts should be made to exclude as much oxygen as possible from the assay systems by flushing with nitrogen, and all operations should be carried out in diffuse light. Use of silicone stopcock grease and rubber or polyethylene should be completely avoided.

B. Sample Preparation

The determination of vitamin E in biological material usually requires several preparatory steps depending on the nature of the material, the pattern of the tocopherols present, and the accuracy of quantitative estimate desired. Plant and animal tissues are first homogenized in a Waring blender or high speed Omni-mixer. The loss of tocopherols during homogenization can be prevented by immersing the blending cup in ice water and by flushing with nitrogen. The homogenates can either be freeze-dried or converted into dry powder by grinding in a mortar with anhydrous sodium sulfate or acetone. Ground products, such as feeds, cereals, and pharmaceutical preparations, and biological fluids, such as plasma and serum, may not require special sample preparation.

C. Extraction

Extraction of lipid material from samples is one of the initial steps in the isolation, purification, and quantitative measurement of tocopherols in complex biological materials. Direct extraction of the total lipid can be accomplished by selecting proper solvent(s) depending on the nature of the sample and the amount of lipid to be extracted. A modified chloroform-methanol procedure [14], using a blender or homogenizer, is most effective for wet samples. Alternatively, dried samples can be satisfactorily extracted with acetone in the Soxhlet apparatus [15] or with peroxide-free diethyl ether in glass-stoppered Erlenmeyer flasks fitted on a mechanical shaker [16].

The total lipid extract is evaporated under nitrogen by warming in a water bath or by swirling in a rotary evaporator. The residue is then dissolved in ethanol for subsequent saponification as may be necessary for further removal of saponifiable lipid before chromatography.

D. Saponification

Saponification is an essential step for the initial extraction of tocopherol-rich fraction either directly from biological material or from solvent extract. Some low-lipid materials such as blood plasma or serum may not require saponification, but, when the amount of free and total tocopherols has to be estimated, saponification of tocopherol esters is necessary. The increase in tocopherol measured after saponification represents the amount of esterified tocopherols such as α-tocopherol acetate.

A variety of techniques used by several investigators and their usefulness in the analysis of tocopherols has been reviewed in detail [7,9]. All methods essentially require refluxing the sample with appropriate solvent, such as ethanol, and freshly prepared or freshly boiled potassium hydroxide solution under controlled conditions of time and temperature so as to prevent loss of tocopherols during saponification. Generally 0.5-1.0 ml of 50-60% solution of potassium hydroxide is used for saponifying 1 g sample within 25-30 min. It is a common practice to exclude air from the reaction system by flushing with nitrogen [17] or with vapors of the solvent being used [18]. Most procedures, however, recommend addition of an antioxidant such as pyrogallol [18,19], β-hydroxyacetanilide [18,20], or sodium ascorbate [21,22]. About 25 mg pyrogallol or 250 mg sodium ascorbate may be sufficient for every 1 g sample to be saponified. Use of ascorbate is preferred to pyrogallol to eliminate the problem of black oxidation products of pyrogallol causing streaking of sample during thin-layer chromatography. If petroleum ether is used as a solvent, p-hydroxyacetanilide can be substituted for pyrogallol, with the advantage that washing the petroleum ether with water may not be necessary as p-hydroxyacetanilide is not extractable by petroleum ether. At the end of the saponification reaction, the flask is cooled and the contents are transferred to a separatory funnel for repeated extraction with an appropriate solvent-containing antioxidant, such as butylated hydroxytoluene (0.00125% of solvent), in petroleum ether or hexane. If hexane is used, the combined extracts are washed with water and dried over anhydrous sodium sulfate. The dried extract is made up to a convenient volume or evaporated in a flash evaporator, and the residues are dissolved in a suitable solvent for subsequent analysis. It is recommended that the conditions for saponification be standardized and recovery tests be carried out for different types of samples to be analyzed.

Pharmaceutical products and standard preparations containing tocopherol esters may not require extensive saponification but can be rapidly hydrolyzed by lithium aluminum hydride [23]. Acid saponification can also be efficiently carried out by refluxing pharmaceutical products with ethanolic sulfuric acid for 3 hr, but this method is only applicable to tocopheryl acetates and not to tocopheryl succinates, which require alkaline hydrolysis [24].

E. Molecular Distillation or Microsublimation

The separation of lipid substances from the samples can also be carried out by molecular distillation [25,26] or microsublimation [27] instead of saponification. The distillation principle in this method can effectively separate tocopherols from most other associated substances, such as chlorophyll, xanthophylls, carotenoids, quinone, ubiquinol, ubichromanol, and sterols, but not vitamin A and β-carotene. However, the conventional molecular distillation equipment [25] is expensive and time consuming and, therefore, has limited use. The microapparatus using a "cold-finger" type condenser [19] has been found to be suitable for preliminary separation of extracts from small samples and provides considerable saving of time and solvents.

The standard saponification procedure, using appropriate precautions as described earlier, is still a method of preference for many investigators, as it provides the advantage of simplicity and speed in the routine assay for vitamin E in most biological materials.

F. Preparatory Column Chromatography

Column chromatography may be a useful step under certain situations when preliminary purification of the unsaponifiable extract or molecular distillate is required before separation of individual tocopherols requiring finer chromatographic techniques. When lipid-rich tissues are being analyzed, initial column chromatography may provide an increased loading capacity of adsorption on a variety of commonly used adsorbants, such as florex [18, 28-30], decalso [31], and celite 545-digitonin [12]. Variable results with respect to the recovery of tocopherols from columns have been reported by the users of activated earth as adsorbants which, however, are quite suited to satisfactory removal of carotenoids, vitamin A, and sterols. Complete removal of sterols may not be possible in some cases and, therefore, precipitation of sterols by freezing extract in methanol solution may be necessary [28, 29] to avoid interference during subsequent analytical procedures. The adsorption characteristics of florex can be improved by treatment with hydrochloric acid and stannous chloride [26] or zinc chloride. The acid is washed off with ethanol and benzene until free from acid. In usual practice, batches of adsorbant material are prepared and poured into chromatography tubes of 14 mm inside diameter and 125 mm in length. The lipid extract to be purified is applied to the column and tocopherols are quantitatively eluted by ethanol for subsequent analysis.

III. CHEMICAL AND PHYSICAL METHODS OF ANALYSIS

A. Colorimetry

The most widely employed method for the analysis of vitamin E in biological materials has been Emmerie and Engel's oxidimetric reaction of tocopherols [32]. The determination is based on the ability of tocopherols to reduce ferric chloride stoichiometrically to ferrous ions forming a red-colored complex with α,α^1-dipyridine, which is measured colorimetrically at 520 nm. This method is applicable to purified extracts from nonspecific reducing substances, but has many limitations such as high blank, unstable color, and variable time required for maximum color development with different tocopherols. α-Tocopherol develops maximum color in 15 sec, whereas ζ-tocopherol takes 2 min or more. Most investigators have used an average time of 30 sec for measuring maximum color development in extracts containing a mixture of tocopherols. Attempts have been made to stabilize the color by adding acetic acid to the reaction system, but its corrosive effect to the spectrophotometer is unavoidable. It should be noted that carotenoids, vitamin A, cholesterol, and other nonspecific reducing substances will interfere with the Emmerie-Engel reaction and that prior chromatographic separation is necessary.

In 1961, Tsen [33] introduced a modified Emmerie-Engel procedure using a new chromogenic reagent bathophenanthroline (4,7-diphenyl-1,10-phenanthroline). The chromophore of this reagent with ferrous iron is quite stable and is $2\frac{1}{2}$ to 3 times more sensitive than that of the α,α^1-dipyridyl reaction. The time required for various forms of tocopherols to develop maximum color intensity is not variable and the reaction is complete within 15-30 sec, thereby eliminating the need for timing each reaction. The background absorbency is very low and many samples can be simultaneously handled for colorimetric assay employing this improved method. The use of orthophosphoric acid in the bathophenanthroline procedure stabilizes the color by preventing the photochemical reduction of the residual iron. The greater sensitivity of this reagent makes it possible to analyze small amounts (1-3 μg) of tocopherols eluted from chromatographic spots on thin-layer plates. However, precautions with respect to protection from light and the use of extra pure chemicals, glass distilled solvents, and clean glassware are absolutely necessary to reduce errors in these colorimetric procedures.

Other more sensitive reagents such as terpyridyl:2,2',2''-tripyridine [34], 2,4,6-tripyridyl-5-triazine [35], and α,α^1-diphenyl-β-picrylhydrazyl [36,37] also offer interesting substitutes for α,α^1-dipyridyl in their special application to microtechniques in clinical chemistry.

B. Spectrophotometry

The concentration of α-tocopherol can be obtained directly by measuring the extinction of the pure ethanol extract of an unknown sample and a standard solution in a spectrophotometer in 1-cm quartz cells at 280, 292, and 301 nm. The following calculations are then applied as per Eqs. (1) and (2):

$$\text{E unknown} = 2.778 \, E_{292} - (1.552 \, E_{280} + 1.626 \, E_{301}) \tag{1}$$

$$\alpha\text{-tocopherol content} = \frac{\text{E unknown}}{\text{E standard}} \tag{2}$$

This method is useful only when the samples to be examined are in pure and concentrated form, since tocopherols have low intensity of absorption in ultraviolet light and their absorption values can be affected by impurities. The spectrophotometric method is not widely used but has been applied by some investigators to measure tocopherols in natural products [38] and pharmaceutical preparations [39].

C. Spectrofluorometry

Spectrofluorometry is an extremely sensitive method for the chemical assay of free and esterified tocopherols. The original fluorescent analysis of Kofler [40] was based on oxidation of tocopherol with nitric acid to form a fluorescent phenazine. Subsequently, saponification and chromatography were used to isolate tocopherols and measure their natural fluorescence [41]. Later, it was discovered by Duggan [23] that, of the several tocopherol compounds, only the free forms exhibited measurable fluorescence whereas tocopherol esters had to be cleaved by ethereal lithium aluminum hydride to form free-fluorescing tocopherols. This provided an excellent device for the analysis of free tocopherols and tocopherol esters in biological materials. Hansen and Warwick modified Duggan's procedure and developed a fluorometric micromethod for measuring free and total tocopherols in human serum [42,43] and in adipose fat tissue [44]. Several adaptations of the basic microfluorometric method are now available for specific application to rat [45] and sheep [46] plasma, and to cerebrospinal fluid [47]. A spectrophotofluorometric technique has also been devised using hydroxyalkoxypropyl Sephadex chromatograph for the determination of tocopherols in extracts of tissues, foods, and pharmaceuticals [48].

All spectrofluorometric assay procedures basically involve measurements of fluorescence on solvent extracts containing tocopherols at 295 and 340 nm, the wavelengths of maximum excitation and emission, respectively. It is important to select a proper solvent for preparing extract of the sample since the fluorescence intensity and wavelength could vary widely among different solvents [49]. The variations are negligible in chlorinated hydrocarbons and are strongest in dioxane [48]. In the case of a tocopherol solution in hexane and ethanol, hydrogen bonding between tocopherol and ethanol can affect tocopherol fluorescence [47]. This solvent effect on fluorescence requires that the standard curve be prepared in the same solvent system

used for the analysis of the sample. The fluorometric procedures are
usually preferred to colorimetric procedures due to the advantages of
simplicity, fastness, accuracy, extreme sensitivity, and the absence of
interference from carotenes, vitamin A, and most other reducing compounds commonly associated with tocopherols in crude lipid extracts. The
interference from chlorophylls present in certain plant materials can be
eliminated by destroying the chlorophylls and reducing the bulk of the lipid
extracts by mild saponification.

D. Column Chromatography

The liquid-solid adsorbant system employed in column chromatography has
been a valid tool for the preliminary separation of interfering compounds
such as carotenoids, vitamin A, ubiquinones, and sterols, but its usefulness in the separation of individual tocopherols, especially β- and γ-
forms, for quantitative estimation is limited [7,9]. However, in recent
years novel applications of chromatographic columns have been evolved
such as in the continuous monitoring of eluant for the detection of individual tocopherols by a spectrofluorometer [48,50]. A major advantage of
liquid-solid column chromatography as against thin-layer chromatography
or gas-liquid chromatography is its enormously greater loading capacity
and naturally high flow rate adaptable to automated analysis. The application of a gradient elution technique can improve the resolution of tocopherols in this system. The adsorbants most commonly used for column
chromatography of tocopherols are deactivated alumina [7,11,51], a mixture of alumina and zinc carbonate [19], and secondary magnesium phosphate [52,53]. Florisil and silicic acid have been used but with limited
success [54]. In recent years, new adsorbants such as Corasil [50] and
hydroxyalkoxypropyl Sephadex [48] have also been used with success. The
tocopherols are separated on these columns into broad groups depending
on the number of methyl groups on the aromatic ring. α-Tocopherol is
most readily separated from other unsaponifiable material using any of
the above mentioned adsorbants, but alumina-zinc carbonate mixture has
been found to be more satisfactory for the separation of α-tocopherol from
small amounts of unsaponifiable extract of a variety of animal tissues [19].
Deactivated secondary magnesium phosphate column partially separates
other tocopherols besides α-tocopherol, but complete separation of all
tocopherols and tocotrienols usually has not been achieved without subjecting the eluate to subsequent paper or thin-layer chromatography [55].

Column chromatographic techniques have recently been improved significantly by using high-pressure/high-speed liquid chromatography for
the quantitative analysis of fat-soluble vitamins [56] and for the separation and quantitative detection of tocopherols in a spectrophotometer or

a spectrofluorometer [50, 57, 58]. Van Niekerk [50] developed a liquid-solid chromatographic method for the direct determination of free tocopherols in plant oils using a Corosil II column eluted under pressure with 5% diisopropyl ether in n-hexane at the flow rate of 1.5 ml/min. Cavins and Inglett [57] provided a method for the optimum separation of the eight naturally occurring vitamin E isomers on an activated Corosil II column eluted by 0.5% tetrahydrofuran in n-hexane at a flow rate of 1 ml/min. Very recently, Abe et al. [58] have reported a high-speed liquid chromatographic method for the determination of a mixture of α-, β-, γ- and δ-tocopherols and naturally occurring tocopherols in vegetable oils on a Jascopack WC-03-500 column as a normal phase partition column and 2% diisopropyl ether in n-hexane as a mobile phase applied at a flow rate of 0.8 ml/min. The above-mentioned high-speed liquid chromatographic methods are quantitative, fast, and easy to apply.

E. Paper Chromatography

Paper chromatography appears to be a simple technique for the separation and identification of individual tocopherols and was developed as an official standard method by the Vitamin E Panel of the Society of Analytical Chemists in England [28]. This method essentially involves a two-dimensional paper chromatography system, employing adsorption on a zinc carbonate-impregnated paper with a solvent mixture such as 30% (v/v) benzene in cyclohexane in the first direction and a reversed-phase partition chromatography in the second direction using 75% ethanol in water. The spots can either be located by the use of an ultraviolet lamp after spraying with fluorescein reagent or by overlaying a template on the unsprayed papers. A template is usually prepared by developing color spots with a dipyridyl-ferric chloride spray and cutting out the marked spots of tocopherols and other reducing materials. The paper used in most assays is Whatman no. 1, but Whatman no. 4 can be used if rapid resolution is desired.

A good separation of most tocopherols, except β- and γ-tocopherols, is usually achieved by two-dimensional paper chromatography, but a total time of 4-5 hr may be required. It is possible that tocopherols may be partially destroyed during this time if the procedure is not carried out under nitrogen. Saponification and partial extraction of high lipid samples may be necessary, but, for the assay of blood serum or plasma, prior saponification is not required. This method is not used very extensively, but some specific applications of interest have been reviewed [7]. Thin-layer chromatography, however, is a method of choice for saving time and when elution of individual spots for the quantitative estimation of individual tocopherols is desired.

F. Thin-Layer Chromatography

Thin-layer chromatography is a widely used method for the separation and quantitative analysis of tocopherols. Several papers on the use of this technique have been published and reviewed [7, 9, 10, 59, 60]. The method is relatively simple and provides many advantages over paper, column, or gas-liquid chromatography.

The usual procedure for thin-layer chromatography involves the following steps: (1) preparation of thin-layer plates; (2) separation of tocopherols; (3) visualization and identification of tocopherols; and (4) elution and measurement of tocopherols.

1. Preparation of Thin-Layer Plates

Impregnated glass-fiber sheets (20 x 20 cm), precoated plastic sheets, or glass plates can be used, but the glass plates are preferred since the thickness of the adsorbent coating to be applied is not limited when sample load has to be increased. The most satisfactory adsorbent or stationary phase is silica gel G, but alumina and magnesium phosphate have also been used. The glass plates are usually coated with silica gel G (250 μm thick) and activated by heating at 100-105°C for about 1 hr. Aqueous sodium fluorescein (0.004%) is often incorporated directly into silica gel G for the visualization of tocopherol spots under ultraviolet light. The activated plates are placed in a rack and stored in a desiccator until used.

2. Separation of Tocopherols

An aliquot of the lipid extract or a standard solution containing tocopherol(s) is dissolved in chloroform or benzene to a desired concentration and spotted rapidly on to the silica gel plate with a suitable applicator such as a micropipette or a microsyringe. The plates are then developed with a mobile phase in a solvent chamber. A wide variety of solvents, either singly or in combination, has been used by several investigators [10], but the proper choice will depend on the nature of the sample, the pattern of tocopherols present, and the degree of separation to be achieved. In one-dimensional chromatography on silica gel G, the use of benzene-methanol (98:2) or cyclohexane-diethyl ether (80:20) solvent systems, have been reported to separate α- and ζ-tocopherols but not β- and γ-tocopherols [60]. Other solvent systems have been developed for the separation of β- and γ-tocopherols on silica gel G [60, 62, 63], but two-dimensional chromatography may be inevitable for the complete separation of all tocopherols from their corresponding tocotrienols and from overlapping components such as retinol, tocopherol quinone, ubiquinone, ubichromenol, and other fat-soluble compounds, if present in a sample.

A widely used two-dimensional, thin-layer chromatography based on the original system of Pennock and co-workers [64, 65] is quite satisfactory for the separation of tocopherols, tocotrienols, and other unsaponifiable compounds on silica gel G. The original method used chloroform for the first dimension and 20% isopropyl ether in light petroleum ether or hexane for the second dimension, but other solvent systems have also been successfully used for the analysis of samples presenting special problems. A more elaborate method involving two-dimensional chromatography followed by rechromatography of one of the final eluates, has been a method of choice for the determination of all tocopherols and tocotrienols and their respective esters [66]. The bulk of the lipid is removed by low-temperature (-70° C) crystallization instead of saponification, and the combined eluate obtained from the β-tocotrienol plus γ-tocopherol spot, after the second dimension run, is hydrogenated and rechromatographed for further separation. The tocotrienol esters, if present, are estimated without any loss by converting to the free form using lithium aluminum hydride reduction.

A typical chromatogram, shown in Fig. 1, illustrates the relative positions of tocopherols and other associated unsaponifiable compounds in animal tissues as separated on silica gel G using benzene-ethanol (99:1) as first solvent and hexane-ethanol (9:1) as second solvent in two-dimensional chromatography [9].

3. Visualization and Identification of Tocopherols

Either sodium fluorescein (0.004%) is mixed into the silica gel or a 0.0025% solution of sodium fluorescein in methanol is lightly sprayed directly on a developed plate for visualization under an ultraviolet lamp with maximum wavelength of 254 nm. Tocopherols on the plate appear as quenched purple spots which can be marked for qualitative identification or for removal from the plate and subsequent quantitative examination. In addition to visualization under ultraviolet light, spraying with various other reagents such as antimony pentachloride [67], phosphomolybdic acid [68], ferric chloride-dipyridine [32], and ferric chloride-bathophenanthroline [33] can also be done to develop visible color spots on thin-layer plates. Ferric chloride-bathophenanthroline spray has been preferred by many because of its increased sensitivity in detecting minute quantities of tocopherols.

4. Elution and Measurement of Tocopherols

The tocopherol spots as located under ultraviolet light can be marked and scraped off the thin-layer plate by a spatula and carefully eluted by ethanol into a glass-stoppered tube through a funnel plugged with glass wool. Alternatively, scrapings from the plate can be transferred into a glass-stoppered centrifuge tube and mixed thoroughly with a known volume of ethanol before

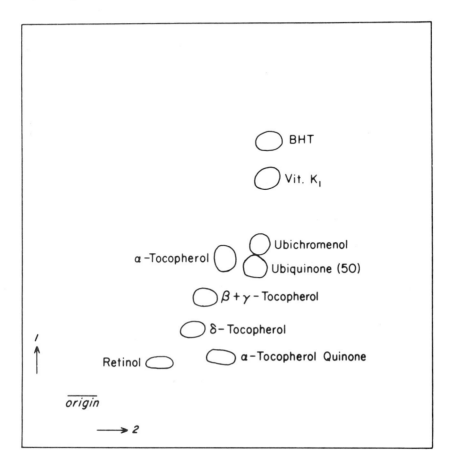

FIG. 1   Relative positions of lipids encountered in animal tissues (except BHT) separated in silica gel G. First solvent, benzene-ethanol 99:1; second solvent, hexane-ethanol 9:1. Spots visualized as purple quenching areas under ultraviolet light (fluorescing background). (From J. G. Bieri in Lipid Chromatographic Analysis, Vol. 2, edited by G. V. Marinetti, New York, Dekker, 1969, p. 472).

centrifuging down the adsorbent material. The eluate can be concentrated to a required volume by evaporating ethanol under a stream of nitrogen, and an aliquot of the eluate can be used for the quantitative measurement of tocopherols by the ferric chloride-bathophenanthroline, Emmerie-Engel colorimetric assay [33], or by the spectrofluorometric procedure [23].

Recently a new microthin-layer chromatoplate (quartz microscope slide) has been used in a rapid direct transmission spectrophotometric procedure for the analysis of tocopherols [69]. The chromatography of tocopherols (1-3 μg) on very thin layers (53 μm) thick) of silica gel (above 325 mesh) has been claimed to provide rapid (about 13 min) high resolution, increased sensitivity, and a decreased shift of the absorption maximum.

G. Gas-Liquid Chromatography

The principles of gas-liquid chromatography for the separation of lipids have been successfully applied to the analysis of vitamin E compounds in biological materials and pharmaceutical products [12]. It is a useful technique for the simultaneous separation and quantitative detection of free tocopherols, tocopherol esters, and their derivatives. The method is quite sensitive, and microgram quantities of different tocopherols can be readily detected. However, the equipment and procedures used for the gas-liquid chromatography are complicated and the working conditions have to be thoroughly standardized for this method to be of use in routine application. In spite of the advantage of increased sensitivity, this method still presents certain drawbacks—separation of β- and γ-tocopherols is not easily achieved, and it becomes absolutely necessary to prepare extracts of the biological materials in extremely pure state to avoid interference from sterols, especially cholesterol, which can only be removed by applying methanol freeze-out technique and/or column chromatography.

The instrument employed for the assay of tocopherols by gas-liquid chromatography is made up of a basic gas chromatographic unit equipped with either a hydrogen flame ionization detector or β-argon ionization detector, and with a suitable Pyrex glass or stainless steel column. The inert support of the column is usually a Gas Chrom, Chromosorb, or Celite that has been silanized. The column is packed with a stationary liquid phase of choice in concentration ranging from 1-10% of the column weight. A variety of silicone-type liquid phases such as SE-30 [67, 70-76], SE-52 [77], QF-1 [71], XE-60 [78], Apiezon N or L [67, 74, 75], and OV-17 or 1 [75, 79] have been used by various investigators, but SE-30 has been a favorite choice for most of the routine analysis of tocopherols. A mixture of liquid phases SE-52 and XE-60 has been successfully used for the separation of most of the tocopherols after their conversion to p-quinones, trimethylsilyl ethers, and the acetate, propionate, trifluoroacetate, and pentafluoropropionate esters [80-83].

The temperature of the column has to be adjusted to a suitable level (range 200-268°C) and the rate of the carrier gas (helium or nitrogen) flow and detector controls are properly regulated to achieve maximum resolution of the tocopherols within the minimum retention time. A suitable size (range 0.5-4.0 μg) sample dissolved in 4-8 μl analytical grade carbon disulfide or tetrahydrofuran is injected rapidly by means of a Hamilton microsyringe through a heated (300°C) injection port. The sample size is previously determined so as to avoid overloading the column and to maintain a linear response in the detector. Cholestane, octacosane, or squalene can be used as internal standard and tocopherol esters of acetate, succinate, or propionate can be injected as reference standards for detecting the relative retention of unknown tocopherol compounds.

A summary of some typical retention times of tocopherols and their derivatives is presented for comparison in Table 2.

H. Electrochemical Method

The original electrochemical technique [84] was based on the observation that oxidation of various tocopherols at the dropping mercury electrodes gave different electrical potentials. This basic polarographic technique using different types of indicator electrodes such as platinum, wax-impregnated graphite, and carbon paste have been used for the analysis of tocopherols in fats, oils, and pharmaceuticals. The electrode system, however, presents several problems that may affect the reliability and reproducibility of polarographic measurements. Surface film formation and adsorption of nonspecific reactants can "poison" the electrode and thereby influence the polarographic measurement of tocopherols. Recently a voltametric method has been described for the measurement of tocopherols in vegetable oils, foods, and pharmaceuticals with a newly developed carbon paste electrode [85]. The samples are saponified and the unsaponifiable fraction is extracted and measured voltametrically. It has been claimed that no elaborate purification of the samples is necessary, as the substances that interfere with standard spectrophotometric procedures are electrochemically inactive in the potential range of operation.

IV. APPLICATIONS OF CHEMICAL AND PHYSICAL METHODS

A. Blood

Measurement of tocopherols in blood has been valuable in our laboratory for the evaluation of vitamin E status of normal human populations [86-90] and patients with malabsorption problems [91]. A variety of methods has been devised and used by workers in this field for the assay of tocopherols in plasma or serum and in red blood cells, but the choice of a suitable method will depend on the size of the sample available and the nature of the assessment being posed to the investigator.

TABLE 2 Relative Retention Time in Minutes of Tocopherols and Their Trimethylsilyl (TMS) Ether Derivatives on Various Liquid Phases Used in Gas–Liquid Chromatography

Compound	Abbreviation	TMS Ether on SE-30	TMS Ether on SE-52 (XE-60 Mix)	Parent Compound on SE-52 (XE-60 Mix)	Parent Compound on OV-1
Tocol	T	0.69	0.80	1.00	—
5-Methyltocol	5-T	0.91	1.07	1.26	—
7-Methyltocol	7-T	0.79	0.91	1.11	—
8-Methyltocol	ζ-T	0.73	0.83	1.08	0.64
5,7-Dimethyltocol	5,7-T	1.16	—	1.36	1.00
5,8-Dimethyltocol	β-T	0.93	—	1.35	0.81
7,8-Dimethyltocol	γ-T	0.95	—	1.39	0.82
5,7,8-Trimethyltocol	α-T	1.37	1.66	1.69	1.18
Tocotrienol	T3	0.91	—	—	—
5-Methyltocotrienol	5-T3	1.21	—	—	—
7-Methyltocotrienol	7-T3	1.05	—	—	—
8-Methyltocotrienol	ζ-T3	0.95	—	—	—
5,7-Dimethyltocotrienol	5,7-T3	1.55	—	—	—
5,8-Dimethyltocotrienol	β-T3	1.21	—	—	—
7,8-Dimethyltocotrienol	γ-T3	1.25	—	—	—
5,7,8-Trimethyltocotrienol	α-T3	1.81	—	—	—
Octacosane (internal standard)		0.57	—	—	—
References		75	81	81	79

1. Plasma or Serum

The analysis of plasma or serum is relatively simple and does not require saponification, as tocopherols in blood are only in free form. Interference from β-carotene in the colorimetric assay of tocopherols in plasma or serum may vary depending on the species, but appropriate corrections can be applied [92]. At times controlled hydrogenation may be necessary to destroy carotenoids if present in high amounts.

The basic steps involved in the measurement of tocopherols in plasma or serum include alcoholic precipitation of protein, extraction of lipids by a suitable hydrocarbon solvent and measurement of total tocopherols either by Emmerie-Engel colorimetric procedures [33, 92] or by spectrofluorometric procedure [23]. For macroanalysis, a colorimetric procedure using bathophenanthroline [33] or a spectrofluorometric method [23] is preferred due to increased sensitivity. For the analysis of blood from infants and small laboratory animals, microcolorimetric [93, 94] and microfluorometric [42, 43] procedures have been developed. Improved fluorometric methods for the microassay of plasma vitamin E in laboratory rats [45] and sheep [46] are also available. The plasma from laboratory rats presents a special problem in that the usual alcohol precipitation and extraction steps as used for the assay of human serum [42, 43] have not been satisfactory for rat plasma. A modified extraction procedure [45] resulted in efficient precipitation of rat plasma proteins which were otherwise interfering with the fluorometric measurement of tocopherols.

Thin-layer chromatography on silica gel G has also been used for the identification and measurement of individual tocopherols in blood serum [79, 95-97], but this technique limits the number of samples that can be analyzed routinely.

2. Red Blood Cells

Measurement of tocopherols in red blood cells may be helpful in understanding the metabolism and transport of tocopherols in blood of normal subjects and patients with abnormal lipid metabolism and abetalipoproteinemia. The original procedure based on Emmerie-Engel tocopherol assay [98] has been recently modified by improving saponification step and by increasing the sensitivity of colorimetric reaction using bathophenanthroline instead of α,α^1-dipyridine [99]. Some earlier methods for determining the distribution of tocopherol in animal erythrocytes were based on indirect measurement of radioactivity after feeding labeled α-tocopherol [100-102]. Thin-layer chromatography and gas-liquid chromatography have been developed for the qualitative and quantitative assay of tocopherols in erythrocytes [79, 103, 104] and are applicable in both animal and human studies. A unique combination of radiolabel techniques, thin-layer chromatography, and gas-liquid chromatography has evolved in solving the problem of determining α-tocopherol in erythrocytes [103] and has been applied successfully to a study of the red cell content of α-tocopherol in normal subjects and patients with abnormal metabolism [104].

3. Platelets

Interest in a procedure for measuring the tocopherol content of platelet cells has recently been generated. It has been suggested that since platelets play a fundamental role in the process of thrombosis, the tocopherol concentration of platelet cells may be a useful index in studying the influence of vitamin E status on platelet function in thrombosis [105] and thrombocytothemia [106]. The method used by Nordöy and Ström [107] for tocopherol in human platelet cells is a modification of a method for red blood cells [99] and involves preparation of platelet-rich plasma by centrifuging blood at 270 g for 15 min at 4°C and recentrifuging platelet-rich plasma at 1200 g for 30 min to obtain a platelet pellet. The pellet is washed twice with a special platelet-washing solution and resuspended in 0.9% saline. The tocopherol content is then determined by subjecting the platelet suspension to a standard procedure of saponification, solvent extraction, thin-layer chromatography, and spectrophotometry using bathophenanthroline reagent [99].

B. Cerebrospinal Fluid

The concentration of tocopherols in biological fluids such as spinal fluid is much lower than in plasma or serum, and a sensitive procedure is required for the assay of vitamin E activity. The spectrophotometric method based on the classic Emmerie-Engel reaction as modified by Tsen [33] and Fabianek et al. [94] and the fluorometric method based on Duggan [23] and later modified by Hansen and Warwick [43, 44] have been adapted for the determination of tocopherols in cerebrospinal fluid [47]. However, the fluorometric procedure is recommended for routine use in the clinical laboratory, because it is more sensitive and it is not necessary to concentrate the sample for the tocopherol analysis.

C. Animal Tissues

1. Liver

The tocopherol concentration in liver is a widely used index for the classic liver storage bioassay in chicks [18, 108, 109] and the assessment of vitamin E status in animals. Unlike plasma or serum, liver contains a large amount of lipid, sterols, and other reducing compounds that may require separation by a series of purification steps for the satisfactory assay of liver tocopherols.

Any of the three basic systems described below can be adopted for the separation and assay of tocopherols distillation: Florex chromatography

[18]; saponification:magnesium in liver and other tissues: molecular phosphate chromatography [109]; and saponification:thin-layer chromatography [9].

a. Molecular Distillation and Florex Chromatography: The liver sample is homogenized and extracted with hot ethanol and Skellysolve B. An aliquot of the lipid extract is distilled under controlled conditions in a molecular still, and the distillate, dissolved in benzene, is chromatographed on a column packed with Florex XXS. An aliquot of the benzene eluate containing tocopherols is evaporated, and the residue is redissolved in a measured volume of ethanol for the determination of tocopherols. This method is suitable for measuring both free and esterified tocopherols but requires a molecular still that is not available in many laboratories.

b. Saponification and Magnesium Phosphate Chromatography: The liver homogenate is extracted with hot ethanol and the resulting extract is saponified by refluxing with ethanolic potassium hydroxide. The unsaponifiable extract in Skellysolve B is placed on a column containing magnesium phosphate which has been properly activated and tested for the efficient separation of α-tocopherol. The total eluate of the 2% solution of diethyl ether in petroleum ether is evaporated under controlled conditions and redissolved in a measured volume of ethanol for the determination of α-tocopherol by the Emmerie-Engel colorimetric procedure.

c. Saponification and Thin-Layer Chromatography: This widely used scheme is relatively simple and has been developed for the assay of tocopherols in animal tissues including liver [9]. A sample of frozen tissue is properly homogenized with ethanol containing pyrogallol. An aliquot of the homogenate is digested and saponified in ethanolic potassium hydroxide. The unsaponifiable material is extracted in hexane containing butylated hydroxytoluene (BHT). An aliquot of hexane extract is evaporated under controlled conditions and redissolved in a small, but known volume of benzene. The benzene extract is quantitatively spotted on thin-layer plate containing silica gel G impregnated with sodium fluorescein. Two-dimensional thin-layer chromatography is carried out using benzene-ethanol (99:1) in the first direction and hexane-ethanol (9:1) in the second direction. The tocopherol spots are immediately visualized and marked under an ultraviolet lamp (254 nm). The identified spots are scraped off and eluted for the quantitative estimation of tocopherols (especially α-tocopherol) by a modified Emmerie-Engel colorimetric procedure using bathophenanthroline reagent.

2. Adipose Tissue

A simple microfluorometric procedure for the assay of tocopherols in adipose tissue has been developed [44]. In this procedure, tissue samples are weighed and homogenized in a glass-tissue grinder and saponified with

5% ethanolic sodium hydroxide solution. The mixture is then extracted with hexane, and the fluorescence of tocopherols is measured in the hexane extract (emission at 340 nm and excitation at 295 nm).

D. Foods and Feeds

Vitamin E is an important nutrient either occurring naturally or added as a supplement in foods and feeds for human and animal consumption. α-Tocopherol is the predominant form of vitamin E in foods but non-α-tocopherols and tocotrienols are also present in foods, feeds, and oils of plant origin [110-113].

1. Natural Tocopherols

The methods commonly used for tocopherol determination in food materials require extensive purification to remove naturally occurring interfering substances such as chlorophylls, xanthophylls, carotenoids, quinones, and other fatty materials. The sample purification has been accomplished by one or more of the procedures such as extraction, molecular distillation or microsublimation, saponification, hydrogenation, and adsorption chromatography, depending on the nature and amount of interfering material present and the degree of purity to be achieved.

The purified extract is then examined for individual and total tocopherols by one or more of the standard methods of analysis. Direct spectrophotometry is of little value for application to food on account of the low intensity of absorption of tocopherols in ultraviolet light. The colorimetric method is sensitive and reliable provided that interfering substances are removed and care is taken to prevent oxidation of tocopherols. Spectrofluorometry provides a very sensitive means of measuring tocopherols, but rigorous purification of solvents is very essential. However, both colorimetry and spectrofluorometry have additional disadvantages in that individual tocopherols cannot be distinguished unless chromatographic procedures are used simultaneously for the separation of individual tocopherols. Two-dimensional paper chromatography has been developed for this purpose by the Analytical Methods Committee of the British Society for Analytical Chemists [28] but is not well adapted to the routine determination of vitamin E in foods. Two-dimensional thin-layer chromatography on silica gel is widely used and is of great value in conjunction with colorimetry or spectrofluorometry in obtaining a rapid and reliable assessment of the forms and amounts of tocopherols present in a variety of foods [114,115], vegetable oils [62,63,65,108,110], edible plant materials such as leaves [117,118], and algae [119,120]. Gas-liquid chromatography offers possibilities for the separation and determination of individual tocopherols simultaneously and with great sensitivity, and has been widely applied to the analysis of foods and fats containing natural vitamin E compounds [75, 76, 121, 123] and foods enriched with α-tocopheryl acetate [7].

The Association of Official Analytical Chemists has adopted, as its official first action, a procedure developed and evaluated by collaborative assay [114]. The steps recommended for the determination of naturally occurring α-tocopherol include extraction with hot ethanol, saponification, isolation of α-tocopherol by thin-layer chromatography, and colorimetry. The recommendation for the determination of supplemental α-tocopheryl acetate in food is to follow extraction, oxidative chromatography, saponification of α-tocopheryl acetate, and colorimetry of α-tocopherol.

In recent years, several new approaches have been devised for the analysis of tocopherols in foods and oils. A fast and easy liquid-solid chromatographic method for the determination of free α-, β-, γ-, and ζ-tocopherol in plant oils has been described [50]. Samples of oil without any preparation are injected directly into a Corasil II column and eluted with a mixture of diisopropyl ether and n-hexane (5:95). The eluate is monitored continuously by a fluorometer, which acts as a specific detector. A similar continuous flow method, involving separation of crude lipid extracts of foods and tissues on hydroxyalkoxypropyl Sephadex column and spectrofluorometric determination of tocopherols in the final eluate, has been designed [48] and successfully used for the examination of vitamin E in Canadian diets [124]. In a recent study conducted in England, vitamin E content of uncooked foods was assessed by applying a bathophenanthroline colorimetric procedure for determining total tocopherols and a gas-liquid chromatographic procedure for determining individual tocopherols [123].

2. Enriched α-Tocopheryl Acetate

Gas-liquid chromatography can be used in the assay of foods and feeds fortified with α-tocopheryl acetate [7]. The procedure may involve separation of lipids by extraction and molecular distillation [25, 26] or microsublimation [27], instead of saponification followed by gas chromatographic determination of free tocopherols and α-tocopheryl acetate simultaneously. As an alternative to gas-liquid chromatography, the molecular distillate or sublimate containing lipid-free tocopherols and tocopheryl acetate can be purified by column chromatography on Florex XXS and the total tocopherol content determined colorimetrically before and after saponification. The increase in tocopherol value after saponification represents the amount of fortified α-tocopheryl acetate content of foods and feeds.

E. Pharmaceuticals

The application of gas-liquid chromatography to the analysis of vitamin E content of biological materials and pharmaceutical products has been

investigated [12]. The method has been thoroughly evaluated in a collaborative study undertaken by the Pharmaceutical Manufacturers Association
at the request of the National Formulary and approved as the official first
action by the Association of Official Analytical Chemists, Washington,
D.C. [76, 125]. Samples of mixed-tocopherol concentrates, multivitamin
tablets, and multivitamin soft gelatin capsules containing α-tocopherol,
α-tocopheryl acetate, and α-tocopheryl succinate were examined by gas-
liquid chromatography. The results of this study indicate that gas-liquid
chromatographic procedure is more specific and reliable than the commonly used Emmerie-Engel colorimetric assay [126, 127] for the analysis of
vitamin E compounds in pharmaceutical products. Specific details regarding sample preparation, extraction-purification, and instrumentation of gas-
liquid chromatography for the assay of vitamin E in pharmaceutical products
can be obtained from the original articles on this subject [12, 76, 125].

A summary of pertinent references illustrating methods available for
the assay of tocopherols in body fluids, animal tissues, foods, and pharmaceuticals is presented in Table 3.

V. BIOLOGICAL METHODS

Bioassay techniques are useful in evaluating the biological activity of
tocopherols and in estimating the vitamin E requirement for humans and
animals. The true biological activity of vitamin E can be determined by its
ability to prevent or reverse specific vitamin E deficiency symptoms. The
manifestations of vitamin E deficiency vary from one species of animal to
another and some of the deficiencies have not been observed in humans.
The most characteristic deficiency symptoms of vitamin E in animals are
sterility (fetal resorption or testicular degeneration), muscular dystrophy,
browning of uterus, encephalomalacia, exudative diathesis, and liver
necrosis. The methods most commonly chosen for the assay of vitamin E
are based on fetal resorption and muscular dystrophy. Erythrocyte
hemolysis, liver storage, and elevation of plasma tocopherol have also
been used. Methods such as the erythrocyte hemolysis test, liver
storage, or elevation of plasma tocopherol are not a direct measure of
biological activity in vivo. They do reflect the relative absorption and
turnover of the test compounds in liver or red blood cells. In general, these tests correlate well with the in vivo methods which measure
the prevention or reversal of specific vitamin E deficiency symptoms (i.e.,
fetal resorption, testis degeneration, muscular dystrophy, encephalomalacia). Therefore, while the hemolysis and liver storage tests are convenient and useful, some caution should be used in interpretation of results
with these methods. The reader is referred to earlier publications [8, 128,
129] for a literature review and more details on the bioassays for vitamin E.

TABLE 3   Summary of References Illustrating Methods for the Assay of Tocopherols in Body Fluids, Animal Tissues, Foods, and Pharmaceuticals

Material	References
A. Blood	
1. Plasma or serum	
a. Macroassay	23, 33, 79, 92, 95-97
b. Microassay	42, 43, 45, 46, 93, 94
2. Red blood cells	79, 98-104
3. Platelet cells	107
B. Cerebrospinal fluid	47
C. Animal tissues	
1. Liver	9, 18, 108, 109
2. Adipose tissue	44
D. Foods, feeds, and oils	
1. Natural tocopherols	
a. Foods and feeds	28, 48, 75, 111, 113-115, 123
b. Oils and fats	50, 57, 58, 62, 65, 66, 110, 116, 121, 122
c. Leaves	117, 118
d. Algae	119, 120
2. Enriched α-tocopheryl acetate	7
E. Pharmaceuticals	12, 76, 125

A. Fetal-Resorption Test

The antisterility assay based on fetal resorption in female rats is a classic biologic method for testing biopotencies of various tocopherols [130-133]. The method is based on measuring the all-or-none response of successfully mated female rats in producing viable offspring. Female rats weighing 40-50 g are reared on a vitamin E-free diet. The depleted rats (about 150 g weight) are mated to fertile males and fertilization ascertained by examining vaginal smears for spermatozoa. Different levels of standard and unknown test doses are fed in food or olive oil over 5 successive days beginning on the fifth day of pregnancy. Nineteen days after confirmed pregnancy, the animals are sacrificed and examined for living fetuses and implantation sites in the uterus. Only those animals having at least four implantation sites are evaluated, and animals having one or more living fetuses are considered positive, while rats with no living young are recorded as negative. Vitamin E activity is determined by calculating the percentage of rats in each test group having positive response and by plotting the calculated probits against dose or log of dose to give the median fertility dose (dose of vitamin E required for a 50% litter efficiency). A ratio of the median fertility values for the standard dose and the test dose is the relative biopotency of the vitamin preparation being tested.

The fetal resorption test in rats is laborious and time consuming, but has the advantage of being more specific than other indirect methods such as hemolysis and liver storage. It has been recently observed that female rats, if maintained on a diet deficient in vitamin E for a prolonged period of time, may fail to conceive in spite of repeated matings [134]. The irreversible sterility observed in these animals is associated with the formation of ceroid pigments in the uterus, which can be measured quantitatively by a sensitive spectrophotofluorometric assay [135].

B. Erythrocyte-Hemolysis Test

Hemolysis of erythrocytes in vitro by oxidizing agents, such as dialuric acid or hydrogen peroxide, has been widely used for evaluating the biological activity of various tocopherols and the status of vitamin E in humans and animals.

1. Hemolysis with Dialuric Acid

The hemolysis test involving protection of erythrocytes from vitamin E-deficient rats against dialuric acid is essentially based on the original method of Rose and György [136] as modified by Friedman et al. [137] and Bruggeman et al. [138]. The test is conducted on male or female rats (about 100 g weight) fed a vitamin E-deficient diet for 3-4 weeks and showing 96-99% hemolysis. Proper test doses are selected to give a range of 20-80% hemolysis. Each test dose is dissolved in 0.2 ml olive oil and administered orally by stomach tube. The hemolysis test with dialuric acid is carried out 40-44 hr after administering test doses, and percentage hemolysis values are calculated [10] for comparing the biopotencies. The method is reasonably simple and precise and agrees well with fetal resorption and chick liver-storage bioassays. Precautions must be taken to eliminate interference by contaminants from unclean glassware and synthetic antioxidants.

2. Hemolysis with Hydrogen Peroxide

A special hemolysis test for the assessment of vitamin E deficiency in humans, based on hemolysis of erythrocytes by hydrogen peroxide instead of dialuric acid, was originally developed by György et al. [139] and later refined by Nitowsky et al. [140] and Horwitt [141]. Most of the steps and precautions to be taken in this bioassay are similar to those described for hemolysis with dialuric acid.

Other simple methods, based on measurement of spontaneous hemolysis in isotonic saline solution [142] and hemolysis in presence of a glucose-glucose oxidase peroxide-generating system using the Fragilograph [143], have also been tried for rapid assessment of vitamin E status in rats.

C. Muscular Dystrophy Test

Muscular dystrophy is a common manifestation of vitamin E deficiency in many species of animals and has been used as a biological index for testing the potency of tocopherols in rats [144], rabbits [145,146], chicks [147-149], and ducklings [150]. In rat and rabbit assay, standard and test doses of vitamin E are given to groups of animals maintained on a vitamin E-deficient diet, and the relative biopotency is assessed by measuring either creatinuria or dystrophic lesions in the thigh musculature. The time of onset of creatinuria has been used as an index of nutritional muscular dystrophy in testing the biopotency of tocopherols [151]. In chick assay, groups of 1 day-old chicks fed a basal vitamin E-deficient diet supplemented with test doses of tocopherols and lesions of muscular dystrophy on a scale ranging from zero, for absence of dystrophy, to four for maximal dystrophy are scored by examining breast muscles [147]. Additional tests for muscular dystrophy based on biochemical measurements, such as the thiobarbituric acid index and the hydrolytic activity of lysosomal enzymes in muscles [149], have also been developed. Serum enzyme activities of aspartate aminotransferase and lactic dehydrogenase have also been useful as alternate biochemical indices of muscular dystrophy in the bioassay of tocopherols [150].

D. Liver-Storage Test

Bioassays based on storage of tocopherols in tissues such as liver have been worked out on the assumption that tocopherol stores in the liver of rats [21,152] and chicks [18,108,109] show a linear response to the level of vitamin E in the diet. There are two commonly used chick liver-storage assays: a 3 day-short assay and a 13 day-long assay. In both assays, groups of 1 day-old chicks are given a tocopherol-low diet and then placed on basal ration supplemented with different levels of tocopherols or test materials for a 3-day or a 13-day period. At the end of the test period, the chicks are sacrificed and the liver tocopherol content is determined chemically. The relative activity of the test materials is determined from the analyses of liver storage in these animals.

E. Other Methods

Other biological methods based on growth [151], encephalomalacia [153], respiratory decline in liver necrosis [154], and testicular degeneration [144] have also been used in a limited number of studies on the biopotency of vitamin E.

F. Standards and Biological Activities

The biological activity of vitamin E is expressed in International Units (IU). Presently 1 IU of vitamin E is considered equivalent to 1 mg of synthetic dl-α-tocopheryl acetate with which the biopotencies of all other forms of tocopherols have been compared. The biopotencies (based on rat anti-sterility test) of commercially available dl-α-tocopherol, d-α-tocopheryl acetate, and d-α-tocopherol are designated to be 1.1, 1.36, and 1.49 IU/mg, respectively [24]. However, l-α-tocopherol (which is prepared specially for research purposes on request), is only about 20-25% as active as d-α-tocopherol [129,138,147] because of its poor storage and retention in the body rather than difference in its absorption [148,155]. A synergistic effect between the d- and l- forms of α-tocopherol has been observed during absorption of a racemic mixture of commonly used dl-α-tocopherol [156]. Other forms such as α-tocotrienol and β-tocopherol present in cereal grains such as barley, oats, and rye are about 40% as active as α-tocopherol [121]. Diets rich in vegetable oils, such as soybean oil, contain considerable amounts of γ-tocopherol [157,158], which is only about 10% as active as α-tocopherol [159]. It has been recommended that in calculating the vitamin E content of mixed diets, values for α-tocopherol should be multiplied by a factor of 1.2 to give a more accurate estimate of their vitamin E activity expressed as α-tocopherol equivalent [2].

VI. RECENT DEVELOPMENTS

Since the time of the writing of this chapter and its submission to the press, several publications have appeared on the methodological aspects of vitamin E. Gutteridge and Stocks [160] have successfully adopted the colorimetric method for the determination of serum tocopherol to automated analysis. Shaikh et al. [161] have developed a high-performance liquid chromatographic procedure for the analysis of supplemental vitamin E in feed, and Vatassery and Hagen [162] have applied the liquid chromatographic method for quantitative determination of α-tocopherol in rat brain. A sensitive, highly reproducible fluorometric method is also now available for the analysis of tocopherol in tissues such as liver, kidney, lung, heart, and red blood cells [163]. For rapid analysis, Waltking et al. [164] have evaluated a polarographic method for the determination of tocopherols in vegetable oils and oil-based products.

ACKNOWLEDGMENTS

Financial support from the National Research Council of Canada and The University of British Columbia is gratefully acknowledged.

REFERENCES

1. Food and Nutrition Board, National Research Council, Recommended Dietary Allowances, Washington, D.C., National Academy of Sciences, 1968.
2. Food and Nutrition Board, National Research Council, Recommended Dietary Allowances, Washington, D.C., National Academy of Sciences, 1974.
3. Committee for Revision, Canadian Dietary Standard, Ottawa, Information Canada, 1975.
4. IUPAC-IUB Commission on Biochemical Nomenclature, Eur. J. Biochem. 46:217 (1974).
5. R. W. Lehman, in Method of Biochemical Analysis, Vol. 2. Edited by D. Glick, New York, Interscience, 1955, p. 153.
6. Methods of Vitamin Assay, 3rd ed. Edited by The Association of Vitamin Chemists, New York, Interscience, 1966, p. 363.
7. R. H. Bunnell, in The Vitamins, Vol. 6. Edited by P. György and W. N. Pearson, New York, Academic, 1967, p. 261.
8. C. I. Bliss and P. György, in The Vitamins, Vol. 6. Edited by P. György and W. N. Pearson, New York, Academic, 1967, p. 304.
9. J. G. Bieri, in Lipid Chromatographic Analysis, Vol. 2. Edited by G. V. Marinetti, New York, Dekker, 1969, p. 459.
10. R. H. Bunnell, Lipids 6:245 (1970).
11. D. L. Laidman and G. S. Hall, in Advances in Enzymology, Vol. 18, Part C. Edited by D. B. McCormick and L. D. Wright, New York, Academic, 1971, p. 349.
12. A. J. Sheppard, A. R. Prosser, and W. D. Hubbard, in Advances in Enzymology, Vol. 18, Part C. Edited by D. B. McCormick and L. D. Wright, New York, Academic, 1971, p. 356.

13. S. R. Ames, in The Vitamins, Vol. 5. Edited by P. György and
    W. N. Pearson, New York, Academic, 1972, p. 225.

14. J. Folch, M. Lees, and G. H. Sloane-Stanley, J. Biol. Chem.
    226:497 (1957).

15. E. E. Edwin, A. T. Diplock, J. Bunyan, and J. Green, Biochem. J.
    75:450 (1960).

16. H. H. Draper and A. S. Csallany, Proc. Soc. Exp. Biol. Med.
    99:739 (1958).

17. G. Klatskin and D. W. Molander, J. Lab. Clin. Med. 39:802 (1952).

18. W. J. Pudelkiewicz, L. D. Matterson, L. M. Potter, L. Webster,
    and E. P. Singsen, J. Nutr. 71:115 (1960).

19. J. G. Bieri, C. J. Pollard, I. Prange, and H. Dam, Acta Chem.
    Scand. 15:783 (1961).

20. R. W. Swick and C. A. Baumann, Anal. Chem. 24:758 (1952).

21. H. R. Bolliger and M. L. Bolliger-Quaife, Vitamin E, Atti 3rd Cong.
    Internatl. (Venice, 1955), Verona, Valdonega, 1956, p. 30.

22. V. N. Krukovsky, J. Agr. Food Chem. 12:289 (1964).

23. D. E. Duggan, Arch. Biochem. Biophys. 84:116 (1959).

24. National Formulary, 12th ed. Washington, D.C., Amer. Pharm.
    Assoc., 1965, p. 406.

25. M. L. Quaife and P. L. Harris, Ind. Eng. Chem. 18:707 (1946).

26. W. J. Pudelkiewicz and L. D. Matterson, J. Biol. Chem. 235:496
    (1960).

27. J. Glavind, H. Heslet, and I. Prange, Z. Vitaminforsch. 13:266 (1943).

28. Analytical Methods Committee, Society for Analytical Chemists,
    Analyst (London) 84:356 (1959).

29. P. W. R. Eggitt and L. D. Ward, J. Sci. Food Agr. 4:176 (1953).

30. F. Brown, Biochem. J. 51:237 (1952).

31. A. T. Diplock, J. Green, E. E. Edwin, and J. Bunyan, Biochem. J.
    76:563 (1960).

32. A. Emmerie and C. Engel, Rec. Trav. Chim. 57:1351 (1938).

33. C. C. Tsen, Anal. Chem. 33:849 (1961).

34. S. Natelson, in Microtechniques of Clinical Chemistry, 2nd ed.
    Springfield, Ill., Thomas, 1961, p. 455.

35. R. G. Martinek, Clin. Chem. 10:1078 (1964).

36. J. Glavind and G. Holmer, J. Amer. Oil Chemists' Soc. 44:539 (1967).

37. W. Boguth and R. Repges, Int. Z. Vitaminforsch. 39:289 (1969).

38. G. Lambertsen and O. R. Braekkan, Analyst 84:706 (1959).

39. F. J. Mulder and K. J. Keuning, Rec. Trav. Chim. 80:1029 (1961).

40. M. Kofler, Helv. Chim. Acta 25:1469 (1942).

41. M. Kofler, Helv. Chim. Acta 26:2166 (1943).

42. L. G. Hansen and W. J. Warwick, Amer. J. Clin. Pathol. 46:133
    (1966).

43. L. G. Hansen and W. J. Warwick, Amer. J. Clin. Pathol. 51:538
    (1969).

44. L. G. Hansen and W. J. Warwick, Clin. Biochem. 3:225 (1970).

45. M. M. Meshali and C. H. Nightingale, J. Pharm. Sci. 63:1084 (1974).
46. G. B. Storer, Biochem. Med. 11:71 (1974).
47. G. T. Vatassery and G. A. Martenson, Clin. Chem. 18:1475 (1972).
48. J. N. Thompson, P. Erdody, and W. B. Maxwell, Anal. Biochem. 50:267 (1972).
49. R. T. Williams and J. W. Bridges, J. Clin. Pathol. 17:371 (1964).
50. P. J. Van Niekerk, Anal. Biochem. 52:533 (1973).
51. R. Strohecker and H. M. Henning, in Vitamin Assay Tested Methods, Weinheim, Verlag Chemie, 1965, p. 283.
52. F. Bro-Rasmussen and W. Hjarde, Acta Chem. Scand. 11:34 (1957).
53. F. Bro-Rasmussen and W. Hjarde, Acta Chem. Scand. 11:44 (1957).
54. M. W. Dicks-Bushnell, J. Chromatog. 27:96 (1967).
55. M. W. Dicks-Bushnell and K. C. Davis, Amer. J. Clin. Nutr. 20:262 (1967).
56. R. C. Williams, J. A. Schmidt, and R. A. Henry, J. Chromatog. Sci. 10:494 (1972).
57. J. F. Cavins and G. E. Inglett, Cereal Chem. 51:605 (1974).
58. K. Abe, Y. Yuguchi, and G. Katsui, J. Nutr. Sci. Vitaminol. 21:183 (1975).
59. E. Stahl (ed.), Dünnschicht-Chromatographic, Berlin, Springer, 1962.
60. H. R. Bolliger, in Dünnschicht-Chromatographic. Edited by E. Stahl, Berlin, Springer, 1962, p. 217.
61. H. D. Stowe, Arch. Biochem. Biophys. 103:42 (1963).
62. M. K. G. Rao, S. V. Rao, and K. T. Achaya, J. Sci. Food Agr. 16:121 (1965).
63. H. G. Lovelady, J. Chromatog. 78:449 (1973).
64. J. F. Pennock, F. W. Hemming, and J. D. Kerr, Biochem. Biophys. Res. Commun. 17:542 (1964).
65. K. J. Whittle and J. F. Pennock, Analyst 92:423 (1967).
66. C. K. Chow, H. H. Draper, and A. S. Csallany, Anal. Biochem. 32:81 (1969).
67. M. Kofler, P. F. Sommer, H. R. Bolliger, B. Schmidli, and M. Vecchi, Vit. Horm. 20:407 (1962).
68. P. P. Nair and N. G. Magar, Indian Chem. Soc. 33:475 (1956).
69. T. Aratani, K. Mita, and F. Mizui, J. Chromatog. 79:179 (1973).
70. N. Nicolaides, J. Chromatog. 4:496 (1960).
71. P. W. Wilson, E. Kodicek, and V. H. Booth, Biochem. J. 84:524 (1962).
72. J. G. Bieri and E. L. Andrews, Iowa State J. Sci. 38:3 (1963).
73. K. K. Carroll and D. C. Herting, J. Amer. Oil Chemists' Soc. 41:473 (1964).
74. H. T. Slover, L. M. Shelley, and T. L. Burks, J. Amer. Oil Chemists' Soc. 44:161 (1967).
75. H. T. Slover, J. Lehmann, and R. J. Valis, J. Amer. Oil Chemists' Soc. 46:417 (1969).
76. B. C. Rudy, F. P. Mahn, B. Z. Senkowski, A. J. Sheppard, and W. D. Hubbard, J. Assoc. Off. Anal. Chem. 55:1211 (1972).

77. P. P. Nair and D. A. Turner, J. Amer. Oil Chemists' Soc. 40:353 (1963).

78. D. A. Libby and A. J. Sheppard, J. Assoc. Off. Agr. Chem. 47:371 (1964).

79. H. G. Lovelady, J. Chromatog. 85:81 (1973).

80. P. P. Nair, I. Sarlos, and J. Machiz, Arch. Biochem. Biophys. 114:488 (1966).

81. P. P. Nair and J. Machiz, Biochem. Biophys. Acta 144:446 (1967).

82. P. P. Nair and Z. Luna, Arch. Biochem. Biophys. 127:413 (1968).

83. W. B. Weglicki, W. Reichel, and P. P. Nair, J. Gerontol. 23:469 (1968).

84. L. I. Smith, L. J. Spillane, and I. M. Kolthoff, J. Amer. Chem. Soc. 64:447 (1942).

85. S. S. Atuma and J. Lindquist, Analyst 98:886 (1973).

86. I. D. Desai, Can. J. Physiol. Pharmacol. 46:819 (1968).

87. I. D. Desai and M. Lee, Can. J. Public Health 62:526 (1971).

88. I. D. Desai and M. Lee, Amer. J. Clin. Nutr. 27:334 (1974).

89. I. D. Desai and M. Lee, Can. J. Public Health, 65:191 (1974).

90. I. D. Desai and M. Lee, Can. J. Public Health, 65:369 (1974).

91. C. W. Darby, A. G. F. Davidson, and I. D. Desai, Arch. Dis. Childhood 48:72 (1972).

92. M. L. Quaife and P. L. Harris, J. Biol. Chem. 156:499 (1944).

93. M. L. Quaife, N. S. Schrimshaw, and O. H. Lowry, J. Biol. Chem. 180:1229 (1949).

94. J. Fabianek, J. Defilippi, T. Rickards, and A. Herp, Clin. Chem. 14:456 (1968).

95. J. G. Bieri and E. L. Prival, Proc. Soc. Exp. Biol. Med. 120:554 (1965).

96. S. Dayton, S. Hashimoto, D. Rosenblum, and M. L. Pearce, J. Lab. Clin., Med. 65:739 (1965).

97. M. K. Horwitt, C. C. Harvey, and E. M. Harmon, Vitamins Hormones 26:487 (1968).

98. R. Silber, R. Winter, and H. J. Kayden, J. Clin. Invest. 48:2089 (1969).

99. H. J. Kayden, C. K. Chow, and L. K, Bjornson, J. Lipid. Res. 14:533 (1973).

100. J. W. Bratzler, J. K. Loosli, V. N. Krukovsky, and L. A. Maynard, J. Nutr. 42:59 (1950).

101. J. Sternberg and E. Pascoe-Dawson, Can. Med. Assoc. J. 80:266 (1959).

102. S. Krishnamurthy and J. G. Bieri, J. Lipid Res. 4:330 (1963).

103. J. G. Bieri, R. K. H. Poukka, and E. L. Prival, J. Lipid Res. 11:118 (1970).

104. J. G. Bieri and R. K. H. Poukka, Int. Z. Vitaminforsch. 40:344 (1970).

105. I. Nafstad, Thrombosis Res. 5:251 (1974).

106. M. Brin, R. Filipski, and L. J. Machlin, Abstr. Int. Cong. Nutr. Kyoto, Japan (1975).
107. A. Nordöy and E. Ström, J. Lipid Res. 16:386 (1975).
108. R. H. Bunnell, Poultry Sci. 36:413 (1957).
109. M. W. Dicks and L. D. Matterson, J. Nutr. 75:165 (1961).
110. D. C. Herting and E. E. Drury, J. Nutr. 81:335 (1963).
111. R. H. Bunnell, J. Keating, A. Quaresimo, and G. K. Parkman, Amer. J. Clin. Nutr. 17:1 (1965).
112. M. W. Dicks, Wyo. Agr. Exp. Sta. Bull. 435 (1965).
113. D. K. Feeter, J. Amer. Oil Chem. Soc. 51:184 (1974).
114. S. R. Ames, J. Assoc. Off. Anal. Chem. 54:1 (1971).
115. I. D. Desai, L. P. O'Leary, and N. Schwartz, Nutr. Rep. Int. 6:83 (1972).
116. J. G. Bieri and R. Poukka Evarts, J. Amer. Dietetic Assoc. 66:134 (1975).
117. P. G. Roughan, Anal. Biochem. 19:461 (1967).
118. C. Bucke, Phytochemistry 7:693 (1968).
119. N. J. Antia, I. D. Desai, and M. J. Romilly, J. Phycol. 6:305 (1970).
120. E. J. Dasilva and A. Jensen, Biochem. Biophys. Acta 239:345 (1971).
121. H. T. Slover, Lipids 6:291 (1971).
122. M. K. G. Rao and E. G. Perkins, J. Agr. Food Chem. 20:240 (1972).
123. A. A. Christie, A. C. Dean, and B. A. Millburn, Analyst (London) 98:161 (1973).
124. J. N. Thompson, J. L. Beare-Rogers, P. Erdödy, and D. C. Smith, Amer. J. Clin. Nutr. 26:1349 (1973).
125. A. J. Sheppard, W. D. Hubbard, and A. R. Prosser, J. Assoc. Off. Agr. Chem. 52:442 (1969).
126. National Formulary, 14th ed. Washington, D.C., Amer. Pharm. Assoc., 1975.
127. United States Pharmacopeia, 18th rev., Easton, Pa., Mack Pub., 1970.
128. M. W. Dicks and L. D. Matterson, Conn. Agr. Exp. Sta. Bull. 362 (1961).
129. S. R. Ames, Lipids 6:281 (1971).
130. K. E. Mason and P. L. Harris, Biol. Symp. 12:459 (1947).
131. M. Joffe and P. L. Harris, J. Amer. Chem. Soc. 65:925 (1943).
132. P. L. Harris and M. I. Ludwig, J. Biol. Chem. 179:1111 (1949).
133. S. R. Ames, M. I. Ludwig, D. R. Nelan, and C. D. Robeson, Biochemistry 2:188 (1963).
134. C. Raychaudhuri and I. D. Desai, Science 173:1028 (1971).
135. I. D. Desai, B. L. Fletcher, and A. L. Tappel, Lipids 10:307 (1975).
136. C. S. Rose and P. György, Amer. J. Physiol. 168:414 (1952).
137. L. Friedman, W. Weiss, F. Wherry, and O. L. Kline, J. Nutr. 65:143 (1958).
138. J. Bruggemann, K. H. Niesar, and C. Zentz, Int. Z. Vitaminforsch. 33:180 (1963).

139. P. György, G. Cogan, and C. S. Rose, Proc. Soc. Exp. Biol. Med. 81:536 (1952).

140. H. M. Nitowsky, M. Cornblath, and H. H. Gordon, Amer. J. Dis. Child. 92:164 (1956).

141. M. K. Horwitt, Amer. J. Clin. Nutr. 8:451 (1960).

142. H. H. Draper and A. S. Csallany, J. Nutr. 98:390 (1969).

143. M. O. Barker, M. Brin, and L. Hainsselin, Biochem. Med. 8:1 (1973).

144. L. J. Filer, R. E. Rumery, and K. E. Mason, in Biological Antioxidants, Trans. 1st Conf., New York, Josiah Macy Found., 1946, p. 67.

145. E. L. Hove and P. L. Harris, J. Nutr. 33:95 (1947).

146. C. D. Fitch and J. F. Diehl, Proc. Soc. Exp. Biol. Med. 119:553 (1965).

147. M. L. Scott and I. D. Desai, J. Nutr. 83:39 (1964).

148. I. D. Desai and M. L. Scott, Arch. Biochem. Biophys. 110:309 (1965).

149. I. D. Desai and M. L. Scott, Proc. 7th Int. Cong. Nutr., Vol. 5, Hamburg, 1966, p. 643.

150. F. C. Jager and J. A. Verbeek-Raad, Int. J. Vit. Res. 40:597 (1970).

151. L. A. Witting and M. K. Horwitt, Proc. Soc. Exp. Biol. Med. 116:655 (1964).

152. K. E. Mason, J. Nutr. 23:71 (1942).

153. H. Dam and E. Sondergaard, Z. Ernahrungswiss. 5:73 (1964).

154. G. P. Rodnan, S. S. Chernick, and K. Schwarz, J. Biol. Chem. 221:231 (1956).

155. I. D. Desai, C. K. Parekh, and M. L. Scott, Biochim. Biophys. Acta 100:280 (1965).

156. F. Weber, V. Gloom, J. Wursch, and O. Wiss, Biochem. Biophys. Res. Commun. 14:186 (1964).

157. J. G. Bieri and R. Poukka Evarts, J. Amer. Dietet. Assoc. 62:147 (1973).

158. J. G. Bieri and R. Poukka Evarts, Amer. J. Clin. Nutr. 27:980 (1974).

159. J. G. Bieri and R. Poukka Evarts, J. Nutr. 104:850 (1974).

160. J. M. Gutteridge and J. Stocks, Lab. Pract. 25:25 (1976).

161. B. Shaikh, H. S. Huang, and W. L. Zielinski, J. Assoc. Off. Anal. Chem. 60:137 (1977).

162. G. T. Vatassery and D. F. Hagen, Anal. Biochem. 79:129 (1977).

163. S. L. Taylor, M. P. Lamden, and A. L. Tappel, Lipids 11:530 (1976).

164. A. E. Waltking, M. Kiernan, and G. W. Bleffert, J. Assoc. Off. Anal. Chem. 60:890 (1977).

4 TOCOPHEROLS IN FOODS

JACK BAUERNFEIND
Hoffmann-La Roche Inc.
Nutley, New Jersey

I. Introduction   100
II. Biogenesis and Life Cycle Trends   101
III. Influence of Harvesting and Weather   102
IV. Genetic Variety   103
V. Inhibitors of Absorption   103
VI. Seasonal Influence in Animal Tissue   104
VII. Influence of Food Processing   104
   A. Drying   105
   B. Organic Acid Treatment   107
   C. Milling   107
   D. Expanding, Puffing, Rolling, and Shredding   110
   E. Irradiation   110
   F. Fumigation   110
   G. Refining, Bleaching, Deacidifying,
      Deodorizing, and Hydrogenating   112
   H. Heating, Cooking, and Baking   113
   I. Dehydration, Canning, and Freezing   115
VIII. Influence of Storage   116
IX. Tocopherol Content of Foods   117
   A. Oils and Fats   118
   B. Nuts and Cereal-Grain Products   120
   C. Milk, Egg, Meat, and Fish   121
   D. Vegetables and Fruits   123
   E. Infant Foods   123
   F. Prepared Convenience Dinners   125
X. Daily Dietary Intake   125
XI. Unresolved Problems   126
XII. Policy of Added Vitamin E to Foods   128

XIII. Summary   132
       Appendix A Tocopherol Content of Foods   133
       Appendix B α-Tocopherol Content of Food   156
       References   160

I. INTRODUCTION

Eight or more compounds in the tocopheryl class, all of which are derivatives of 6-chromanol, are widely distributed in nature. A recognized series [1, 2] is made up of four compounds with a tocol structure bearing a saturated isoprenoid C-16 side chain and four compounds with a trienol structure bearing three double bonds in the C-16 side chain (Fig. 1). The structure having the highest vitamin E activity for animals and humans is α-tocopherol. It is not the one which is always most abundant

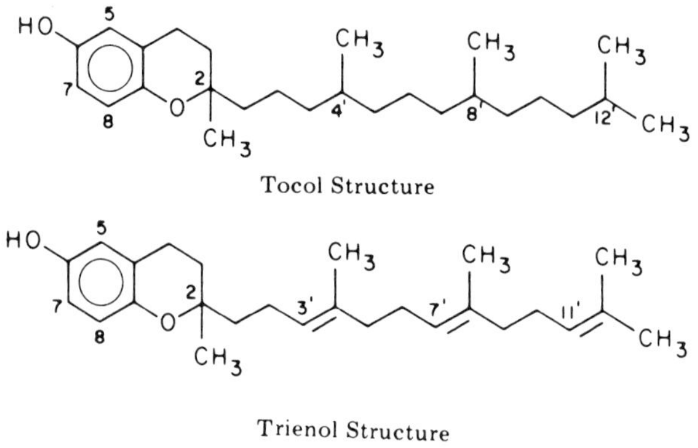

Tocol Structure

Trienol Structure

Position of Methyls	Trivial Name (Abbreviations)	
	Tocol Structure	Trienol Structure
5,7,8	α-tocopherol (α-T)	α-tocotrienol (α-T-3)
5,8	β-tocopherol (β-T)	β-tocotrienol (β-T-3)
7,8	γ-tocopherol (γ-T)	γ-tocotrienol (γ-T-3)
8	δ-tocopherol (δ-T)	δ-tocotrienol (δ-T-3)

FIG. 1   Formulas of eight members of the tocopheryl series. (From Ref. 2, with permission.)

of the tocopheryl series in a variety of foods. Attempts are now being made to include a vitamin E contribution from the non-α-tocopherols when they occur in significant quantities [3] in diets. Studies on the biological activities of the various tocopherols have been recorded over the years in the literature [4-9].

Of the tocol structures, α-tocopherol is least resistant to oxidation [10-12]. α-Tocopherol is the predominant form of the tocopherols in human tissues [13-15]. Tocopherols are not synthesized by mammals, and, therefore, they become a part of mammalian tissue primarily through the ingestion of plant life by humans and animals. d-α-Tocopherol, dl-α-tocopherol, and their esters have been available from commercial sources for some decades and are alternate or additional sources of dietary tocopherols.

II. BIOGENESIS AND LIFE CYCLE TRENDS

The tocopherols occur mainly in the unesterified form in a variety of plant life such as nuts, seeds, oils, fruits, vegetables, and grasses. Nuts, seeds, some grains, and vegetable oils are superior sources. Their distributional pattern in plant foods is modified by species, variety, stage of maturity, season, time, and manner of harvesting, processing procedures, and storage time. Animal tissue and animal products are usually low-to-poor sources and are influenced by the dietary consumption of tocopherols by the animal. Based upon incomplete data, the biogenesis of tocopherols in plant life is judged to be through the intermediate of the trienol structure by hydrogenation. The α-form, as an alternate route, can arise as successive methylations of mono- and disubstituted tocols. This hypothesis has arisen from the change in concentration of the tocol and trienol structures during the developing stages of the plant life. The tocopherols are believed to play a developmental role in the life of the plant and are not merely exogenous substances [16-18]. The germinating capacity of grain is related to tocopherol content [19].

Green [20] studied the changes in the various tocopherols in corn (maize), wheat, barley, and peas from seed to harvest. Whereas α-tocopherol is synthesized in young growing plants, other tocopherols are predominant in the seeds. Green proposed that tocopherols are interconvertible in plants and that, during germination and growth, the α-form is synthesized from other tocopherols by transmethylation. Chattopadhyay and Banerjee [21] had previously observed that the total tocopherol content of plants increases during germination. The total tocopherol content of leafy plants changes during the stages of maturation [22] in their life cycle. The biogenesis of the tocopherols has been recently reviewed by Glover [23].

III. INFLUENCE OF HARVESTING AND WEATHER

The level of α-tocopherol in grasses generally falls as development
approaches seed maturity. The level in alfalfa (lucerne) and in timothy
falls some 20-65%, depending on whether the crop is harvested at the grass
stage or at the full flowering stage, as related by Kivimae and Carpena
[24]. Decreases from 79 to 90% have been reported by Brown [22] in different grasses covering the early-to-late maturing stages. Brown [22]
noted the α-tocopherol content was high in young grasses, but fell to a low
value in late maturity (Fig. 2). Grass stems are poor in content, the
leafy portions of the plant containing 20-50 times the stem values of the
tocopherols. Significant losses occur in the drying of grass, and, therefore, hay and silage are highly variable sources of vitamin E. Earlier,

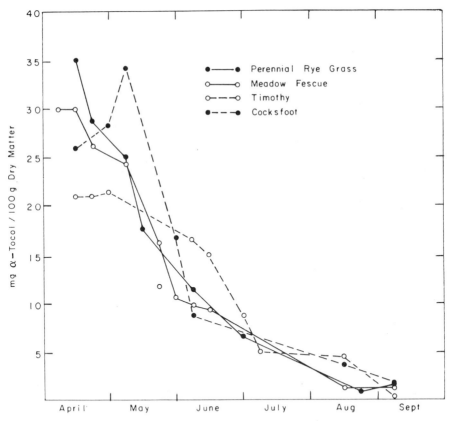

FIG. 2   Effect of stage of growth on α-tocopherol content of grasses.
(From Refs. 22 and 44.)

Maxim and Gondos [25] and Albonico and Fabris [26] observed a decrease
of 34-65% in tocopherol content, again depending on whether alfalfa and
clover were harvested at the leafy or postflowering stage. The seasonal
influence on the tocopherol level in forage grasses in the United Kingdom
were reported by Booth [27] where substantial differences occurred. In
these observations, mixed factors such as weather conditions, season, as
well as stage of growth were probably at work. The tocopherol level of
sunflower and grape seed oil are also influenced by the time of harvesting
and unfavorable environmental conditions [24]. Much rain and humidity
during harvest cause substantial damage to the grains. This results in a
fall in germinating power, an increase in peroxide content, and a lowered
tocopherol content.

IV. GENETIC VARIETY

Hjarde et al. [28], measuring total and α-tocopherol content of red clover,
noted that, while the levels were influenced by the stage of the growing
cycle, they were less influenced by cultivar differences and growing sites.
Brown [22] recorded little difference on the effects of genetic variety on
tocopherol level in different cultivars of alfalfa. On the other hand, Cabell
and Ellis [29] observed a 35% variation among nine different cultivars of
wheat and a 58% variation in corn cultivars. With different cultivars of
white, red, and yellow corn, Cattaneo et al. [30] showed that the total
tocopherol varied about ±10% within the cultivars and an overall variation
of about 30%. Among four cultivars of wheat, Antonijevic et al. [31]
found tocopherol levels which varied by 29%. Feldheim [32] reported on
the total tocopherol content of three varieties of ripe paprika: 10 samples
of one ranged from 0.45 to 8.24 mg/100 g, five samples of another variety
0.30-0.58 mg/100 g, and three samples of a third variety 1.0-8.2 mg/
100 g, thus illustrating a variable influence of cultivars on tocopherol content. It appears that plant genetics is a variable factor of influence on the
tocopherol level in plant food. Current data suggest a lesser influence on
grasses and forages, but marked influence of the stage of growth on
tocopherol levels of these plants. Perhaps critical comparisons have not
yet clearly measured a genetic influence. With grain-bearing plants,
genetic variety appears to constitute a major influence on tocopherol level.

V. INHIBITORS OF ABSORPTION

An important factor is availability of the tocopherol content in plant foods
to humans or animals, as cited by Bunnell et al. [33]. Only one-third of
the tocopherol from alfalfa meal appeared to be utilized by the chick, as

measured by liver storage [34,35]. In 1966, Olson et al. [36] isolated a compound from alfalfa lipids which inhibited tocopherol deposition. Inhibitors of vitamin E absorption have also been reported to exist in certain legumes, namely, kidney beans [37,38] and peas [39]. Absorption from the gut of tocopherol in the feed is inhibited, as judged by a reducation in tocopherol level in the plasma, when kidney beans are included in the ration of mature sheep [40].

Nitrates present in plant foods can be microbially converted to nitrites. Nitrites are also added to whole and comminuted meats in the curing process as a means of preservation. The feeding of nitrites (0.3% as potassium nitrite) in the diet of rats has been reported to precipitate a deficiency of vitamin E [41]. Feeding potassium nitrite to hens [42] decreased the α-tocopherol content of eggs by 40%. Feeding sodium nitrite to chickens [43] was also reported to lower α-tocopherol stores in the avian liver.

VI. SEASONAL INFLUENCE IN ANIMAL TISSUE

The tocopherol content of milk is higher in summer and lower in winter [44]. Not surprisingly, seasonal variations have also been observed [45-47] in butter. Veijo et al. [48] of Finland reported α-tocopherol values of 0.68-1.91 mg in winter butter and 1.72-3.84 mg/100 g in summer butter. Kanno et al. [49], in Japan, confirmed the seasonal influence (Fig. 3) on the tocopherol content of bovine milk fat. They found 3.4 mg α-tocopherol in summer and 2.2 mg/100 g butter fat in winter. No other tocopherols were present except a trace of γ-tocopherol, 0.2 mg in summer and 0.1 mg/100 g in winter. Lueck and Mueller-Mulot [50], employing thin-layer chromatography, determined the α-tocopherol content of South African butter from 27 factories. An average α-tocopherol content of 5.8 mg/100 g of butter fat was found, with a range of 4.4-7.2 mg.

The variation of α-tocopherol content of milk fat over the seasons is a reflection of the amount of dietary α-tocopherol in the cow's ration. The grasses of the green pastures in the early stage of growth are high in α-tocopherol content. This is reflected in the milk and butter fat of cows or other milk-producing animals. When the season of dry pastures or the feeding of dry forage, silage, and dry concentrates occurs, and when no attempt is made to maintain or control ample α-tocopherol levels in the ration by a dietary supplementation program, the tocopherol values of the milk and milk by-products such as cream, butter, cheese, ice cream, etc., decrease.

VII. INFLUENCE OF FOOD PROCESSING

The tocopherols are subject to destruction by oxygen, forming quinones, dimers, and trimers. Oxidation is accelerated by exposure to light, heat,

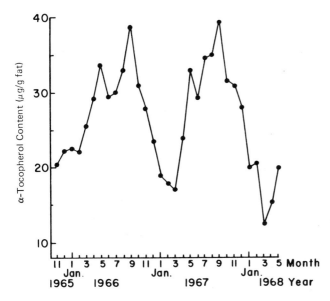

FIG. 3   Variation of α-tocopherol content of milk fat over the seasons. (From Ref. 48, with permission.)

alkali, and the presence of certain trace minerals such as iron (Fe^{3+}) and copper (Cu^{2+}). Ferrous and cuprous ions and ground-state copper do not react with tocopherol [51]. If ascorbic acid and/or chelating agents are present, they will protect tocopherols from the metal-activated oxidation. The tocopherols are more stable in acid than in alkali to oxidation. In the absence of oxygen they are relatively heat- and light-stable and relatively stable to alkali. Esterification of tocopherols by acylation of the free phenolic hydroxy increases their stability to oxygen. Exposure of tocopherols to hydroperoxides and peroxides formed in the development of oxidative rancidity in fats also lowers tocopherol content. During the handling and processing procedures, foods are usually exposed to one or more of these destructive influences. Refined and processed foods are thus variable and usually less predictable sources of vitamin E than whole fresh foods [52].

A. Drying

Natural drying by exposure to the sun reduced the level of tocopherols in clover and corn leaves to a zero value in 4-5 days [53]. When the drying was undertaken in the shade, the level fell more slowly. Thafvelin and Oksanen [54] observed the effects of methods of drying on tocopherol, linolenic acid, and peroxide values in timothy grass, red clover, and tufted hair grass (Deschampsia caespitosa) when dried in the sun or artificially. Dried on hay poles, the tocopherol loss was about the same (about 48%) as when dried in cocks; dried in swaths, the loss was about 60%. The extent of destruction of vitamin E during haymaking was found to be directly dependent on the method of drying and on the length of the drying period. During forage cutting and drying, changes occur in fatty acid composition [54, 55]. Apparently environmental factors, such as brightness of sunlight, amount of tissue bruising, time of curing, method of drying, etc., relate to the degree of tocopherol losses which may be experienced [22, 54, 56].

Artificial drying and silage making are superior to normal haymaking in the preservation of tocopherols of grasses [22]. Based on a U.S. survey [57] in 1961, the average value for dehydrated alfalfa (20.1 mg/100 g) was almost double that for sun-cured products (11.5 mg/100 g). Bunnel et al. [33] reported alfalfa to be the richest source of α-tocopherol fed to livestock. In an examination of 12 dehydrated alfalfa meals, the α-tocopherol level ranged from 2.8 to 14.1 mg/100 g. The variation is deduced to have been influenced by the time interval between cutting and drying, conditions and length of storage, etc. In a 1968 study, losses of α-tocopherol during commercial-scale dehydration [58] in alfalfa production ranged from 5 to 33%, and larger losses (54-73%) occurred during storage (Table 1). These losses are further detailed in a comprehensive 1970 report [59].

TABLE 1   Stability of α-Tocopherol During Storage of Dehydrated Alfalfa Meal

Meals[b]	Moisture (%)	α-Tocopherol content (mg/100 g)[a]		
		Initial	12 Wk	Loss (%)
1	12.2	13.7	3.7	73
2	9.2	17.2	4.9	72
3	7.1	12.9	3.7	71
4	2.5	13.8	6.3	54
5[c]	2.5	13.8	9.0	35
6	8.3	18.1	7.6	55

[a] Dry basis, average of duplicate analyses.
[b] Stored 12 weeks at 90°F.
[c] Added 0.15% ethoxyquin.
Source: From Ref. 58.

At harvest time, ripe grains are not always sufficiently dry to be put into storage, and, hence, artificial drying or other preservation methods must be put into effect or else the grains mold. Moldy and low-weight grains may be low in α-tocopherol content [60, 61]. Adams et al. [61] recorded vitamin E deficits in 16 samples of lightweight corn to amount to 21% below values for normal sound corn. Artificial drying of corn can be effectively carried out when well controlled without destruction of vitamin E or unsaturated fatty acids. Overdrying, particularly at high temperature, will lead to some destruction of these nutrients in corn [62]. Inconsistent results were obtained by Pond et al. [63]. Young et al. [64] reported a small decrease of α-tocopherol content in the artificial drying of corn.

B. Organic Acid Treatment

Another approach to the preservation of high-moisture grain is the addition of organic acids as an antifungal agent. When 1% propionic acid was added to moist barley grain by Madsen et al. [65] and the grain stored for 6 months, the propionic acid-treated barley contained 0.3 mg tocopherols compared with 3.3 mg/100 g for untreated and dried barley. Subsequent tests [66] were set up which confirmed the findings of low vitamin E levels in high-moisture barley treated with propionic acid following some months of storage. Jensen et al. [67] observed substantially reduced levels of vitamin E and the carotenes in organic acid treatment of high-moisture corn (maize). This was not the case when propionic acid was applied to corn grain dried artificially. A rapid and large decrease (Fig. 4) in the natural α-tocopherol content of acid-treated corn during storage was reported by Young et al. [64]. The decline of α-tocopherol content of naturally dried corn appeared to be inversely related to the dry matter of the corn. Komoda and Harada [68] have recorded that the addition of water to raw soybeans resulted in extensive oxidation of the tocopherols within 7 days. A rapid rise in peroxide value of high-moisture grain compared with dry grain [69] may account for the destructive action of α-tocopherol in most grains. dl, α-Tocopheryl acetate added to high-moisture corn was stable in storage trials [64].

C. Milling

Hand dissection of four hybrid samples of corn kernels into its components and assay by Gram et al. [70] have revealed their distribution of the tocopherols. The endosperm tocopherol content varied from 27% in normal dent corn to 11% in high-lysine corn and represented all of the measurable trienol structures found in the corn kernel. The germ fraction containing

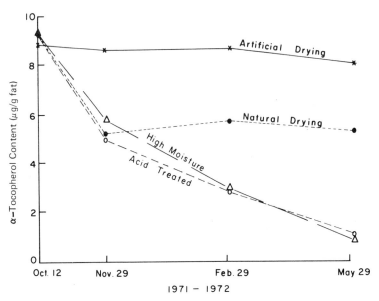

FIG. 4   Stability of α-tocopherol in stored corn.   (From Ref. 64, with permission.)

only tocol structures contributed 70% in the normal dent and 86% in the high-lysine samples of the total tocopherol content of the whole kernel.   In wheat kernels the absence of trienols from the embryo and the tocols in the germ and aleurone layer, tissues capable of active metabolism, were reported [71].   No evidence for the existence of tocopheryl esters in the kernel could be found.

In the fractionation of the wheat kernel in the milling process, Binnington and Andrews [72] were some of the first to indicate that white flour was relatively low in vitamin E activity and that the germ, and, secondly, the bran-containing portions were the richer sources.   The degree of milling was recognized as important.   Hentzler et al. [73] reported wheat flours of 100, 50, and 30% extraction (whole wheat to refined white flour) to contain progressively less tocopherol.   Milling rye [74] and triticale [75] also results in flour fractions of lower tocopherol content. Moran [76] has reviewed the nutritional significance and loss of nutrients in the milling process; Frazer et al. [77] and Thomas et al. [78] reported on the distribution of vitamin E in the milling and processing of grain.

The baking quality of flour improves upon months of storage.   This is believed to be due to oxidative changes.   Hence flours are treated with oxidants, such as chlorine dioxide, to imitate aging and thereby achieve rapid flour improvement. Further destruction of vitamin E occurs during wheat, rye, or barley milling into flour at the bleaching or improving stage [74] with benzoyl peroxide or nitrogen trichloride treatment. The effect of nitrogen trichloride and chloride dioxide treatment on the tocopherols of wheat flour has been confirmed by others [74, 77, 79-82]. Chlorine dioxide-treated flour fed to rats was ineffective [83] as a vitamin E source, the animal developing vitamin E deficiency symptoms (Fig. 5). Flour improvement by added ascorbic acid did not appear to cause loss of tocopherol in white flour or to decrease the tocopherol content of bread, although some tocopherol destruction occurs by the aeration process of bread-making [79, 84].

Wet milling of corn was investigated by Howland et al. [85]. Commercial wet milling appears to have little effect on the content of α- and γ-tocopherols in corn-germ oil. The tocopherol composition of corn-germ oil from hand-dissected germ was about the same as that of the germ recovered from a wet milling plant. According to Grams et al. [86], the respective recoveries of α- and total tocopherols were 68 and 73% after dry milling and 18 and 27% after wet milling. Tocopherols were highly concentrated in the germ products from both dry milling (19.6 mg/100 g) and wet milling (8.5 mg/100 g). The explanation for the contrasting results of Grams et al. [86] given by Howland et al. [85] was that their data were taken on samples from a commercially operating wet milling plant whose plant extraction processes gave higher recovery values.

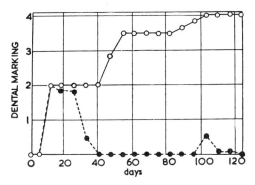

FIG. 5   Vitamin E deficiency symptoms, as judged by dental depigmentation observations, in rats fed either a diet containing untreated white flour (open circles, solid line) or white flour treated with chlorine dioxide (solid circles, broken line). Maximum marking for normal brown upper incisors = 4; marking for completely white incisors = 0. (From Ref. 80, with permission.)

D. Expanding, Puffing, Rolling, and Shredding

Herting and Drury [87] have pursued a study of the tocopherol content of cereal grains and processed cereals utilizing two-dimensional thin-layer chromatography. Although α-, β-, and γ-tocopherol and α-tocotrienol values were reported on some products, the authors state that the α-tocopherol values were of primary interest in their study. Virtually any type of processing resulted in less vitamin E in the processed product. For corn products, losses of 35% for white corn meal to 98% for corn flakes were reported. For wheat products the losses ranged from 22% for puffed wheat to 92% for white flour. While rice products also showed large losses in milled, expanded, and shredded products, it was interesting to note that oatmeal products, such as the rolled long- or short-cooking type suffered no loss in processing. This is due to the mild processing involved, mainly dehulling, crimping, and partial cooking. Corn, wheat, and rice grain processing can involve removal of grain fractions, flaking, shredding, puffing, expanding, and parboiling. When different commercial brands of breakfast cereals were examined by Herting and Drury [87], a wide variation in α-tocopherol content was evident as in three brands of corn flakes with values ranging from 0.03 to 0.15 mg/100 g; in three brands of shredded wheat, 0.09-0.31 mg/100 g; in three brands of rolled oats 0.94-1.81 mg/100 g; and in four brands of puffed rice, 0.05-0.12 mg/100 g. According to Sechi and Rossi-Manaresi [88], well-milled white rice (essentially the endosperm) retains only a trace of the total tocopherol level originally present in the brown rice.

E. Irradiation

Vitamin E destruction as a result of irradiation with electrons was compared in foods by Diehl [89]. Losses were highest in products with a high-fat content. Exclusion of atmospheric oxygen reduced the loss caused by irradiation. Kung et al. [90] reported tocopherol destruction to the extent of 29-61% in fluid milk irradiated with gamma rays at 80,000-480,000 roentgen. Kraybill [91] noted 10-30% destruction of tocopherol when dairy products were irradiated with 80,000 roentgens per hour. Destruction of tocopherol in irradiated meat has also been observed [92,93]. The tocopherol content of Manitoba wheat, English wheat [94], and German oats [95] decreased with increasing radiation (Table 2). If the dosage levels can be controlled to achieve a desired goal such as for insect control, it may be possible to hold tocopherol destruction to a minimal value.

F. Fumigation

The effects of fumigation and storage on the tocopherols in wheat grain, milling fractions, and baked products were investigated by Slover and

TABLE 2   Influence of Irradiation on the Tocopherol Content of Oats and Wheat

Irradiation (krad)	Total tocopherol (mg/100 g)		Total tocopherol (mg/100 g)		α-Tocopherol (mg/100 g)	α-Tocotrienol (mg/100 g)
	Manitoba wheat[a]		English wheat[a]		Oats[b]	Oats
0	2.70		2.96		0.58	1.25
50	—		—		0.52	1.20
100	2.20		2.73		—	—
500	—		—		0.37	0.64
1,000	1.67		2.60		—	—
5,000	1.10		2.07		—	—
10,000	0.58		1.83		—	—

[a] See Ref. 94.
[b] See Ref. 95.

Lehmann [96] by a gas chromatographic separation technique [97]. Wheats were fumigated periodically with methyl bromide, ethylene dichloride, carbon tetrachloride, and phosphine over a 3-year period. The amount of α-tocopherol, α-tocotrienol, β-tocopherol, and β-tocotrienol did not change significantly as a result of fumigation.

G. Refining Bleaching, Deacidifying, Deodorizing, and Hydrogenating

Crude oils are removed from plant sources by a pressure or solvent process, after which they undergo a series of processing steps to become refined oils for food preparation and table use. Two principal reactions have been considered by Frankel et al. [98] to control the fate of tocopherols in autoxidizable fats: the reaction between tocopherol and formed reactive hydroperoxides and the spontaneous oxidation of tocopherol by atmospheric oxygen, of which the former reaction is the more important. Tocopherol destruction is accelerated by light, alkali, and certain high-valence trace metals and can occur during the refining process. Losses cited [99] in refining vary from 0 to 30%, in bleaching from 14 to 48%, in deodorizing 14-35%, in deacidifying 5-20%, and in hydrogenating from 5 to 70%. These data resulted from compiled reports on different oils, by different workers, probably using different processing variables. In 1975, Juillet [100] reviewed losses of tocopherol resulting from the processing of oil and mentioned that the extent of the losses varies with the methodology employed (Table 3). Deodorizing and bleaching were cited as stages where substantial losses can occur. Kivimae and Carpena [24] cite data of higher losses for batch processing of soybean oil than for centrifugal refining, and hence confirm the generalization that specific losses depend on the nature of the refining process. Jakubowski et al. [101] recorded tocopherol

TABLE 3   Modification of the Tocopherol Content of Oils During Refining[a]

Type of oil	Unrefined	Deacidified	Bleached	Deodorized	Destearinated
Coconut	3-5	—	—	3	—
Corn	119	—	—	95	—
Olive	110	105	95	95	20
Soybean	152-212	—	—	110-175	—
Palm	50-52	—	—	35-40	—

[a] Figures given are in milligrams of total tocopherols per 100 grams.
Source: From Ref. 100.

losses of 10 and 17% in the refining of rapeseed and soybean oil, respectively. Refining techniques reduce the tocopherol content of palm, coconut, and peanut oils [102]. In fish oils, Einset et al. [103] noted that the rate of autoxidation was inversely correlated with tocopherol content. Corn oil and cottonseed oil [60] also show appreciable losses of tocopherols during the refining process. Other variables are age of oils at the time of assay and the stability of the tocopherols contained therein. The removal of α-tocopherol in the processing of crude plant oils [104] is suggested by the higher tocopherol content in the sludge or "foots" from vegetable oil processing. This is the commercial source of d-α-tocopherol obtained by extraction and/or molecular distillation. Some d-α-tocopherol is prepared by further methylation of d, β-, d, γ-, and d, δ-, or by hydrogenation of d, α-tocotrienol.

H. Heating, Cooking, and Baking

Some form of heating is applied to many types of foods during processing or in preparation of food for table use. Chow and Draper [12] investigated the stability of natural tocopherols (tocols, trienols) in corn and soybean oil heated at 70°C and aerated at 100 ml/min. In corn oil, α-tocopherol and α-tocotrienol were destroyed faster than γ-tocopherol and γ-tocotrienol. At an equivalent concentration of 0.02% in stripped corn oil, the order of antioxidant activity of the natural tocopherols was $\gamma > \delta > \beta > \alpha$. Tocopherol oxidation and peroxide formation occurred more rapidly in corn than in soybean oil. Previously, Parkhurst et al. [11] had reported an order of $\gamma > \delta > \alpha$ in a lard system and a temperature of 97°C. The exact order of antioxidant activity is influenced by their concentration [105, 106]. Chow and Draper [12] commented that the marked differences in stability of raw and refined oils have been attributed to variations in the amount of antioxidants present and in fatty acid composition, but other organic and inorganic constituents are probably involved. Owing to these differences in the rate of oxidation of the various tocopherols in oils, vitamin assays for total tocopherols underestimate the rate of loss in biological activity [12].

Frying readily destroys tocopherol. Ramanujan and Anantakrishan [107] heated peanut oil to 175°C for 30 min and found a loss of 32%, but upon adding 0.02% of propyl gallate or butylhydroxyanisole in other trials, this loss was reduced to 11%. Sesame oil heated to 175°C for 30 min lost 40% of its tocopherol content. Antioxidants added to this oil were less successful in delaying tocopherol destruction.

Significant losses of tocopherol occur according to Bunnell et al. [108] during the storage of food cooked in vegetable oils, while there may be little loss of tocopherol in foods during deep-fat frying in fresh vegetable oil. In heating vegetable oils to high temperature, α-tocopheryl acetate

TABLE 4 Stability of the Natural Tocopherols in Vegetable Oils versus Added α-Tocopheryl Acetate Under Stress of Heat

Type of oil	Initial natural tocopherol (mg/100 g)	Natural tocopherol destroyed (%)	Added dl,α-tocopheryl acetate (mg/100 g)	Tocopheryl acetate destroyed (%)
Deodorized, unhydrogenated corn oil	100	97	100	13
Deodorized, hydrogenated corn oil	105	99	100	19
Deodorized, unhydrogenated cotton-seed oil	91	97	100	19
Deodorized, hydrogenated cotton-seed oil	80	99	100	8
Deodorized, unhydrogenated soybean shortening oil	101	96	100	12
Deodorized, hydrogenated soybean shortening oil	73	99	100	13
Stabilized safflower oil	59	97	100	6
Unstabilized safflower oil	36	98	100	5

Source: From Ref. 100.

added to cooking oils is vastly more stable than the unesterified tocopherols naturally present in the oils (Table 4).

LeCoq [109] demonstrated that one-third of the tocopherol was lost
when wheat germ was heated at 100°C on a water bath for 1 hr; direct
heating to 120-150°C caused a higher loss (89%) after 45 min. The baking
process destroys a portion of the tocopherols whether the bread is made
from milled or bleached flours. Slover and Lehmann [96] found losses of
β-tocotrienols of 18.2% for bread and 9.9% for rolls. In another baking
trial [80], 36% of the total tocopherols was destroyed; of the tocopherols
observed α-tocopherol was most easily destroyed. In baking rye breads,
less destruction of tocopherol was noted in the under crust (10%) than in
the upper crust (40%) in conventional baking; less tocopherol was lost in
the upper crust (20%) by infrared baking [110]. Menger [84] reported
losses of tocopherol during backing of various types of breads to range
from 5 to 50%. Sharman and Richards [111] studied commercial English
breads and observed that when white bread was fed to rats as a sole diet,
red cell hemolysis occurred, whereas whole meal bread or wheat germ-
enriched white bread gave protection, the α-tocopherol activity of the
various breads correlating with the hemolysis data.

Booth and Bradford [112] employing two-dimensional chromatography
[113] examined the α-tocopherol content of several vegetables, namely,
brussel sprouts, cabbages, carrots, leeks, and yew, and reported cooking
losses (cooking in water) of less than 10%. Brubacher [114] on the other
hand, analyzing a few vegetables (potatoes and beans), noted somewhat
higher losses (20% or more). The study of Bunnell et al. [108] revealed
that the ordinary cooking processes employed in preparing food for consumption did not involve large losses of tocopherol.

I. Dehydration, Canning, and Freezing

Various methods of processing meat products have an influence on the
α-tocopherol content of meat. Dehydration caused 36-45% loss of
α-tocopherol in chicken and beef, but little or none in pork [93]. Losses
of 41-65% of α-tocopherol were recorded due to canning processes.
Losses of tocopherol in the production of canned beans, corn, and peas
are indicated as severe, over 50% [52,108]. Processing losses of tocopherol of peas as reported by Aczel [115] were small. Blanching of almonds
caused a loss of about 20% of initial tocopherol content according to Tappel
et al. [116], while 80% destruction occurred during the roasting of the nuts.
In the production of nonfat dry milk, the butterfat is first removed and,
hence, condensed milk and dried products resulting therefrom are essentially devoid of α-tocopherol [117]. While tocopherols are stable during
the freezing process, the low-storage temperatures, as first noted by
Bunnell [108], do not prevent the oxidation of the tocopherols, and hence,

substantial losses can occur with time. There is great loss of tocopherol in potato chips stored at room temperature and in french-fried potatoes and potato chips in frozen storage (Table 5). Despite good commercial packaging, large losses of tocopherol occur and are believed to be due to the action of hydroperoxides.

VIII. INFLUENCE OF STORAGE

Harris [44] has reviewed the influences of storage and processing on the retention of vitamin E in foods. Some loss of tocopherols during storage of wheat grain and milling fractions were expected both as a result of oxidation and as a secondary effect of fatty acid oxidation [96]. Mere shelf storage of cereal grains gradually lowers tocopherol levels. Rothe et al. [118] noted an approximate 50% reduction in tocopherols of white and whole grain flour and about 25% loss in wheat germ as a result of 80-day storage of these products at 37°C. Whole wheat flour lost 35% of its tocopherol upon storage for 38 days and 60% of its tocopherol after storage for 80 days.

TABLE 5   Stability of Tocopherol in Fried Foods

Storage time and temperature	Total tocopherol (mg/100 g)	Percent loss
Tocopherol content of oil extracted from potato chips		
After manufacture	75	—
Stored chips, 2 weeks, 23°C	39	48
Stored chips, 1 month, 23°C	22	71
Stored chips, 2 months, 23°C	17	77
Stored chips, 1 month, -12°C	28	63
Stored chips, 2 months, -12°C	24	68
Tocopherol content of oil extracted from french-fried potatoes		
After manufacture	78	—
Stored fried, 1 month, -12°C	25	68
Stored fried, 2 months, -12°C	20	74

Source: From Ref. 108.

Whole wheat meal lost 90% of its tocopherol content upon 4 months of storage [119]. Wheat germ stored at 4°C or 20°C for 6 months lost about 10% of its tocopherol [120], while, in an earlier study [121], wheat germ lost 75% of its tocopherol in storage 1-2 months. An approximate 36% loss of α-tocopherol in corn stored for 12 weeks was recorded by Kodicek et al. [122]. In 1963, Herting and Drury [60] reported a 35% loss of α-tocopherol in the storage of ground corn for 6 months at room temperature. Livingston et al. [58] observed α-tocopherol decreases of 54-73% in alfalfa stored 12 weeks at 90°F and of 5-33% during commercial scale alfalfa dehydration. Akopyan [123] revealed heavy losses of tocopherol in clover meal (55%), sweet clover meal (67%), and cocksfoot meal (100%) after over 1 year of storage. The loss of tocopherol is temperature-related [124]: in trials with rye grass stored for 6 weeks at 3°C, a loss of 8% was recorded; at 60°C the loss rose to 49%. About 95% of the original tocopherol content was destroyed [122] in stored tortillas (12 weeks at room temperature). Ground, dried tortillas lost 80% of their tocopherol after 6 months' storage, while the ground white corn they were made from lost only 30% of its tocopherol after the same storage period. Storage of oils results in considerable destruction of tocopherol depending on the oil, time, temperature, and concentration of antioxidants [99, 125]. Tocopherol content in castor oil was reduced 90% by storage at 10°C for 1 year, while that in coconut oil was only reduced 25% by similar storage. Safflower oil lost 45% of its tocopherol content after 6 months' storage at 10°C, 55% after 3 months' storage at room temperature, and 70% after storage at 37°C for 3 months. Peanut oil lost 80% of its tocopherol content during storage at 10°C for 1 year; a loss between 62 and 88% was recorded after 4 months in storage when the temperature rose from 10° to 43°C.

Tocopherols are apparently nature's choice of an antioxidant [44, 126], as is indicated by a high correlation between total tocopherol level and combined linoleic and linolenic acids in a number of oil-bearing plants. The tocopherols of the plant oils are destroyed by heat and during storage. While added synthetic antioxidants stabilize fats against oxidation, they may not protect the original tocopherol levels, thus altering the α-tocopherol/polyunsaturated fat ratio; hence, oils may be overrated as α-tocopherol sources [127].

IX. TOCOPHEROL CONTENT OF FOODS

A 192-page review with 434 references on the vitamin E content of foods and feeds was written by Dicks [99], which included all literature up to and partially including 1965. Much of this compilation deals with total tocopherol contents of foods. Where available, α-tocopherol values were also reported. Some years later, Ames [52] compiled vitamin E values of foods. Recognizing that most non-α-tocopherols have little nutritional significance

Ames limited his tabulation to the mean α-tocopherol content, and the range of contents for a variety of food products. Wherever possible, the values selected from the literature for the tabulation were obtained by reliable analytical procedures.

In the past decade there has been further activity in the development and refinement of the assay of individual tocopherols. There is, however, no universally adopted method for all tocopherols in foods. It is timely to show what values have been reported during the past decade for the individual tocopherols in foods for comparative purposes within and without classes of foods. An eventual objective should be the acquisition of a complete understanding of the distribution and significance of the known tocopherols in our commonly used food products. Slover and co-workers in a series of papers [96,97,128-131] have been reporting the individual tocopherol content of many foods and are working toward the development [132, 133] of an overall analytical method which can be applied more universally.

The nomenclature of the tocopherols by Pennock et al. [1] and the eight tocopherols designated as α-, β-, γ-, and δ-tocols (or tocopherols) and α-, β-, γ-, and δ-trienols (or tocotrienols) have been employed as designations in Appendix A, which tabulates the tocopherol content in foods. The table must be used with caution as the data have been obtained by different methodologies and by different investigators. Added to variation in the natural tocopherol content of food are further influences of harvesting, processing, and storage variables. Hence, while reference to food composition tables may give one a relative concept of tocopherol values, the best estimate of tocopherol content will be an analysis of the food sample in question. Since α-tocopherol is the principal tocopherol contributing vitamin E activity, Appendix B has also been prepared to indicate many foods containing 1 milligram or more of α-tocopherol per 100 grams of food. Data taken from three reviews on the tocopherol content of foods in the appendix cover the past 35 years. The foods have been arranged in decreasing order of α-tocopherol content.

Initially, foods were assayed for vitamin E activity by the biological method using animals. This approach gave way to total tocopherol evaluation by chemical analyses. More recent advances in chromatography permit analysis of a variety of tocopherols and tocotrienols which are presented in this report. There have been past reviews and compilations on the subject of food vitamin E or tocopherol values [9,14,19,24,60,100,134,135].

A. Oils and Fats

Vegetable oils are generally much richer than animal fats in tocopherol content [14]. Taeufel and Serzisko [136] reported more γ- and δ-tocopherol than α-tocopherol in soybean oil, but in olive oil, rye-germ oil, rice-germ oil, and sunflower oil, α-tocopherol was the primary tocol. α- and

β-Tocopherol made up the principal tocopherols in wheat germ oil. Herting and Drury [60] employed column chromatography on $MgHPO_4$ to determine the α-tocopherol content of 60 samples of fats and oils from 17 different plants. While total tocopherols ranged from 0.2-2.4 mg/100 g in coconut oil to 165.6-189.7 mg/100 g in wheat germ oil, α-tocopherol varied from none to little in coconut oil, cocoa butter, castor bean oil, and linseed oil up to 84.8-127.6 mg/100 g in wheat germ oil. The α-tocopherol content relative to total tocopherols, was reported as 0% in castor bean and linseed oil to about 90% in safflower oil. Herting and Drury [60] reported the percentage of α-tocopherol in total tocopherols to be relatively constant for each plant source except corn. Total tocopherols of 125 corn inbreds showed a 5-fold range in content and a 10-fold variation when related to oil content [137].

The four tocotrienols related to α-, β-, γ-, and δ-tocopherol were reported to have been found in palm oil by Pennock et al. [1]. Latex from the rubber tree, Hevea brasiliensis, was found to contain substantial amounts of free and esterified α-, γ-, and δ-tocotrienols shortly thereafter by Dunphy et al. [138] and Whittle et al. [139]. Sturm et al. [140] have determined α-, γ-, and δ-tocopherol content in peanut oils from 17 individual varieties. A two-dimensional thin-layer chromatographic system has been used to separate the tocols and trienols before assaying them with the Emmerie-Engel reaction by Whittle and Pennock [141] to measure tocopherol content of vegetable oils. Chow et al. [142], in tocopherol estimation, substituted a low-temperature crystallization technique for the usual partially destructive saponification step prior to thin-layer chromatography techniques and reported high-tocopherol recoveries. The tocopherol in sunflower seed oil is predominantly α-tocopherol [143]. Vegetable oils, in contrast to seeds, generally have simpler tocopherol patterns and contain primarily the tocol structures [130]. Few oils have α-tocopherol as the major form. The γ-tocol predominates in many oils; β-tocol is in wheat germ oil and δ-tocol is in soybean and peanut oils. The tocopherols in the common vegetable oils have been studied by Fedeli et al. [144]. Sunflower seed oil contains 50-70 mg/100 g of total tocopherols [145]. Using gas chromatography, mass spectrometry, and thin-layer chromatography to estimate β- and γ-tocopherol separately, Govind and colleagues [146] quantitated the tocol and trienol structure content of some plant oils. Oats contain mostly α-tocotrienol (58.3% of the total tocopherols present) and barley also is high (57.1%). Coconut oil has mostly γ-tocotrienol (53.6%). Wheat germ contains primarily α- and β-tocol structures. Soybean oil is high in γ-tocol (61.9%) with some δ- (26.6%) and α-tocol (11.5%).

In contrast to a variety of tocopherols in margarine the only form in butter is α-tocopherol. For butter, a mean α-tocopherol value of 1.65 mg/100 g was found by Ward [147]. A value of 1.36 mg/100 g was obtained for Dutch, 1.96 for Danish, and 1.65 for New Zealand butters.

The vitamin E content of margarine varies greatly, according to the oils from which it is made and treatment which the oils receive in refining, deodorizing, and hydrogenating. Some oils are rich in tocopherols such as soybean, cottonseed, and corn; others like coconut, palm-kernel, and whale are low. Ward [147], using two-dimensional chromatography [113], reported the α-tocopherol content of 13 samples of British margarines to range from 0.69 to 5.58 mg/100 g and a total tocopherol range of 1.76-10.0 mg/100 g. American margarines were higher with an α-tocopherol range of 3.3-15.8 mg/100 g, presumably because of greater use of corn, cottonseed, and soybean oils. Hydrogenation of oils significantly lowered tocopherol content. For example, Ward [147] reported peanut oil at a total tocopherol level of 20.3 mg/100 g and the hydrogenated product to contain 3.3 mg. The total tocopherol content of six commercial German margarines varied between 13.7 and 31.5 mg/100 g margarine [131]. By the use of column and paper chromatography and spectrophotometry, Lambertsen et al. [148] recorded an average α-tocopherol value of 5.2 mg (range 2.0-9.0) and a γ-tocopherol value of 8.9 mg (range 1.0-27.0) per 100 g for Norwegian margarines. After 7 months of storage, average losses of 20% α-tocopherol and 14% γ-tocopherol were found. According to Zemanovic and Mastenova [149] no tocopherol loss occurs during the manufacture of margarine if proper precautions are taken. Most margarines contain more γ- than α-tocopherol, a characteristic of some vegetable oils such as corn oil [128]. When the ratio of α-tocopherol to polyunsaturated fatty acid (PUFA) content is examined, all the margarines studied had ratios of less than 0.6 mg α-tocopherol/g of PUFA, a preferred ratio. Carpenter and Slover [128] further reported a wide variation in PUFA, the amount of trans-unsaturation, positional isomers, tocopherol content, triglyceride structures, and α-tocopherol/PUFA ratios (actually from 0.1 to 0.5 g).

From Appendix A the α-tocopherol content in milligrams per 100 grams for oils and fats are as follows: butter, 2.2 (range 1.0-3.3); coconut, 0.45 (0.4-0.5); corn, 15.9 (2.3-29.4); cottonseed, 44.0 (32-56); lard, 1.20; margarine (hard), 10.7 (3.2-19.9); margarine (soft), 13.9 (4.1-32.7); margarine (whipped), 3.2; olive, 10.1 (0.8-24.0); palm, 21.1 (18.8-25.6); peanut, 18.9 (10.7-33.9); rapeseed, 23.6 (18.4-23.8); safflower, 39.6 (34.2-45.8); soybean, 7.9 (3.4-11.5); sunflower, 48.7; and wheat germ 119.4 (110-133). Some oils contain appreciable levels of other tocopherols. Margarines contain γ-, in addition to α-tocopherol, and at times, some δ-tocopherol.

B. Nuts and Cereal-Grain Products

Filberts and almonds are rich in α-tocopherol; pecans and coconuts are poor sources, and peanuts and brazil nuts are intermediate [150]. Seeds and grains are the source of high-potency oils, and, hence, these seeds and grains themselves are the important plant sources of the tocopherols. α-Tocopherol is widely distributed among the cereal grains. Slover [130] reported a consensus that barley contained α-tocotrienol and β-tocopherol in addition to α-tocopherol. Oats also contain α-tocotrienol and α-tocopherol. α-Tocopherol and β-tocotrienol were present in rye. Wheat germ, with 7-11% fat and 5-46 mg/100 g total tocopherols (55-66% of which is α-tocopherol) is an excellent source of tocopherol [99]. Whole rye and whole rice are fair sources of tocopherols. Other grains and most of the processed grain flours are poor sources of tocopherol. Total tocopherol contents of pulses reported by Nazir and Magar [151] were judged to be low for their class of plant products. Corn is variable [47,60] in α-tocopherol content, ranging from 5 to 47%. Variability existed in both total tocopherol content and in the ratio of α- to γ-tocopherol. Slover et al. [131] observed variations in the α- and β-tocopherol and α- and β-tocotrienol content in different wheat samples.

Baked grain products have two sources of tocopherols, one from the grain fraction involved and another from the vegetable shortening, margarine, or butter added. Wide variability in these products is due to variation in food-refining methods, recipes of manufacture, and heating, storage, and handling procedures. Depending on the recipe and cooking method, cookies, pies, and snack foods can be fairly good α-tocopherol sources [108]. Slover and Lehman [96] and Slover et al. [131] studied the tocopherol content of wheat and wheat products, and baked products resulting therefrom. The trienols were less stable to heat stress than the tocols. Baked products often contained γ- and δ-tocopherols as a result of vegetable fats or oils added in the recipe.

Herting and Drury [87] reported large losses in the processing of grains into breakfast products. While commercial manufacturers of cereals often replace vitamins and some minerals, vitamin E is usually not included.

C. Milk, Egg, Meat, and Fish

The α-tocopherol content of cow's milk varies with the season. The tocopherol in animal fats is primarily in the α-form. It is highest in June to October, the period of fresh grass pasture consumption, and lowest in December to March, when dry forages and concentrates are consumed. An average value may be 18 mcg/g lipid (range 4-30) corresponding to 0.62 mg/quart (range 0.15-1.06), significantly less than that found in human milk [117]. The same authors noted a range of α-tocopherol values of 10-25 mcg/g lipid or 0.38-0.95 mg/quart of reconstituted milk in the assay of five brands of evaporated milk. Most significant in their evaluation of products is their report on the very low α-tocopherol content of nonfat or skim milk. Because of the removal of the milk fat from this product, it only contains about 0.02 mg α-tocopherol/quart, a fact that should be conveyed to consumers who have switched from whole fluid milk products to fat-free milk products.

Human milk is much richer in vitamin E than cows' milk [152]. For example, human milk was found to contain 6 times the α-tocopherol content of cows' milk [153]. Quaife [154] reported a range of 76-1800 mcg of total tocopherols per gram of lipid in 15 human milk samples within 1 week after parturition, reflecting in a large part a difference in past dietary intake. This level dropped to 37-58 mcg/g lipid in four samples taken 1-8 months after parturition. Harris et al. [155] cites an average value of 72 mcg/g lipid in 10 samples of raw human milk and 49 mcg/g lipid in another composite sample. Woodruff [156], in a study of 20 human milk samples, found an average value of about 50 mcg of α-tocopherol per gram of lipid. In 1969, Herting and Drury [117], using thin-layer chromatography [157], reported α-tocopherol values of 38 (range 20-64 for eight samples), 44 and 42 (range 22-60 for nine samples) per gram of lipid for frozen fresh, pasteurized, and lyophilized human milk, respectively. Hence, human milk would appear to have about 40 mcg/g lipid or about 1.14 mg/quart (3% fat) of α-tocopherol, which is believed to be the chief tocopherol in milk. Interestingly enough, human milk also varies in tocopherol content according to the season [158]. The mean tocopherol values in summer were 1.13-1.47 mg and in winter 0.57-0.86 mg/100 g. Pasteurization produced a loss of a quarter of the vitamin E content; heating at 100°C destroyed 20% of the α-tocopherol content, whereas 72-78°C had little or no effect [153].

The vitamin E content of cows' milk can be raised by administering supplementary amounts of vitamin E according to Hamed and Decker [159]. Vitamin E administration also slightly improved the vitamin A content of milk, presumably because of some protective or sparing activity by vitamin E.

Egg yolks are a fairly good dietary source of vitamin E for humans. From Appendix B, the α-tocopherol content in mg/100 g is 2.60 (range 1.6-3.9) as reported by Ames [52] and 2.75 (range 1.6-3.9) as reported by Dicks [99], while whole egg contained 0.46 mg/100 g from this review and 1.10 and 1.04 from the previous compilations.

Vitamin E content of milk has been observed as highly influenced by diet, which is undoubtedly true of meats as well; only recently has this subject been studied. Fish, meat, and poultry supply low-to-moderate amounts of α-tocopherol, with fish the highest of the three [108,160]. Yamanchi et al. [161] have recently reported on the α- and γ-content of skeletal muscles of livestock. Appendix A shows the α-tocopherol content for some meats and fish; most values are less than 1 mg/100 g of tissue.

D. Vegetables and Fruits

Some vegetables can be fairly good sources of tocopherol, containing
1-15 mg α-tocopherol per 100 g [99]. Examples are: dandelion leaves,
kale, green leafy tops of leeks, mustard leaves, nettle leaves, parsley
leaves, spinach leaves, sweet potatoes, turnip leaves, and yarrow leaves.
Kale is high in tocopherols, while mangolds, fodder beets, and swedes are
very low [22]. Booth and Bradford assayed a variety of fruits and vegetables [162, 163]. Most of the tocopherols of the apple and cucumber were in
the skin. Blackberries contained more γ- and δ- than α-tocopherol and
more tocopherols were found in wild berries than in cultivated types.
Tocopherols other than α were not found in significant amounts in vegetables. In broccoli and cauliflower, there was only a small amount in the
flower, more in the small leaf, and much more in large leaves; likewise,
cabbage had barely detectable levels in the colorless heart but higher levels
in outer green leaves. Hence, tocopherol values in cabbage are variable.
In celery, pale green edible stalks were higher in tocopherol than white
stalks. Outer leaves of lettuce contained more than the inner leaves.
Brussels sprouts were richer in tocopherol content during times of slow
growth than during rapid growth. September-sown garden cress was higher
than that grown in March. Parsley and watercress leaves were higher in
content than the stalks. Most fruits and vegetables, particularly those
processed, do not contribute significant amounts of α-tocopherol to the
diet [108]. Fresh, frozen, and canned peas contain 0.55, 0.25, and
0.02 mg/100 g α-tocopherol, respectively. This indicates destruction
in the canning and storage process. Home cooking for immediate consumption has only a small destructive effect [112].

Tocopherols [99] are more concentrated in the leaves of plants than in
the roots or stems. They are more prevalent in green leaves than in pale
leaves and more concentrated in large or mature leaves than in small or
immature leaves. Hence, it can be said that tocopherol concentration is
high in dark green, leafy tissue, moderate in fast-growing leaves, high in
slow-growing leaves, and low in roots and colorless tissues.

E. Infant Foods

All infants, especially the premature, begin neonatal life with very low
levels of tissue tocopherol. This level rises only after continued breast-
feeding or ingestion of artificial formulas containing an adequate vitamin E
level, or after receiving parenteral vitamin E after birth. Oski and
Barness [164] were the early investigators to point out that artificial infant
formulas contained widely varying amounts of vitamin E, and that some did
not contain a sufficient amount to prevent a vitamin E deficiency state

characterized by symptoms such as hemolytic anemia and low serum vitamin E levels.

Infant formulas exist in two commercial forms, liquids and powders. Six infant formulas and 10 infant cereals were analyzed [165] for total tocopherol content [165] and found to contain 0.08-3.1 and 0.03-1.8 mg/100 g; the α-tocopherol contents were 0.08-1.1 and 0.03-0.5 mg/100 g, respectively. These food products were also analyzed for unsaturated fatty acids and the ratio of α-tocopherol (milligrams) to polyunsaturated acids (grams) determined. Ratios for infant formulas and infant cereals were 0.2-0.3 and 0.02 to 0.3, respectively. These products are considered to be unsatisfactory sources of tocopherol for infant consumption. A wide range of values was evident. In 1969, when 12 formulas in the United States became nutrified with added vitamin E, an examination of these and others for α-tocopherol content revealed a much closer set of values [117]. For nine products prepared from a milk base, the products varied from 120 to 201 mcg/g lipid or 2.71 to 6.80 mg/quart on a reconstituted basis. These were noted to have an α-tocopherol (milligrams) to PUFA (grams) ratio varying from 0.32 to 0.96. On the other hand, for hypoallergenic infant formulas, usually made from nonmilk products (three of which were fortified with vitamin E), the reported α-tocopherol values were 94-224 mcg/g lipid or 2.30-7.67 mg/quart but the α-tocopherol to PUFA range of values was low at 0.19-0.42.

Desai et al. [166] investigated the proprietary infant formulas and substitute products available in Canada. The individual tocopherols were separated by a two-dimensional thin-layer chromatographic technique [141] and quantified by spectrophotometric estimation using the Emmerie-Engel procedure. Thirty samples of infant formulas, 15 based on cows' milk and 15 on noncows' milk were examined. The milk-based formulas contained primarily α-tocopherol, whereas γ- and δ-tocopherols, less biologically active forms, were the tocopherol structures in the nonmilk-based formulas. A significant observation is that about 60% of these infant formulas had an α-tocopherol to PUFA ratio of less than 0.4, a minimum value judged to have some significance in a preferred relationship between these nutrients. PUFA intake is one determinant of vitamin E needs according to previous investigators [167-172]. Secondly, only about 7% of the cows' milk-based formulas and 20-50% of the nonmilk-based proprietary infant formulas met the criteria of the daily infant need for vitamin E, namely, 5 IU as set by the NAS-NRC Food and Nutrition Board.* Ford et al. [173] compared dried milk preparations on sale in seven European countries and found marked differences in vitamin E content (α- and γ-tocols and trienols); four of these products for infants were based on

---

*National Academy of Sciences—National Research Council Food and Nutrition Board.

cows' milk and contained 0.70-0.83 mg/100 g and three products of non-milk base contained 4.77-10.21 mg/100 g.

Infant foods of one national commercial brand and selected products of a second brand obtained from two local supermarkets in Idaho during the years 1969-1971 were assayed for tocopherol content with primary emphasis on α-tocopherol [174]. Strained nuts contained 0.23-1.33 mg/100 g of α-tocopherol; strained desserts, 0.17-0.31; strained meat dishes, 0.13-0.73; egg yolk, 0.60; infant cereals [117], 0.04-0.49; and strained vegetables, 0.12-1.55. Fruits and vegetables were regarded as good in terms of vitamin E/PUFA ratios but not in terms of absolute content of vitamin E. Peaches, apricots, squash, and spinach were regarded as good sources in terms of both their content of vitamin E and the vitamin E/PUFA ratios [174].

F. Prepared Convenience Dinners

With the advent of home freezers in the United States, frozen dinners were developed which, upon heating, become immediately ready for consumption. These may be a meat-vegetable stew, or meat, fish, chicken, or turkey separated from potatoes, noodles, or rice, and one or more vegetables. Some contain fruit or a pudding, some a soup. Thompson et al. [175] assayed 24 different prepared frozen dinners for α-tocopherol content in milligrams per dinner, and reported a mean of 1.19 (range 0.29-3.49). In a paper the following year they [176] reported on five additional prepared frozen dinners which ranged from 0.39 to 4.46 mg of α-tocopherol per dinner. DeRitter et al. [177] assayed 14 prepared frozen dinners in a frozen condition and after heating (ready-to-serve), and observed a 15% loss of α-tocopherol during the heating process.

X. DAILY DIETARY INTAKE

In 1950 Harris et al. [134] estimated the average α-tocopherol intake per capita in the United States to be about 14 mg/day, of which over 50% was contributed by oils and fats. In 1963, Harris and Embree [169] arrived at a similar figure, namely, 15 mg/day based on 1960 per capita food consumption in the United States and food composition tables for α-tocopherol. Bunnell et al. [108] did an extensive investigation on the α-tocopherol content of food as consumed with an assay procedure using column chromatography on $MgHPO_4$. The daily intake of α-tocopherol, considering typical breakfast, luncheon, and dinner menus in the United States and using analytic data on foods, was estimated to be between 2.6 and 15.4 mg with an overall daily average of 7.4 mg. Ikehata et al. [178] reported on the daily intake of vitamin E in Japanese diets, and, based on limited data,

a value of 5.3 mg was recorded. Analysis of whole daily diets of normal
subjects and of diets prepared in hospitals to resemble home diets of
ambulant hospital patients showed that the majority of diets in Great
Britain [179] have a vitamin E content of 5 mg/day despite being generally
satisfactory in calories, protein, and fat content. The authors [179]
measured α-, β-, and γ-tocopherol content of the diet, but, since
γ-tocopherol contributed insignificantly to the total vitamin E content, it
was excluded from the calculations. Low daily vitamin E intakes have also
been indicated to occur in the Dominican Republic. The composite daily
diet of Canadians was estimated to contain approximately 7 mg of
α-tocopherol by Thompson et al. [175], which agrees fairly closely with
the values of 7.4 mg by Bunnell et al. [108] and a 9 mg value reported by
Bieri and Poukka-Evarts [3] for a typical diet in the United States. The
latter investigators published a study [3] in 1973 wherein meals obtained
from an NIH cafeteria were analyzed by two-dimensional thin-layer
chromatography and α-, γ-, and δ-tocopherol and total tocopherol values
were reported. The authors commented on the basis of present data that
about 9 mg of α-tocopherol and additional quantities of γ-tocopherol were
consumed daily. It was suggested that the contribution of γ-tocopherol to
the total vitamin E activity should be considered and that the recommended
allowance be more explicit on the permissible variation of intake of
vitamin E, depending on the type and amount of fat consumed.

Currently the vitamin E daily allowances of humans as recommended
in the 1974 NAS-NRC Food and Nutrition Board publication [186] are: for
infants, 4-5 IU; children (age 1-14 yr), 7-10 IU; males (15-51+ yr), 15 IU;
females (15-51+ yr), 12 IU; and pregnant and lactating women, 15 IU. The
current U.S. Food and Drug Administration (FDA) vitamin E daily allowances [187] used in the nutritional labeling of commercially produced foods
and vitamin supplements are: for infants, 10 IU; adults and children,
30 IU; and pregnant and lactating women, 30 IU.

XI. UNRESOLVED PROBLEMS

It is difficult to obtain precise estimates of vitamin E intake for individuals
based on tabular data [175,179,188]. Smith et al. [179] examined the diets
of 40 ambulant patients in a metabolic ward. The diets were prepared in
the hospital diet kitchen and were based on the patients' normal dietary
intake when at home. In addition, 10 diets from the staff of the hospital
were collected under home conditions. Vitamin E contents of the diets
were calculated using food composition tables and the authors' unpublished
analytical values. Of the diets analyzed, 7 of the 10 normal subjects' diets
and 29 of the 40 patients' diets contained less than 5 mg tocopherol per
day. There was poor correlation between analytical and calculated values
(Fig. 6). Estimated values were frequently higher than analytical values.

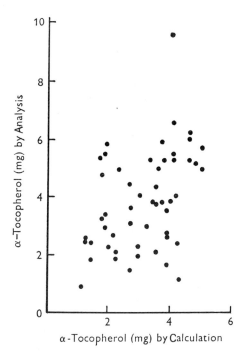

FIG. 6   Correlation between α-tocopherol content of diets by analysis and α-tocopherol content by calculation using food composition tables. (From Ref. 179, with permission.)

The authors point out the labile nature of vitamin E. Thompson et al. [175] doubt whether tabulated vitamin E values of foods are going to have much practical value in diet evaluations. Perhaps the use of tabular values may be of greatest help when applied to relatively large populations. Anyone interested in precise values of the tocopherol content for vitamin E intakes of individuals must currently resort to analytical assay of the diets in a ready-to-eat condition.

Another aspect that must be resolved is whether any substantial value can be attributed to the non-α-tocopherols in foods in practical, ready-to-eat meals. The paper of Bieri and Poukka-Evarts [4] on α-tocopherol metabolism, biological activity, and significance in human vitamin E nutrition supplies some revealing data on the potential value of γ-tocopherol in the human diet based on animal studies. It raises questions which further research must resolve before concluding that γ-tocopherol provides 20% of the vitamin E activity in the overall human diets in this country. This paper is evidently the basis for the statement in the NAS-NRC 1974 Recom-

mended Dietary Allowances publication [186] that, "at present, it may be assumed that the non-α-tocopherol compounds contribute additional vitamin E
activity equivalent to about 20% of the indicated α-tocopherol content of a
mixed diet." Even though significant γ-tocopherol values [189, 190] can be
attained in some tissues of animals by feeding mixtures of γ- and α-tocoph-
erols in a ratio of 2:1 to 4:1 or by feeding vegetable oils, the fact that quite
variable ratios of γ to α are found in such important rat tissues as liver,
kidney, testis, heart, etc., is cause for need of further understanding
before invoking changes in the method of assessing vitamin E intakes in the
human diet. In the above rat studies, the most responsive storage tissue
for γ-tocopherol was adipose tissue, which today is not believed to be a
readily available reservoir of vitamin E [191]. Even though γ-tocopherol
has been shown to be in human plasma [15] to the extent of 15% of α-
tocopherol, γ-tocopherol disappears more quickly from the circulation
than does the α-form. This would seem to be evidence of lack of preference for it by the organism. When γ-tocopherol elicits vitamin E activity,
is it first converted [192] by methylation to α-tocopherol? Likewise, is
the reason that α-tocopherol is suspected of being more highly active than
γ-tocopherol because it is more easily converted to α-tocopherol by
physiological hydrogenation? Do the non-α-tocopheryl compounds function
primarily by sparing α-tocopherols? Is γ-tocopherol reasonably constant
in supplying partial vitamin E activity or are certain dietary and/or species
requirements influencing factors? When testing the vitamin E activity of
γ-tocopherol, the biological response [5] was low and variable depending
on conditions employed.

Rather than having the general figure of 20% added to the α-tocopherol
content of mixed diets throughout the United States as an estimate of additional vitamin E value from non-α-tocopherols, it would seem more
prudent to declare that, where chemical assays of mixed diets show a substantial level of certain non-α-tocopherols, these diets should be granted a
certain percentage of vitamin E activity beyond that supplied by α-tocoph-
erol. Animals have been eating a mixed diet of plant and cereal grain
origin containing most of the tocopherols for centuries, and yet animal
tissues and their by-products contain α-tocopherol as the primary tocopherol [99, 147, 193]. We need further enlightenment on the metabolism of
the non-α-tocopherols in humans before assigning meaningful nutritional
import.

XII. POLICY OF ADDED VITAMIN E TO FOODS

In 1974 a fortification policy [194] for cereal-grain products was proposed
by the NAS-NRC Food and Nutrition Board. These products meet the
criteria for carriers of nutritional fortification for most nutrients. It suggests therefore, that nutrients be added to all cereal-grain products,

wherever technically feasible, as a means of supplementing the intake of those nutrients for which significant numbers of the population appear to be at risk of deficiency. Nutrients recommended for fortification of cereal-grain products are: vitamin A, thiamin, riboflavin, niacin, pyridoxine, folic acid, iron, calcium, magnesium, and zinc. Since vitamin E, like some of the other nutrients listed, is substantially lowered [87, 195] in the processing of cereal-grain products (Table 6), and since application forms of α-tocopheryl acetate are available to make fortification [196] of cereal products feasible (Table 7), the reason vitamin E was not included in the above list must be that it is not yet judged to be at risk in a significant number of the population. An NAS-NRC Food and Nutrition Board Committee on Nutritional Misinformation prepared a release [197] on supplementation of human diets with vitamin E, which states that the wide distribution of vitamin E in vegetable oils, cereal grains, and animal fats makes a deficiency very unlikely. Premature infants or individuals with impaired absorption of fats may require supplemental vitamin E, but they should, in any event, be under the care of a physician. The release [198] by the American Medical Association (AMA) Council on Foods and Nutrition on general policies on the improvement of the nutritive quality of foods does not specifically mention vitamin E.

In 1966, Rubin and Cort [199], and a few years later, Harris [200], discussed supplmentary vitamin E in the diet and the suitability of including α-tocopheryl acetate in the present formulation of thiamin, riboflavin, niacin, and iron now added to white flour. Herting and Drury [87] cited the

TABLE 6   Losses of Vitamins in the Refining of Whole Wheat:
Concentrations in Wheat, White Flour, Germ, and Millfeeds

Nutrient	Wheat (μg/g)	Flour (μg/g)	Germ (μg/g)	Millfeeds (μg/g)	Loss in flour (%)
Thiamin	3.5	0.8	22.0	17.0	77.1
Riboflavin	1.5	0.3	5.5	4.2	80.0
Niacin	50.0	9.5	80.0	150.0	80.8
Vitamin B_6	1.7	0.5	12.0	7.2	71.8
Pantothenic acid	10.0	5.0	25.0	22.0	50.0
Folacin	0.3	0.1	1.5	1.1	66.7
α-Tocopherol	16.0	2.2	125.0	38.0	86.3

Source: From Ref. 196.

TABLE 7   Stability of Added Vitamins in Cereal-Grain Products

			Months of storage (23°C)		
	Claim	Found	2	4	6
A. Flour					
Vitamin A (IU)	7500.0	8200.0	8200.0	8020.0	7950.0
Vitamin E (IU)[a]	15.0	15.9	15.9	15.9	15.9
Pyridoxine (mg)	2.0	2.3	2.2	2.3	2.2
Folacin (mg)	0.30	0.37	0.30	0.35	0.3
B. Yellow Corn Meal					
Vitamin A (IU)		7500.0	7500.0		6800.0
Vitamin E (IU)[a]		15.8	15.8	15.9	
Pyridoxine (mg)		2.8	2.8	2.8	
Folacin (mg)		0.30	0.30		0.29
Thiamin (mg)		3.5			3.6

	Claim	Found after baking	5 Days of bread storage (23°C)
C. Bread			
Vitamin A (IU)	7500.0	8280.0	8300.0
Vitamin E (IU)[a]	15.0	16.4	16.7
Pyridoxine (mg)	2.0	2.4	2.5
Folacin (mg)	0.3	0.34	0.36

[a] As dl, α-tocopheryl acetate.
Source: From Ref. 197.

extensive loss of vitamin E during the processing of cereal-grains and suggested the advisability of restoring nutritive value by nutrification of the finished cereal products. Stability performance of α-tocopheryl acetate added to processed cereal products of corn, wheat, and rice has been demonstrated by Cort et al. [196] and others [201,202].

In 1967, the American Academy of Pediatrics [203] suggested that certain infant formulas might be supplemented with vitamin E using the vitamin E content of human milk as a guide. Dicks-Bushnell, investigating the vitamin E content of infant formulas and cereals, and Davis [165] echoed this recommendation. Since that time, many U.S. formulas have added α-tocopheryl acetate. In 1972 Desai et al. [116] strongly recommended that all proprietary infant formulas based on either modified cows' milk or simulated nonmilk, fat-based products and all other substitutes, including cows' milk and milk products used for infant feeding, be supplemented with a sufficient amount of α-tocopheryl acetate to meet all criteria of vitamin E adequacy for infant nutrition. Primarily Herting and Drury [117], determining that nonfat dry milk supplies practically no vitamin E, pointed out that use of this form of milk, unsupplemented with vitamin E in developing countries, should be questioned since, presumably, some is used for feeding young infants. Attention was directed to the increasing use of nonfat milk in this country and the advent of imitation and filled milks for which standards had not yet been set. In a 1972 follow-up paper of earlier work, Davis [204] stated that baby foods generally do not supply much vitamin E and expressed concern that the vitamin E intake of infants consuming most formulas would be below recommended levels. The formula would be an excellent and logical vehicle for the administration of vitamin E supplements for infants.

Foods other than processed cereal products have been considered for nutrification with added α-tocopheryl acetate. The case for nutrifying margarine with added α-tocopheryl acetate was considered by Bunnell et al. [185] in 1971. In Europe, several manufacturers are adding α-tocopheryl acetate to margarine. In 1974, Bauernfeind and Cort [2] discussed the tocopherols in food technology applications. Tocopherols, such as α or γ, in combination with ascorbyl compounds, such as ascorbyl palmitate, when used as additives to chicken or pork fat function as well or better than added commercial synthetic antioxidants. Where natural antioxidants are desired, a tocopherol-ascorbate incorporation into food merits evaluation [205-208].

XIII. SUMMARY

As sources of food tocopherols, four of the tocol structure and four of the trienol structure have been considered. α-Tocopherol has the highest vitamin E activity for humans and animals and is the predominant tocopherol in their tissues. Tocopherol content of foods depends upon stage of life cycle, agronomic factors, genetic factors, season, weather, harvesting methods, processing procedures, storage environment, and time periods of storage. Inhibitors exist in foods and feeds that influence the absorption of vitamin E in the body. Tocopherols are sensitive to oxygen and oxidative reactions, especially in the presence of catalysts, heat, alkali, and certain radiation. The influence of processing procedures has been detailed, as well as the effect of storage conditions on tocopherol content. Two things stand out, namely, the lability of tocopherols and the great variability of their content in foods. An attempt has been made for the first time to compile the content of individual tocopherols in individual foods based on available literature reports for the period 1965-1975.

A few reports have appeared on the vitamin E intake of populations based on analyses of diets consumed or calculations made from tables of α-tocopherol content of foods when the daily meal pattern is known. These show a daily intake of 5-9 mg α-tocopherol, whereas recommended allowances indicate a higher desired intake. Some unresolved problems are cited, such as the pitfall of using present food composition tables for vitamin E assessment of diets and the nutritional significance of the non-α-tocopherols in the human diet. Some scientists declare that, in the absence of widely recognized symptomology of vitamin E deficiency in the human population, present tocopherol intakes under current life-styles are adequate. This is an issue that a future decade of vitamin E research and its evaluation must resolve. A technology currently exists for the addition of α-tocopheryl acetate to foods as a nutrient and/or of α-tocopherol as an antioxidant to foods and dietary supplements.

APPENDIX A   Tocopherol Content of Foods (mg/100 g) (Literature Values 1965-1975)

Item	Number of samples	Tocopherols[a]									Source
		α-T	α-T3	β-T	β-T3	γ-T	γ-T3	δ-T	δ-T3	TOT	
Breakfast Cereals											
Corn flakes A	1	0.08	–	–	–	0.16	–	–	–	–	87
Corn flakes B	1	0.15	–	–	–	0.59	–	–	–	–	87
Corn flakes C	1	0.03	–	–	–	0.13	–	–	–	–	87
Corn flakes	1	0.12	–	–	–	–	–	–	–	0.43	108
Corn flakes	1	0.17	–	0.31[b]	–	–	–	–	–	–	184
Corn grits	1	0.30	–	–	–	0.84	–	–	–	–	87
Corn, puffed	1	0.09	–	–	–	0.33	–	–	–	–	87
Corn, shredded	1	0.08	–	–	–	0.26	–	–	–	–	87
Hominy grits	1	0.31	–	–	–	–	–	–	–	1.17	108
Oat cereal, dry	1	0.60	–	–	–	–	–	–	–	3.43	108
Oatmeal	1	2.27	–	–	–	–	–	–	–	3.23	108
Oatmeal, rolled A	1	1.33	0.53	–	–	0.19	–	–	–	–	87
Oatmeal, rolled B	1	0.94	0.25	–	–	0.12	–	–	–	–	87
Oatmeal, rolled C	1	1.81	0.32	–	–	0.06	–	–	–	–	87
Oatmeal, 1 min.	1	2.04	0.69	–	–	0.07	–	–	–	–	87
Oatmeal, instant	1	1.86	0.49	–	–	–	–	–	–	–	87
Oatmeal, boiled, milk	1	0.57	–	0.11[b]	–	–	–	–	–	–	184
Oatmeal, boiled, water	1	0.19	–	0.05[b]	–	–	–	–	–	–	184

[a] Tocopherols: alpha-tocol (α-T), alpha-trienol (α-T3), beta-tocol (β-T), beta-trienol (β-T3), gamma-tocol (γ-T), gamma-trienol (γ-T3), delta-tocol (δ-T), delta-trienol (δ-T3), and total tocopherols (TOT).
[b] β- plus γ-tocols.

133

APPENDIX A (continued)

Item	Number of samples	Tocopherols[a]									Source
		α-T	α-T3	β-T	β-T3	γ-T	γ-T3	δ-T	δ-T3	TOT	
Breakfast Cereals (continued)											
Oats, shredded	1	0.08	–	–	–	0.08	–	–	–	–	87
Rice cereal, dry	1	0.04	–	–	–	–	–	–	–	0.28	108
Rice, expanded	1	0.01	–	–	–	0.02	–	–	–	–	87
Rice, expanded, toasted	1	0.23	–	0.31[b]	–	–	–	–	–	–	184
Rice, expanded, toasted B	1	0.22	–	0.34[b]	–	–	–	–	–	–	184
Rice, grits	1	0.04	–	–	–	0.11	–	–	–	–	87
Rice, puffed A	1	0.07	–	–	–	0.10	–	–	–	–	87
Rice, puffed B	1	0.07	–	–	–	0.13	–	–	–	–	87
Rice, puffed C	1	0.05	–	–	–	0.08	–	–	–	–	87
Rice, shredded	1	0.02	–	–	–	0.02	–	–	–	–	87
Rice and wheat cereal A	1	0.33	–	0.18[b]	–	–	–	–	–	–	184
Rice and wheat cereal B	1	0.28	–	0.08[b]	–	–	–	–	–	–	184
Wheat cereal, whole	1	1.17	0.33	0.57	2.40	–	–	–	–	–	131
Wheat and barley cereal	1	0.61	–	–	–	–	–	–	–	2.45	108
Wheat biscuit A	1	1.35	–	2.04[b]	–	–	–	–	–	–	184
Wheat biscuit B	1	1.06	–	0.22[b]	–	–	–	–	–	–	184
Wheat bran flakes	1	1.13	–	2.34[b]	–	–	–	–	–	–	184
Wheat flakes	1	0.72	–	1.65[b]	–	–	–	–	–	–	184
Wheat flakes	1	0.42	–	0.65	1.28	–	–	–	–	–	131
Wheat flakes A	1	0.25	–	0.62	–	–	–	–	–	–	87
Wheat flakes B	1	0.54	0.14	1.70	–	–	–	–	–	–	87

134

	n	α-T	α-T3	β-T	β-T3	γ-T	γ-T3	δ-T	δ-T3	TOT	Ref
Wheat, flake cereal	1	0.62	0.25	0.35[b]	1.22	—	—	—	—	—	129
Wheat, puffed A	1	0.68	0	1.84	—	—	—	—	—	—	87
Wheat, puffed B	1	0.47	0	1.71	—	—	—	—	—	—	87
Wheat, puffed	1	1.17	—	1.62[b]	—	—	—	—	—	—	184
Wheat, shredded A	1	0.17	0	0.96	—	—	—	—	—	—	87
Wheat, shredded B	1	0.31	0.20	0.49	—	—	—	—	—	—	87
Wheat, shredded C	1	0.09	0	—	—	—	—	—	—	—	87
Wheat, shredded	1	0.39	0.28	0.31	1.36	—	—	—	—	—	131
Cereal Grain Products											
Barley	5	0.40	1.30	0.30	0.70	0.05	0.20	0.01	—	—	130
Barley	1	0.20	1.10	0.40	0.30	0.03	0.20	0.01	—	—	130
Barley	1	0.08	0.67	0.05	0.48	0.05	0.23	trace	—	—	129
Barley, pearled	1	0.04	0.51	trace	0.32	trace	0.12	—	—	—	129
Buckwheat flour	1	0.32	—	—	—	7.14	—	0.45	—	—	129
Bulgur	1	0.06	0.14	0.12	1.08	—	—	—	—	—	129
Corn	11	0.60	0.20	—	0.40	3.80	0.50	trace	—	—	130
Corn, yellow	1	0.60	0.30	—	—	4.50	0.50	—	—	—	130
Corn	1	0.61	0.31	—	—	3.94	0.53	trace	—	—	129
Corn	1	0.70	—	—	—	—	—	—	—	—	176
Corn, yellow	17	1.99	—	—	—	—	—	—	—	—	33
Corn, yellow	10	1.53	—	—	—	5.10	—	—	—	—	87
Cornmeal, yellow	1	0.64	—	—	—	—	—	—	3.43	—	33
Cornmeal, yellow	1	0.42	—	—	—	0.90	—	—	—	—	87
Corn, white	1	0.98	—	—	—	3.10	—	—	—	—	87

[a] Tocopherols: alpha-tocol (α-T), alpha-trienol (α-T3), beta-tocol (β-T), beta-trienol (β-T3), gamma-tocol (γ-T), gamma-trienol (γ-T3), delta-tocol (δ-T), delta-trienol (δ-T3), and total tocopherols (TOT).

[b] β- plus γ-tocols.

APPENDIX A (continued)

Cereal Grain Products (continued)

| Item | Number of samples | Tocopherols[a] | | | | | | | | | Source |
		α-T	α-T3	β-T	β-T3	γ-T	γ-T3	δ-T	δ-T3	TOT	
Cornmeal, white	1	0.64	—	—	—	1.75	—	—	—	—	87
Millet	1	0.05	—	trace	—	1.30	—	0.40	—	—	130
Milo	12	1.22	—	—	—	—	—	—	—	—	33
Oats	6	0.70	0.70	0.20	0.10	0.30	—	—	—	—	130
Oats	1	0.50	1.10	0.10	0.20	—	—	—	—	—	130
Oats	4	2.05	—	—	—	—	—	—	—	—	33
Oats	4	1.54	0.30	—	—	0.05	—	—	—	—	87
Oats, steel cut	1	0.09	0.22	0.07	0.08	—	—	—	—	—	129
Oats, rolled	1	0.65	1.35	0.11	0.15	—	—	—	—	—	129
Oats, stored 6 yrs.	1	0.42	0.17	—	—	0	—	—	—	—	87
Rice	5	0.30	trace	—	—	0.30	0.50	0.04	—	—	130
Rice	1	0.35	—	—	—	0.38	—	—	—	—	87
Rice, brown	1	0.60	—	—	—	0.33	0.87	trace	—	—	129
Rice, brown	2	1.35	—	—	—	—	—	—	—	—	33
Rice, brown	3	0.26	—	—	—	0.40	—	—	—	—	87
Rice, brown, boiled	1	1.35	—	1.04[b]	—	—	—	—	—	—	184
Rice, brown, parboiled	3	0.15	—	—	—	0.33	—	—	—	—	130
Rice, white	1	0.10	trace	—	—	0.10	0.20	trace	—	—	130
Rice, white	1	0.16	0.07	—	—	0.10	0.22	trace	—	—	129
Rice, white	1	0.10	—	—	—	0.27	—	—	—	—	87
Rice, white, fried	1	0.06	—	0.15[b]	—	—	—	—	—	—	184

	n	α-T	α-T3	β-T	β-T3	γ-T	γ-T3	δ-T	δ-T3	TOT	
Rice, white, boiled	1	0.09	—	0.10[b]	—	—	—	—	—	—	184
Rice, white, steamed	1	0.15	—	0.11[b]	—	—	—	—	—	—	184
Rice meal	1	0.10	—	—	—	0.27	—	—	—	—	87
Rye	4	0.80	1.30	0.40	0.90	0.60	—	—	—	—	130
Rye	1	1.60	1.50	0.40	0.80	—	—	—	—	—	97
Rye	1	1.45	1.42	0.56	0.86	—	—	—	—	—	129
Rye flour, light	1	0.35	0.14	0.13	0.13	—	—	—	—	—	129
Rye flour, medium	1	0.79	0.85	0.56	0.98	—	—	—	—	—	129
Rye flour, dark	1	1.41	2.89	0.60	1.78	—	—	—	—	—	129
Sesame	1	—	—	—	—	22.70	—	—	—	—	97
Soybean meal, solvent process											
44% protein	1	0.30	—	—	—	—	—	—	—	—	33
50% protein	1	0.30	—	—	—	—	0.08	—	—	—	33
Wheat	9	1.00	0.40	0.90	2.50	—	—	—	—	—	130
Wheat	1	1.40	0.50	0.70	3.30	—	—	—	—	—	130
Wheat	1	1.00	0.40	0.70	2.80	—	—	—	—	—	97
Wheat	1	1.10	0.33	0.78	2.87	—	—	—	—	—	96
Wheat	1	0.95	0.29	0.73	2.94	—	—	—	—	—	129
Wheat, hard	5	1.35	0.47	0.73	3.28	—	—	—	—	—	131
Wheat, soft	4	1.24	0.50	0.65	3.04	—	—	—	—	—	131
Wheat, durum	2	0.99	0.67	0.48	3.67	—	—	—	—	—	131
Wheat, whole	4	1.11	—	—	—	—	—	—	—	—	33
Wheat, whole	9	0.87	0.12	2.20	—	—	—	—	—	—	87
Wheat meal	1	0.11	0	1.32	—	—	—	—	—	—	87
Wheat germ, stabilized	1	11.65	—	9.16[b]	—	—	—	—	—	—	184
Wheat bran	1	1.63	1.10	1.01	5.37	—	—	—	—	—	97

[a] Tocopherols: alpha-tocol (α-T), alpha-trienol (α-T3), beta-tocol (β-T), beta-trienol (β-T3), gamma-tocol (γ-T), gamma-trienol (γ-T3), delta-tocol (δ-T), delta-trienol (δ-T3), and total tocopherols (TOT).
[b] β- plus γ-tocols.

APPENDIX A   (continued)

Item	Number of samples	Tocopherols[a]									Source
		α-T	α-T3	β-T	β-T3	γ-T	γ-T3	δ-T	δ-T3	TOT	
Cereal Grain Products (continued)											
Wheat bran	1	1.74	1.05	1.27	6.40	—	—	—	—	—	96
Wheat bran	2	1.71	—	—	—	—	—	—	—	—	33
Wheat middlings	4	2.68	—	—	—	—	—	—	—	—	33
Wheat mill run	4	3.17	—	—	—	—	—	—	—	—	33
Wheat shorts	1	4.72	0.81	3.54	4.81	—	—	—	—	—	96
Wheat flour, whole	1	0.82	0.27	0.66	2.20	—	—	—	—	—	129
Wheat flour, low-grade	1	1.20	0.22	0.93	2.43	—	—	—	—	—	96
Wheat flour, hard	1	0.02	—	0.05	0.57	—	—	—	—	—	131
Wheat flour, durum	1	0.03	0.25	0.15	1.78	—	—	—	—	—	131
Wheat flour, all purpose	1	0.03	0.05	0.03	0.29	—	—	—	—	—	131
Wheat flour, patent, white	1	0.28	0.14	0.20	2.18	—	—	—	—	—	96
Wheat flour, unbleached	1	0.15	0.08	0.12	1.47	—	—	—	—	—	129
Wheat, WURLD	1	—	—	0.10	0.66	—	—	—	—	—	129
Cereal-Grain Baked Products											
Biscuit mix	10	0.30	—	trace	0.12	1.77	—	0.55	—	—	131
Bread dough	1	0.40	0.13	—	1.32	1.12	—	0.44	—	—	96
Bread	1	0.36	0.15	—	1.08	1.24	—	0.53	—	—	96
Bread, white, conventional	10	0.04	—	0.02	0.18	0.24	—	0.11	—	—	131
Bread, white, conventional	5	0.01	—	0.02	0.10	—	—	—	—	—	131
Bread, white, continuous	10	trace	—	0.01	0.11	0.06	—	0.04	—	—	131

138

Food	n	α-T	β-T	α-T3	β-T3	γ-T	γ-T3	δ-T	δ-T3	TOT	Ref
Bread, white, continuous	5	0.02	0.03	0.09	0.19	–	0.36	–	–	–	131
Bread, white	1	0.10	–	–	–	–	–	–	–	0.23	108
Bread, white, sliced A	1	0.12	0.27[b]	–	–	–	–	–	–	–	184
Bread, white, sliced B	1	0.18	0.46[b]	–	–	–	–	–	–	–	184
Bread, white, sliced C	1	0.13	0.53[b]	–	–	–	–	–	–	–	184
Bread, white, unsliced	1	0.19	0.22[b]	–	–	–	–	–	–	–	184
Bread, white milk, sliced A	1	0.28	0.63[b]	–	–	–	–	–	–	–	184
Bread, white milk, sliced B	1	0.11	–	–	–	–	–	–	–	–	184
Bread, white milk, sliced C	1	0.06	0.29[b]	–	–	–	–	–	–	–	184
Bread, whole wheat	10	0.16	0.15	0.58	0.38	–	0.21	–	–	–	131
Bread, whole wheat	1	0.45	–	–	–	–	–	–	–	2.20	108
Bread, whole wheat	1	1.10	0.09[b]	–	–	–	–	–	–	–	184
Bread, whole wheat, malt	1	0.67	0.73[b]	–	–	–	–	–	–	–	184
Bread, whole wheat, extra protein	1	0.29	1.32[b]	–	–	–	–	–	–	–	184
Bread, brown, milk, sliced	1	0.34	0.61[b]	–	–	–	–	–	–	–	184
Bread, rye, dark	1	1.24	1.13[b]	–	–	–	–	–	–	–	184
Bread, rye, light	1	0.12	0.22[b]	–	–	–	–	–	–	–	184
Bread, rye and wheat A	1	0.50	0.09[b]	–	–	–	–	–	–	–	184
Bread, rye and wheat B	1	0.38	0.10[b]	–	–	–	–	–	–	–	184
Cake, soft wheat flour	6	1.16	trace	0.17	6.59	–	2.12	–	–	–	131
Cake, butter, plain A	1	1.11	1.45[b]	–	–	–	–	–	–	–	184
Cake, butter, plain B	1	0.14	0.22[b]	–	–	–	–	–	–	–	184
Cake, butter, plain C	1	0.35	0.27[b]	–	–	–	–	–	–	–	184
Cake, butter, rich A	1	3.82	0.36[b]	–	–	–	–	–	–	–	184

a Tocopherols: alpha-tocol (α–T), beta-tocol (β–T), alpha-trienol (α–T3), beta-trienol (β–T3), gamma-tocol (γ–T), gamma-trienol (γ–T3), delta-tocol (δ–T), delta-trienol (δ–T3), and total tocopherols (TOT).
b β– plus γ–tocols.

APPENDIX A (continued)

Item	Number of samples	Tocopherols[a]									Source
		α-T	α-T3	β-T	β-T3	γ-T	γ-T3	δ-T	δ-T3	TOT	
Cereal-Grain Baked Products (continued)											
Cake, butter, rich B	1	0.73	—	0.49[b]	—	—	—	—	—	—	184
Cake, butter, rich C	1	0.98	—	0.53[b]	—	—	—	—	—	—	184
Cake, pound	1	1.10	—	—	—	—	—	—	—	7.40	108
Cake, sponge A	1	0.19	—	0.33[b]	—	—	—	—	—	—	184
Cake, sponge B	1	0.30	—	0.31[b]	—	—	—	—	—	—	184
Cake, cheese	1	0.86	—	0.60[b]	—	—	—	—	—	—	184
Cake, chocolate	1	0.42	—	0.35[b]	—	—	—	—	—	—	184
Cupcakes, chocolate	1	0.14	—	—	—	—	—	—	—	0.42	108
Cookies, cream, chocolate	1	1.29	—	—	—	—	—	—	—	2.81	108
Cookies, oatmeal, peanut	1	6.00	—	—	—	—	—	—	—	7.67	108
Cookies, shortbread	1	0.46	—	—	—	—	—	—	—	1.33	108
Cookies, shortbread	1	1.32	—	0.69[b]	—	—	—	—	—	—	184
Cookies, wafer type	1	0.53	—	—	—	—	—	—	—	1.43	108
Cookies, chocolate chip	1	0.79	—	1.47[b]	—	—	—	—	—	—	184
Cookies, chocolate, cream	1	0.91	—	3.95[b]	—	—	—	—	—	—	184
Cookies, chocolate, marshmellow	1	0.49	—	—	—	—	—	—	—	—	184
Cookies, plain, homemade	1	1.36	—	0.27[b]	—	—	—	—	—	—	184
Cookies, wheat and soy meal	1	3.45	—	5.97[b]	—	—	—	—	—	—	184
Crackers, soft flour	1	0.39	0.09	0.25	1.05	0.10	—	0.03	—	—	131
Crackers, club	1	0.80	—	—	—	—	—	—	—	1.17	108

Food	Amount	α-T	β-T	γ-T	δ-T	α-T3	β-T3	γ-T3	δ-T3	TOT	Ref.
Crackers, low fat	1	1.03	–	1.65[b]	–	–	–	–	–	–	184
Crackers, low fat, sesame	1	0.90	–	–	–	–	–	–	–	–	184
Crackers, medium fat	1	0.36	–	0.83[b]	–	–	–	–	–	–	184
Crackers, medium fat, cheese	1	1.12	–	1.06[b]	–	–	–	–	–	–	184
Crackers, high fat, cheese	1	6.34	–	6.87[b]	–	–	–	–	–	–	184
Crackers, bran	1	0.23	–	0.66[b]	–	–	–	–	–	–	184
Crackers, wheat	1	1.37	–	1.43[b]	–	–	–	–	–	–	184
Crackers, wheat and rye	1	1.13	–	0.97[b]	–	–	–	–	–	–	184
Crumpets, toasted	1	0.11	–	0.17[b]	–	–	–	–	–	–	184
Doughnuts	10	0.95	–	–	0.48	2.94	–	0.97	–	–	131
Doughnuts, pink icing	1	0.37	–	0.51[b]	–	–	–	–	–	–	184
Macaroni	2	0.02	0.02	0.02	0.24	–	–	–	–	–	131
Pancakes	1	1.08	–	0.82[b]	–	–	–	–	–	–	184
Pie, apple, baked	1	2.50	–	–	–	–	–	–	–	15.7	108
Pie, apple, homemade	1	1.15	–	0.32[b]	–	–	–	–	–	–	184
Pie, bluberry, baked	1	3.12	–	–	–	–	–	–	–	17.7	108
Pie, loganberry, baked	1	1.08	–	0.35[b]	–	–	–	–	–	–	184
Pie, rhubarb and apple	1	0.52	–	0.15[b]	–	–	–	–	–	–	184
Pudding, plain, steamed	1	0.91	–	0.44[b]	–	–	–	–	–	–	184
Pudding, instant chocolate milk	1	0.08	–	0.06[b]	–	–	–	–	–	–	184
Pudding, chocolate mousse, cream	1	0.37	–	0.08[b]	–	–	–	–	–	–	184
Pudding, orange souffle	1	0.41	–	0.04[b]	–	–	–	–	–	–	184
Rolls, dough	1	1.03	0.29	–	1.32	4.23	–	1.64	–	–	96
Rolls	1	1.08	0.29	–	1.19	4.92	–	1.69	–	–	96

[a] Tocopherols: alpha-tocol (α-T), alpha-trienol (α-T3), beta-tocol (β-T), beta-trienol (β-T3), gamma-tocol (γ-T), gamma-trienol (γ-T3), delta-tocol (δ-T), delta-trienol (δ-T3), and total tocopherols (TOT).
[b] β- plus γ-tocols.

APPENDIX A   (continued)

Item	Number of samples	Tocopherols[a]									Source
		α-T	α-T3	β-T	β-T3	γ-T	γ-T3	δ-T	δ-T3	TOT	
Cereal-Grain Baked Products (continued)											
Rolls, hamburger	10	0.06	–	0.01	0.17	0.40	–	0.17	–	–	131
Scones, plain	1	1.33	–	0.75[b]	–	–	–	–	–	–	184
Snacks, potato chips	1	6.40	–	–	–	–	–	–	–	11.40	108
Snacks, pretzel sticks	1	0.15	–	–	–	–	–	–	–	0.77	108
Spaghetti, boiled	1	0.03	–	0.17[b]	–	–	–	–	–	–	184
Spaghetti, meat, tomato, cheese	1	0.25	–	0.33[b]	–	–	–	–	–	–	184
Spaghetti, canned, complete	1	0.43	–	0.24[b]	–	–	–	–	–	–	184
Tarts, chocolate, homemade	1	1.17	–	0.68[b]	–	–	–	–	–	–	184
Tarts, coconut and raspberry	1	0.57	–	0.42[b]	–	–	–	–	–	–	184
Tarts, lemon and orange	1	0.36	–	0.33[b]	–	–	–	–	–	–	184
Fruit Products											
Apples, fresh	1	0.31	–	–	–	–	–	–	–	0.51	108
Bananas, fresh	1	0.22	–	–	–	–	–	–	–	0.42	108
Bananas	1	0.49	–	–	–	–	–	–	–	–	176
Cantaloupe, fresh	1	0.14	–	–	–	–	–	–	–	0.31	108
Fruit punch	1	0.15	–	0.08[b]	–	–	–	–	–	–	184
Grapefruit juice	1	0.04	–	–	–	–	–	–	–	0.18	108
Mango, green	1	0.26	–	–	–	0.27	–	–	–	–	130
Mango, ripe	1	0.98	–	–	–	–	–	–	–	–	130

	n	α-T	α-T3	β-T	β-T3	γ-T[b]	γ-T3	δ-T	δ-T3	TOT	Ref
Muskmelon	1	10.10	—	—	—	—	—	—	—	—	130
Orange juice	1	0.04	—	—	—	—	—	—	—	0.20	108
Strawberries, fresh	1	0.13	—	—	—	—	—	—	—	0.29	108
Strawberries, frozen	1	0.21	—	—	—	—	—	—	—	0.40	108
Infant Formulas											
Milk-base formula 1[c,d]	1	7.25	—	—	—	—	—	—	—	7.25	166
Milk-base formula 2[d]	1	0.72	—	—	—	—	—	—	—	0.77	166
Milk-base formula 5[d]	1	0.46	—	—	—	—	—	—	—	0.46	166
Milk-base formula 10[d]	1	0.33	—	—	—	—	—	—	—	0.33	166
Milk-base formula 15[d]	1	0.03	—	—	—	—	—	—	—	0.03	166
Liquid formula LB[c,e]	2	3.99	—	—	—	6.70	—	0	—	—	117
Liquid formula LC[c,e]	1	6.80	—	—	—	3.11	—	1.36	—	—	117
Powder, formula PD[c,e]	4	4.58	—	—	—	13.03	—	0	—	—	117
Non-milk formula 1	1	4.42	—	—	—	12.40	—	2.92	—	19.75	166
Non-milk formula 5	1	4.69	—	—	—	6.90	—	0.65	—	12.25	166
Non-milk formula 10[c]	1	8.00	—	—	—	0.32	—	—	—	8.30	166
Non-milk formula 15	1	0.26	—	—	—	0.16	—	—	—	0.42	166
Hypoallergenic, liquid LA[c,e]	1	7.67	—	—	—	11.55	—	4.59	—	—	117
Hypoallergenic, liquid LC[e]	1	3.32	—	—	—	15.29	—	1.84	—	—	117

a Tocopherols: alpha-tocol (α–T), alpha-trienol (α–T3), beta-tocol (β–T), beta-trienol (β–T3), gamma-tocol (γ–T), gamma-trienol (γ–T3), delta-tocol (δ–T), delta-trienol (δ–T3), and total tocopherols (TOT).

b β– plus γ–tocols.

c Nutrified with α–tocopheryl acetate.

d Tocopherol content in milligrams per liter (reconstituted).

e Tocopherol content in milligrams per quart (reconstituted).

APPENDIX A (continued)

Item	Number of samples	Tocopherols[a]									Source
		α-T	α-T3	β-T	β-T3	γ-T	γ-T3	δ-T	δ-T3	TOT	
Infant Cereals											
Cereal, barley A	1	0.04	—	0.42[b]	—	—	—	—	—	1.02	165
Cereal, barley B	1	0.16	—	–	—	—	—	—	—	0.26	165
Cereal, oatmeal A	1	0.29	—	1.21[b]	—	—	—	—	—	1.62	165
Cereal, oatmeal B	1	0.08	—	0	—	—	—	—	—	0.08	165
Cereal, rice A	1	0.49	—	0.80	—	—	—	—	—	1.63	165
Cereal, rice B	1	0.03	—	0	—	—	—	—	—	0.03	165
Infant Strained Fruits											
Applesauce	2	0.52	—	trace[b]	—	—	—	trace	—	0.52	174
Apricots	2	0.70	—	0.13[b]	—	—	—	–	—	0.83	174
Bananas	2	0.23	—	–	—	—	—	–	—	0.23	174
Pears	2	0.55	—	0.07[b]	—	—	—	0.07	—	0.69	174
Peaches	2	1.33	—	0.07[b]	—	—	—	–	—	1.40	174
Plums	2	0.38	—	0.05[b]	—	—	—	0.20	—	0.63	174
Prunes	2	0.38	—	0.07[b]	—	—	—	–	—	0.45	174
Infant Strained Desserts											
Chocolate custard	2	0.23	—	–	—	—	—	—	—	0.23	174
Cottage cheese, pineapple	2	0.17	—	–	—	—	—	—	—	0.17	174
Fruit dessert	2	0.31	—	–	—	—	—	—	—	0.31	174

144

Infant Strained Vegetables

	n	α-T	α-T3	β-T	β-T3	γ-T	γ-T3	δ-T	δ-T3	TOT	
Beets	2	0.12	—	trace[b]	—	—	—	—	—	0.12	174
Carrots A	2	0.84	—	0.23[b]	—	—	—	—	—	1.07	174
Carrots B	3	0.40	—	0.09[b]	—	—	—	trace	—	0.49	174
Corn, creamed	3	0.16	—	0.09[b]	—	—	—	0.11	—	0.36	174
Beans, green	2	0.16	—	0.09[b]	—	—	—	—	—	0.26	174
Peas A	3	0.15	—	0.62[b]	—	—	—	0.10	—	0.86	174
Peas, creamed B	4	trace	—	0.52[b]	—	—	—	0.22	—	0.74	174
Spinach, creamed	4	1.55	—	0.08[b]	—	—	—	trace	—	1.63	174
Squash A	2	0.36	—	0.48[b]	—	—	—	—	—	0.84	174
Squash B	3	0.35	—	0.13[b]	—	—	—	—	—	0.48	174
Sweet potato A	4	0.50	—	trace	—	—	—	—	—	0.50	174
Sweet potato B	3	0.38	—	0.24	—	—	—	0.09	—	0.71	174
Vegetable, garden	3	0.61	—	0.41	—	—	—	0.18	—	1.20	174
Vegetable, mixed	2	0.22	—	0.05	—	—	—	0.11	—	0.38	174
Infant Strained Meat Dishes											
Beef	2	0.73	—	—	—	—	—	—	—	0.73	174
Beef, noodles, vegetables	2	0.33	—	0.06[b]	—	—	—	—	—	0.39	174
Beef liver	2	0.32	—	—	—	—	—	—	—	0.32	174
Chicken	2	0.30	—	0.14[b]	—	—	—	0.09	—	0.53	174
Chicken, noodles	3	0.15	—	0.06[b]	—	—	—	0.06	—	0.27	174
Ham	2	0.45	—	trace	—	—	—	—	—	0.45	174
Turkey	4	0.34	—	—	—	—	—	—	—	0.34	174

[a] Tocopherols: alpha-tocol (α-T), alpha-trienol (α-T3), beta-tocol (β-T), beta-trienol (β-T3), gamma-tocol (γ-T), gamma-trienol (γ-T3), delta-tocol (δ-T), delta-trienol (δ-T3), and total tocopherols (TOT).

[b] β- plus γ-tocols.

APPENDIX A   (continued)

Item	Number of samples	Tocopherols[a]									Source
		α-T	α-T3	β-T	β-T3	γ-T	γ-T3	δ-T	δ-T3	TOT	
Infant Strained Meat Dishes (continued)											
Turkey, rice, vegetables	3	0.13	—	trace[b]	—	—	—	—	—	0.13	174
Veal	2	0.22	—	trace[b]	—	—	—	—	—	0.22	174
Egg yolk	3	0.60	—	0.59[b]	—	—	—	0.47	—	1.66	174
High beef, vegetables	2	0.52	—	0.06[b]	—	—	—	—	—	0.58	174
High chicken, vegetables	3	0.23	—	0.08[b]	—	—	—	0.16	—	0.47	174
High ham, vegetables	2	0.22	—	0.11[b]	—	—	—	—	—	0.33	174
High turkey, vegetables	2	0.14	—	—	—	—	—	—	—	0.14	174
High veal, vegetables	2	0.13	—	trace[b]	—	—	—	—	—	0.13	174
Meat, Fish											
Bacon	1	0.53	—	—	—	—	—	—	—	0.59	108
Bacon	1	0.37	—	—	—	—	—	—	—	—	176
Beef, ground, fried	1	0.37	—	—	—	—	—	—	—	0.63	108
Beef steak, broiled	1	0.30	—	—	—	—	—	—	—	0.55	108
Bologna	1	0.06	—	—	—	—	—	—	—	0.49	108
Chicken breast, broiled	1	0.37	—	—	—	—	—	—	—	0.58	108
Chicken breast	1	0.42	—	—	—	—	—	—	—	—	176
Chicken, frozen, baked A	1	0.04	—	—	—	—	—	—	—	0.16	108
Chicken, frozen, baked B	1	0.16	—	—	—	—	—	—	—	1.10	108
Chicken, frozen, baked C	1	0.38	—	—	—	—	—	—	—	1.39	108
Chicken, fried	1	0.58	—	—	—	—	—	—	—	—	176

Food	n	α-T	α-T3	β-T	β-T3	γ-T	γ-T3	δ-T	δ-T3	TOT	Ref.
Haddock filet, broiled	1	0.60	—	—	—	—	—	—	—	1.20	108
Haddock	1	0.43	—	—	—	—	—	—	—	—	176
Ham steak, fried	1	0.28	—	—	—	—	—	—	—	0.52	108
Lamb chop, broiled	1	0.16	—	—	—	—	—	—	—	0.32	108
Liver, broiled	1	0.63	—	—	—	—	—	—	—	1.62	108
Liver, uncooked	1	0.50	—	—	—	—	—	—	—	—	182
Liverwurst	1	0.35	—	—	—	—	—	—	—	0.69	108
Pork chop, fried	1	0.16	—	—	—	—	—	—	—	0.60	108
Pork chop	1	0.24	—	—	—	—	—	—	—	—	176
Salami	1	0.11	—	—	—	—	—	—	—	0.68	108
Salmon steak, broiled	1	1.35	—	—	—	—	—	—	—	1.81	108
Sausage, fried	1	0.16	—	—	—	—	—	—	—	0.32	108
Scallops, frozen, baked	1	0.60	—	—	—	—	—	—	—	6.20	108
Shrimp, frozen, baked	1	0.60	—	—	—	—	—	—	—	6.60	108

Milk and Egg Products

Food	n	α-T	α-T3	β-T	β-T3	γ-T	γ-T3	δ-T	δ-T3	TOT	Ref.
Butter	1	3.30	—	—	—	—	—	—	—	3.20	182
Butter	1	1.00	—	—	—	—	—	—	—	1.00	108
Butter	20	1.68	—	—	—	0.14	—	—	—	—	48
Butter	1	2.65	—	—	—	—	—	—	—	—	176
Butter, summer	Many	—	—	—	—	—	—	—	—	2.90	49
Butter, winter	Many	—	—	—	—	—	—	—	—	1.91	49
Cheese	1	0.86	—	—	—	—	—	—	—	—	176
Eggs	1	0.46	—	—	—	—	—	—	—	1.43	108
Eggs dried	1	9.50	—	—	—	—	—	—	—	9.50	182

a Tocopherols: alpha-tocol (α-T), alpha-trienol (α-T3), beta-tocol (β-T), beta-trienol (β-T3), gamma-tocol (γ-T), gamma-trienol (γ-T3), delta-tocol (δ-T), delta-trienol (δ-T3), and total tocopherols (TOT).

b β- plus γ-tocols.

APPENDIX A   (continued)

Item	Number of samples	Tocopherols[a]									Source
		α-T	α-T3	β-T	β-T3	γ-T	γ-T3	δ-T	δ-T3	TOT	
Milk and Egg Products (continued)											
Ice cream, chocolate A	1	0.36	–	–	–	–	–	–	–	1.02	108
Ice cream, chocolate B	1	0.37	–	–	–	–	–	–	–	1.10	108
Ice cream, vanilla	1	0.06	–	–	–	–	–	–	–	0.39	108
Milk chocolate bar	1	1.10	–	–	–	–	–	–	–	4.20	108
Milk, whole fluid	1	0.04	–	–	–	–	–	–	–	0.09	108
Milk, freeze dried	1	0.70	–	–	–	–	–	–	–	0.70	182
Milk, fluid, spring[c]	10	0.56	–	–	–	–	–	–	–	–	117
Milk, evaporated[c]	5	0.39	–	–	–	–	–	–	–	–	117
Milk, dry, nonfat	3	0.02	–	–	–	–	–	–	–	–	117
Nuts											
Almonds	2	27.40	0.50	0.30	–	0.90	–	–	–	–	130
Almonds	1	23.00	–	–	–	–	–	–	–	–	129
Almond meal	1	31.70	0.50	0.30	–	0.90	–	–	–	–	97
Cashews	1	0.19	–	–	–	3.84	–	0.17	–	–	129
Peanuts	1	9.70	–	–	–	6.60	–	–	–	–	130
Peanuts	1	11.35	–	–	–	8.38	–	–	–	–	129
Peanuts, dry roasted	1	7.70	–	–	–	–	–	–	–	11.70	108
Peanuts, cocktail	1	6.70	–	–	–	–	–	–	–	11.20	108
Peanut butter	9	6.20	–	–	–	9.40	–	–	–	–	Unpub.
Pecans	1	1.20	–	–	–	19.10	–	–	–	–	130

	No.	α-T	α-T3	β-T	β-T3	γ-T	γ-T3	δ-T	δ-T3	TOT	
Pecans	1	1.01	—	—	—	19.78	—	—	—	—	129
Poppyseed	1	1.80	—	—	—	9.20	—	—	—	—	130
Sunflower seeds, raw	1	49.50	2.73	—	—	—	—	—	—	—	129
Walnuts, English	1	0.40	—	—	—	15.80	—	—	—	—	130
Walnuts, English	1	0.62	—	—	—	17.23	—	1.52	—	—	129
Oils and Fats											
Barley, stored	1	35.21	67.36	4.59	12.25	4.59	12.25	0	0	153.10	142
Castor	1	trace	—	nil	—	23.04	—	21.96	—	45.00	181
Coconut	1	0.50	0.50	0.10	1.90	0.60	—	—	—	—	130
Coconut	1	0.40	0.30	0.15	1.50	0.45	—	—	—	2.80	146
Corn	8	11.20	—	5.00	—	60.20	—	1.80	—	—	130
Corn A	1	7.90	—	—	—	44.70	—	0.40	—	—	97
Corn B	1	16.20	—	—	—	60.30	—	—	—	—	97
Corn	1	17.00	—	66.00[b]	—	—	—	5.00	—	—	176
Corn	1	11.90	—	39.50[b]	—	—	—	0	—	51.40	182
Corn	1	6.00	—	trace	—	43.70	—	2.00	—	51.70	141
Corn A	1	26.00	—	87.00[b]	—	—	—	trace	—	113.00	183
Corn B	1	26.00	—	92.00[b]	—	—	—	trace	—	118.00	183
Corn, mazola	1	2.32	0	0	0	43.52	0	0.46	0	46.30	142
Corn, fresh A	1	5.11	1.70	0	0	70.63	6.80	0.85	0	85.10	142
Corn, fresh B	1	29.43	14.72	0	0	94.83	24.52	0	0	163.50	142
Cottonseed	9	38.90	—	—	—	38.70	—	—	—	—	130
Cottonseed	1	32.00	—	—	—	31.30	—	—	—	—	97

[a] Tocopherols: alpha-tocol(α-T), alpha-trienol(α-T3), beta-tocol(β-T), beta-trienol(β-T3), gamma-tocol(γ-T), gamma-trienol(γ-T3), delta-tocol(δ-T), delta-trienol(δ-T3), and total tocopherols (TOT).

[b] β- plus γ-tocols.

[c] Tocopherol content in milligrams per quart (reconstituted).

APPENDIX A (continued)

Item	Number of samples	Tocopherols[a]									Source
		α–T	α–T3	β–T	β–T3	γ–T	γ–T3	δ–T	δ–T3	TOT	
Oils and Fats (continued)											
Cottonseed	1	56.00	–	38.00[b]	–	–	–	trace	–	94.00	183
Cottonseed A	1	48.90	–	–	–	29.60	–	–	–	78.50	141
Cottonseed B	1	47.00	–	–	–	27.50	–	–	–	74.50	141
Cottonseed		50.97	–	–	–	41.03	–	–	–	92.00	181
Cottonseed	1	34.00	–	27.00[b]	–	–	–	0	–	–	176
Cottonseed, old	1	4.00	–	16.00[b]	–	–	–	0	–	–	176
Lard	1	1.20	0.70	–	–	0.70	–	–	–	–	97
Margarine A, hard	1	3.40	–	–	–	14.40	–	3.50	–	–	128
Margarine B, hard	1	6.80	–	–	–	18.30	–	3.80	–	–	128
Margarine C, hard	1	6.90	–	–	–	22.70	–	3.50	–	–	128
Margarine D, hard	1	15.00	–	–	–	53.60	–	2.00	–	–	128
Margarine E, hard	1	8.80	0.50	0.60	trace	0.80	trace	0.40	–	–	128
Margarine F, hard	1	10.90	–	–	–	–	–	–	–	–	185
Margarine G, hard	1	19.00	–	–	–	–	–	–	–	–	185
Margarine H, hard	1	3.16	–	–	–	–	–	–	–	–	185
Margarine I, hard	1	11.00	–	–	–	–	–	–	–	–	185
Margarine J, hard	1	19.90	–	–	–	–	–	–	–	–	185
Margarine K, hard	1	11.80	–	–	–	–	–	–	–	–	185
Margarine L, hard	1	12.30	–	–	–	–	–	–	–	–	185
Margarine M, whipped	1	3.20	–	–	–	15.10	–	3.00	–	–	128
Margarine N, soft	1	4.10	–	–	–	10.30	–	2.70	–	–	128

150

Product	n	α-tocol	α-T3	β-tocol	β-T3	γ-tocol	γ-T3	δ-tocol	δ-T3	TOT
Margarine O, soft	1	5.80	–	–	–	40.40	–	12.60	–	128
Margarine P, soft	1	6.60	–	–	–	21.10	–	1.90	–	128
Margarine Q, soft	1	11.70	–	–	–	29.00	–	8.10	–	128
Margarine R, soft	1	7.60	–	2.40[b]	–	–	–	0	10.00	182
Margarine S, soft	1	22.20	–	–	–	–	–	–	–	185
Margarine T, soft	1	32.70	–	–	–	–	–	–	–	185
Margarine U, soft	1	22.20	–	–	–	–	–	–	–	185
Margarine V, soft	1	10.10	–	–	–	–	–	–	–	185
Margarine W, soft	1	21.00	–	–	–	–	–	–	–	185
Margarine X, soft	1	9.30	–	–	–	–	–	–	–	185
Margarine Y, soft	1	13.10	–	–	–	–	–	–	–	185
Margarine, corn oil	1	13.20	–	–	–	–	–	–	46.70	108
Margarine, soy and cotton	1	13.00	–	–	–	–	–	–	59.50	108
Mayonnaise A, cottonseed	1	6.00	–	–	–	–	–	–	9.00	108
Mayonnaise B, polyunsaturated	1	24.00	–	–	–	–	–	–	50.00	108
Mayonnaise C	1	8.60	–	–	–	–	–	–	42.00	108
Mustardseed	1	8.60	–	–	–	17.60	–	5.80	–	130
Neem	1	–	–	trace	–	57.92	–	59.08	117.00	181
Olive	4	5.10	–	–	–	–	–	–	–	130
Olive	1	0.80	–	–	–	–	–	–	–	97
Olive	1	24.00	–	trace[b]	–	–	–	trace	24.00	183
Olive	1	10.40	–	0[b]	–	0	–	0	10.40	182
Palm	4	25.60	14.30	–	3.20	31.60	28.60	7.00	6.90	130
Palm 1	1	20.70	12.10	trace	3.80	–	26.60	7.30	70.50	141

[a] Tocopherols: alpha-tocol (α-T), alpha-trienol (α-T3), beta-tocol (β-T), beta-trienol (β-T3), gamma-tocol (γ-T), gamma-trienol (γ-T3), delta-tocol (δ-T), delta-trienol (δ-T3), and total tocopherols (TOT).

[b] β– plus γ-tocols.

Item	Number of samples	Tocopherols[a]									Source
		α–T	α–T3	β–T	β–T3	γ–T	γ–T3	δ–T	δ–T3	TOT	
Oils and Fats (continued)											
Palm 2	1	20.40	14.90	trace	2.40	—	30.20	—	6.90	74.80	141
Palm 3	1	20.00	14.70	trace	2.90	—	26.80	—	7.10	71.50	141
Palm 4	1	18.80	15.20	trace	3.00	—	28.10	—	6.70	71.80	141
Peanut	11	13.00	—	—	—	21.60	—	2.10	—	—	130
Peanut, Spanish	4	10.70	—	—	—	22.60	—	1.30	—	—	140
Peanut, Virginia	7	16.40	—	—	—	22.00	—	1.10	—	—	140
Peanut, runner	6	16.60	—	—	—	26.60	—	1.50	—	—	140
Peanut	1	18.60	—	—	—	13.80	—	—	—	—	97
Peanut	1	23.00	—	31.00[b]	—	—	—	trace	—	54.00	183
Peanut	1	33.85	—	—	—	59.61	—	—	—	93.00	181
Peanut	1	8.23	—	20.0–31.0[b]	—	—	—	0.10–0.20	—	34.0–54.0	140
Rapeseed	5	18.40	—	—	—	38.00	—	1.20	—	—	130
Rapeseed, refined	1	28.00	—	49.00[b]	—	—	—	0	—	—	176
Rapeseed	1	23.80	—	—	—	42.40	—	1.10	—	67.30	141
Safflower	3	38.70	—	—	—	17.40	—	24.00	—	—	130
Safflower	1	34.20	—	—	—	7.10	—	—	—	—	97
Safflower	1	45.84	—	—	—	19.49	—	23.67	—	—	181
Sesame	2	13.60	—	—	—	29.00	—	—	—	—	130
Sesame		25.67	—	—	—	40.59	—	—	—	66.00	181
Shortening	1	9.90	—	—	—	66.20	—	23.00	—	—	97
Soybean	14	10.10	—	—	—	59.30	—	26.40	—	—	130

		α-T	α-T3	β-T	β-T3	γ-T	γ-T3	δ-T	δ-T3	TOT
Soybean	1	10.30	—	—	—	55.50	—	23.90	—	146
Soybean, refined	1	12.00	—	94.00[b]	—	—	—	31.00	—	176
Soybean A	1	4.20	—	—	—	25.20	—	5.30	—	97
Soybean B	1	9.40	—	trace	—	63.00	—	23.20	—	97
Soybean	1	3.40	—	—	—	32.60	—	20.40	56.40	141
Soybean	1	11.52	—	78.00[b]	—	59.33	—	25.15	96.00	181
Soybean A	1	7.00	—	61.00[b]	—	—	—	24.00	109.00	183
Soybean B	1	6.00	—	0	—	—	—	26.00	93.00	183
Soybean	1	5.24	0	—	0	79.85	0	45.82	130.00	142
Sunflower	10	48.70	—	—	—	5.10	—	0.80	—	130
Walnut	1	56.30	—	—	—	59.50	—	45.00	—	130
Wheat germ	3	133.00	2.60	71.00	18.10	26.00	—	27.10	—	130
Wheat germ	1	115.30	2.60	66.00	8.10	—	—	—	—	97
Wheat germ		110.03	8.48	80.77	12.72	—	—	—	212.00	146
Vegetables										
Asparagus	1	1.80	—	0.50	—	0.07	—	—	—	130
Asparagus, frozen	1	1.40	—	0.07	—	0.12	—	—	—	129
Beans, fresh	1	0.02	—	—	—	0.09	—	—	—	129
Beans, canned	1	0.03	—	—	—	—	—	—	0.05	108
Beans, frozen, cooked	1	0.11	—	0.07[b]	—	—	—	—	0.25	108
Beans, baked, canned	1	0.30	—	—	—	—	—	—	1.00	182
Beans, baked, Boston	1	0.14	—	—	—	—	—	—	1.14	108
Beans, kidney, red	1	trace	—	—	—	3.44	—	trace	—	129
Beans, lima, dry	1	trace	—	—	—	7.15	—	0.53	—	129

[a] Tocopherols: alpha-tocol (α-T), alpha-trienol (α-T3), beta-tocol (β-T), beta-trienol (β-T3), gamma-tocol (γ-T), gamma-trienol (γ-T3), delta-tocol (δ-T), delta-trienol (δ-T3), and total tocopherols (TOT).
[b] β- plus γ-tocols.

APPENDIX A (continued)

Vegetables (continued)

| Item | Number of samples | Tocopherols[a] | | | | | | | | | Source |
		α-T	α-T3	β-T	β-T3	γ-T	γ-T3	δ-T	δ-T3	TOT	
Beans, navy, dry	1	0.47	–	–	–	–	–	–	–	1.68	108
Broccoli, fresh	1	0.46	–	–	–	0.18	–	–	–	–	129
Cabbage	1	0.11	–	–	–	–	–	–	–	–	176
Cabbage, fresh, white	1	0.02	–	–	–	trace	–	–	–	–	129
Cabbage, fresh, red	1	trace	–	–	–	–	–	–	–	–	129
Carrots	1	0.51	0.04	0.01	0.08	–	–	–	–	–	130
Carrots	1	0.11	–	–	–	–	–	–	–	0.21	108
Carrots, fresh	1	0.57	0.04	0.02	trace	–	–	–	–	–	129
Cauliflower, fresh	1	0.04	–	–	–	0.05	–	–	–	–	129
Celery	1	0.38	–	–	–	–	–	–	–	0.57	108
Corn, fresh	1	0.06	0.20	–	–	0.40	0.40	–	–	–	130
Corn, canned	1	0.04	0.12	–	–	0.16	0.30	trace	–	–	129
Corn, canned	1	0.05	–	–	–	–	–	–	–	0.09	108

Food		α-T	α-T3	β-T	β-T3	γ-T	γ-T3	δ-T	δ-T3	TOT	
Corn, frozen	1	0.03	0.14	–	–	0.09	0.38	trace	–	–	129
Corn, frozen, cooked	1	0.19	–	–	–	–	–	–	–	0.48	108
Lettuce	1	0.50	–	0.70b	–	–	–	–	–	1.20	182
Lettuce	1	0.37	–	–	–	–	–	–	–	–	176
Lettuce	1	0.06	–	–	–	–	–	–	–	0.17	108
Peas, fresh	1	0.55	–	–	–	–	–	–	–	1.73	108
Peas, canned	1	0.02	–	–	–	–	–	–	–	0.04	108
Peas, frozen, uncooked	1	0	–	0.60b	–	–	–	–	–	0.60	182
Peas, dried	1	0.30	–	–	6.4	–	–	0.6	–	–	130
Potatoes, raw	1	0.05	–	–	–	–	–	–	–	0.09	108
Potatoes, baked	1	0.03	–	–	–	–	–	–	–	0.06	108
Potatoes, boiled	1	0.04	–	–	–	–	–	–	–	0.06	108
Potatoes, fried, french	1	0.12	–	–	–	–	–	–	–	0.36	108
Potatoes, fried, french	1	0.27	–	–	0.13	–	–	–	–	–	176
Spinach, fresh	1	1.79	–	–	–	–	–	–	–	–	129
Spinach, canned	1	0.02	–	–	–	–	–	–	–	0.06	108
Tomatoes, fresh	1	0.40	–	–	–	–	–	–	–	0.85	108

a Tocopherols: alpha-tocol (α-T), alpha-trienol (α-T3), beta-tocol (β-T), beta-trienol (β-T3), gamma-tocol (γ-T), gamma-trienol (γ-T3), delta-tocol (δ-T), delta-trienol (δ-T3), and total tocopherols (TOT).
b β- plus γ-tocols.

APPENDIX B α-Tocopherol Content of Food (mg/100 g)[a]

Item	Bauernfeind compilation (1965–1975)		Ames review[b]		Dicks' compilation (1940–1965)[c]	
	Mean	Range	Mean	Range	Mean	Range
Wheat germ	119.44	110.30–133.00	—	—	156.20	85.00–209.00
Rice germ oil	—	—	—	—	98.00	92.00–104.00
Rye oil	—	—	—	—	97.00	—
Wheat oil	48.70	—	—	—	52.00	—
Sunflower oil	49.50	—	—	—	—	—
Sunflower seeds, hulled	—	—	—	—	40.86	22.40– 55.00
Cottonseed oil	43.97	32.00– 56.00	35.80	10.20–54.00	40.80	10.20– 76.00
Rice bran oil	—	—	—	—	44.50	26.40– 58.00
Safflower oil	39.58	34.20– 45.80	34.80	22.60–45.80	41.34	22.60– 82.00
Barley oil	35.21	—	—	—	37.30	34.00– 42.00
Wheat bran oil	—	—	—	—	27.50	20.00– 35.00
Almonds	27.20	23.00– 27.40	15.00	—	15.00	—
Sesame oil	25.67	—	25.70	24.40–27.30	25.00	24.00– 26.00
Corn germ oil	—	—	—	—	23.00	—
Rapeseed oil	23.57	18.40– 23.80	18.20	15.10–22.50	19.30	15.00– 23.00
Palm oil	21.10	18.80– 25.60	29.00	16.00–40.00	17.30	5.60– 30.00
Filberts	—	—	21.00	—	21.00	—
Cod liver oil	—	—	—	—	—	—
Peanut oil	18.88	10.70– 33.90	15.60	7.00–36.70	21.40	9.70– 32.20
Corn oil	15.90	2.30– 29.40	18.70	14.70–23.60	16.00	11.00– 30.00
Margarine, soft	13.87	4.10– 32.70	—	—	11.66	5.00– 24.00
Grapeseed oil	—	—	—	—	13.00	—

Food						
Mayonnaise	12.97	6.00– 24.30	—	—	—	—
Wheat germ (meal)	11.65	—	12.50	5.80–16.30	12.50	5.30– 18.20
Margarine, hard	10.75	3.16– 19.90	11.60	3.30–15.80	6.46	0.50– 16.00
Peanuts	10.52	9.70– 11.40	—	—	9.55	4.60– 14.50
Olive oil	10.08	0.80– 24.00	13.50	7.80–22.00	10.40	3.10– 22.00
Rice bran	—	—	—	—	8.10	—
Soybean oil	7.92	3.40– 11.50	12.90	6.40–24.20	12.90	6.40– 30.00
Peanuts, roasted	7.20	6.70– 7.70	6.40	4.50– 7.70	—	—
Brazil nuts	—	—	6.50	—	—	—
Sweet potatoes	—	—	—	—	6.50	4.00– 10.00
Herring oil	—	—	—	—	6.00	2.00– 6.00
Potato chips	6.40	—	4.30	2.10–64.00	4.50	—
Peanut butter	6.20	3.20– 8.60	—	—	2.14	—
Cookies, oatmeal–peanut	6.00	—	6.00	—	—	—
Corn germ	—	—	5.50	3.80– 7.30	5.40	3.40– 7.40
Blackberries, wild	—	—	—	—	3.50	—
Dandelion greens	—	—	—	—	3.18	1.30– 5.00
Margarine, whipped	3.20	—	—	—	—	—
Egg yolk	—	—	2.60	1.60– 3.90	2.75	1.60– 3.90
Turnip greens	—	—	—	—	2.24	—
Broccoli	—	—	2.00	1.10– 3.80	2.40	1.00– 3.80
Butter	2.16	1.00– 3.30	1.90	1.00– 2.60	1.90	1.40– 2.60
Parsley	—	—	1.80	1.20– 2.60	1.98	1.10– 3.00
Poppyseeds	1.80	—	—	—	—	—
Spinach	1.79	—	2.50	1.30– 4.70	2.74	1.30– 4.60

a Foods containing 1 mg or more of α-tocopherol per 100 g.
b From Ref. 52.
c From Ref. 99.

APPENDIX B (continued)

Item	Bauernfeind compilation (1965–1975)		Ames review[b]		Dicks' compilation (1940–1965)[c]	
	Mean	Range	Mean	Range	Mean	Range
Oatmeal	1.70	0.90– 2.30	0.90	0.10– 2.30	0.70	0.50– 0.80
Wheat bran	1.69	1.60– 1.70	1.50	0.10– 4.90	1.38	0.30– 4.40
Pies, mixed	1.66	0.52– 3.12	2.80	2.50– 3.10	0.97	0.20– 2.70
Asparagus	1.60	1.40– 1.80	2.50	–	2.50	–
Crackers, wheat	1.37	–	–	–	–	–
Salmon, broiled	1.35	–	1.35	–	–	–
Rye grain	1.28	0.80– 1.60	1.20	0.70– 1.70	1.20	0.70– 1.70
Rye bread, dark	1.24	–	–	–	–	–
Milo grain	1.22	–	–	–	–	–
Lard	1.20	–	1.70	0.20– 3.00	1.20	0.20– 2.30
Cookies, mixed	1.18	0.50– 3.50	–	–	3.06	2.00– 5.00
Pecans	1.10	1.00– 1.20	1.50	–	1.50	–

Wheat grain	1.10	0.90– 1.40	1.20	0.50– 1.80	1.18	0.50– 2.00
Water cress	—	—	—	—	1.13	0.60– 1.80
Crackers, rye and wheat	1.10	—	1.10	—	—	—
Chocolate bar, milk	1.10	—	1.70	1.30– 2.10	—	—
Corn grain	1.01	0.40– 2.00	1.10	—	1.40	0.20– 2.10
Cakes, mixed	0.93	0.10– 3.80	1.10	—	3.49	2.59– 4.39
Herring	—	—	1.00	0.30– 1.60	1.10	0.30– 1.60
Brussel sprouts	—	—	1.00	0.40– 2.00	1.00	0.40– 2.00
Parsnips	—	—	1.00	—	1.00	—
Currants, black	—	—	—	—	1.00	—
Rice, brown	0.73	0.13– 1.40	1.30	1.20– 1.30	1.20	0.33– 2.10
Bread, whole wheat	0.53	0.20– 1.10	—	—	1.52	—
Walnuts	0.51	0.40– 0.60	1.50	—	—	0.76– 1.23
Eggs, whole	0.46	—	1.10	0.80– 1.20	1.04	0.76– 1.23
Coconut	0.45	0.40– 0.50	0.60	0.00– 1.60	1.73	0.20– 3.60

a Foods containing 1 mg or more of α-tocopherol per 100 g.
b From Ref. 52.
c From Ref. 99.

REFERENCES

1. J. F. Pennock, F. W. Hemming, and J. D. Kerr, Biochem. Biophys. Commun. 17:542 (1964).
2. J. C. Bauernfeind and W. M. Cort, in Encyclopedia of Food Technology. Edited by A. Johnson and M. Peterson, Westport, Conn., AVI Publishing Co., 1974, pp. 337-375.
3. J. G. Bieri and R. Poukka-Evarts, J. Amer. Diet. Assoc. 62:147 (1973).
4. J. G. Bieri and R. Poukka-Evarts, Amer. J. Clin. Nutr. 27:980 (1974).
5. J. G. Bieri and R. Poukka-Evarts, R. J. Nutr. 104:850 (1974).
6. J. Bunyan, D. McHale, J. Green, and S. Marcinkiewicz, Br. J. Nutr. 15:253 (1961).
7. G. Brubacher and H. Weiser, Wiss. Veroeffent. Deut. Ges. Ernaehrung. 16:50 (1967).
8. B. Century and M. K. Horwitt, Fed. Proc. 24:906 (1965).
9. H. H. Draper, in Fat-Soluble Vitamins. Edited by R. A. Morton, New York, Pergamon, 1970, pp. 333-393.
10. M. H. Stern, C. D. Robeson, L. Weisler, and J. G. Baxter, J. Amer. Chem. Soc. 69:869 (1947).
11. R. M. Parkhurst, W. A. Skinner, and P. A. Sturm, J. Amer. Oil Chem. Soc. 45:641 (1968).
12. C. K. Chow and H. H. Draper, Internatl. J. Vit. Nutr. Res. 44:396 (1974).
13. M. L. Quaife and M. Y. Dju, J. Biol. Chem. 180:263 (1949).
14. W. Lange, J. Amer. Oil Chem. Soc. 27:414 (1950).
15. J. G. Bieri and E. L. Prival, Proc. Soc. Exp. Biol. Med. 120:554 (1965).
16. J. Bruinsma, Chem. Weekbl. 59:599 (1963).
17. G. S. Hall and D. L. Laidman, Biochem. J. 101:5P (1966).
18. T. Baszynski, Acta Soc. Bot. Pol. 30:307 (1961).
19. W. Feldheim and B. Thomas, Ernaehrung 2:97 (1957).
20. J. Green, J. Sci. Food Agr. 9:801 (1958).
21. H. Chattopadhyay and S. Banerjee, Food Res. 17:402 (1952).
22. F. Brown, J. Sci. Food Agr. 4:161 (1953).
23. J. Glover, in Fat-Soluble Vitamins. Edited by R. A. Morton, New York, Pergamon, 1970, pp. 199-208.
24. K. Kivimae and C. Carpena, Acta Agr. Scand. Suppl. 19:161 (1973).
25. V. Maxim and M. Gondos, Bucharest. Inst. Ceret. Zootch. Lucrarile Sti. 19:135 (1961).
26. F. Albonico and A. Fabris, Agrochim. 2:147 (1958).
27. V. H. Booth, J. Sci. Food Agric. 15:342 (1964).

28. W. Hjarde, W. Hellstrøm, and E. Akerberg, Acta Agric. Scand. 13:3 (1963).
29. C. A. Cabell and N. R. Ellis, J. Nutr. 23:633 (1942).
30. P. Cattaneo, G. Karman de Sutton, and J. A. Burguete, Rev. Argent. Grasas Aceites 2:87 (1960).
31. D. Antonijevic, B. Vajic, and R. Dragoniv, Zavod za zdraystvenu zastitu NR Srbije-Beograd. 1:127 (1962).
32. W. Feldheim, Z. Lebens. Untersuch. Forsch. 104:24 (1956).
33. R. H. Bunnell, J. P. Keating, and A. J. Quaresimo, J. Agric. Food Chem. 16:659 (1968).
34. R. H. Bunnell, Poultry Sci. 36:413 (1957).
35. W. J. Pudelkiewicz and L. D. Matterson, J. Nutr. 71:143 (1960).
36. G. Olson, W. J. Pudelkiewicz, and L. D. Matterson, J. Nutr. 90:199 (1966).
37. I. D. Desai, Nature (London) 209:810 (1966).
38. H. F. Hintz and D. E. Hogue, J. Nutr. 84:3 (1964).
39. S. H. Sanyoi, Calcutta Med. J. 50:409 (1953).
40. G. C. Bandyopadhyay, Diss. Abstr. Int. 31(6):3090-B (1970).
41. B. L. O'Dell, Z. Erek, L. Flynn, G. B. Garner, and M. E. Muhrer, J. Animal Sci. 19:1280 (1960).
42. V. Lautner, Biol. Chem. Vyz. Zvirat 8:37 (1972).
43. J. Lazar, J. Kovac, and A. Kaliska, Folia Veterinaria 17:35 (1973).
44. R. S. Harris, Vit. Horm. 20:603 (1962).
45. C. Anglin, J. H. Mahon, and R. A. Chapman, J. Dairy Sci. 38:333 (1955).
46. W. A. McGillivary, J. Sci. Technol. 38A:466 (1956).
47. S. K. Searles and J. G. Armstrong, J. Dairy Sci. 53:150 (1970).
48. A. Veijo, J. Nordland, and M. Antila, Suomen Kamstilehti 38:7B (1965).
49. C. Kanno, K. Yamauchi, and T. Tsugo, J. Dairy Sci. 51:1713 (1968).
50. H. Leuck and W. Mueller-Mulot, S. Afr. J. Dairy Sci. 3:153 (1971).
51. W. M. Cort, in Nutritional Evaluation of Food Processing. Edited by R. H. Harris and E. Karmas, Westport, Conn., AVI Publishing Co., 1975, pp. 383-392.
52. S. R. Ames, in The Vitamins, Vol. V, 2nd ed. Edited by W. H. Sebrell, Jr. and R. S. Harris, Academic Press, New York, 1972, p. 233.
53. G. O. Akopyan, Izv. Akad. Naukarmyan. SSR Ser. Biol. 11:95 (1958).
54. B. Thafvelin and H. E. Oksanen, J. Dairy Sci. 49:282 (1966).
55. J. Vander Veen and H. S. Olcott, J. Agric. Food Chem. 15:682 (1967).
56. V. H. Booth, Phytochemistry 3:273 (1964).
57. L. W. Charkey, A. K. Pyke, and R. E. Carlson, J. Agric. Food Chem. 9:70 (1961).

58. A. L. Livingston, J. W. Nelson, and G. O. Kohler, J. Agric. Food Chem. 16:492 (1968).

59. A. L. Livingston, R. E. Knowles, and G. O. Kohler, USDA-ARS Technical Bulletin No. 1414, Washington, D.C., U.S. Government Printing Office, March, 1970.

60. D. C. Herting and E. E. Drury, J. Nutr. 81:335 (1963).

61. C. R. Adams, H. J. Eoff, and C. R. Zimmerman, Feedstuffs, Sept. 8, 1975, p. 24.

62. C. K. Chow and H. H. Draper, J. Agric. Food Chem. 17:1316 (1969).

63. W. G. Pond, W. H. Allaway, E. F. Walker, Jr., and L. Krook, J. Animal Sci. 33:996 (1971).

64. L. G. Young, A. Lun, J. Pos, R. P. Forshaw, and D. Edmeades, J. Animal Sci. 40:495 (1975).

65. A. Madsen, H. P. Mortensen, and E. Larson, Forsogslab. Arbog. 65 (1970).

66. A. Madsen, H. P. Mortensen, W. Hjarde, E. Leerbeck, and T. Leth, Acta Agric. Scand. Suppl. 19:169 (1973).

67. A. H. Jensen, D. H. Baker, P. B. Lynch, and B. G. Harmon, Proceedings of the Illinois Pork Industry Day, University of Illinois, 4-11 Dec. 1973.

68. M. Komada and I. Harda, J. Amer. Oil. Chem. Soc. 46:18 (1969).

69. J. F. Connoly and T. A. Spillane, Irish J. Agric. Res. 7:261 (1968).

70. G. W. Grams, C. W. Blessin, and G. E. Inglett, J. Amer. Oil Chem. Soc. 47:337 (1970).

71. G. S. Hall and D. L. Laidman, Biochem. J. 108:46 (1968).

72. D. S. Binnington and J. S. Andrews, Cereal Chem. 18:618 (1941).

73. H. R. R. Hentzler, A. Gorter, and M. Elkelen, Voeding 10:112 (1949).

74. C. Engel, Z. Vit. Forsch. 12:220 (1942).

75. K. Lorenz and P. Limjaroenrat, Leben. Wissenschaft. Technol. 7:86 (1974).

76. T. Moran, Nutr. Abstr. Rev. 29:1 (1959).

77. A. C. Fraser, J. R. Hickman, H. G. Sammons, and M. J. Sharratt, J. Sci. Food Agric. 1:464 (1956).

78. B. Thomas, W. Feldheim, and M. Rothe, Ernaehrung 2:603 (1957).

79. T. Moran, J. Pace, and E. E. McDermott, Nature (London) 171:103 (1953); 174:449 (1954).

80. T. Moore, I. M. Sharman, and R. J. Ward, J. Sci. Food Agric. 8:97 (1957); Proc. Nutr. Soc. 16:xix (1957).

81. E. L. Mason and W. L. Jones, J. Sci. Food Agric. 9:524 (1958).

82. A. C. Frazer and J. G. Lines, J. Sci. Food Agric. 18:203 (1967).

83. T. Moore, I. M. Sharman, and R. J. Ward, Br. J. Nutr. 12:215 (1958).

84. D. Menger, Brot Gebaeck 8:167 (1957).

85. D. W. Howland, J. J. Pienkowski, and R. A. Reiners, Cereal Chem. 50:661 (1973).

86. G. W. Grams, C. W. Blessin, and G. E. Inglett, Cereal Chem. 48:356 (1971).

87. D. C. Herting and E. E. Drury, J. Agric. Food Chem. 17:785 (1969).

88. A. M. Sechi and R. Rossi-Manaresi, J. Vitaminol. 4:114 (1958).

89. J. F. Diehl, Z. Lebensm. Unters. Forsch. 142:1 (1970).

90. H. C. Kung, E. L. Gaden, Jr., and C. G. King, J. Agric. Food Chem. 1:142 (1953).

91. H. F. Kraybill, Assoc. Food Drug Off. U.S. Q. Bull. 20:171 (1956).

92. C. E. Poling, W. D. Warner, F. R. Humberg, E. F. Reber, W. M. Urban, and E. E. Rice, Food Res. 20:193 (1955).

93. M. H. Thomas and D. H. Calloway, J. Amer. Diet. Assoc. 39:105 (1961)

94. K. H. Tipples and F. W. Norris, Cereal Chem. 42:437 (1965).

95. J. Washuettl, Ernaehrung. Umsch. 16:474 (1969).

96. H. T. Slover and J. Lehmann, Cereal Chem. 49:412 (1972).

97. H. T. Slover, J. Lehmann, and R. Valis, J. Amer. Oil Chem. Soc. 46:417 (1969).

98. E. N. Frankel, D. D. Evans, and P. M. Cooney, J. Agric. Food Chem. 7:438 (1959).

99. M. W. Dicks, Agric. Exp. Sta. Bull. 435, University of Wyoming, Laramie, December, 1965.

100. M. T. Juilet, Fette Seifen Anstrichm. 77:101 (1975).

101. A. Jakubowski, A. Pilak, and K. Pilak, Food Sci. Technol. Abstr. 3:12N, 546 (1971).

102. J. K. B. A. Ata and A. Cobbina, Ghana J. Agric. Sci. 6:45 (1973).

103. E. Einset, H. S. Olcott, and M. E. Stanby, Comm. Fisheries Rev. 19:35 (1957).

104. T. Rupel, Vitamin E Manufacture, Park Ridge, Noyes Data Corp., N.J., 1969, pp. 1-114.

105. C. H. Lea and R. J. Ward, J. Sci. Food Agric. 10:537 (1959).

106. R. N. Moore and W. G. Bickford, J. Amer. Chem. Soc. 29:1 (1952).

107. R. A. Ramanujan and C. P. Anantakrishnak, Indian J. Dairy Sci. 11:179 (1958).

108. R. H. Bunnell, J. P. Keating, and A. J. Quaresimo, J. Agric. Food Chem. 16:659 (1965).

109. R. LeCoq, C. Rd. Soc. Biol. (Paris) 138:836 (1944).

110. B. Gassmann and R. Schneeweiss, Nahrung 3:42 (1959).

111. I. M. Sharman and P. J. Richards, Br. J. Nutr. 14:85 (1960).

112. V. H. Booth and M. P. Bradford, Int. J. Vit. Res. 33:276 (1963).

113. J. Green, S. Marcinkiewicz, and P. R. Watt, J. Sci. Food Agric. 6:274 (1955).

114. G. Brubacher, Int. J. Vit. Res. 36:409 (1966).

115. A. Aczel, Ind. Obst. Gemueseverwentung. 57:317 (1972).

116. A. L. Tappel, F. W. Knapp, and K. Urs, Food Res. 22:287 (1957).

117. D. C. Herting and E. E. Drury, Amer. J. Clin. Nutr. 22:147 (1968).

118. M. Rothe, W. Feldheim, and B. Thomas, Ernaehrung. 3:386 (1958).

119. J. Muehlefluh, Med. Ernaehrung. 4:20 (1963).

120. S. Nordfeldt, N. Olson, G. Anstrand, and V. Hellstroem, Kungl. Lantbrukshoegsk. Ann. 28:181 (1958).

121. F. Grandel and H. Neumann, Muehlenlab. 10:1 (1940).

122. E. Kodicek, R. Brande, S. K. Kon, and K. G. Mitchell, Br. J. Nutr. 13:363 (1969).

123. G. O. Akopyan, Izv. Akad. Nauk armyan SSR Ser. Biol. 15:29 (1962).

124. G. O. Kohler, E. Beier, and C. C. Bolze, Poultry Sci. 34:468 (1955).

125. D. J. Nazir and N. C. Magar, Indian J. Appl. Chem. 24:18 (1961).

126. E. L. Hove and P. L. Harris, J. Amer. Oil Chem. Soc. 38:405 (1951).

127. K. Schwartz, Proc. Soc. Exp. Biol. Med. 99:20 (1958).

128. D. L. Carpenter and H. T. Slover, J. Amer. Oil Chem. Soc. 50:372 (1973).

129. H. T. Slover and J. Lehmann, J. Amer. Oil Chem. Soc. 49:313A (1972).

130. H. T. Slover, Lipids 6:291 (1971).

131. H. T. Slover, J. Lehmann, and R. J. Valis, Cereal Chem. 46:635 (1969).

132. H. T. Slover, R. J. Valis, and J. Lehmann, J. Amer. Oil Chem. Soc. 45:552 (1968).

133. J. Lehmann and H. T. Slover, Lipids 6:35 (1971).

134. L. Harris, M. L. Quaife, and W. J. Swanson, J. Nutr. 40:367 (1950).

135. H. Thaler, Proceedings of a Symposium on Tocopherols, Darmstadt, Dr. Dietrich Steinkopff Verlag, 1967, pp. 177-188.

136. K. Taeufel and R. Serzisko, Ernaehrung. 6:333 (1961).

137. F. W. Quackenbush, J. G. Firch, A. M. Brunson, and L. R. House, Cereal Chem. 40:250 (1963).

138. P. J. Dunphy, K. J. Whittle, J. F. Pennock, and R. A. Morton, Nature (London) 207:521 (1965).

139. K. J. Whittle, P. J. Dunphy, and J. F. Pennock, Biochemistry 100:318 (1966).

140. P. A. Sturm, R. M. Parkhurst, and W. A. Skinner, Anal. Chem. 38:1244 (1966).

141. K. J. Whittle and J. F. Pennock, Analyst 92:423 (1967).

142. C. K. Chow, H. H. Draper, and A. S. Csallany, Anal. Biochem. 32:81 (1969).
143. T. C. Rao and S. V. Rao, J. Oil Technol. Assoc. India 6:45 (1974).
144. E. Fedeli, F. Camurati, and G. Jaciosi, Revista Italiana delle Sostanze Grasse 48:565 (1971).
145. E. Kurucz and M. J. Peredy, Symp. Int. Oxyd. Lipides, Catal. Met. 3rd Corps Gras Paris Inst. Publ., 1974, pp. 193-207.
146. M. K. Govind Rao and E. G. Perkins, J. Agric. Food Chem. 20:240 (1972).
147. R. J. Ward, Br. J. Nutr. 12:231 (1964).
148. G. Lambertsen, H. Myklestad, and O. R. Braekkan, J. Food Sci. 29:164 (1964).
149. J. Zemanovic and E. Mastenova, Prum. Potravin 19:111 (1968).
150. G. Lambertsen, H. Myklestad, and O. R. Braekkan, J. Sci. Food Agric. 13:617 (1962).
151. D. Nazir and N. G. Magar, Indian J. Chem. 1:278 (1963).
152. H. H. Williams, JAMA 175:104 (1961).
153. K. P. Millar and A. D. Sheppard, N.Z. J. Sci. 15:3 (1972).
154. M. L. Quaife, J. Biol. Chem. 169:513 (1947).
155. P. L. Harris, M. L. Quaife, and P. O'Grady, J. Nutr. 46:459 (1952).
156. C. W. Woodruff, M. C. Bailey, J. T. Davis, N. Rogers, and J. G. Coniglio, Amer. J. Clin. Nutr. 14:83 (1964).
157. D. C. Herting and E. E. Drury, J. Chromatogr. 30:502 (1967).
158. H. D. Herre, Monats. Kinderheil 113:95 (1965).
159. M. Y. Hamed and P. Decker, Int. J. Vit. Res. 30:41 (1959).
160. R. G. Ackman and M. G. Cormier, J. Fish. Res. Board Can. 24:357 (1967).
161. K. Yamanchi, N. Kadotani, and T. Ohaski, Nippon Chikusan Gakkai-Ho 45:625 (1974).
162. V. H. Booth and M. P. Bradford, Br. J. Nutr. 17:575 (1963).
163. V. H. Booth, Analyst 88:627 (1963).
164. F. A. Oski and L. A. Barness, J. Pediatr. 70:211 (1967).
165. M. W. Dicks-Bushnell and K. C. Davis, Amer. J. Clin. Nutr. 20:262 (1967).
166. I. D. Desai, L. P. O'Leary, and N. Schwartz, Nutr. Repts. Internat. 6:83 (1972).
167. M. K. Horwitt, Amer. J. Clin. Nutr. 8:451 (1960).
168. M. K. Horwitt, Vit. Horm. 20:541 (1962).
169. P. L. Harris and N. D. Embree, Amer. J. Clin Nutr. 13:385 (1963).
170. S. A. Hashim and R. H. Asfour, Amer. J. Clin. Nutr. 21:7 (1968).
171. C. D. Fitch and J. S. Dinning, J. Nutr. 79:69 (1963).
172. L. J. Machlin and R. S. Gordon, Proc. Soc. Exp. Biol. Med. 103:659 (1960).

173. J. E. Ford, J. W. G. Porter, K. J. Scott, S. Y. Thompson, J. Le Marquand, and A. S. Truswell, Arch. Dis. Childhood 49:874 (1974).

174. K. C. Davis, J. Food Sci. 38:442 (1973).

175. J. N. Thompson, J. L. Beare-Rogers, P. Erodody, and D. C. Smith, Amer. J. Clin. Nutr. 26:1349 (1973).

176. J. N. Thompson, P. Erdody, and W. B. Maxwell, Anal. Biochem. 50:267 (1972).

177. E. DeRitter, M. Osadca, J. Scheiner, and J. Keating, J. Amer. Dietet. Assoc. 64:391 (1974).

178. N. Ikehata, H. Tanaka, and C. Kamishima, Vitamins (Kyoto), 38:253 (1968).

179. C. L. Smith, J. Kelleher, M. S. Losowsky, and N. Morrish, Br. J. Nutr. 26:89 (1971).

180. W. H. Sebrell, Jr., K. W. King, R. E. Webb, C. H. Daza, R. A. Franco, S. C. Smith, E. L. Severinghaus, F. X. Pi-Sunyer, B. A. Underwood, M. Flores, M. C. Conner, T. Townsend, J. M. Pezzotti, and B. Castillo, Arch. Latinamer. Nutr. 22:77 (1972).

181. M. K. Govind-Rao, S. Venkob-Rao, and T. K. Achaya, J. Sci. Food Agric. 16:1 (1965).

182. A. A. Christie, A. C. Dean, and B. A. Millburn, Analyst 98:161 (1973).

183. H. D. McBride and D. H. Evans, Anal. Chem. 45:446 (1973).

184. S. Nobile, J. M. Woodhill, and P. E. Rosevear, Food Tech. Aust. 27:342 (1975).

185. R. H. Bunnell, B. Borenstein, and G. W. Schutt, J. Amer. Oil Chem. Soc. 48:175A (1971).

186. NAS-NRC Recommended Dietary Allowances, 8th ed., Washington, D.C., Printing and Publication Office, National Academy of Sciences, 1974.

187. Fed. Regis., no. 138, 38:20714, 2 August 1973.

188. Nutr. Rev. 30:55 (1972).

189. I. R. Peake, H. G. Windmueller, and J. G. Bieri, Biochim. Biophys. Acta 260:697 (1972).

190. I. R. Peake and J. G. Bieri, J. Nutr. 101:1615 (1971).

191. M. Brin, L. J. Machlin, J. Keating, J. Nelson, R. Filipski, and O. N. Miller, Fed. Proc. 35:740 (1976).

192. H. Schmandke, Int. Zeitschr. Vitaminforsch. 34:400 (1964).

193. I. Kaludin, Ernaehrung 9:29 (1964).

194. NAS-NRC, Proposed Fortification Policy for Cereal-Grain Products, Washington, D.C., Printing and Publishing Office, National Academy of Sciences, 1974.

195. H. A. Schroeder, Amer. J. Clin. Nutr. 24:562 (1971).

196. W. M. Cort, B. Borenstein, J. H. Harley, M. Osadca, and J. Scheiner, Food Technol. 30:52 (1976).
197. Nutr. Rev. 31:327 (1973).
198. JAMA 225:1116 (1973).
199. S. H. Rubin and W. M. Cort, in Protein Enriched Cereal Foods for World Needs. Edited by M. Milner, St. Paul, Minn., Assoc. Cereal Chemists, 1969, pp. 220-233.
200. R. S. Harris, J. Agric. Food Chem. 16:149 (1968).
201. E. DeRitter, Food Technol. 30(1):48 (1976).
202. S. H. Rubin, W. M. Cort, A. Emodi, and L. Scialpi, presented at the 60th Annual Meeting of Cereal Chemists, Kansas City, 25-27 October 1975.
203. Pediatrics 40:916 (1967).
204. K. C. Davis, Amer. J. Clin. Nutr. 25:933 (1972).
205. W. M. Cort, J. Amer. Oil Chem. Soc. 51:321 (1974).
206. W. M. Cort, J. W. Scott, and J. H. Harley, Food Technol. 29(11):46 (1975).
207. W. M. Cort, Food Technol. 28(10):60 (1974).
208. H. Klaeui, in Proceedings of the University of Nottingham Residential Seminar on Vitamins. Edited by M. Stein, London, Churchill Livingston, 1971, pp. 110-143.

5 BIOCHEMISTRY

Part 5A/ Absorption   170

Part 5B/ Transport and Metabolism   193

Part 5C/ Biogenesis   268

Part 5D/ Nutrient Interrelationships   272

Part 5E/ Biochemical Function   289

    Section 1   Vitamin E: Its role as a biological
                  free radical scavenger and its
                  relationship to the microsomal
                  mixed-function oxidase systems   289

    Section 2   Role in nucleic acid and protein
                  metabolism   318

    Section 3   The role of vitamin E in
                  mitochrondrial metabolism   332

Part 5F/ Hormonal Status in Vitamin E Deficiency   348

Part 5G/ Role in Function and Ultrastructure of Cellular
    Membranes   372

Part 5A/ Absorption

HUGO E. GALLO-TORRES
Hoffmann-La Roche Inc.
Nutley, New Jersey

I.	Introduction	170
II.	Intestinal Absorption	171
	A. Methods for Investigation of Intestinal Absorption of Vitamin E	171
	B. Lymphatic Absorption	175
	C. Site of Absorption	176
	D. Efficiency of Absorption	179
	E. Effect of Bile and Pancreatic Juice	180
	F. Effect of Other Dietary Lipids	181
III.	Intestinal Transport	183
IV.	Overall Process of Intestinal Absorption	185
V.	Summary	188
	References	189

I. INTRODUCTION

The gastrointestinal absorption of nutrients has been studied with a number of techniques of continuously increasing sophistication. Only a few of these procedures have been applied to the intestinal absorption of tocopherols [1-24], and the physicobiochemical mechanism of absorption of vitamin E is poorly defined. Interactions usually observed between vitamin E and other nutrients at different tissues can also be demonstrated in the intestine. A number of malabsorption states involve malabsorption of vitamin E [11, 22, 25-32]. Additionally, decreased absorptive capacity has been implicated as a limiting factor in the repair of hemolytic anemia related to vitamin E deficiency in premature infants [33]. Thus, understanding of the digestion-absorption process of vitamin E is also of practical importance owing to possible therapeutic implications in primary or secondary deficiency states.

II. INTESTINAL ABSORPTION

A. Methods for Investigation of Intestinal Absorption of Vitamin E

The methods so far applied to study of vitamin E absorption (in vivo) and transport (in vitro) are listed in Table 1. The rat has been the experimental subject in the majority of studies, and observations in humans have been scant. dl-α-Tocopheryl acetate has been the substance most frequently employed in the assessment of absorption. Only a few reports refer to experiments designed to study absorption of free tocopherol or derivatives other than the acetate ester. Most of the methods are not suitable for an adequate calculation of the efficiency of absorption of tocopherol. Also evident from this table is the large number of variables used by different authors, which makes quantitative comparisons difficult.

It is important to consider the influence of different techniques on the interpretation of absorption data. Intestinal balance studies, tissue distribution measurements, and tolerance curves do not lend themselves to investigation of absorption mechanisms. Where blood levels are used as the criterion, rapid removal of α-tocopherol by body tissues could lead to low estimates of absorption [41, 42]. The concentration to tocopherol in tissues varies widely, depending upon the time elapsed after a single oral administration. Plasma or serum tocopherol concentrations are the consequence of the influx and outflow of the vitamin within the varying pools of different tissues. Additionally, use of these methods may provide results which are affected by factors unrelated to the actual mucosal transfer mechanisms. Among such factors are motility of the gastrointestinal (GI) tract, blood flow, and tissue metabolism. Therefore, results obtained with these methods are a combination of the effects of absorption, tissue uptake, turnover, and intermediary metabolism.

The gastric emptying rate may complicate the results in intact nonanesthetized animals. Intestinal motility and enterohepatic circulation are also factors influencing the fecal excretion of tocopherol. Recently, polar metabolites of α-tocopherol have been found in the bile from rats administered either free tocopherol, dl-α-tocopheryl acetate, or dl-α-tocopheryl nicotinate [43]. Misleading conclusions could be reached using ratios of the luminal concentration of tocopherol (or total lipid) to a water-soluble reference substance, since aqueous and particulate phases may move at different rates [44]. In anesthetized animals, gastric emptying and intestinal motility are avoided, although variations in blood flow and anesthetic effect are present [45]. Results should, therefore, be interpreted with caution.

Gut preparations without an intact blood supply may not be suitable for studies involving tocopherol (or lipid) absorption [46, 47]. The exposure of cut surfaces of preparations in vitro to the bathing medium may influence

TABLE 1   Methods for Investigation of Intestinal Absorption of Vitamin E[a]

Method	Species
In vivo	
Prevention of degeneration in the testis	Rat
Plasma (serum) tocopherol concentration	Cirrhotic humans
	Normal humans
Plasma and tissue concentration	Rat, chicken
Liver tocopherol content	Rat
Plasma tocopherol concentration after direct instillation into the large intestine	Pigs, patients with mid-transverse colostomies
Serum tocopherol concentration in addition to red cell hemolysis	Children with biliary obstruction
Excretion in the feces	Human with muscular dystrophy
	Patients with steatorrhea
	Patients without steatorrhea
	Monkey
Ligated intestinal loops	Normal and dystrophic chicks
Collection of thoracic duct lymph	Patients with gastric carcinoma and lymphatic leukemia
	Rat

Chemical form investigation	Efficiency of absorption[b] (%)	Reference
Nonsaponifiable fraction of wheat germ oil	Und[c]	34
d,l-α-Tocopheryl acetate	Und	35
d-α-Tocopheryl acetate	Und	37
[5-methyl-^{14}C]d,α-Tocopherol	40	1
d,l-α-Tocopherol	Und	38
Multivitamin preparation	Nearly 0	39
d,l-α-Tocopheryl acetate	Und	31
α-Tocopherol	50	36
α-Tocopheryl quinone		
α-Tocopherol hydroquinone diacetate		
[5-methyl-^{3}H]d,l-α-Tocopherol	31-83	11
[5-methyl-^{3}H]d,l-α-Tocopherol	51-86	40
d-α-Tocopheryl acetate	44	40
d-α-^{3}H-Tocopheryl acetate	Und	2
l-α-^{3}H-Tocopheryl acetate		
(randomly labeled)		
[5-methyl-^{3}H]d,l-α-Tocopherol	21	
d,l-α-Tocopheryl-3,4-^{14}C acetate	25(6 hr), 29(16 hr)	3
d,l-α-Tocopheramine-3,4-^{14}C	63	
N-[methyl-^{3}H]d,l-γ-Tocopheramine	91	
d,l-α-Tocopheryl-1',2'-^{3}H-acetate	10(12 hr)	8
d,l-3,4-[^{3}H]-α-Tocopheryl nicotinate	20	9

TABLE 1   (continued)

Method	Species
In vivo (continued)	
Disappearance from small intestinal loops	Rat
Preintestinal disappearance	Ruminants
Collection of portal vein plasma	Rat
In vitro	
Intestinal perfusion	Hamster
Intestinal slices	Rat
Everted sacs	Rat

[a] Methods are arranged in accordance with their first report in the literature.
[b] Unless otherwise specified, these figures represent the percentages of administered compound "absorbed" in 24 hr.
[c] Und = undetermined.

the uptake and binding of substances and the oxygen consumption of the cells. Also, the ability to accumulate tocopherol will depend on the anatomic site (see Part 5C). With intestinal slices, only gut uptake and accumulation can be estimated; it is not possible to measure transfer into the serosal fluid. In the everted sac, the vitamin generally has to pass through submucosal and smooth-muscle layers before reaching the serosal fluid. Although some transfer may occur via the lymphatic vessels; kinetic measurements are affected. Eversion could also alter permeability to some solutes.

Although no single method or parameter is entirely satisfactory for characterizing the intestinal absorption of vitamin E, analysis of the thoracic duct lymph is probably the only direct way of studying the extent and the forms in which this and other related compounds are absorbed from the intestine. For studies in the rat, a technique has been reported

Chemical form investigation	Efficiency of absorption[b] (%)	Reference
α, β, γ or δ-Tocopherol	32, 18, 30, and 2, respectively (6 r)	7
α-Tocopherol	Poor	14
d,l-α-Tocopheryl-1',2'-[^{3}H] acetate	Negligible	20
d,l-α-Tocopheryl acetate	Und	12
[5-methyl-^{3}H] d,l-α-Tocopherol	Und	17
[5-methyl-^{3}H]α-Tocopherol	Und	24

which incorporates the standardization of lymph flow, making it useful in the assessment of small differences in the rate of absorption to tocopherol and other lipid-soluble materials [8,9,15,19,20,23,49-50].

In the present review, the term absorption is mostly used to define the whole sequence of events taking place between the introduction of tocopherol or its esters into the gastrointestinal tract and the appearance of the compound in its original or derivative form in the thoracic duct lymph or portal vein blood. The term transfer is only used in reference to studies in vitro.

B. Lymphatic Absorption

Using rats with cannulated intestinal lymphatics, Johnson and Pover [51] found evidence for the absorption of radiotocopherols into the intestinal lacteals. Blomstrand and Forsgren [3] studied two subjects, one with gastric carcinoma and the other with lymphatic leukemia. Following catheterization of the thoracic duct by the Werner procedure [52], the patients were given [5-methyl-^{3}H] dl-α-tocopherol, dl-α-tocopheryl-[3,4-^{14}C]acetate, dl-α-tocopheramine-3,4-^{14}C, or N-[methyl-^{3}H]dl-γ-tocopheramine in a formula meal. Thus, it was demonstrated that, in humans, the lymphatic pathway is also the major route for absorption of vitamin E or its derivatives. Most of the material recovered in the lymph was identical to the administered tocopherol or tocopheramine. Tocopheryl acetate was split and appeared in the lymph as unesterified tocopherol. Studies in rats with cannulated thoracic ducts have confirmed that vitamin E esters must be hydrolyzed before their entry into the lacteals [8,9]. Rats with intact enterohepatic circulation were given a saline emulsion containing protein, carbohydrate, monolein, 2 mg of dl-α-tocopheryl acetate, and 50 μCi of dl-α-tocopheryl-[1',2'-^{3}H]acetate. Most of the vitamin E appearing in the lymph was in the nonesterified form; however, small quantities of tocopheryl-p-quinone or acetate were found. Maximum absorption of radio-active tocopherol was observed at 2-4 hr and at 8-10 hr (Fig. 1). Such biphasic kinetics have been repeatedly observed. Administration of unesterified tocopherol also results in biphasic kinetics in the lymph [16,23]. This could be due either to emptying of the gut or, more likely, to enzyme-substrate mobilization for production of chylomicrons and very low density lipoproteins (VLDL) [23]. Unlike cholesterol [49,50] or vitamin A [53], vitamin E is not reesterified during the absorption process. In this respect, α-tocopherol behaves like vitamin D [54-56] or vitamin K [57,58]. Information is not available in the literature indicating if the hydrolysis of vitamin E esters is intracavital (luminal), intracellular, or whether it occurs at the level of the brush border membrane.

C. Site of Absorption

Information on the intestinal site of absorption of tocopherol in humans is limited. The vitamin does not seem to be absorbed from the large intestine of patients with midtransverse colostomies [39]. Although earlier studies suggested that no part of the GI tract is responsible for α-tocopherol absorption [2,59], more recent observations [60] strongly suggest that, in the rat, the region of greatest uptake is at the junction of the upper and middle thirds of the small intestine (Fig. 2). Administration of radiotocopherol via the duodenum rather than in the rumen or abomasum resulted in higher radioactivity in the blood and tissues of sheep. Hidiroglou and Jenkis thus concluded that in this species, the jejunum is the main site of absorption of vitamin E [61]. In apparent agreement with these findings, the studies of Hollander and his coworkers [24] indicate that all concentrations tested, the mean absorption rate of α-tocopherol

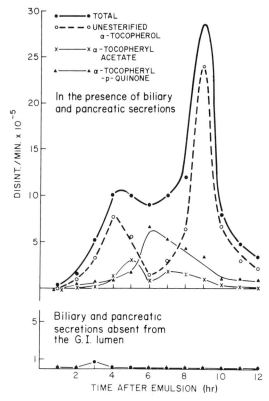

α - TOCOPHERYL ACETATE

SP. ACT. 356 μC/mg
PURITY: >99.0%

FIG. 1 Kinetics of appearance of radiotocopherol and related compounds in the thoracic duct lymph of rats at hourly intervals in the presence of biliary and pancreatic secretions (upper graph) and in their absence (lower graph). In both instances, an emulsion was administered containing protein, carbohydrate, monoolein and dl-α-tocopheryl-1′, 2′-^{3}H$_2$-acetate (from Gallo-Torres, ref. 8).

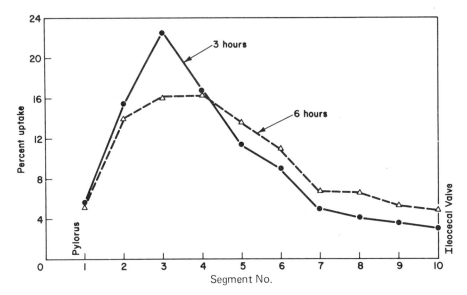

FIG. 2   Site of intestinal absorption of vitamin E in the rat. Overnight
fasted rats were administered, by intragastric emulsion, 2 mg of
<u>dl</u>-α-tocopheryl acetate and 50 μCi of <u>dl</u>-α-tocopheryl-1',2'-^{3}H$_2$-acetate.
Groups of animals were killed by a blow to the head either 3 or 6 hr after
dosing. The small intestine was separated from the stomach and the
cecum. It was rinsed with 20 ml of 0.15 M NaCl and its length measured.
The gut was then divided in 10 portions of equal size, beginning at the
duodenum and ending at the terminal ileum. After mincing in 1 ml water,
the lipids in each portion were extracted and the radioactivity was counted
by standard procedures. The region of greatest uptake is at the junction
of the upper and middle thirds of the small intestine (from Gallo-Torres,
ref. 60).

by the medial small gut segment is consistently greater than absorption of
the vitamin by the proximal and distal segments of the gut. All the above
findings suggest that the medial small intestine of mammals—perhaps
through unique physicobiochemical properties of the luminal absorptive
cell membrane—possesses greater functional absorptive surface when
compared with the proximal and distal small bowel. These considerations
could be of practical importance in cases such as surgical ablation of
certain segments of the gut. It should nevertheless be mentioned that the
site of maximum transport by an isolated segment of intestine in vitro may
not necessarily correspond to a maximum absorption site in vivo. The

site of absorption of vitamin E may depend on factors such as administered dose, relationships between rate of absorption, and rate of transit, as well as type and amount of gut contents.

D. Efficiency of Absorption

The few available reports in the literature indicate that absorption of dietary vitamin E is incomplete (see Table 1). As previously stated, the efficiency of absorption depends to a large extent upon the experimental conditions of the study. In the above-mentioned study by Blomstrand and Forsgren [3], in patients with cannulated thoracic duct the 24-hr recovery of the labeled tocopherols administered was as follows: [5-methyl-^{3}H]dl-α-tocopherol, 21%; dl-α-tocopheryl-3, 4-^{14}C]acetate, 29% (in 16 hr); dl-α-tocopheramine-3, 4-^{14}C, 63%; and N-[methyl-^{3}H]dl-γ-tocopheramine, 91%. Several investigators have taken these data as evidence to indicate that unesterified vitamin E is absorbed less efficiently than any of its derivatives. However, attention should be called to the fact that this study was carried out in a very limited number of patients to whom compounds of varying specific activity were administered at 24-hr intervals. The sequence in which the compounds were dosed is of importance. Continuous drainage of thoracic duct lymph for 24 or more hours could produce dehydration and changes in the conditions required to obtain critical micellar concentrations in the gut lumen, thereby influencing the above results. Analysis of lymph in other species has also confirmed the incompleteness of α-tocopherol absorption. Thus, 12 hr after their intragastric dosage, about 10-20% of the administered dl-α-tocopheryl acetate or dl-α-tocopheryl nicotinate was recovered—mostly as free tocopherol—in the thoracic duct lymph of rats [8,9]. An even lower recovery was reported by Hashim and Schuttringer [62].

Klatskin and Molander [63] found that in humans as much as 64% of the daily intake is excreted in the feces. In a study by Simon and colleagues [64], the amount of α-tocopheryl succinate absorbed from the GI tract did not exceed 10% of the oral dose. Other reports have confirmed that the absorption of α-tocopherol is limited [5, 11, 36, 40, 65, 66], although the net absorption varied with the experimental conditions. Low efficiency of absorption of other tocopherols has also been reported. Thus, Pearson and McBarnes [7] studied the disappearance, from small intestinal loops of rats, of tocopherols, each dissolved in 0.2 ml glyceryl trioleate. The "percent absorption" (magnitude of disappearance) of α-, γ-, β, and δ-tocopherol from the loops was: 32, 30, 18, and 1.8, respectively. These differences in the relative rates of intestinal absorption could partially explain the apparent paradox between the in vitro antioxidant potencies of the β- and δ-tocopherol and their biopotencies.

E. Effect of Bile and Pancreatic Juice

That bile is necessary for optimal absorption of vitamin E was suggested
about four decades ago [34, 67]. More recently, Forsgren [4] reported
extremely small percentages of orally administered tocopherol in lymph
from the thoracic duct of patients with biliary obstruction. More detailed
experiments demonstrated that bile salts as well as pancreatic juice are
necessary for the transfer of tocopherol from the intestinal mucosa for the
lacteals [8]. As shown in Table 2, when both bile and pancreatic juice
flowed normally into the duodenum, more than 10% of the administered
radioactivity appeared in the lymph during the 12 hr following gastric
intubation. Essentially, the same results were obtained when whole bile
was substituted by a sodium taurocholate solution. Only neligibile amounts
of radioactivity were detected in the thoracic duct lymph when the mixed
secretion of bile and pancreatic juice were diverted from the intestine.
The infusion of either pancreatic juice or bile, separately, resulted in a
better absorption than that observed when the two secretions were absent
from the intestine (Table 2). Nevertheless, absorption was poorer than
that obtained when the two secretions were both present in the intestinal
lumen. Using an in vitro system, Akerib and Sterner [12] confirmed that
the transfer of vitamin E by the intestinal mucosal cell is dependent upon
the presence of bile salts in the medium. In vivo experiments reported by
Mac Mahon et al. [13, 68] have also confirmed the necessity of bile for
tocopherol absorption.

Thus, a normal flow of bile and pancreatic juice in some manner
creates conditions—perhaps through pancreatic lipase or other digestive

TABLE 2   Effect of Bile and Pancreatic Juice on the Lymphatic Appearance of Vitamin E

Secretion in duodenum		Percent of administered radioactivity[a]
Biliary + pancreatic	Present	> 10.0
	Absent	< 0.1
Only pancreatic		1.5
Only biliary		1.3

[a] Cumulative percentage recovered in the lymph in the 12 hr following
intragastric administration of an emulsion containing radiotocopheryl
acetate.

Source: From Gallo-Torres [19].

enzymes—essential for the hydrolysis in vivo and in vitro of vitamin E esters. The proposition that bile salts solutions dissolve α-tocopherol [8,9,15,19] was recently confirmed [24,69]. The ability of bile salt solutions to dissolve vitamin E would be merely a reflection of their detergent properties [50,68-71]. Above a critical concentration, bile salt molecules aggregate to form micelles [71,72]. These polymolecular aggregates behave like macromolecules with respect to osmotic activity, dialysis, or sedimentation. Bile salts alone form micelles which, however, are stabilized by phospholipids. These amphiphilic compounds are arranged so as to form an ionic surface inside which there is a lipid-like droplet capable of dissolving truly lipophilic compounds, such as tocopherol. Definite differences appear to exist among several species of animals with regards to bile acid composition; it is not unlikely that these differences could explain the differences in absorption of vitamin E among several species.

F. Effect of Other Dietary Lipids

Schmandke and Schmidt [38] measured the concentration of liver tocopherol 24 hr after the oral administration of 2 mg of dl-α-tocopherol in either 0.5 ml neat's-foot oil or in 0.5 ml of an aqueous 3% solution of Tween-80. They concluded that the vitamin is twice as well absorbed from orally administered aqueous solution as compared to oily solutions. Other studies have lended support to this conclusion. Of great importance is the microenvironment in which tocopherol finds itself before uptake into the intestinal mucosa. It has been established that certain dietary polyunsaturated fatty acids (PUFA) interact with vitamin E, especially in the intestine [15,73-76]. This is of practical importance because the dietary levels of PUFA, especially arachidonic and linoleic acid may be the principal determinants of the requirement of vitamin E in humans [77,78]. In lymph cannulated rats, it was demonstrated that intragastrically administered glycerides (either mono- or triolein) stimulate absorption of vitamin E to a greater degree than an equivalent amount of unsaturated fatty acid. As shown in Table 3, increase of the linoleic acid content in the emulsion led to a comparative decrease in the absorption of tocopherol to such a point that only 7% was absorbed when the emulsion contained 32% of the fatty acid. The finding that high concentrations of PUFA in the lumen lead to a decreased absorption of vitamin E was traced to a depression of intestinal uptake [12]. Alderson et al. [14] provided further demonstration of the reduction of vitamin E absorption by PUFA. These investigators evaluated the effects of corn oil on the preintestinal disappearance of tocopherol in abomasal fistulated steers. The percentage disappearance, as estimated from changes in the ratio of tocopherol to the marker chromic oxide when the animals received the corn oil ration, was 23.4%, a figure significantly lower than the value of 36.4% recorded with the control animals.

TABLE 3   Effect of Increasing Amounts of Lipids on the Lymphatic Appearance of Vitamin E

Emulsifying agent	Percent of lipid in the emulsion	Percentage of administered dose recovered in the lymph[a]
Linoleic acid	4	10
	16	12
	32	7
Monoolein	4	11
	16	18
	32	23
Triolein	4	12
	16	17
	32	25

[a] These rounded-off figures represent average values obtained in the lymph collected during the 12 hr following intragastric administration of tocopheryl acetate.

Source: From Gallo-Torres [19].

Other factors seem to facilitate tocopherol absorption from the intestine, and recently, evidence has been presented [20] that the chain length of the triglyceride could greatly affect the interaction of its hydrolytic products with the bile salt solution in the intestinal contents (Table 4). This would affect the concentration of tocopherol in its micellar phase and its subsequent uptake and absorption. As shown in Figures 3-5, the absorption of tocopherol is enhanced by solubilization in medium-chain triglycerides as compared to long-chain triglycerides. Absorption does not occur through the portal vein (Table 5) [20]. It is generally accepted that the absorption of tocopherol is more efficient when fat, i.e., glycerides or phospholipids, is included in the diet [77-80]. However, some reports appear to contradict this concept. Thus, Panos et al. [81], as well as Barness et al. [82], observed rapid response to daily doses of 25-50 mg of vitamin E in premature infants fed a fat-free diet for 6 weeks. These findings suggest that, in the immature gut, the absorption of tocopherol is less dependent upon the intraluminal presence of lipids than in the fully developed intestine.

TABLE 4   Radioactivity in Systemic Blood 4 hr after the Administration of 40 μCi (or 4.0 μg) d-α-[5-methyl-^{3}H] Tocopherol in Triglycerides of Different Chain Length

Long-chain triglyceride			Medium-chain triglyceride		
Rat no.	Body wt (g)	dpm x 10^6	Rat no.	Body wt (g)	dpm x 10^6
1	242	6.2[a]	11	240	6.9[a]
2	230	5.1	12	230	5.7
3	234	6.7	13	234	7.4
4	236	7.3	14	232	7.9
5	228	4.8	15	228	5.8
6	218	2.1	16	218	5.4
7	218	4.5	17	218	7.9
8	212	5.3	18	200	6.6
		5.2 ± 1.6[b]			6.7 ± 1.0[b]

[a] Rounded figures; value calculated for the whole animal, assuming that in the rat, blood represents 6% of the body weight [24].
[b] Mean ± SEM. The two means are significantly different by Student's t-test (P = 0.01).

III. INTESTINAL TRANSPORT

Few reports have been concerned with the molecular events taking place during the uptake and transport of vitamin E. Using perfused intestines of golden hamsters [83], Akerib and Sterner [12] confirmed that vitamin E transport is dependent upon the presence of bile salts. Also confirmed was the fact that the presence of unsaturated fatty acids significantly reduces the amount of vitamin E that can be transported through the intestinal barrier. Making use of rat small intestinal slices, Pearson and Legge [17] demonstrated that the uptake of α-tocopherol was greatly reduced in the absence of a micellar phase, thereby confirming suggestions resulting from work using in vivo preparations [8, 68]. More recent

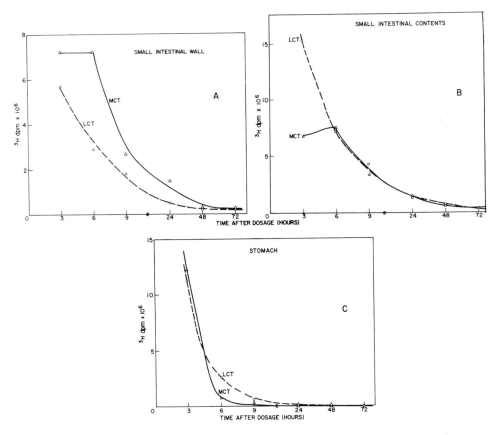

FIG. 3   A.   The influence of the chain length of solubilizing triglyceride
on the appearance of radioactivity in the wall of the small intestine of rats
after administration of a trace dose (2 μg) of d-α-[5-methyl-^{3}H]-tocopherol.
B.   Total radioactivity remaining in the lumen of the small intestine of rats
after the administration of ^{3}H-radiovitamin E in an emulsion containing
either a long or a medium-chain triglyceride.   C.   The effect of triglycerides of different chain length on the disappearance of ^{3}H-α-tocopherol
from the stomach of rats.   (From Brin and Gallo-Torres, ref. 20.)

investigations with the use of everted small intestinal sacs [24] from rats
have suggested that the rate of absorption of vitamin E by the medial portion of the small bowel was significantly higher than the rate of absorption
of tocopherol by the proximal and distal small bowel segments (Fig. 6).
These results are in complete agreement with the previously mentioned

observations that the region of greatest uptake is at the junction of the upper and middle thirds of the small gut [60]. In experiments in vitro, the rate of absorption of vitamin E followed a linear relationship to the concentration. Saturation kinetics were not observed in these experiments. Further, the rate of absorption of α-tocopherol by the various regions of the small bowel did not change significantly with the addition of metabolic inhibitors and uncouplers as compared to baseline experiments. These experimental results suggest that the transport of α-tocopherol by the gut may take place by nonsaturable passive diffusion processes which are not carrier mediated, that is, they are not dependent on energy.

IV. OVERALL PROCESS OF INTESTINAL ABSORPTION

The digestion-absorption of dietary vitamin E (either in its free or in its esterified form) requires the normal functioning of the pancreas and of the GI tract, as well as adequate secretion of bile. The extent of hydrolysis of different α-tocopheryl esters seems to depend upon their chemical structure. It would appear that hydrolysis is not a prerequisite for the absorption of vitamin E esters [86], although digestion of tocopheryl esters

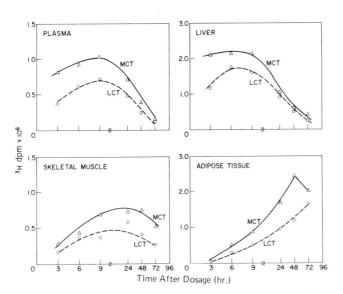

FIG. 4   Distribution of radioactivity in the tissues of rats after single administration of ^{3}H-α-tocopherol in an emulsion containing either MCT (Δ) or LCT (O). (From Brin and Gallo-Torres, ref. 20.)

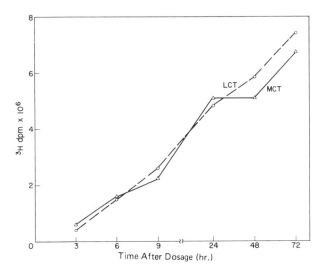

FIG. 5   Excretion of ^{3}H-radioactivity in the urine of rats after administration of vitamin E in an emulsion containing triglycerides of different
chain length. (From Brin and Gallo-Torres, ref. 20.)

certainly improves absorption. Bile salts and phospholipids efficiently
solubilize tocopherol by the formation of micelles. Pancreatic enzymes,
perhaps through a lipase, efficiently hydrolyze esters of vitamin E, and
the main product of hydrolysis is free tocopherol. The first stage of normal vitamin E absorption represents a partition between a luminal
phospholipid-bile salt mixed-micellar phase and the lipid phase of the
epithelial cell. Thus, intraluminal microenvironment is of paramount
importance to determine uptake and ultimate absorption of liposoluble
vitamins. When tocopherol is absorbed, it first leaves the intestinal lumen
and penetrates the gut mucosal cell through the brush border. Information
is not available as to whether only tocopherol is taken up or if the intestine
takes up the entire bile salt-phospholipid tocopherol complex. The transfer of this vitamin across the epithelial cell may require several stages,
most of them poorly understood, although they may involve diffusion processes. Unesterified vitamin E is probably absorbed by a process in
which the tocopherol presented to the luminal side of the intestinal mucosal
cell readily displaces a similar molecule already present in the lipoproteins
of the cell membrane and thereby penetrates the cell. The vitamin subsequently leaves the other side of the cell, enters the fluid of the lamina
propria, and from this penetrates the lymphatic capillaries to be carried
away from the intestine via the chylomicrons.

The suggestion that small amounts of tocopherol may be transported from the intestine via the portal vein was based on indirect evidence and has not been properly substantiated. However, in birds, the vitamin and its esters are absorbed entirely by the portal route. No compartmentalization seems to exist in the chicken with regard to absorption of lipid-like materials between portal blood vessels and lymphatic vessels. But these two routes of absorption are well differentiated in mammals [82] and tocopherol is absorbed primarily, if not solely, through lymphatic pathways. Recent studies indicate that lymphatic absorption of α-tocopherol parallels that of free cholesterol irrespective of infusion media at the time of maximum absorption [23]. Although these two substances are absorbed into the lymph at the same rate, they are distributed differently into the lymph VLDL. The lipoproteins of the intestinal mucosal and liver cytosol seem to be identical with VLDL of serum [21]. In lymph, free cholesterol is associated more closely with polar VLDL constituents and is partitioned more like the phospholipids than the nonpolar triglycerides and cholesterol esters. Tocopherol, on the other hand, is partitioned more like the triglycerides and cholesterol esters, the nonpolar constituents of the lymph VLDL. This suggests that free cholesterol is localized more to the surface of the VLDL, while tocopherol is distributed throughout the particle with the majority located in the core of the VLDL. The observed lower vitamin E absorption with PUFA may be due to the fact that unsaturated fatty acids have greater space-occupying requirements on VLDL than saturated fats. This would leave less room for other lipid materials such as tocopherol on the carrier lipoproteins [84]. However, further investigations are necessary to clarify these concepts.

TABLE 5   Ratios of Portal/Systemic (P/S) Radioactivity in the Blood of Rats Given d-α-[5-methyl-^{3}H] Tocopherol in Either Medium or Long-Chain Triglycerides

Minutes after stomach intubation (solubilizing triglyceride appears in parenthesis)	P/S ratio
67 (MCT)[a]	0.68
73 (LCT)	0.90
78 (LCT)	0.63
87 (MCT)	0.88
94 (LCT)	0.86
100 (MCT)	0.99

[a] MCT = medium-chain triglyceride; LCT = long-chain triglyceride.

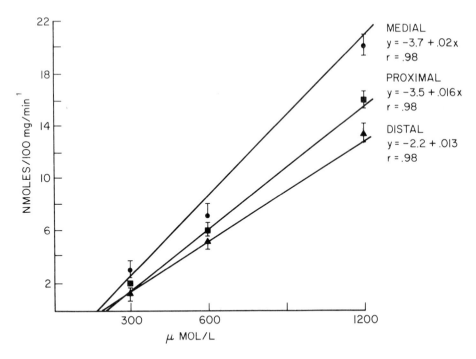

FIG. 6   Transport rate of α-tocopherol in the face of incremental increases of the concentration of the vitamin in the incubation solution.
Everted rat small bowel sacs were incubated in a micellar medium, and
transport rates were measured at incubation solution concentrations of
α-tocopherol of 300, 600, and 1200 μM.   The mean rate of transport of
vitamin E at each concentration was calculated and plotted against the
incubation solution concentration of tocopherol.   The transport rate of the
vitamin followed a linear relationship to the concentration in the incubation medium.   The lack of saturation kinetics observed in this range of
concentrations suggests that transport of vitamin E takes place by a passive noncarrier-mediated diffusion process.   (From Hollander et al.
ref. 24.)

V. SUMMARY

    1. Our present understanding is that in mammals α-tocopherol
absorption takes place mainly through lymphatic pathways where it is
transported as part of a lipoprotein complex.

2. Tocopheryl esters are predominantly hydrolyzed in the gut lumen. Little absorption of vitamin E esters occurs. Although hydrolysis is not a prerequisite for the absorption of tocopheryl esters, it certainly improves absorption.

3. The available information indicates that the efficiency of absorption of tocopherol and/or its esters is relatively poor (20-40%, depending upon the dose fed and the experimental conditions). More information seems desirable on the quantitative aspects of vitamin E absorption in animals as well as in humans.

4. Both biliary and pancreatic secretions are essential for adequate absorption of vitamin E. This information is of practical importance because the lack of either bile or pancreatic flow resulting from either disease processes or poor dietary stimulation would tend to reduce absorption. Absorption is probably maximal when vitamin E is consumed with other lipid-containing foods.

5. Vitamin E is better absorbed from orally administered aqueous solutions than oily solutions. Long-chain triglycerides stimulate absorption to a greater degree than an equivalent amount of unsaturated free fatty acids. Absorption is in turn enhanced by solubilization in medium-chain triglycerides. Linoleic acid, a polyunsaturated fatty acid, decreases the absorption of vitamin E. Thus, the absorption of tocopherol is intimately related to the simultaneous digestion and absorption of dietary lipids.

6. The intimate mechanism of tocopherol absorption is poorly understood. Intestinal transport may occur through a passive diffusion process.

7. Data are needed on the interrelations, during the process of absorption, between vitamin E and other nutrients such as vitamin A, carotinoids, ascorbic acid, vitamin K and isoprenoid-containing substances, and cholesterol.

REFERENCES

1. S. Krishnamurthy and J. G. Bieri, J. Lipid Res. $\underline{4}$:330 (1963).
2. I. D. Desai, C. K. Pareth, and M. L. Scott, Biochim. Biophys. Acta $\underline{100}$:280 (1965).
3. R. Blomstrand and L. Forsgren, Int. J. Vit. Nutr. Res. $\underline{38}$:328 (1968).
4. L. Forsgren, Acta Chir. Scand. (Suppl.) 399 (1969).
5. W. J. Pudelkiewicz and N. Mary, J. Nutr. $\underline{97}$:303 (1969).
6. J. Kelleher, T. Davis, and M. S. Losowsky, Biochem. J. $\underline{114}$:74P (1969).
7. C. K. Pearson and M. McC. Barnes, Int. J. Vit. Nutr. Res. $\underline{40}$:19 (1970).

8. H. E. Gallo-Torres, Lipids 5:379 (1970).
9. H. E. Gallo-Torres, Int. J. Vit. Nutr. Res. 40:505 (1970).
10. C. K. Pearson and M. McC. Barnes, Br. J. Nutr. 24:581 (1970).
11. J. Kelleher and M. S. Losowsky, Br. J. Nutr. 24:1033 (1970).
12. M. Akerib and W. Sterner, Int. J. Vit. Nutr. Res. 41:42 (1971).
13. M. T. Mac Mahon, G. Neale, and G. R. Thompson, Eur. J. Clin.
    Invest. 1:288 (1971).
14. N. E. Alderson, G. E. Mitchell, Jr., C. O. Little, R. E. Warner,
    and R. E. Tucker, J. Nutr. 101:655 (1971).
15. H. E. Gallo-Torres, F. Weber, and O. Wiss, Int. J. Vit. Nutr.
    Res. 41:504 (1971).
16. I. R. Peake, H. G. Windmueller, and J. G. Bieri, Biochim. Biophys.
    Acta 260:679 (1972).
17. C. K. Pearson and A. M. Legge, Biochim. Biophys. Acta 288:404
    (1972).
18. T. Davies, J. Kelleher, C. L. Smith, B. E. Walker, and M. S.
    Losowsky, J. Lab. Clin. Med. 79:824 (1972).
19. H. E. Gallo-Torres, Acta Agric. Scand. (Suppl.) 19:97 (1973).
20. M. Brin and H. E. Gallo-Torres, Fed. Proc. 33:671 (1974).
21. O. V. Rajaram, P. Fatterpaker, and A. Sreenivasan, Biochem. J.
    140:509 (1974).
22. D. P. R. Mueller, J. T. Harries, and J. K. Lloyd, Gut 15:966
    (1974).
23. L. K. Bjornson and H. E. Gallo-Torres, Fed. Proc. 34:913 (1975).
24. D. Hollander, E. Rim, and K. S. Muralidhara, Gastroenterology
    68:1492 (1975).
25. H. M. Nitowsky, M. Cornbath, and H. H. Gordon, Amer. J. Dis.
    Child. 92:164 (1956).
26. H. Braunstein, Gastroenterology 40:224 (1961).
27. H. J. Binder, D. C. Herting, V. Hurst, S. C. Finch, and H. M.
    Spiro, Engl. J. Med. 273:1289 (1965).
28. M. S. Losowsky and P. J. Leonard, Gut 8:539 (1967).
29. M. T. Mac Mahon and G. Neale, Clin. Sci. 38:197 (1970).
30. J. T. Harries and D. P. R. Mueller, Arch. Dis. Child. 46:341 (1971).
31. J. T. Harries and D. P. R. Mueller, Gut 12:579 (1971).
32. M. S. Losowsky, B. E. Walker, and J. Kelleher, Nutrition in
    steatorrhea, in Malabsorption in Clinical Practice, London,
    Churchill Livingstone, 1974, pp. 56-57.
33. S. Gross and D. K. Melhorn, J. Pediatr. 85:753 (1974).
34. J. D. Greaves and C. L. A. Schmidt, Proc. Soc. Exp. Biol. Med.
    37:40 (1937).
35. G. Klatskin and D. W. Molander, J. Clin. Invest. 31:159 (1952).
36. H. Rosenkrantz, A. T. Milhorat, and M. Farber, Metabolism 2:556
    (1953).

37. J. Pomeranze and R. J. Lucarello, J. Lab. Clin. Med. 42:700 (1956).
38. H. Schmandke and G. Schmidt, Int. J. Vit. Nutr. Res. 35:138 (1965).
39. M. F. Sorrell, O. Frank, A. D. Thomson, H. Aquino, and H. Baker, Nutr. Rep. Int. 3:143 (1971).
40. J. G. Bieri and R. H. Poukka Evarts, Proc. Soc. Exp. Biol. Med. 140:1162 (1972).
41. U. Gloor, J. Würsch, U. Schwieter, and O. Wiss, Helv. Chim. Acta 49:2303 (1966).
42. I. R. Peake and J. G. Bieri, J. Nutr. 101:1615 (1971).
43. H. E. Gallo-Torres, unpublished work (1979).
44. K. Y. Lee, D. M. Hurley, and W. J. Simmonds, Bioch. Biophys. Acta 337:214 (1974).
45. R. J. Levin, Brit. Med. Bull. 23:209 (1967).
46. S. Bennett-Clark, J. Lipid Res. 12:43 (1971).
47. C. Sylvén, Biochim. Biophys. Acta 203:365 (1970).
48. R. Blomstrand and J. Gurtler, Int. J. Vit. Nutr. Res. 41:189 (1971).
49. H. E. Gallo-Torres and O. N. Miller, Proc. Soc. Exp. Biol. Med. 130:552 (1969).
49a. H. E. Gallo-Torres, O. N. Miller, and J. G. Hamilton, Biochim. Biophys. Acta 176:605 (1969).
50. H. E. Gallo-Torres, O. N. Miller, and J. G. Hamilton, Arch. Biochem. Biophys. 143:22 (1971).
51. P. Johnson and W. F. R. Pover, Life Sci. 4:115 (1962).
52. B. Werner, Acta Chir. Scand. (Suppl.) 355 (1965).
53. D. L. Yeung and M. J. Veen-Baigent, Can. J. Pharmacol. 753 (1972).
54. D. Schachter, J. D. Finkelstein, and S. Kowarski, J. Clin. Invest. 43:787 (1964).
55. R. Blomstrand and L. Forsgren, Acta Chem. Scand. 21:1662 (1967).
56. N. H. Bell and P. Bryan, Amer. J. Clin. Nutr. 22:425 (1969).
57. R. Blomstrand and L. Forsgren, Acta Chem. Scand. 21:1662 (1967). (1968).
58. M. J. Shearer, A. Mc Burney, and P. Barkhan, Vitamin K: Studies on the absorption and metabolism of Phylloquinone (vitamin K$_1$) in man, in International Symposium on Fat-Soluble Vitamins, Section IV, New York, Academic, 1974, pp. 513-542.
59. J. Stenberg and E. Pascoe-Dawson, Can. Med. Assoc. J. 80:266 (1959).
60. H. E. Gallo-Torres, unpublished work (1979).
61. M. Hidiroglou and K. J. Jenkis, Ann. Biol. Anim. Bioch. Biophys. 14:667 (1974).

62. S. A. Hashim and G. R. Schuttringer, Amer. J. Clin. Nutr. 19:137 (1966).

63. G. Klatskin and D. W. Molander, J. Lab. Clin. Med. 39:802 (1952).

64. E. J. Simon, C. S. Gross, and A. T. Milhorat, J. Biol. Chem. 221:797 (1956).

65. M. Y. Dju, M. L. Quaife, and P. L. Harris, Amer. J. Physiol. 160:259 (1950).

66. W. J. Pudelkiewicz and L. D. Matterson, J. Nutr. 71:143 (1960).

67. K. M. Brinkhous and E. D. Warner, Amer. J. Pathol. 17:81 (1941).

68. M. T. Mac Mahon and G. R. Thompson, Eur. J. Clin. Invest. 1:161 (1970).

69. Y. I. Takahashi and B. A. Underwood, Lipids 9:855 (1974).

70. A. F. Hofmann, Biochem. J. 89:57 (1963).

71. A. F. Hofmann and D. Small, Ann. Rev. Med. 18:333 (1967).

72. A. F. Hofmann and B. Borgström, J. Clin. Invest. 43:247 (1964); A. F. Hofmann, Gastroenterology 50:56 (1966).

73. F. Weber, U. Gloor, and O. Wiss, Fet. Seif. Anstrichmittel. 64:1149 (1962).

74. F. Weber and O. Wiss, Helv. Physiol. Pharm. Acta 21:131 (1963).

75. F. Weber, H. Weiser, and O. Wiss, Z. Ernahrungs. 4:245 (1964).

76. O. Wiss and F. Weber, Z. Ernahrungs. (Suppl.) 4:152 (1965).

77. H. Dam, J. Nutr. 28:297 (1944).

78. M. K. Horwitt, Interrelations between vitamin E and polyunsaturated fatty acids in man, in Vitamins and Hormones, Vol. 30, New York, Academic, 1962, pp. 541-558.

79. H. Patrick and C. L. Morgan, Science 98:434 (1943).

80. A. Scharf and C. A. Slanetz, Proc. Soc. Exp. Biol. Med. 57:159 (1944).

81. T. C. Panos, B. Stinnett, G. Zapata, J. Eminias, B. V. Marasigan, and A. G. Beard, Amer. J. Clin. Nutr. 21:15 (1968).

82. L. A. Barness, F. A. Oski, M. L. Williams, G. Morrow, III, and S. B. Arnaud, Amer. J. Clin. Nutr. 21:40 (1968).

83. R. Schneider, K. Burdett, and W. F. R. Pover, Life Sci. 8:123 (1969).

84. G. B. J. Glass, Routes for absorption, in Introduction to Gastrointestinal Physiology, Englewood Cliffs, N. J., Prentice-Hall, 1968, p. 146.

85. N. Spritz and M. A. Mishkel, J. Clin. Invest. 48:78 (1969).

86. T. Nakamura, Y. Aoyama, T. Fujita, and G. Katsui, Lipids 10:627 (1975).

Part 5B/ Transport and Metabolism

HUGO E. GALLO-TORRES

Hoffmann-La Roche Inc.
Nutley, New Jersey

	I.	Introduction	193
	II.	Transport from Lymph to Blood	194
	III.	Tissue Distribution	197
		A. Significance of Plasma Tocopherol Concentration	197
		B. Tocopherol in the RBC	200
		C. Tocopherol Content of Human Tissues	201
		D. Distribution in Animal Tissues	203
		E. Distribution in Organs After Oral Administration	206
		F. Relationship of Tissue Uptake to Oral Dose	213
		G. Distribution After Parenteral Administration	214
	IV.	Mobilization	226
	V.	Metabolism	231
		A. Chemical Reactions	231
		B. Occurrence of α-Tocopherol Metabolites In Vivo and In Vitro	237
	VI.	Excretion	250
		A. Excretion in Urine, Feces, and Skin	250
		B. Biliary Excretion	250
	VII.	Overall Metabolism of Vitamin E	252
	VIII.	Summary	256
		References	257

I. INTRODUCTION

The topic of tocopherol absorption was discussed in detail in Part 5A. The present discussion will address itself to lymphatic and plasmatic transport, tissue uptake, distribution, storage, mobilization, metabolism, and excretion of the vitamin. As discussed further on, a number of factors other than absorption from the intestine may influence blood levels of vitamin E. Accordingly, "appearance in the blood" seems a more accurate term than "absorption" to describe blood levels of vitamin E after its oral administration.

In general, this text has been restricted to established observations which have been made in more than one laboratory. However, certain new results, some of which may not have been yet confirmed at the time of writing are also included. The reader is asked to bear in mind the tentative nature of this material, included for the purpose of providing a comprehensive survey of the literature presently available. For additional information about various aspects of vitamin E bioavailability, the reader is referred to excellent monographs by Mason in 1949 and 1954 [1,2], Wiss et al. in 1962 [3], Roels in 1967 [4], and the more recent, excellent review by Draper in 1970 [5]. Reports on international symposia have also appeared [6-11].

II. TRANSPORT FROM LYMPH TO BLOOD

Vitamin E passes as the free tocopherol from the gut wall to the systemic circulation via the lymphatic system (see Part 5A). The transfer from intestinal cell to lymph occurs simultaneously by at least two processes: the concomitant transfer of dietary lipids and the formation of the lipid-carrying particle that appears in the lymph; the latter involves the synthesis of proteins. Vitamin E circulates in the lymph as tocopherol bound to nonspecific lipoproteins, and it is distributed according to the fat composition of each fraction. The reesterification of fatty acids back to triglycerides and of cholesterol back to cholesterol esters are also processes which accompany the extrusion of vitamin E into the lacteals. In the rat, various dietary fats may have different effects upon the size and distribution of lymph particles [12]. In a human subject studied by Blomstrand and Forsgren [13], the chylomicrons, isolated from pooled samples representing the main peak of the absorbed radioactivity, contained about 77% of the chromatographed radioactivity after the oral administration of labeled tocopheryl acetate.

Further elucidation of the distribution of α-tocopherol within the lymph very low-density lipoproteins (VLDL) was done in animals with catheterized abdominal thoracic ducts [14]. Rats were infused with either saline or a liquid diet containing corn oil. On the day after surgery, the animals were given a single, oral dose of emulsion containing proteins, carbohydrates, triolein, and 100 μg of [5-methyl-^{3}H] d-α-tocopherol. Perfusion with saline or corn oil was continued, and lymph samples were collected each hour for 20-50 hr. On agarose gel electrophoresis (Fig. 1),

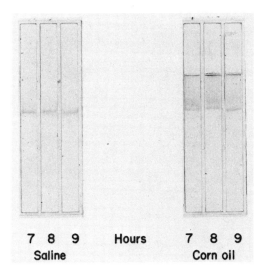

7 8 9   Hours   7 8 9
Saline   **Corn oil**

FIG. 1   Agarose gel electrophoresis of lymph lipoproteins in rats infused either with saline or corn oil.

rat lymph from saline-infused rats showed one major lipoprotein band with a mobility similar to that of rat plasma VLDL, while rat lymph from corn oil-infused rats showed the VLDL band plus a large chylomicron band which remained at the origin of the gel. Examination of the distribution of α-tocopherol within the lymph VLDL was then attempted. The distribution scheme shown in Fig. 2 was used. In the schematic representation of the distribution of lipids after disruption of the lymph VLDL

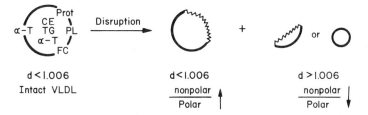

FIG. 2   Disruption scheme of lymph VLDL used to examine the distribution of tocopherol with respect to other lipids.

TABLE 1 Lipid Distribution[a] of Rat Lymph VLDL After Disruption by Repeated Freeze-Thaw Cycles and Subsequent Centrifugation

	Phospholipid	Free cholesterol	α-Tocopherol	Cholesterol esters	Triglyceride	Total cholesterol	Total lipid
d < 1.006	75	80	94	97	92	93	89
d > 1.006	25	20	6	3	8	7	11
d < 1.006	51	64	92	96	86	91	78
d > 1.006	49	36	8	4	14	9	22

[a] Percentage of the lipid on the original intact particle.

Source: From Bjornson and Gallo-Torres [14].

shown in Table 1, distribution of tocopherol is compared with that of cholesterol. It would appear that tocopherol is distributed throughout the molecule with the majority located in the core of the VLDL, while free cholesterol is localized more to the surface of the VLDL. The fact that the vitamin is distributed throughout the lipoprotein suggests that all the lipids are being protected by the antioxidant activity of tocopherol during the process of lymphatic transport. In agreement with previous work, free cholesterol and cholesterol esters partitioned differently after lymph VLDL disruption; the nonpolar cholesterol ester was located in the core of the lipoprotein, that is, at a site similar to that of free tocopherol. Consequently, free cholesterol of the lipoproteins exchanges very rapidly with the free cholesterol in the plasma membranes and other lipoproteins. On the other hand, α-tocopherol exchanges less readily than free cholesterol. Similarly, in a recent study of α-tocopherol and free cholesterol exchange between rat plasma and red blood cells (RBC), high-density lipoprotein (HDL) and RBC, and VLDL and RBC it was also demonstrated that in all cases α-tocopherol exchanged less rapidly than free cholesterol [15]. These findings suggest that tocopherol would alter cell membrane systems less rapidly than cholesterol.

The lymph lipoproteins carry tocopherol to the general circulation from which the vitamin is taken up by the liver and virtually all extrahepatic tissues.

III. TISSUE DISTRIBUTION

A. Significance of Plasma Tocopherol Concentration

A number of studies have demonstrated that orally administered vitamin E appears rapidly in plasma and tissues [3, 16-35]. Plasma levels depend upon the interplay of a number of factors, such as the concentration of triglycerides, phospholipids, cholesterol and lipoprotein carriers, rate of removal from the plasma, and retention rates in individual tissues [36]. The values in plasma and other tissues also depend on the sensitivity and specificity of the chosen analytical method. Many reports on plasma tocopherols have made use of the molecular distillation-Florex chromatography method of Quaife and Harris [37]. This procedure, based on the Emmerie-Engel color reaction has been repeatedly modified [38-42]. It has the disadvantage of nonspecificity; frequently, total reducing substances are measured rather than α-tocopherol specifically. Correction is required for carotenes and polyunsaturated fatty acids which tend to reduce the color formation. As a result, many literature values for the concentration of tocopherol in plasma and tissues overestimated the actual content and must, therefore, be cautiously interpreted [43-53].

One of the most reliable methods to study tissue distribution of vitamin E is the determination of specific radioactivity in tissues and fluids after administration of labeled compounds. It has been repeatedly suggested that expressing vitamin E content as milligrams of tocopherol per gram of fat is a better index than using the customary milligrams per gram of fresh tissue. Additional valuable information on the distribution of the vitamin may be obtained by macro- or microradioautography (see Sec. G.2).

Transport of tocopherol in plasma is similar to its lymphatic transport and is associated with lipoproteins [54-63]. Most investigations indicate that there is no specific lipoprotein carrier of the vitamin in the plasma (or other tissues), although this concept has been recently questioned [64, 65]. Determinations of the concentrations of α-tocopherol, LDL, cholesterol, and the distribution of the vitamin between LDL and HDL were carried out by Davies et al. [59] on the sera of fasted normal subjects and hospital in-patients with a wide variety of clinical conditions. These studies confirmed the correlation between α-tocopherol and cholesterol concentrations (r = 0.587). A very close correlation (r = 0.925) was shown between the total serum α-tocopherol and that portion carried by the LDL which, under fasting conditions, transports the major part of the serum vitamin E. A lower correlation (r = 0.527) was seen between the total α-tocopherol and that carried by the HDL, which is the minor portion of the total. Oral administration of α-tocopheryl acetate to normal subjects produced large increases in the serum levels of α-tocopherol but did not affect concentrations of LDL tocopherol. These studies emphasize the importance of determining the concentration of LDL to obtain an accurate dynamic picture of the levels of α-tocopherol in the serum.

Distinct differences were recently observed by Bjornson et al. [66] between the plasma transport of tocopherol and carotene. They determined the concentrations and distributions of major lipids (triglycerides, phospholipids, cholesterol), tocopherol, and carotenoids in the plasma lipoprotein fractions (VLDL, LDL, and HDL) or normal human subjects, patients with hypolipoproteinemia, and patients with erythropoietic protoporphyria treated with oral α-tocopherol and/or β-carotene. In general, the percent distribution of tocopherol was most closely correlated with the distribution of total lipids in the individual lipoproteins, while the major portion of β-carotene was present in the LDL, irrespective of the lipid distribution in the lipoproteins. In further evaluations, the α-tocopherol and β-carotene concentrations of plasma and RBC in·patients treated with tocopherol and carotene were determined regularly for a 1-year period. Plasma and RBC tocopherol concentrations exhibited a rapid, parallel increase in response to tocopherol supplementation. On the other hand, the plasma and RBC carotene concentrations showed a much slower and nonparallel increase in response to carotene administration. When carotene supplementation was stopped, the elevated carotene levels in both plasma and RBC persisted for several months. The elevated plasma carotene level persisted longer than the raised RBC carotene levels. These results strongly suggest that α-tocopherol and β-carotene are transported differently in the peripheral circulation and that these compounds differ markedly in their tissue storage and mobilization.

Another example of the close correlation between α-tocopherol and lipoproteins is provided by patients with a-β-lipoproteinemia, a condition in which chylomicron formation is blocked and the major carrier protein is absent from the serum. In children who have not been treated, vitamin E cannot be detected in the serum and red cell hemolysis is considerably raised [67].

Changes in the concentration of plasma tocopherol depend upon a variety of factors [23, 26, 29, 32-34, 58, 68-96], such as age and pregnancy, whether the sample is taken during fasting or at different times after feeding, and the nutritional status (e.g., protein deficiency) of the subject. Certain evidence suggests that plasma vitamin E levels rise during pregnancy [97-101]. This information is of importance because of the possible role of vitamin E deficiency in the etiology of disorders of the newborn. Many workers have reported very low blood levels, especially in premature infants [102-104]. The time taken to attain normal adult levels is short in infants who are breast-fed, but longer time is required for those on artificial milk feeding [100, 101, 105-107].

Experiments designed to clarify whether or not the vitamin E status of infants at birth is related to that of the mother have not yielded uniform results. Straumfjord and Quaife [98] concluded that there was no correlation between the levels in the plasma of the mother and infant. Minkowski et al. [108] reported that the plasma level of the infant at birth could be influenced by injecting vitamin E into the mother prior to delivery. In another study by Leonard et al. [89], it was shown that as the plasma vitamin E level in the mothers increased, there was an increase in the plasma level in the infants. Thus, although tocopherol is a substance that crosses the placental barrier with difficulty [109], the maternal vitamin E levels during pregnancy can nevertheless influence the vitamin E levels in fetus.

The most important factor influencing the plasma vitamin E concentration appears to be the content of total lipid (triglycerides, cholesterol, and phospholipids), as well as β-lipoprotein carrier of the plasma. In normal subjects the plasma tocopherol level increases progressively from the third to the seventh decade, irrespective of sex [88]. Hoppner et al. [85] conducted a survey of serum tocopherol levels of 125 Canadians and found the mean serum tocopherol level to be 1.29 ± 0.34 mg/100 ml (range 0.70-2.5 mg/100 ml); serum tocopherol levels of subjects 25 years old and younger were significantly lower than those over 25 years of age. In another study [61] comprising 815 healthy adults, a highly significant correlation was found between the tocopherol content of plasma and the

β-lipoprotein content of serum. These correlations have been recently confirmed [110]. Plasma vitamin E levels that exceed the usual averages have been observed in hypothyroidism [111], diabetes mellitus [112], hypercholesterolemia [88], and heart disease [113]. These conditions are usually associated with high serum lipids.

The vitamin E tolerance test has been found to be abnormal in diseases associated with malabsorption [35]. This test may give more information than fasting vitamin E levels alone. In conditions associated with low serum lipids, low plasma tocopherol levels have been found. These conditions include certain liver diseases [114], a-β-lipoproteinemia [32,67], protein malnutrition [115], cystic fibrosis [32,67,75], and other gastrointestinal disorders [34,90,116]. The low concentration of vitamin E in plasma is usually associated with an increased susceptibility of erythrocytes to oxidative hemolysis.

Serum tocopherol levels decreased with hypolipidemic treatment (clofibrate) and returned to high values when therapy was discontinued [78]. This may be of practical importance in cardiovascular diseases [117-130]. In a recent study [62], the use of oral contraceptives resulted in a slightly increased plasma cholesterol level (by approximately 7%) and a decreased plasma tocopherol level as well as β-lipoproteins (by approximately 20%). Thus, the usual high correlation which exists between vitamin E and β-lipoproteins is less evident as a result of oral contraceptive administration.

B. Tocopherol in the RBC

As previously mentioned, vitamin E is also transported in the erythrocyte [86]. Silber et al. [131] showed that, in the rat erythrocyte, uptake and efflux are independent of energy, but sensitive to temperature. The vitamin is localized to the cell membrane [63]. Rapid exchange between erythrocytes and plasma appears to take place, with an hourly fraction tocopherol efflux of 26%. The vitamin is transferred from the RBC to the LDL. The dynamics of vitamin E transport have been described in detail by Kayden and Bjornson [132]. In rats, the fatty acid composition of RBC lipids was not influenced by the vitamin E content and only moderately by the linoleic acid content of the diet [133]. In another report [134], the total polyunsaturated fatty acids (PUFA) of RBC from a-β-lipoproteinemic patients ranged from 31 to 42% of total fatty acids, a value lower than the 40 to 48% seen in normal subjects. The RBC from a-β-lipoproteinemic patients appeared to be capable of maintaining a normal α-tocopherol content even though the plasma level was greatly depressed. The molar ratio of α-tocopherol to PUFA in the RBC from a-β-lipoproteinemic subjects was 1:850. It would be of interest to determine the molar ratio of vitamin E to other membrane components, such as lecithin and cholesterol.

It is not clear whether the red cell vitamin E status is indicative of the vitamin E status of the other tissues in the body [134]. Oski and Barness [104] described "vitamin E deficient erythrocytes" or pyknocytes; these morphological alterations have also been reported in grossly premature infants with vitamin E deficiency [135]. Vitamin E may influence hematopoiesis [136]. Also of interest is the work of Ahkong et al. [137] who found α-tocopherol to be a mild "fusogenic" compound; that is, it has the ability to induce fusion of hen erythrocytes in vitro. However, it is not known whether the vitamin alone or in combination with other substances (such as vitamin A, lysophosphatidylcholine, or unsaturated fatty acids) is involved either directly or indirectly in membrane fusion occurring in vivo under physiological or pathological conditions. Diplock and Lucy [138] have proposed that α-tocopherol may participate in the stabilization of biological membranes by formation of specific complexes with some molecules of polyunsaturated phospholipids.

C. Tocopherol Content of Human Tissues

Determination of tocopherol content of human tissues was initially carried out with a nonspecific analytical procedure in which the colorimetric reaction depends upon the oxidation-reduction potential of the specimens. Vitamin E in human tissues was determined in two subjects by Quaife and Dju in 1949 [139] and by Mason et al. in 1952 [140,141]. Data from the latter report have been summarized in Table 2. The average level of tocopherol(s) (α, γ, δ) in 20 human fetuses (2-6 months' gestation age) analyzed in toto was 0.31 mg/100 g fresh tissue. In 10 other fetuses (3-6 months), values were 0.57 for skeletal muscle, 0.57 for liver, and 0.60 for visceral organs. The average tocopherol content of 19 placentas (2 months to term) was 0.71 g/100 g. There was no tendency for tocopherols to increase or decrease in fetal tissue or placenta. In 17 premature infants, the average tocopherol values were: lung, 0.51; skeletal muscle, 0.63; heart, 0.85; kidney, 0.87; liver, 1.14; and adipose tissue, 214 mg/100 g; corresponding values for six full-term infants were significantly lower. In one full-term stillbirth, analyzed in toto, tocopherol concentration was 0.56 mg/100 g, and total tocopherols 20.15 mg. In 16 infants (3 days to 3 years), the average tocopherol content of muscle, liver, and adipose tissue was 0.51, 0.83, and 2.41 mg/100 g, respectively. In five individuals 13-17 years of age, the corresponding values were 1.24, 1.30, and 9.25 mg/100 g. In 10 individuals 61-93 years of age, the average tocopherol levels were: liver, 0.92; heart, 1.0; skeletal muscle, 1.58; and adipose tissue, 9.92 mg/100 g. The concentration of the vitamin in pituitary, testes, and adrenals was considerable higher. These studies indicate that during early and middle adult life tocopherols increase somewhat in liver and skeletal muscle; during these periods, the vitamin

TABLE 2   The Content of Tocopherol[a] in Human Organs and Tissues, as
a Function of Age

Organ or tissue	Human fetuses (2-6 months)	Placenta (2 months to term)	Premature infants
In toto	0.3		
Skeletal muscle	0.6		0.6
Liver	0.6		1.1
Visceral organs	0.6		
Placenta (2 months to term)		0.7	
Lungs			0.5
Heart			0.9
Kidneys			0.9
Adipose tissue			
Reference	139-141	139-141	139-141

[a] Rounded figures, in milligrams of tocopherol per 100 grams of wet tissue.

increases markedly in adipose tissue. Vitamin E content in tissues from
older humans does not change when compared with those in younger people.
In 1958, the same group of investigators [142, 143] suggested that it was
best to express vitamin E levels as milligrams of tocopherol per gram of
fat rather than per gram of tissue.

In 1975, determination of tocopherol(s) by modern methods in the
tissues of three presumably normal subjects who died suddenly showed
tocopherol concentrations in liver, muscle, and adipose tissue in about the
same range as in 1949 and 1958, but concentrations in the heart were twice
as high and in the lung 3 times higher than earlier [144]. Modern methods
of analysis were also used to determine tocopherol concentrations in the
livers from 101 victims of sudden or rapid deaths from unnatural causes in
New York City [145]. In this study (see Table 2) the range of values for
α-tocopherol was similar to that of Dju et al. [139-143], but the mean value
was considerably lower, which could be due, at least in part, to the direct
determination of tocopherol by modern procedures. A steady increase with

Full-term stillbirth	Infants (3 days to 3 yr)	Children (13-17 yr)	Adults (61-93 yr)	Adults
20.2 0.6 mg/100 g				
	0.5	1.2	1.6	
	0.8	1.3	0.9	1.1
			1.0	
	2.4	9.3	9.9	
139-141	139-141	139-141	139-141	145

age was also observed in both lipid and α-tocopherol per gram of liver, but the rate of accumulation of lipid exceeded that of the vitamin. Liver concentrations did not seem to be related to ethnic background or cause of death. Table 3 summarizes the recent report by Mino and colleagues [146], who determined vitamin E in human liver extracts by means of a floridin column using the ratio of the tocopherol band area to the total scanning values of thin-layer chromatography (TLC) analysis by simultaneous densitometry. This procedure showed a steady increase in the levels of tocopherol throughout fetal life. This is possibly related to a gradual improvement of tocopherol transport across the placenta. Values after birth, but especially in adults, were higher than during fetal life.

D. Distribution in Animal Tissues

Studies in animals have confirmed that vitamin E is distributed throughout the body [25, 26, 30, 147-167]. However, some of these studies made use of

TABLE 3 Tocopherol Level in the Human Liver in Fetuses, Infants, and Adults

Age	Cause of death	Percent of densitometrically determined tocopherol band to total scanning values	Tocopherol in liver (μg/g wet wt)
Gestation			
3 mo.	Artificial interruption	53.0	1.0
	Artificial interruption	59.0	1.5
	Artificial interruption	62.5	3.0
	Average ± SD	58.1 ± 3.9	1.8 ± 0.8
4 mo.	Artificial interruption	77.5	1.7
	Artificial interruption	70.3	1.8
	Artificial interruption	65.8	3.2
	Artificial interruption	71.9	1.1
	Artificial interruption	64.1	1.8
	Artificial interruption	68.0	3.0
	Artificial interruption	75.0	1.0
	Artificial interruption	61.2	3.5
	Average ± SD	69.3 ± 5.2	2.2 ± 0.9
5 mo.	Artificial interruption	72.0	1.7
	Artificial interruption	73.2	2.0
	Artificial interruption	75.0	2.4
	Artificial interruption	62.1	3.9
	Artificial interruption	62.5	5.8
	Average ± SD	69.0 ± 5.0	3.2 ± 1.5

6 mo.	Artificial interruption	80.2	3.8
	Artificial interruption	65.6	4.3
	Artificial interruption	63.0	4.6
	Artificial interruption	59.0	4.9
	Average ± SD	66.9 ± 8.0	4.4 ± 0.4
10 mo.	Asphyxia	83.5	5.7
Afterbirth			
3 days	RDS, prematurity	91.9	6.1
4 mo.	Down, heart failure	64.0	6.4
6 mo.	Heart failure	66.7	7.4
1 yr	Heart failure	64.7	8.3
	Average ± SD	71.8 ± 11.6	7.0 ± 0.9
18 yr	Traffic accident	81.7	37.6
34 yr	Traffic accident	57.0	11.9
39 yr	Head injury	63.3	18.2
40 yr	Traffic accident	65.0	21.6
42 yr	Head injury	60.0	18.0
42 yr	Head injury	53.0	17.9
	Average ± SD	63.3 ± 9.1	20.9 ± 8.0
68 yr	Stomach cancer	74.3	16.3

Source: Adapted from Ref. 146, p. 67, by courtesy of the Vitamin Society of Japan.

nonspecific procedures such as the Emmerie-Engel colorimetric reaction, which has several disadvantages. This method does not detect minute amounts of vitamin E or its metabolites. In addition, compounds devoid of vitamin E activity may react and produce false high values. A better picture can now be obtained with the use of vitamin E radiolabeled with either ^{14}C or ^3H. Determination of radioactivity in tissues after administration of labeled tocopherols is an accurate and quantitatively reliable technique to describe organ distribution. The use of semiquantitative, macroradioautographic procedures allow quick comparisons to be made, but additional valuable information may be obtained by microradioautography, especially when used in conjunction with electron microscopy and subcellular fractionation. Finally, it is important to differentiate between experiments describing the fate of "physiological" doses of tocopherol and those in which massive ("pharmacological") doses are employed.

E. Distribution in Organs After Oral Administration

A study of the distribution of vitamin E in tissues of normal rats was carried out by administering via the intragastric route dl-α-tocopheryl-1',2'-$\left[^3H_2\right]$acetate in an emulsion containing protein, carbohydrate, and purified triolein [161]. To prevent coprophagy, the rats were confined to Bollman restraining cages and allowed to drink a 0.85% solution of NaCl ad libitum for the duration of the experiment. In agreement with findings by others [3,11,43], considerable variations were found in the concentration of radioactivity in the tissues at different times after dosing (Figs. 3 and 4). With the possible exception of the liver, all organs appear to extract labeled tocopherol from the plasma for a period of up to 48 and even 96 hr (not depicted) after administration. When expressed in terms of ^3H disintegration per minute (dpm) per gram of wet tissue, uptake was found to be lowest in skeletal muscle. Values for the heart, adipose tissue, and kidneys, although higher than the skeletal muscle, did not differ significantly from each other. A pronounced uptake was noted in the spleen. Radioactivity in the liver did not change with time but was higher than in the spleen throughout the experiment. Ovarian uptake was high, but the values for the adrenal gland were higher than those in all other tissues examined. An increasing ratio of adrenal/blood radioactivity with time was observed. Thus, 3, 6, 12, 24, and 48 hr after administration of the emulsion, the corresponding ratio was 3, 6, 12, 32, and 32. This increment with time in the adrenal/blood radioactivity ratio has been observed by other investigators such as Weber et al. [26] who showed that 24 hr after oral administration of l-α- or d-α-tocopherol to rats, the concentration of these two isomers in the adrenal gland were, respectively, 32 and 37 times higher than in the blood. These findings are also in accord with those of Mellors and Barnes [153] who demonstrated that after oral

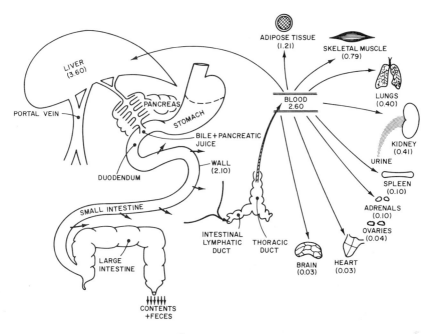

FIG. 3   Distribution of total ^{3}H-radioactivity in the different organs of
rats after acute intragastric administration of tritium-labeled vitamin E.
An emulsion containing protein, carbohydrate, monoolein, and <u>dl</u>-α-1',2'-
[3]H-tocopheryl acetate was given, by stomach tube, to rats fasted overnight.
The animals were killed 12 hr after dosage, and the total radioactivity in
the organs was determined. The figures in parentheses represent the percentages of administered radioactivity recovered 12 hr after administration of emulsion.

administrations of 5-methyl-[^{14}C]α-tocopherol to rats, the spleen and
adrenal lipids had a relatively high uptake of radioactivity. Regardless of
what ester of vitamin E is fed, the most abundant compound appearing in
the adrenal is free tocopherol which increased with time. Thus, in animals
dosed respectively with vitamin E acetate or nicotinate 3 hr after feeding,
75% and 67%, respectively, of the chromatographed radioactivity from the
samples was associated with unesterified tocopherol [161]. This proportion of free tocopherol was even higher 48 hr postprandially, when the
corresponding fractions reached as much as 82 and 90%. The high incorporation of tocopherol in the adrenal suggests that vitamin E may have
some specific function in the adrenal gland. More information is required

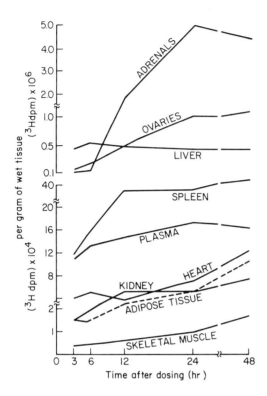

FIG. 4   Appearance of total radioactivity in the tissues of rats after the oral administration of labeled tocopheryl acetate. The experimental conditions were those described in Fig. 3.

on the affect of α-tocopherol on the adrenal function and its relationship with other vitamins (such as ascorbic acid, vitamin A, and pyridoxine), which concentrate in this organ. Kitabchi (Part 5F.) suggests that tocopherol may stimulate the steroid hydroxylase system in this organ and may be involved in the modulation of membrane-bound, adrenocorticotropic hormone (ACTH)-simulated adenyl cyclase.

    It is possible that some of the proposed biological activities of vitamin E (such as its possible "antiinflammatory action," its effect on cardiovascular disease, or in peptic ulcer disease, etc.) may take place only when the vitamin reaches adequately high concentrations at the target tissue or site of action. For this reason, many investigators have looked for vitamin E derivatives capable of producing high tissue concentrations

of this vitamin. In one such study, it was found that after its oral administration, dl-α-tocopheryl nicotinate (TN) appeared in the liver and plasma
of chickens in high concentrations and primarily as the ester fed (see
Table 4). In the liver, the concentration of the vitamin was twice as high
with TN (mostly as the esterified ester) than with tocopheryl acetate (TA)
(mostly as free tocopherol) (see Fig. 5). In all other tissues, however,
including the plasma, radioactivity after TA was higher than after TN.
High concentration of vitamin E in the liver of chickens given TN is probably due to the fact that in birds, the vitamin is absorbed almost entirely
via the portal vein. No compartmentalization seems to exist in the chicken
in regard to absorption of lipid-like materials between portal blood vessels
and lymphatic vessels, whereas these two routes of absorption are very
well differentiated in mammals [168,169]. A comparison was carried out
of the distribution of total radioactivity in rat tissue lipids after the oral
administration of labeled TN or TA [161]. In this species, total radioactivity was higher in the tissues of animals receiving TN rather than TA
only at 12 hr after dosing, but not at most other time intervals studied.
Since equimolar concentrations of the ester were administered, these

TABLE 4   Plasma and Liver Tocopherol Levels of Chicks at Various
Time Intervals After a Single Oral 16 IU Dose with d,l-α-Tocopheryl
Nicotinate

	Hours after dosage	Plasma		Liver, total
		Free	Total	
d,l-α-Tocopheryl acetate	2	2.1[a]	–	2.4
	4	4.2	–	8.6
	8	5.9	–	7.7
	16	3.7	–	5.6
	24	2.3	–	4.4
	40	2.8	–	3.9
d,l-α-Tocopheryl nicotinate	2	0.1	1.2	2.3
	4	0.6	1.6	13.0
	8	0.6	2.9	22.6
	16	1.7	2.9	22.2
	24	1.7	3.1	17.7
	40	1.8	3.4	11.5

[a] In milligrams per deciliter (rounded figures).

Source: From R. H. Bunnell et al., unpublished observations.

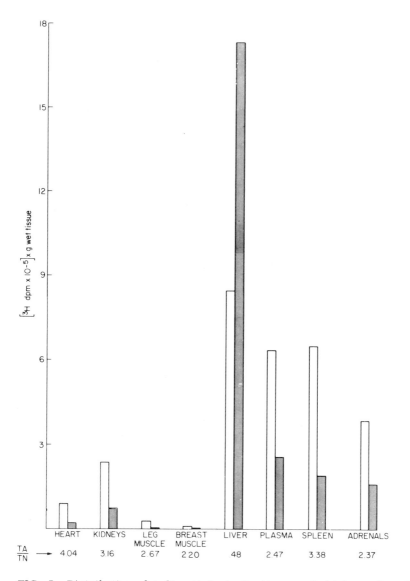

FIG. 5   Distribution of radioactivity in the tissues of chickens after the oral administration of either tocopheryl acetate (open bars) or tocopheryl nicotinate (hatched bars).

results suggest that tissues of mammals have either a lower affinity for TN or that an ester (such as TN) has a faster turnover than free tocopherol (arising from TA administration).

Findings on tocopherol distribution in other animal species have been in general agreement with those reported for the rat and chick. Hidiroglou et al. [156] studied the distribution of a single dose of $[^3H]$ dl-α-tocopherol in 16 sheep fed a dystrophy-producing hay alone or supplemented with cod-liver oil. As in the rat, radioactivity distributed itself throughout all organs of the sheep, and the relative sensitivity of tissues for vitamin E uptake was similar in both species. During the experimental period, which lasted for 5 days after administration of the vitamin, radioactivity was higher in the rumen liquor of cod liver oil-fed sheep than in those which received only hay. This correlated quite well with a higher fecal excretion of vitamin E when emulsified in cod-liver oil. These findings are in complete agreement with the reported inhibition of intestinal absorption (and therefore tissue uptake) produced by unsaturated fatty acids [162].

Engelhardt [167] examined the plasma and tissue levels of radioactivity in harp seal after intragastric administration of labeled tocopherols under various conditions. In this study, the d-α form showed much higher plasma maxima and retention than dl-α-tocopherol. Also, plasma concentration peaks occurred somewhat later but were greater when the vitamin was fed with Tween-80 than with herring and corn oil, respectively (Fig. 6). Greater plasma levels occurred with the use of herring oil than with corn oil, which suggests that, as in the case of the rat, linoleic acid decreases the bioavailability of tocopherol [162]. Seals previously maintained on a vitamin E-deficient diet showed greater plasma maxima than seals not so deprived. It is possible that the stress of vitamin E deficiency may result in increased bioavailability of the vitamin. A detailed examination of dose-derived tissue tocopherol in the vitamin E-deprived seals, carried out at 1, 3, and 7 days after intragastric intubation revealed that the greatest tracer-labeled dietary tocopherol concentration (microgram per gram of tissue) was in the spleen (see Table 5). As in studies in other species, liver, adrenals, pituitary, lymph gland, and testis were high in tracer concentration. The next highest grouping was formed by pancreas, lung, and kidney. This group was followed by the muscle tissues (diaphragm, intercostal, tongue, heart, ventricle, and uterus) as well as thyroid gland, salivary gland, epididymis, prostate gland, retina, and blubber. Finally, very low, labeled vitamin E concentration was found in all brain tissue, hypaxial and scapular muscle, ovary, and rib marrow. Unfortunately, comparisons with values in other species are precluded because the percent of administered radioactivity found in individual organs was not mentioned in this report.

The chain length of the triglyceride in which orally administered tocopherol is emulsified influences the subsequent tissue uptake of the vitamin. In rats, intestinal absorption of vitamin E is enhanced when the vehicle is medium-chain triglycerides (MCT) rather than long-chain triglycerides (LCT) [33,170,171]; such an improvement in absorption takes place by a mechanism which may involve factors other than simple solubilization [172]. These findings may be of practical importance, since it is possible that combining vitamin E with MCT may provide formulations useful in the nutritional management of a variety of disorders characterized by low vitamin E in plasma and tissues due to intestinal malabsorption [173].

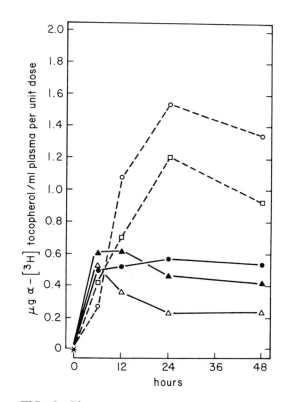

FIG. 6   Plasma concentrations of labeled tocopherol after injection of a single dose, comparing the effect of feeding the vitamin in Tween-80 to two seals and in herring oil to three seals. This figure was taken from Englehardt (ref. 167, p. 602) by courtesy of The National Research Council, Canada.

TABLE 5   Levels of d-α-[³H] Tocopherol in Harp Seal (Phoca groenlandica) Tissues as Related to Time Postingestion

Tissue	Concentration (µg/g tissue)		
	1 day	3 days	7 days
Spleen	94.5	6.3	8.5
Liver	47.0	1.5	6.1
Adrenal gland	10.2	3.0	–
Pituitary gland	19.2	–	3.0
Parathyroid gland	5.7	–	2.3
Lymph gland	9.3	1.0	3.5
Testis	–	–	3.1
Pancreas	4.2	0.5	1.4
Lung	5.9	0.5	1.6
Kidney	8.8	0.8	1.9
Muscle, diaphragm	1.8	0.3	0.8
Muscle, intercostal	1.3	0.3	0.5
Muscle, tongue	2.5	0.2	1.1
Muscle, heart	2.8	0.4	1.0
Uterus	2.1	0.4	–
Thyroid gland	1.7	–	0.7
Salivary gland	3.1	0.4	0.7
Epididymis	–	–	0.6
Prostate gland	–	–	0.8
Retina	–	0.4	1.1
Blubber	0.6	0.1	0.5
Cerebrum	0.7	0.1	0.2
Cerebellum	1.3	0.1	0.4
Medulla oblongata	0.5	0.1	0.2
Muscle, hypaxial	0.9	0.2	0.4
Muscle, subscapular	1.1	0.1	0.4
Ovary	2.8	0.1	–
Rib marrow	0.5	0.1	–

Source: Reprinted from ref. 167, p. 605, by courtesy of the National Research Council of Canada.

F. Relationship of Tissue Uptake to Oral Dose

The amount of tocopherol dispersed in tissue is directly related to the logarithm of the dose administered. This relationship has been shown for the plasma, liver, testes, muscle, and spleen in the rat [174]. This is also true over a wide range of intakes for the lung (Fig. 7) [175] and in the chicken for muscle tissue [176] (see Fig. 8). In addition, recent findings by Machlin and Filipski demonstrate that dietary vitamin E accumulates in platelets at a concentration as high as that in adrenals. The tocopherol content in platelets was closely related to the plasma tocopherol (Fig. 9). In humans, administration of vitamin E has been shown to increase vitamin E levels of adipose [177] and muscle tissue [78].

G. Distribution After Parenteral Administration

Information on the fate of vitamin E after parenteral administration is scarce. This accounts, at least in part, for the poor understanding of the bioavailability of this vitamin. In some instances, administration of high levels of vitamin E may not result in a sufficient concentration in a target tissue to obtain some described physiological effect. For instance,

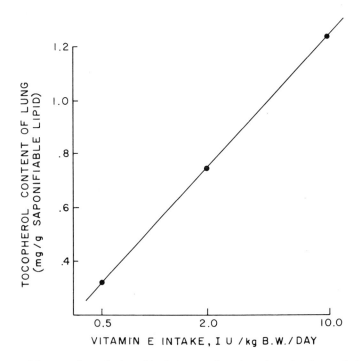

FIG. 7   The relationship between the vitamin E intake and the tocopherol content of lung (rats).

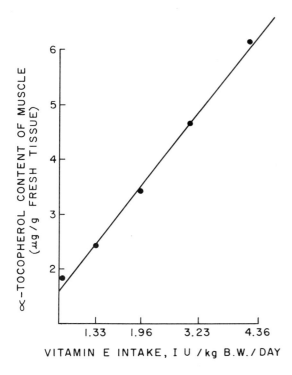

FIG. 8 The relationship between the vitamin E intake and the tocopherol content of the muscle (chickens).

vitamin E is used in open heart surgery, during which the blood is oxygenated under higher oxygen tension in an extracorporeal apparatus. This stresses lipid antioxidant reserves of the red cell membrane, resulting in excessive, undesirable oxidative hemolysis of the erythrocyte and a drop in plasma tocopherol to levels well below the acceptable minimum of 0.5 mg/100 ml. High levels of the vitamin are needed in the blood to prevent hemolysis. Parenteral administration of commercial preparations of dl-α-tocopherol in micellar aqueous dispersions, however, does correct the rapid decline of the free tocopherol levels in the blood in this situation, whereas dispersions of dl-α-tocopheryl acetate does not (Horwitt, unpublished observations). This illustrates the need for information on the fate of various preparations of vitamin E after parenteral administration.

A study of tissue uptake and distribution of vitamin E after parenteral administration involved the intravenous injection of dl-α-tocopheryl-1', 2'- $\left[{}^3H_2\right]$ acetate in normal rats [178]. The radioactive compound and the

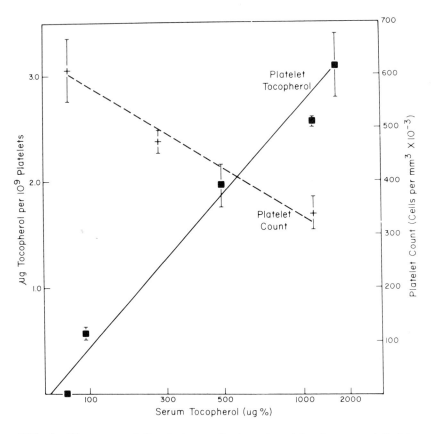

FIG. 9   Close correlation between the tocopherol in plasma and that in platelets.

suitable unlabeled carrier were dissolved in an aqueous suspension containing Emulphor-EL 620, which is the solubilizing agent most commonly found in commercial preparations. The animals were killed at different time intervals, and the radioactivity in the extracted lipids from all tissues was analyzed at the times indicated in Fig. 10. The amount of radioactivity in the plasma declined rapidly. There was a varied rate of uptake for different tissues examined. Total radioactivity in the spleen was higher than in any other organ, while that in the lungs was almost as high as in the spleen and did not vary with time. In the liver, it showed a slow decline, which started 12 hr after the intravenous injection. All other tissues examined (adrenals, ovaries, adipose tissue, small

intestine, etc.) showed a linear uptake which increased with time, just as
in the case of the oral administration. Low concentration of radioactivity
was seen in small intestine, adipose tissue, and skeletal muscle, but these
tissues showed a linear uptake which increased with time, so that the
values at 48 hr were considerably higher than at 3 hr. Linear uptake was
also seen in the ovaries and in the adrenals. In both organs the radioactivity concentration was greater than the plasma and by 48 hr approximated that seen in the lungs and spleen (Fig. 10). The figure shows clearly
the increasing ratio with time of adrenal/blood radioactivity. Thus, 0.5,
3, 6, 12, 24, and 48 hr after injection, the corresponding ratios were 0.4,
5, 16, 17, 48, and 60, demonstrating the enormous capacity of the adrenals
to accumulate intravenously administered vitamin E, just as in the case of
oral dosage with vitamin E.

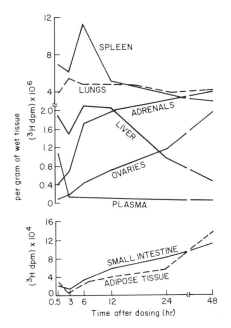

FIG. 10   Total radioactivity of plasma, liver, lungs, spleen, and other
tissues after i.v. injection of dl-α-tocopheryl-1',2'-^{3}H$_2$-acetate to
normal rats. The ester of tocopherol, dissolved in an Emulphor-EL 620-
containing suspension, was injected into the femoral vein. Animals were
killed at specified time intervals, and the total radioactivity in the organs
was analyzed by standard procedures.

TABLE 6 The Percent Distribution of Radioactivity in Rat Tissues After Administration of 50 μCi of Tritiated Esters of Tocopherol

Tissue	d,l-3,4-[³H₂]α-Tocopheryl nicotinate Time after injection (hr)						d,l-α-Tocopheryl-1',2'-[³H₂]acetate Time after injection (hr)					
	0.5	3	6	12	24	48	0.5	3	6	12	24	48
Liver	39.15[a]	52.54	45.90	49.01	56.70	43.51	34.00	53.29	62.24	66.36	45.49	24.50
Spleen	42.70	37.20	41.63	40.90	29.68	36.10	12.21	23.06	16.81	10.09	9.28	6.04
Plasma[b]	6.49	0.93	1.05	0.97	1.83	1.77	40.28	7.88	5.46	6.48	6.00	6.69
Lungs	4.86	4.41	4.46	4.11	3.57	2.53	1.26	2.72	2.11	2.15	2.76	3.23
Skeletal muscle[c]	3.17	1.84	3.01	2.43	3.23	6.62	5.11	5.09	3.77	6.65	13.78	18.02
Heart	1.62	1.06	1.46	0.42	0.44	0.40	2.63	4.13	3.63	0.42	1.20	1.17
Adipose tissue[d]	0.80	1.03	1.24	0.88	2.65	6.33	2.30	1.54	3.25	4.70	13.28	30.15
Stomach[e]	0.44	0.20	0.30	0.14	0.22	0.35	1.06	1.19	0.97	0.43	1.39	0.85

Kidneys	0.39	0.28	0.34	0.19	0.24	0.28	0.45	0.36	0.29	0.37	0.85	1.26
Small intestine[e]	0.21	0.30	0.38	0.32	0.77	1.10	0.45	0.39	0.81	1.31	2.78	3.50
Adrenals	0.08	0.10	0.13	0.14	0.36	0.53	0.07	0.18	0.37	0.55	1.59	2.28
Ovaries	0.05	0.05	0.09	0.08	0.28	0.42	0.05	0.10	0.26	0.32	1.45	2.09
Brain	0.03	0.04	0.03	0.03	0.04	0.05	0.07	0.06	0.05	0.06	0.15	0.22
Pituitary	< 0.01	< 0.01	< 0.01	< 0.01	< 0.01	< 0.01	< 0.01	< 0.01	< 0.01	< 0.01	< 0.01	< 0.01
Percent of administered dose	56	58	50	56	45	48	70	48	52	50	32	28

[a] Percentage of the total ^{3}H-radioactivity recovered in whole organ or tissue at specified time.
[b] Values calculated for the whole animal, considering that, in the rat, total blood represents about 6% of the body weight.
[c] Calculations done on the assumption that the skeletal muscle represents about 40% of the body weight in the rat.
[d] In order to obtain these values, 13.6% of the body weight was attributed to the adipose tissue.
[e] These values include the luminal contents at the time of killing.

Source: Reprinted from ref. 178 by courtesy of Verlag Hans Huber, Bern, Switzerland.

Studies of the radioactivity in the whole organ (Table 6) clearly show that for vitamin E acetate (and the resulting free tocopherol) the liver is a site for temporary storage, whereas the adipose tissue and skeletal muscle become qualitatively more important as time lapses. However, this may depend upon the chemical nature of the compound injected (Table 6), since α-tocopheryl nicotinate may be taken up by organs the reticuloendothelial system (see Sec. G.3).

Shiratori [179] reported an experiment in which tritium-labeled α-tocopherol was incorporated into chylomicra by feeding dl-α-[5-methyl-^{3}H]tocopherol to thoracic duct-cannulated rats. The [^{3}H]α-tocopherol in chylomicra was injected i.v. into normal male rats. Distribution of label measured in skin, viscera, and carcass at 2, 24, 96 hr, and 10 days demonstrated a rapid uptake and prolonged retention in the dermal tissues of the skin (not including subcutaneous tissue and hair) when compared to viscera and carcass. Such relative distribution in skin increased from 10.3% at 2 hr to 40.1% of the recovered dose at 20 days. At all times examined, radioactivity in skin was higher than in either subcutaneous fat or epididymal fat. Shiratori's studies suggest that skin has storage capacity for tocopherol. It is, therefore, possible that significant amounts of vitamin E may be secreted or excreted through the skin, a fact which had been ignored by most other researchers.

With respect to distribution of vitamin E after parenteral administration to other species, Caravaggi [180] found that, in contrast with nonruminants, α-tocopherol appears rapidly in the blood after instrmuscular injection of sheep with dl-α-tocopheryl acetate. A maximum level more than 30 times higher than that prior to administration was reached 10 hr after injection. In this species, massive amounts given orally resulted in two- to fourfold increases; these findings are similar to those observed in the case of nonruminants. In another investigation, Tikriti [181] compared the distribution of orally and parenterally administered 5-methyl [^{14}C] d-α-tocopheryl acetate (25 μCi) in an open lactating Holstein cow by frequent sampling and analyses of blood, milk, subcutaneous fat/ and urine for 8 days. Three weeks were allowed for the elimination of radioactivity between experiments. The animal was sacrificed 30 hr after a second administration (intramuscular) of 40 μCi, and the tissues were extensively sampled. Levels of radioactivity in milk, plasma, adipose tissue, and urine after intramuscular injection were several times higher than those after oral administration. The uptake and depletion in various excreta and tissues were similar for both routes. Of the administered radioactivity, 10.5% was found at the site of injection (100 cm^2) when the animal was killed; 22.4, 9.6, 9.1, 6.6, and 0.6% were contained in the plasma, liver, udder, lung, and spleen, respectively, and 4.5% was accounted for in body fat, amounting to about 10% of the cow's weight. The pancreas and adrenals were relatively high in activity; the heart, kidneys, ovaries and uterus were intermediate, and relatively low radioactivity was found in the bile, brain, muscle, intestines, spinal cord, and tongue. These findings on the tocopherol distribution in the cow are in general agreement with those reported for the rat.

Newmark et al. [182] found that when properly formulated, micellar-type aqueous dispersions of tocopheryl acetate were administered i.v. or i.m. to dogs, the rate-limiting step in the bioavailability of the free tocopherol was the rate of hydrolysis of the acetate ester. In this study, similar dispersions of free tocopherol yielded blood levels of tocopherol manyfold higher than those obtained with the acetate ester after intravenous injection; and also yielded much greater increases in blood levels of free tocopherol after intramuscular injection than the acetate ester formulation, particularly in the early period after the dose. This suggests that in blood of nonruminants the hydrolysis of vitamin E to the corresponding free tocopherol takes place rather slowly (see Sec. V). Bauernfeind et al [183] reviewed some biopharmaceutical factors in intramuscular administration of vitamin E to children.

2. Distribution in Subcellular Particles

The studies of Mellors and McC. Barnes [153] suggested that, in the liver and spleen cells, radioactivity from orally administered [5-methyl-^{14}C]α-tocopherol was associated mainly with the structural components, such as mitochondria and microsomes. More recently, Bonetti and Novello [184] studied the distribution of labeled vitamin E in subcellular particles. Tritium-labeled tocopherols, emulsified in 0.5 ml saline-1% Tween-80, was injected i.v. to male rats fed either a stock diet or a liver necrogenic diet [185]. No difference in vitamin E distribution was observed in tissues of rats fed the necrogenic diet, supplemented with vitamin E, selenium, or both. The pattern of tocopherol distribution at different times in crude mitochondria, microsomes, 105,000 g supernatant, and liver homogenate is depicted in Fig. 11. Crude mitochondria had higher specific labeling than other fractions during the entire experimental period. In this sub-cellular particle, the specific labeling decreased more than 50% in 24 hr and then remained almost constant. In microsomes, the plateau was reached earlier between the sixth and twelfth hour. The cell sap had a lower specific labeling that decreased until 6 hr and then remained con-stant. These data suggest that tocopherol rapidly entered the liver cell and did not remain in the cell sap but that the vitamin was bound mainly to mitochondria and also to microsomes. One part of the vitamin is rapidly metabolized or released; the other part varies in percentage for each substructure and is more stable. Therefore, there appear to be at least two compartments in the cell fraction, one in which the tocopherol (or some metabolite) is loosely bound, the other involves tighter binding of the

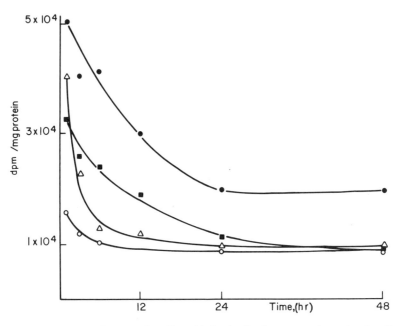

FIG. 11   Distribution of radioactivity in the homogenate and subcellular
fractions of livers of vitamin E-deficient rats. Mitochondria were obtained by centrifuging 600 g supernatant at 8000 g for 15 min. Microsomes
were sedimented at 105,000 g for 1 hr from 15,000 g supernatant. This
figure was taken from Bonetti and Novello [184] by courtesy of Verlag Hans
Huber, Bern, Switzerland.

vitamin. It remains to be demonstrated whether these two compartments
have different functions.

Bonetti and Novello [184] prepared inner and outer membranes from
purified mitochondria. The specific labeling for crude inner membranes
plus matrix, outer membranes, and soluble fraction were, respectively,
14.4, 26.3, and 10.4 dpm/μg protein with one method and 6.9, 57.3, and
34.8 dpm/μg with another procedure. These data suggest that, irrespective of the method employed, the labeling is strongly bound to membranes,
outer membranes being more labeled than inner membranes. Microsomes
were further fractionated in smooth and rough endoplasmic reticulum by
centrifugation on a layer of 1.3 M sucrose and 3 mM $MgCl_2$. The initial
specific labeling of the fraction was 82 dpm/μg protein; after centrifugation, rough and smooth fractions had a specific activity of 52 and 96 dpm/
μg, respectively. To investigate the binding of tocopherol to microsomes,

labeled fractions were treated with deoxycholate at different concentrations; the solubilization of a large part of the radioactivity was obtained with concentration higher than 0.5% (w/v). The solubilized radioactivity was not lost after dialysis for 24 hr against 0.25 M sucrose, and under these conditions a precipitate was formed that accounted for up to 45% of the solubilized radioactivity. It would be of interest to confirm the very rapid incorporation of vitamin E into membranes as well as the higher affinity for tocopherol by outer membranes when compared with inner membranes.

3. Vitamin E and the Reticuloendothelial System (RES)

Striking differences were found in the rate of disappearance from the plasma and in the tissue distribution of intravenously injected $\underline{d},\underline{1}$-3, 4-[^{3}H$_2$]$\alpha$-tocopheryl nicotinate (TN) and $\underline{d},\underline{1}$-1', 2'-[^{3}H$_2$]$\alpha$-tocopheryl acetate (TA) [178]. The half-time clearance of these esters demonstrated that TN removal from the blood had an exponential character, and it was much faster than removal of TA (Fig. 12). Such rapid removal of TN from the bloodstream was accompanied by rapid deposition of this vitamin E ester in the spleen, lungs, and liver, suggesting that TN undergoes phagocytosis by the cells of the RES [186]. This hypothesis was recently tested by Frigg and Gallo-Torres [187], who examined by light microscopic autoradiography the cellular distribution of total radioactivity after intravenous injection to rats of either ^{14}C- or ^{3}H-labeled TN. The animals were decapitated, and the organs were immediately removed and processed according to the method described by Eckert [188]. The sections were stained in Harris' hematoxyline and eosine and embedded in Kaiser's glycerine gelatine.

As shown in Fig. 13a, radioactivity in the liver was confined to definite areas of 5-40 μm diameter in the perilobular zone. These represented either individually labeled cells (Fig. 13b) with an irregular boundary, corresponding to Kupfer cells, or clusters of macrophages. The majority of parenchymal hepatic cells and other tissue elements were devoid of radioactivity. The tendency of α-tocopheryl nicotinate to accumulate in an annular pattern at the periphery of the hepatic lobules may be due to the fact that the peripheral Kupffer cells are exposed to the highest concentration of the compound. The older and more centrally located cells are not exposed to such a high concentration. This intrahepatic distribution of the radioactive material is dependent upon the efficiency of the phagocytosis which, in turn, is influenced by the perfusion rate of the blood into the hepatic tissue. The morphological appearance of the splenic tissue was normal. High amounts of radioactivity were found to be localized in circular areas in the red pulp surrounding the white pulp (perifollicular zone; Fig. 13c). This activity was related to reticular cells with phagocytic properties (free histiocytes and macrophages). These cells, one example of which is given in Figure 13d, belong to the RES and are known to have a high phagocytic activity. Other tissue elements of the spleen were devoid of radioactivity. The number of silver grains were higher in the splenic than in the hepatic tissue, probably because the spleen is especially well equipped for phagocytosis. The unique structure of the microcirculation of the red pulp [189, 190] is not duplicated in any other organ. This could explain why the spleen is the main site of accumulation of the injected material. As in the spleen and liver, the radioactivity in the lungs was confined to alveolar macrophages (Fig. 13e). The size and shape of these labeled cells were about the same as that seen in the other organs.

Sections of the ileocecal lymph nodes did not contain detectable radio-activity. It is not surprising that lymph nodes do not remove i.v. injected α-tocopheryl nicotinate to an appreciable extent, because these organs specialize in removing particles injected into the lymphstream and not those injected into the bloodstream [191].

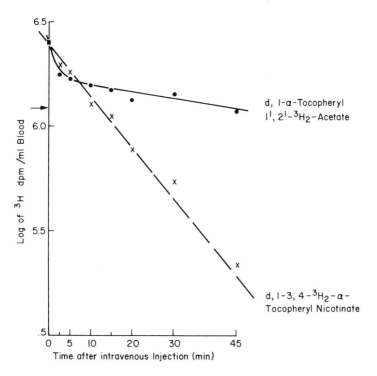

FIG. 12   Removal rate of tritiated α-tocopheryl nicotinate (x . . . . . . x) or α-tocopheryl acetate (● —— ●) from the blood after i.v. injection in rats. The esters of tocopherol, dissolved in an emulsion containing Emulphor-EL 620, were injected into the femoral vein. Serial blood samples were with-drawn from a tail cut. The arrow represents the concentration of radio-activity corresponding to the intravascular half-time clearance value.

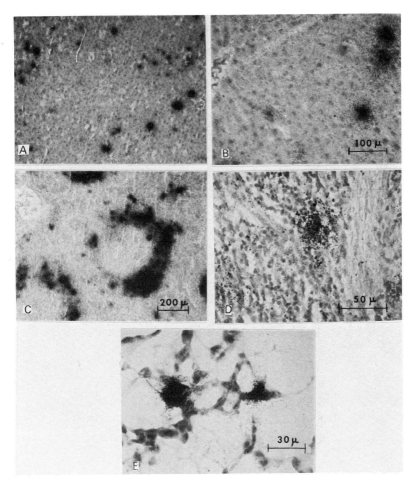

FIG. 13. Vitamin E and the reticuloendothelial system (RES). A and B. Microradioautographs of the liver of a rat 30 min after an i.v. injection of 25 mg of d,l-α-tocopheryl nicotinate-7-^{14}C, demonstrating a distinct cell distribution of the material in the perilobular zone. A, lower magnification; B, x 320. Exposure time: 16 days. C. Microautoradiography of the spleen of a rat injected with 25 mg ^{14}C-α-tocopheryl nicotinate. Thirty minutes after injection, the silver grains are specifically localized in circular areas which clearly outline the perifollicular zones and are more abundant in the red pulp; x 131. Exposure time: 15 days. D. Spleen macrophage of a rat injected i.v. with 30 mg ^{3}H-tocopheryl nicotinate and killed 6 hr after dosage; x 880. Exposure time: 77 days. E. Localization of ^{3}H-α-tocopheryl nicotinate to areas of the lung identified as alveolar macrophages. The rat was killed 6 hr after i.v. administration of 30 mg of the radioactive vitamin E derivative; x 1112. Exposure time: 77 days.

The above-described data confirmed the hypothesis that after its i.v. injection, α-tocopheryl nicotinate undergoes phagocytosis by the cells of the RES throughout the body in a manner similar to that reported for carbon particles [192]. The rate of removal of vitamin E esters from the bloodstream depends upon certain physicochemical factors such as the dose, nature, and dimension of the suspended particles as well as upon certain biological factors such as blood flow, size of liver and spleen, and, possibly, species of the animal. The clearance of TN is similar to that of other substances, although the accumulation of the radioactivity in the RES is not exactly the same as that found with colloidal carbon or with trypan blue. This difference could be due to RES-cell specificity that is, definite cells are responsible for the phagocytosis of certain particles [193].

It is not known whether the RES participates in the physiological handling of orally administered liposoluble vitamins. Vitamin A administered i.v. is taken up by the RE cells (unpublished observations), suggesting that phagocytosis by the RES of intravenously administered liposoluble vitamins is a general, and perhaps a quantitatively, important phenomenon. These considerations become of practical interest in those cases in which fat-soluble vitamins are given i.v., such as parenteral hyperalimentation and also during the possible involvement of vitamin E and other liposoluble vitamins in immunological processes.

IV. MOBILIZATION

There is little information on the rates at which the various tissues are depleted in the absence of dietary vitamin E. Knowledge of the kinetics of storage and mobilization of vitamin E in body tissues is of paramount importance in understanding the physiological role of this vitamin. Also relevant is the feasibility of using the tocopherol concentration in body tissues to determine the relative potency of vitamin E from various dietary sources or pharmaceutical preparations. Some tissues, such as the adipocyte, liver, and muscle are considered to be the major storage depots for tocopherol. It is not known, however, whether these tissue reserves can be released and made available to needed tissues when dietary sources are low or absent.

In rats and rabbits fed a deficient diet, liver vitamin E decreased rapidly for several weeks, then reached a plateau, whereas the muscle concentration of the vitamin declined much more slowly [194]. In calves, Grifo et al. [148] found that the sensitivity of body tissues to graded amounts of tocopherol in the ration was in the following descending order: heart, liver, perinephritic fat, and trapezius muscle. Expressing tocopherol concentration on a per gram lipid basis resulted in appreciable change in sensitivity as compared to wet basis.

When normal human volunteers were fed a diet low in vitamin E [195], it took 5 months for the average plasma levels to decrease from the initial value of 1.01 to about 0.5 mg/100 ml. Plasma levels remained stable thereafter. In additional studies [112, 126], human adipose tissue was obtained from a group of 12 subjects who had been ingesting large amounts of polyunsaturated fat for 15 months or more, and from a group of 31 hospitalized control subjects. The average tocopherol content of the adipose tissue did not differ appreciably between the two groups, suggesting that high PUFA intake does not result in an increased utilization of the tocopherol being stored in the adipose tissue. Witting et al. [196] found that the whole-body concentration of α-tocopherol of rats depleted from the time of weaning, fell precipitously for 4 weeks, then declined at a much slower rate. The type of dietary fat, either saturated or unsaturated, did not have significant influence on the rate of tocopherol depletion.

Other studies have confirmed that the rate of depletion of vitamin E upon withdrawal from the diet varies considerably from tissue to tissue, being relatively rapid in plasma and liver, slower from skeletal and heart muscle, and very slow from adipose tissue. Thus, Bieri [173] determined the depletion of α-tocopherol in six tissues in rats periodically for 6 weeks. In both young and mature rats, plasma, liver, and heart concentrations fell to one-half or less of the initial values in 1-2 weeks and then underwent a much slower decline. In the young, growing rat, vitamin E concentration in depot fat, testis, and muscle decreased significantly during the rapid growth period, then assumed the slower decline characteristic of mature rats. On the basis of these findings, Bieri [173] concluded that all of these tissues (except depot fat) contain a labile pool of α-tocopherol, which mobilizes rapidly, and a fixed component which is retained for long periods. In his view, body stores of α-tocopherol do not maintain the plasma concentration until the latter has fallen to one-half or less of the "normal" value.

In Bieri's studies, the concentration of tocopherol in adipose tissue decreased. However, since the total amount of fat was not measured, a decrease in tocopherol concentration in the fat might have reflected dilution due to increased lipid deposition and not bioavailability. A recent report by Machlin et al. [197] indicates that vitamin E in adipose tissue represents a tissue depot with an extremely low turnover and that this tocopherol may not be bioavailable. The study was done in male guinea pigs, with a starting weight of 170-220 g. All animals received a basal diet containing 200 mg/kg dl-α-tocopheryl acetate for 3 weeks. Two groups of animals fed either a lard or a corn oil diet were sacrificed and the tocopherol content of tissues determined. The remaining guinea pigs were transferred to diets devoid of vitamin E and groups of five were sacrificed at 1, 2, 4, 5, or 8 weeks and their tissues analyzed for tocopherol. In agreement with Bieri's findings in the rat [173] the depletion of tocopherol from plasma and

TABLE 7   Depletion of Tocopherol from Guinea Pig Tissues[a]

| | No. of animals | Body wt | Microgram per gram | | |
			Plasma	Fat	Liver
Zero time	10	367 ± 22^{b}	7.3 ± 0.6	29.8 ± 3.1	56.9 ± 7.3
1 week (8/21)	10	399 ± 11	3.0 ± 0.2	25.3 ± 1.8	10.6 ± 1.0
2 weeks (8/28)	10	438 ± 19	2.3 ± 0.2	21.1 ± 2.0	6.3 ± 0.8
4 weeks (9/11)	8	513 ± 35	0.0 ± 0.0	18.6 ± 3.9	4.0 ± 0.6
6 weeks (9/11)	8	666 ± 14	1.5 ± 0.3	15.5 ± 2.7	3.7 ± 0.5
8 weeks (10/6)	8	632 ± 33	0.1	9.0 ± 0.7	2.8 ± 0.3

[a] Figures in these and other columns represent the mean $\pm$ SEM.

Source: This report was presented at the 1976 Federation Meetings (Machlin et al., Fed. Proc. 35, 1976).

liver was relatively rapid; heart and muscle tissues were depleted at a much slower rate (Table 7). The tocopherol concentration of the adipose tissue decreased over an 8-week period in those animals on a vitamin E-free diet. However, this decrease was a consequence of dilution by lipid deposition, because the total amount of tocopherol in the fat mass did not change. Since definite, light microscopic myopathic lesions were found in some guinea pigs sacrificed at 6 or 8 weeks after the beginning of the depletion period (Fig. 14); the studies reported by Machlin et al. [196] strongly suggest that adipose tocopherol is not available to the animal in quantities sufficient to protect other tissues from the pathological consequences of vitamin E depletion. It should nevertheless be mentioned here that neither Bieri [173] nor Machlin et al. [197] made reference to the concentration of selenium in their diets. This information is considered of importance because Cheeke and Shull [198] have suggested that selenium may prolong the retention time of the initial reserves of vitamin E.

tissue		Microgram per gram tissue			
Muscle	Heart	Fat	Liver	Muscle	Heart
7.9 ± 0.7	19.6	113.3 ± 19.1	849.5 ± 129.0	882	28.2
9.1 ± 0.5	23.8	107.1 ± 15.4	167.8 ± 13.0	1092	28.5
6.5 ± 0.6	15.6	100.8 ± 16.2	107.2 ± 13.0	858	20.6
4.5 ± 0.8	9.1	112.6 ± 28.5	67.8 ± 9.6	705	12.1
3.3 ± 0.4	6.1	148.6 ± 28.8	73.7 ± 8.5	650	11.0
2.3 ± 0.2	4.1	89.3 ± 17.8	54.5 ± 5.4	445	6.8

Therefore, in terms of storage of vitamin E, the adipose tissue contains one of the largest pools of nonexchangeable tocopherol in humans as well as lower animals. It is generally assumed that vitamin E in tissues exists as a structural component of membranes. It is not known, however, whether adipose tissue accumulates the vitamin in amounts proportional to those required for cellular membrane elements. Therefore, it will be of interest to determine the tocopherol to phospholipid and/or triglyceride molar ratio in adipose tissue and compare it to the molar ratio of other mammalian cell or membrane, especially that of red blood cells. Possibly, the tocopherol in depot fat is localized in the central oil droplet of the lipid-storing adipocyte, hence, its characteristic of an extremely slow exchangable pool, not bioavailable for practical purposes. Further experimentation is needed to elucidate these relationships.

Although both α- and γ-tocopherol are absorbed to the same extent [27], the γ-tocopherol is eliminated from the tissues at a much more rapid

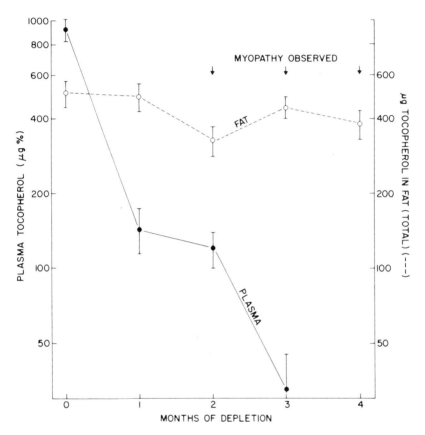

FIG. 14   Depletion of adipose tocopherol in guinea pigs.   Myopathy was observed in some animals killed at 6 or 8 weeks after the beginning of the depletion period.

rate [27, 30].   Evidently the absence of the methyl group at position 5 is quite critical for optimal retention of tocopherol in most tissues.   The high biological activity of α-tocopherol compared with other isomers may be primarily related to the pharmacokinetic properties of the vitamin; that is its ability to be retained in tissues, presumably bound to certain membrane components, may be necessary for maximal activity.

V. METABOLISM

A. Chemical Reactions

In this review, a summary of the reaction products of tocopherol occurring
in vitro will be followed by a discussion of the possible existence of some
of these compounds in body tissues. The most common reaction which
vitamin E undergoes is one of oxidation. Kinetic measurements have indicated that tocopherol can act as a hydrogen donor in a hydrogen-transferring
system, where the hydrogen of the 6-OH group is the active species [199].
In these reactions, tocopherol was oxidized either reversibly or irreversibly,
and the end products depended upon the polarity of the solvent in which the
oxidation process was carried out.

The oxidation of tocopherol in nonpolar solvents could be useful in the
understanding of the reactions of the vitamin in products such as oils and
anhydrous fats. Using the stable free-radical 1,1-diphenyl-2-picrylhydrazyl
(DPPH·) as the oxidizing agent, Boguth [199] demonstrated that, in chloroform or benzene solution, the vitamin reacts with DPPH quantitatively after
a long period of time by formation of the corresponding hydrazine DPPH:H.
In agreement with Blois' findings [200], 1 mol of α-tocopherol was capable
of reducing 2 mol DPPH· . The first fast-reaction step of α-tocopherol is

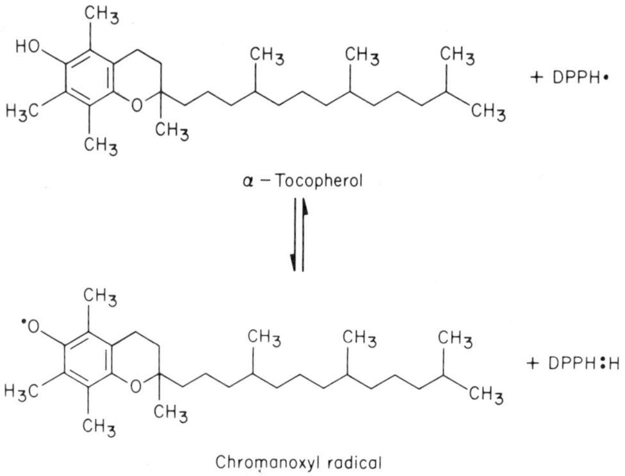

FIG. 15   Formation of chromanoxyl radical.

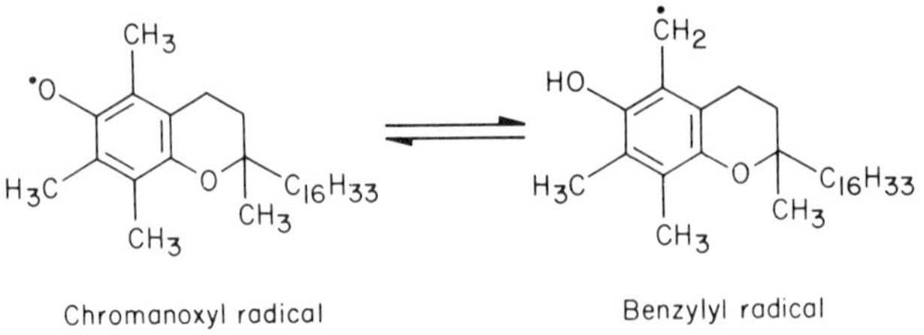

FIG. 16. Conversion of chromanoxyl into benzylyl radical.

based upon the loss of a hydrogen atom by formation of the chromanoxy radical (0·) (Fig. 15). The reversibility of this reaction enables tocopherol to transfer hydrogen, that is, to function as a catalyst. That the first oxidation step occurs at the 6-OH group had been demonstrated by Skinner and Alaupovic [201]. This information is of practical importance, because esters of tocopherol do not react with oxidizing agents. A 1,4-radical rearrangement of the chromanoxy radical into a benzylic radical is possible (Fig. 16). Since benzylyl radicals are highly reactive, this process continues to the formation of dimers, which are further oxidized by DPPH'' (Fig. 17). Boguth and Blahser [202] and Repges and Sernetz [203] presented evidence that the tocopheryl radical disappears in a second-order reaction, during which it reacts with a second tocopheryl radical by disproportionation. The intermediate o-quinone methide (Fig. 18) is quite unstable and is

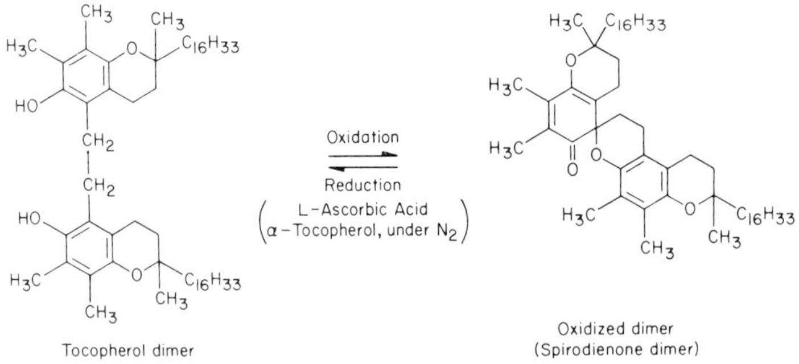

FIG. 17. Oxidation-reduction of tocopherol dimer.

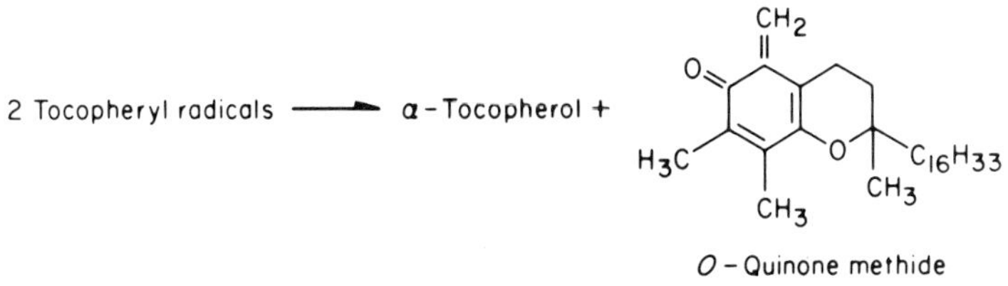

2 Tocopheryl radicals ⟶ α-Tocopherol +

O - Quinone methide

FIG. 18 Disappearance of tocopheryl radical by disproportionation, with the formation of o-quinone methide.

dimerized to the spirodiene ether. In this process, small amounts of trimers are also found [204, 205]. Because reactions in nonpolar media do not occur in cells, the described oxidation products of vitamin E in nonpolar solvents are thought not to occur in vivo. However, some of these compounds may occur in body tissues, and this will be discussed in detail below.

Of greater biologic significance is the oxidation of α-tocopherol in the presence of polar solvents such as water or other nucleophilic agents (R-OH). The first essential step in this reaction is the formation of an 8a-hydroxy or an 8a-alkoxy-α-tocopherone, the stability of which depends upon the pH of the medium, the nature of the solvent, and the alkoxy substituent itself [206, 207] (see Fig. 19). Boguth [199] discussed the formation of 5-benzoyloxymethyl-8-tocopherol during the oxidation of α-tocopherol with benzoyl peroxide ($C_6H_5COO\cdot$). This reaction would comprise (1) the formation of an adduct of the vitamin with $C_6H_5COO\cdot$, which then rearranges into 5-benzoyloxymethyl-α-tocopherol; (2) decomposition of the adduct into benzoic acid and the chromanoxy radical, which first disproportionates into α-tocopherol and the corresponding o-quinone methide and, subsequently, adds benzoic acid to produce 5-benzoyloxymethyl-α-tocopherol; and (3) 1, 4-radical, rearrangement of the phenoxy radical into the isomeric 5-benzyl radical and subsequent reaction with $C_6H_5COO\cdot$. Whatever the mechanism, the reversibility of this first reaction permits the transfer of protons and electrons through an intermediate carbonium ion without the formation of a tocopheryl quinone [207]. Upon subsequent hydrolysis, the tocopherones are irreversibly converted into quinones, but reduction regenerates the tocopherol. When the oxidizing agent is ferric chloride in the presence of dipyridyl, the first product of oxidation of α-tocopherol is a metastable epoxide which ascorbic acid can reduce back to the vitamin. On being left to stand the epoxide can irreversibly give a tocopheryl quinone. Tocopheryl quinones (TQ) can be reduced to the corresponding quinols by zinc and acetic acid (see Fig. 20). Also of relevance

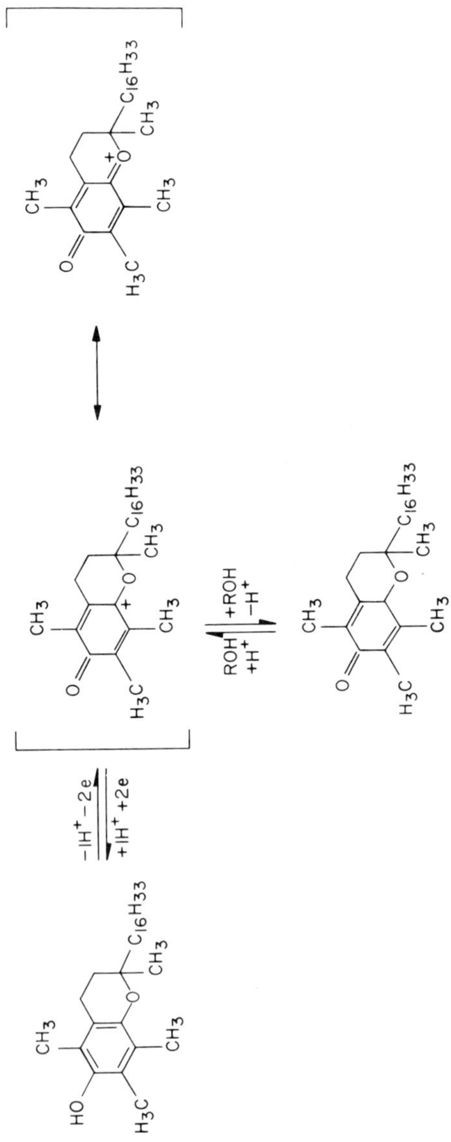

FIG. 19   Initial steps in the oxidation of α-tocopherol in the presence of nucleophilic agents.

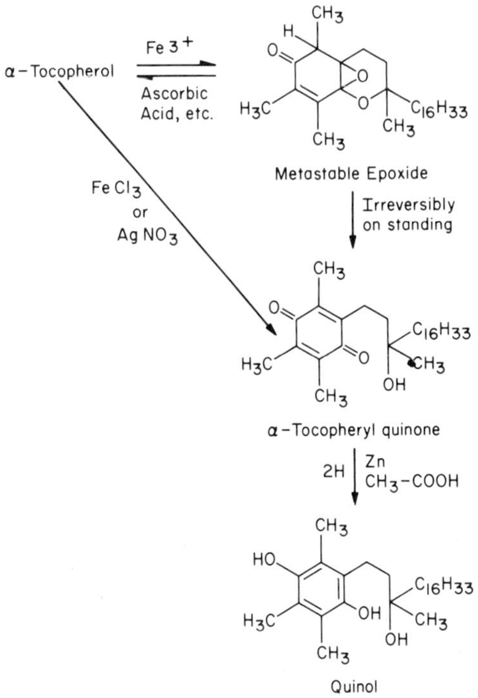

FIG. 20   Formation of tocopheryl quinone (TQ).   Further oxidation of TQ to quinol.

is the oxidation of α-tocopherol to TQ by CCl_4-ethanol solvent [208].   This information is of interest because antioxidants in general, and vitamin E in particular, are capable of conferring protection against the hepatotoxic effect of CCl_4 presumably through RES participation (see Sec. G.3).

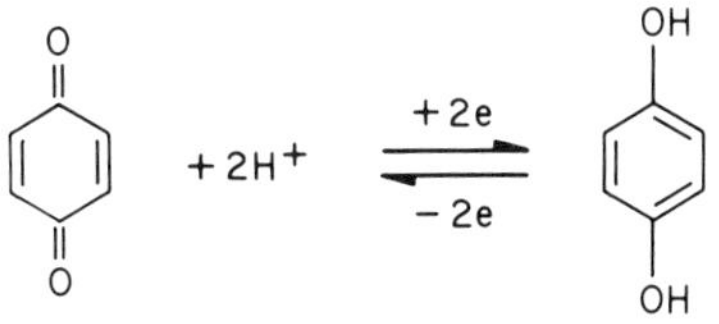

FIG. 21   Characteristic reactions of all quinones, including α-tocopheryl quinone.

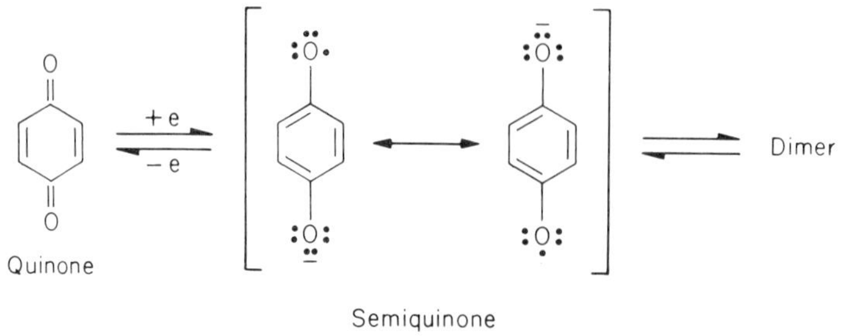

FIG. 22 Oxidation-reduction of quinone, resonance species of semiquinone, and the formation of dimers.

The most characteristic and important reaction of quinones (conjugated cyclic diketones, rather than aromatic compounds) is reduction to the corresponding di-OH aromatic compounds (Fig. 21). The reduction of quinones requires two electrons, and it is of course possible that the electrons could either be transferred together or one at a time. The product of a single electron transfer leads to what is appropriately called a semiquinone with both a negative charge and an odd electron. As indicated before, some semiquinone radicals undergo reversible dimerization reactions to form peroxides (Fig. 22).

When α-tocopherol is oxidized by means of alkaline ferricyanide, a dimer is formed (Fig. 23), the structure of which has been the subject of

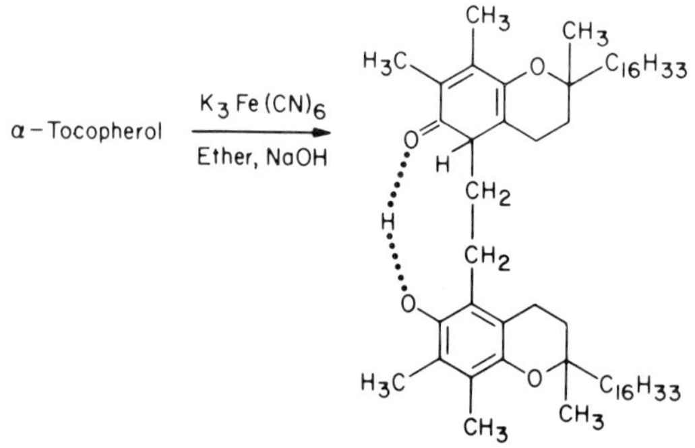

FIG. 23 Product resulting from the oxidation of α-tocopherol with $K_3Fe(CN)6$ (in vitro).

much controversy. The dimer was designated as di-α-tocopherone by Csallany and Draper [209, 210], and regarded as spirenone ether by Nelan and Robeson [211]. When none of these two structures seemed to fit the data of Strauch et al. [212], Csallany [213] carried out a reappraisal of the dimeric structure. (See Sec. B.2.)

B. Occurrence of α-Tocopherol Metabolites In Vivo and In Vitro

Many studies have been carried out with the hope that further elucidation of vitamin E metabolism in vivo may help to clarify its basic physiologic function. More than half a century of this work has sometimes led to contradictory conclusions. The following is a discussion of the possible occurrences of metabolites in tissues.

1. α-Tocopheryl Quinone

Good evidence has been obtained for the existence of α-tocopheryl quinone (TQ) in plants [214]. More than three decades ago, Scudi and Buhs [215] reported that dog plasma contained "3 parts of TQ to 1 part of tocopherol," but Hines and Mattill [216] were unable to find TQ in liver, muscle, or urine. There have been many references to the occurrence of TQ in animal tissues [153, 159-162, 186, 217-225]. However, since this compound can readily form in vitro, it is difficult to establish to what degree this metabolites is an artifact resulting from isolation procedures. To avoid these problems, it is customary to add antioxidants to the tissue under study. Among those frequently used are butylated hydroxytoluene (BHT), butylated hydroxyanisole (BHA), and vitamin C. In autoxidizing lipids, ascorbic acid and α-tocopherol form a synergistic antioxidant combination. These findings have led Tappel [226] and Witting [227] to suggest that vitamin E in biologic systems might form a redox complex with vitamin C. In agreement with this, Green and his associates [228] demonstrated a pronounced protective effect of ascorbic acid on the decay of d-α-tocopherol labeled with ^{14}C and ^{3}H in the 5-methyl group (see Table 8). Consequently, organs such as the adrenals, which accumulate large amounts of both vitamins, should offer maximal protection to lipids against peroxidation. Whether this is indeed true is not known. Also, it is often overlooked that the first steps of the oxidation reactions of tocopherol are, to a marked degree, reversible. It is thus possible that the addition of antioxidants to the tissues being used for in vitro studies or obtained from in vivo work may give rise to what is usually called "unoxidized tocopherol," when in reality the vitamins exist in tissues as an unstable chemical entity ("semioxidized"). Findings obtained under these conditions are quite reproducible, but in reality, they may represent "isolation artifacts." A final solution to this dilemma may require new isolation and identification procedures.

TABLE 8   Recovery and Isotopic Ratio of [5-Methyl-^{14}C, ^{3}H]α-Tocopherol Present With and Without Ascorbic Acid During the Autoxidation of Lard at 75° [a]

Time (hr)	Without ascorbic acid				With ascorbic acid			
	^{14}C (dps)	^{3}H (dps)	^{3}H/^{14}C ratio	Tocopherol recovery (%)	^{14}C (dps)	^{3}H (dps)	^{3}H/^{14}C ratio	Tocopherol recovery (%)
3	40.8	211	5.17	74	56.1	317	5.65	101
21	21.2	139	6.56	38	58.9	323	5.48	106
44	4.6	24	5.22	8	52.1	291	5.59	94

[a] Each value is the mean of two analyses of 200-mg samples of lard containing 0.284 mg α-tocopherol with a specific activity of: ^{14}C, 195 dps/mg; ^{3}H, 1107 dps/mg (^{3}H/^{14}C ratio, 5.68).

Source: From Ref. 228, by permission of Cambridge University Press.

Other compounds with isoprenyl units appear to be metabolized in a similar manner to α-tocopherol. These naturally occurring substances include: phylloquinone (vitamin K_1), menaquinone-4 (vitamin K_2), ubiquinone-45 (coenzyme Q_9), hexahydroubiquinone-4 (phythylubiquinone), hexahydro-plasto-quinone-4 (phythylplastoquinone), β-, γ-, and ξ-tocopherols, and the tocopheramines and their substitution products. The striking similarity between the metabolism of these substances and that of tocopherols is discussed in Sec. B.4.

The most sensitive method of detecting TQ and other vitamin E metabolites has been the use of ^{14}C-labeled α-tocopherol. Csallany et al. [219] injected 5-methyl-[^{14}C]α-tocopherol into vitamin E-deficient rats. The livers were removed, minced, and ground to dryness in anhydrous sodium sulfate. The dried liver was extracted with acetone and the concentrated extract cooled to -70°C to remove by filtration a bulk of the lipids which carried little radioactivity. The chromatographic procedures were examined for artifacts: no oxidation products were found when [^{14}C]-tocopherol was subjected to the separation steps. About 9% of the injected radioactivity was recovered in the liver extract; TQ accounted for 19% of the recovered liver radioactivity and unchanged α-tocopherol for 25%; another metabolite accounted for more than half of the radioactivity (see Sec. B.2). These results were in contrast to those of Alaupovic et al. [253] who reported the isolation of three unidentified metabolites but no α-tocopheryl-p-quinone from the livers of rats and pigs given intraperitoneal doses of α-tocopherol. Also, Krishnamurthy and Bieri [25] reported that, after oral administration of [^{14}C]α-tocopherol to vitamin E-deficient rats and chickens, the radioactivity in tissues was almost exclusively α-tocopherol, with no evidence for a significant accumulation of TQ or other metabolites. In the liver of rats administered [^{14}C]α-tocopherol i.p., 80% of the recovered radioactivity was in the form of unchanged tocopherol and 11% was presented as TQ [221].

Weber et al. [230] studied the distribution of radioactive vitamin E in control and corn oil-fed rats. Total radioactivity in liver, brain, kidney, heart, and blood was significantly lower in the corn oil-fed rats than in the controls; no tocopherol metabolites could be found in these organs in either group. Depot fat was the exception: in coconut oil-fed rats, the main portion of the label was present as unchanged α-tocopherol and only small amounts as TQ. A diet with 10% linoleic acid methyl ester led to depot fat with a 10-fold increase of PUFA compared with the control rats; in this group, the portion of TQ was very large and there was little unchanged tocopherol left (Fig. 24). Similar results were obtained whether the ^{14}C-labeled tocopherol was injected or given orally. These observations suggest that TQ is formed in significant amounts when the PUFA content of depot fat is sufficiently high to cause in situ oxidation of vitamin E. Only traces of [^{14}C]TQ were found when [^{14}C]d-α-tocopherol was

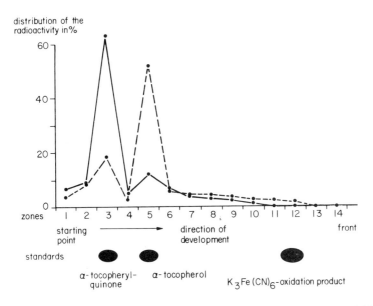

FIG. 24   Thin-layer chromatography of rat adipose tissue, 24 hr after the
intragastric administration of 2 mg ^{3}H-d-α-tocopheryl acetate. Note the
high concentration of α-tocopheryl quinone in animals fed with a 10%
methyl-linoleate diet. Source: From ref. 230.

incubated with methyl linoleate in an air oven at 60°C for 70 hr in a 1:2
(w/w) ratio. This procedure resulted in dimers and trimers of tocopherol
and a large amount of highly polar products. These compounds may represent decomposition products of TQ, which is known to be less stable than
the dimer or trimer [231]. Other studies in thoracic duct-cannulated rats
have demonstrated that the intestine is unable to oxidize tocopherol to a
great extent [159,160], even in the presence of large amounts of PUFA [162].

Recently, Aristarkhova et al. [224] used a chemiluminescent procedure
to study the changes in natural antioxidants after the administration of large
amounts of tocopheryl acetate. The quantity of total natural antioxidants in
the tissues increased about 40 times. This amount far exceeded that associated with free tocopherol, which increased only 10 times. These results
strongly suggest that, through redox reactions, natural antioxidants may
interchange in the body. An interesting finding in this study was that the
increase in the utilization of tocopherol correlated quite well with the
kinetics of accumulation of TQ (see Fig. 25). These results demonstrated
that an increase in the antioxidant activity of lipids leads to a concomitant

change in their oxidation potential, the end result being an increase in the rate of generation of free radicals. This is presumably a regulatory mechanism to maintain the antioxidant activity of lipids in a level of steady state. More recently, Shimasaki and Privett [225] reported on the oxidation of vitamin E, as well as changes in lipid and fatty acid composition of rat blood components incubated in vitro with hydroperoxides obtained from autoxidized methyl linoleate. Among the reaction products was tocopheryl quinone as well as unidentified substances isolated in the nonsaponifable fraction of lipid extract of hemolyzed RBC (see Fig. 26). These investigators observed little reaction of linoleate hydroperoxide with vitamin E or lipids of the serum. These results indicate that the strong antioxygenic action of vitamin E in vivo is due to its structural orientation in membranes.

Although TQ appears to participate in photosynthetic electron transport in chloroplasts [215], it is not clear what function, if any, this compound may have in animal tissues. Demonstration of its activity depends upon the bioassay employed, as well as the dose administered. Thus, TQ administered even in large doses, failed to substitute for vitamin E in the rat fertility test [232, 233], suggesting that it is not cyclized in vivo to the chromanol form in this species; this conclusion was substantiated by isotope techniques [234]. In agreement with these findings, Proll and

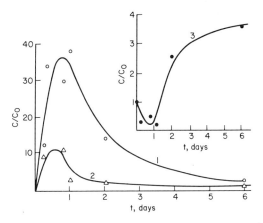

FIG. 25 Changes in the relative amounts of esterified, free and oxidized tocopherol in association with liver lipids of mice after i.p. administration of tocopheryl acetate (200 mg/kg body wt). 1, esterified tocopherol; 2, free tocopherol; 3, tocopheryl quinone. This figure was taken from Aristarkhova et al. (ref. 224, p. 705), by permission of Pergamon Press, Elmsford, New York.

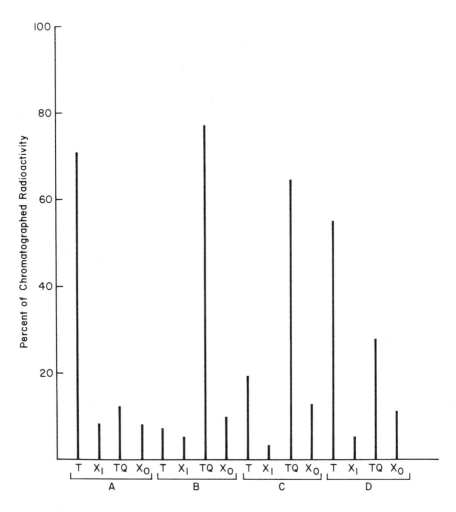

FIG. 26 Distribution of radioactivity in components separated by thin-
layer chromatography from the nonsaponifiable fraction of the incubation
of 1 ml suspension of erythrocytes containing: ^{3}H-labeled tocopherol
either in buffer alone (A); 4 mg LOOH in buffer for 15 min at 37°C (B); in
buffer with 4 mg LOOH and 10 μg ^{3}H-labeled vitamin E (C); or 4 mg LOOH
in buffer containing 10 μg ^{3}H-labeled vitamin E for 15 min at 37°C (D).
The specific activity used in C and D was 220,000 ^{3}H-labeled tocopherol
per milligram. Abbreviations: T, free tocopherol; X_1, unidentified substance arising from membrane or area corresponding to same; TQ,
α-tocopheryl quinone; Xo, unidentified spot at origin of plate. This figure was modified from Shimasaki and Privett [225].

Schmandke [235] tested in rats eight metabolites of α-tocopherol, including the quinone, dimer, and Simon metabolites for vitamin E efficiency by the hemolysis test. The intravenously administered compounds were given in equimolar as well as fivefold higher doses related to tocopherol given. None of the metabolites showed an effect on the hemolysis rate of vitamin E-deficient rats. However, Bunyan et al. [236] examined TQ and also α-tocopheryl hydroquinone (THQ) for activity in the gestation-resorption test in the rat and found 0.4 and 0.6%, respectively, of the potency of d-α-tocopheryl acetate. This amount was more than could be accounted for by traces of α-tocopherol that might have been present in the products. The effect of TQ in in vitro systems was considerably higher than the apparent activity observed in vivo. Moreover, Mackenzie et al. [237] found that both TQ and THQ are able to prevent and cure the creatinuria, paralysis, and loss of weight caused by vitamin E deficiency in rabbits. West and Mason [238] established that in hamsters, d-α-tocopheryl hydroquinone has a capacity to protect against experimental muscular dystrophy due to vitamin E deficiency. In vivo THQ may have a short half-life, since further studies have demonstrated that this compound maintains fertility and alleviates dystrophy in rats if administered by daily injections [239, 240]. Mauer and Mason [241] have recently concluded that d-α-tocopheryl hydroquinone has antisterility activity in the vitamin E-deficient male hamster and rat, approximating one-fifth that of d-α-tocopheryl acetate. Taken as a whole, these studies allow the conclusion that both the quinone and the hydroquinone possess some vitamin E activity; THQ has antioxidant properties and is more active than TQ. Consequently, it is important to gather a clear picture of the metabolic fate of these compounds.

Quinones are known to be reduced in rat liver preparations [242], and Henniger and Crane [243] reported reduction of TQ in the presence of reduced nicotinamide adenosine diphosphate (NADPH) in spinach chloroplasts. These findings are in good agreement with those of Chow et al. [234] who demonstrated that intraperitonially injected [^{14}C] d-α-tocopheryl quinone is reduced to the hydroquinone form in rat liver (see Fig. 27). [^{14}C] TQ was the only radioactive compound recovered in significant amounts in the liver extract of animals injected with either [^{14}C] TQ or [^{14}C] THQ. Internal standards demonstrated that the quinone was stable to the extraction and chromatographic procedures used, but that the hydroquinone was completely converted to the quinone in the course of the isolation procedure. Hence, it was not possible to determine directly whether the oxidized or reduced form is the predominant species present in the liver in situ. However, TQ was excreted as a conjugate of the hydroquinone in the feces and of α-tocopheronic acid in the urine. Also, a large fraction of the radioactivity in the feces of [^{14}C] THQ-injected rats was present as a conjugate which apparently was formed from the reduced compound in the liver. These investigations suggested that TQ was present

α-Tocopheryl-p-quinone   α-Tocopheryl-p-hydroquinone

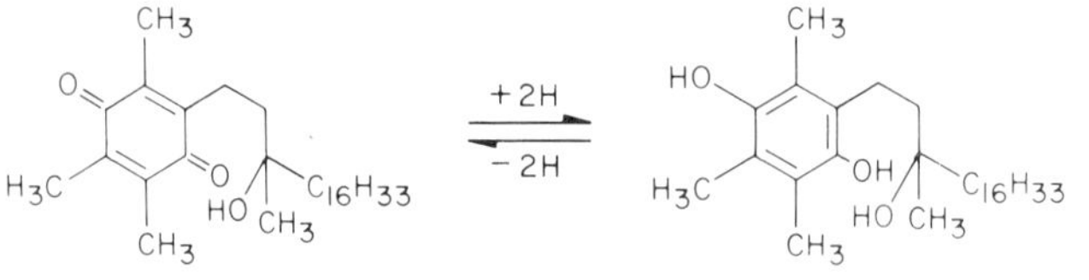

FIG. 27   The formation of α-tocopheryl hydroquinone from α-tocopheryl quinone. This conversion was first demonstrated by Chow et al. [234].

mainly in the reduced state in the liver and kidneys; neither TQ nor THQ appeared to be converted back to α-tocopherol in vivo. The observation that the quinone is readily reduced in mammalian tissues is not in agreement with the reported low biological activity of TQ when compared to that of THQ. Chow et al. [234] proposed that the progressive enzymatic reduction of TQ is closely coupled with conjugation of the hydroquinone. It is possible that parenterally administered THQ may exert an antioxidant effect in the peripheral tissues before it is deactivated by conjugation in the liver and degradation in the kidneys. According to this hypothesis then, TQ is reduced to THQ, conjugated in the liver, and excreted in the bile. In the kidney TQ undergoes reduction, conjugation and oxidative degradation of the side chain to form a conjugate of tocopheronic acid which is excreted in the urine. In the view of Chow et al. [234] therefore, TQ is reduced to THQ. Theoretically, however, THQ could be converted back to the quinone, and it is possible that these compounds may normally exist in equilibrium, which is disrupted by the usual isolation procedures.

2.   Dimers, Trimers, and Other Adducts

As indicated above, dimeric and trimeric oxidation products of tocopherol have been reported in the literature. It should be mentioned that tocopherol is capable of forming adducts with other molecules as well but these are seldom mentioned in the literature. For example, 5-benzoyl-oxymethyl-dl-α-tocopherol and the 5-alkoyloxymethyl derivatives have been synthesized. Adducts with dihydropyran and tetracyanoethylene were prepared by Skinner and Parkhurst [244], who also synthesized cyclic 5-methyleneoxy-6-oxy-7,8-dimethyl tocol phosphate [245]. Nilsson et al. [246] prepared a styrene adduct. Other adducts were prepared by Komoda and Harada [247]. More recently, Gardner et al. [248] found an adduct of vitamin E and linoleic acid hydroperoxide. Porter et al. [249,250] have reported that a similar reaction operates in the formation of adducts of oxidizing tocopherol and linoleic acid or soybean lecithin. Therefore, the possibility cannot be excluded that in vivo vitamin E may form adducts which have not yet been identified.

As previously discussed, in addition to identifying TQ as a metabolite of vitamin E in the liver, Csallany et al. [219] found an unidentified polar metabolite which accounted for more than half of injected 5-methyl-[^{14}C]α-tocopherol. After further purification [251], they assumed that metabolite might be an oxidation product of α-tocopherol. Therefore, α-tocopherol was oxidized with alkaline potassium ferricyanide and the main oxidation product was isolated. This was shown by chromatography in several different systems and by carrier crystallization of the bromobenzoic acid esters of the reduced products, to be identical with the liver metabolite. Subsequent studies [252] of the isolation ferricyanide oxidation product of α-tocopherol by chromatography on neutral alumina showed that it contained two components, one of which was identical with the liver metabolite. The molecular weight of the compound was approximately twice that of α-tocopherol. This finding, along with the observation that the reduction product of the unknown compound had two hydroxyl groups, strongly suggested that the unknown was a dimer of oxidized vitamin E. The occurrence of this metabolite had been suggested by the work of Alaupovic et al. [253], who following the administration of ^{14}C-labeled tocopherol to rats and pigs, detected an unidentified metabolite which they designated compound O. The formation of dimers has been denied by some investigators, but their existence has been reported by other laboratories. Weber and Wiss [220] found that dimer and quinone were formed from α-tocopherol during the autoxidation of unsaturated lipids. Green et al. [228] observed the formation of quinone, dimer, and unidentifiable products during the decay of radioactive tocopherol in the process of the autoxidation of methyl linoleate. Csallany et al. [231] presented evidence that, under appropriate conditions, oxidation products analogous to dimers (and trimers) are formed in vitro in the presence of autoxidizing methyl linoleate or of methyl linoleate hydroperoxide. On the other hand, Strauch et al. [212] reported that dimers and trimers were not demonstrable after oral administration of α-tocopherol to rats. Thus, there is no uniformity of opinion regarding the existence of dimers and trimers in mammalian tissues under physiological conditions.

Also, there appears to be conflicting proposals relative to the final structure of the dimer. The metabolite results from divalent oxidation of α-tocopherol, loss of the 7-methyl group, and subsequent dimerization. The structure of the spirenone ether proposed by Nelan and Robeson [211], although confirmed independently by Schudel et al. [254], did not fit with a number of the observations of Csallany and Draper [210], who showed evidence that the material isolated by Nelan and Robeson was probably a mixture. Csallany and Draper [210] concluded that the condensation mechanism included the formation of a central double bond. However, Strauch et al. [212] reported molecular weight data obtained by mass spectroscopy that were inconsistent with both their proposed structure, as well as that of Csallany and Draper. It was, however, admitted that artifacts formed during gas chromatography may have interfered with the findings of Strauch et al. [255]. The most extensive characterization of the dimeric oxidation product has been carried by Csallany [213], who in 1971, carried out a reinvestigation on the structure of a dimer of α-tocopherol isolated from rat liver. She demonstrated by near infrared spectroscopy, silylation, and deuterium labeling that the dimer contains a previously undetected hydroxyl group. In her view, dimerization entails the formation of a nine-membered chelate ring through strong intramolecular hydrogen bonding; the resulting compound has a molecular weight of 858. A structure was proposed that was compatible with these new findings and with most of the published data from other investigators. The postulated revised structure can be seen in Fig. 28.

3. Simon's Metabolites

These compounds were the first metabolites of vitamin E to be firmly identified. In 1956, Simon and his coworkers [256, 257] characterized two metabolites from the urine of rabbits and humans given large doses of α-tocopherol. One metabolite was a hydroxy acid and the other its lactone. Structure determinations revealed that oxidation had broken the chroman ring to produce a quinone (as in TQ), while the hydrocarbon side chain had been shortened from 16 carbons to three carbons and oxidized to a carboxylic acid. Chemical, spectroscopic, and analytical evidence was presented for the formulation of their chemical structures as 2-(3-hydroxy-3-methyl-5-carboxypentyl)-3, 5, 6-trimethyl-1, 4-benzoquinone and its γ-lactone. These compounds are commonly referred to as Simon's metabolites on

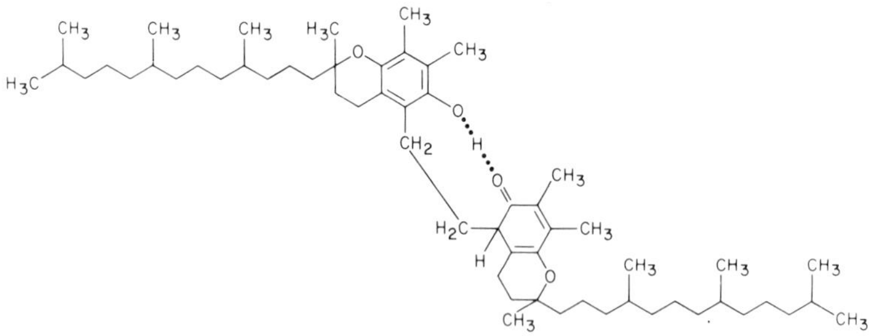

FIG. 28   The structure of tocopherol dimer, as proposed by Csallany [213].

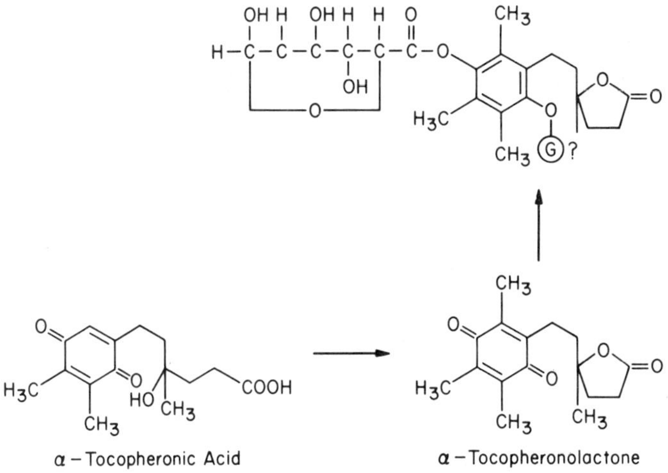

FIG. 29 Simon's metabolites of vitamin E. Notice conjugation in the glucuronic acid (G).

account of their long chemical names. Green et al. [258] gave these substances the trivial names of tocopheronic acid and tocopheronolactone (see Fig. 29).

The existence of these metabolites has been confirmed by many investigators. Simon's metabolites have also been shown in urine of rats [242]; their urinary excretion is influenced neither by feeding a diet rich in linoleate or by administering the d- or the l-form of tocopherol [220]. These results suggest that the oxidation of tocopherol to Simon's metabolites is not dependent upon the configuration of the asymmetric C_2. The major portion of these urinary metabolites is present as a conjugate with glucuronic acid, but it is not yet known whether it contains one of two glucuronic acid molecules. The intimate mechanism for the formation of Simon's metabolites is not known in detail. Simon and coworkers postulated that the first step is the formation of a phenolic glucuronide of α-tocopherol or of the corresponding hydroquinone after rupture or the chromane ring. This would be followed by an extensive degradation of the side chain first by α-oxidation and then by β-oxidation, until a side chain of seven carbon atoms is reached. On the last step, the lactonization of the OH group in γ-position with the terminal carboxyl group would take place. Thus, according to Simon et al. [256, 257], the quinone is an intermediate in the formation of α-tocopheronic acid, a view that has been disputed by Schmandke and Schmidt [259]. Other experiments on the metabolism of labeled tocopherol have indicated that when the dose administered

is within physiological limits, such as 1 or 2 mg for each rat, the amount
of radioactivity excreted in the urine within 48 hr is small, usually less
than 1% of the administered dose. Therefore, it is thought that these
urinary metabolites represent an extremely minor pathway of the metabolism of α-tocopherol. Other considerations suggest that Simon's metabolites are merely detoxification products. Conjugation with glucuronic
acid is a well-established means of detoxification of phenolic compounds.
Moreover, Simon's metabolites have never been detected in the tissues.
Furthermore, with one exception, these excretory compounds do not seem
to possess biological activity for intact animals. Uchiyama et al. [260]
reported that α-tocopheronolactone, injected i.p. into rats, at a dose of
10 mg per animal, exerted antiinflammatory activity to the same extent as
hydrocortisone acetate against dextran- and carrageenin-induced paw
edemas. This interesting report awaits further confirmation.

4. Comparison with Other Isoprenyl-Containing Compounds

A comparison of the distribution and metabolism of vitamin E to that of
other naturally occurring compounds with isoprenyl units in the side chain
has been carried out by the group at Hoffmann-La Roche in Basel. The
distribution pattern of hexahydroubiquinone-4, phylloquinone, menaqui-
none-4, α-tocopherylquinone, and α-tocopherol in the body of rats was
similar inasmuch as, a few hours after oral administration, a rather high
accumulation of the substances in the liver took place with subsequent
decreases in favor of higher concentrations in other organs. This transfer of the substances from the liver to other organs was not observed for
ubiquinone-9. On the contrary, the small amounts of ubiquinone-9 originally present in other organs were transferred to the liver, so that, after
24 hr, 97% of the total amount of ubiquinone-9 was localized in the liver.
Only α-tocopherol was accumulated selectively in the adrenals, whereas
menaquinone-4 reached much higher concentrations in the heart muscle
than did the others. α-Tocopherylquinone, phylloquinone, and menaqui-
none-4 were metabolized in the rat in the same manner as α-tocopherol,
i.e., by shortening of the side chains to seven carbon atoms by ω- and
β-oxidation and introduction of a hydroxy group, so that γ-lactones were
formed. These metabolites thus bear analogy to the metabolite of
α-tocopherol isolated by Simon and coworkers, differing only in the quinone part of the molecule. All the metabolites are excreted in the urine
as conjugates, presumably glucuronides. They can be isolated after acid
hydrolysis as the corresponding γ-lactones. A schematic representation
of these similarities is given in Fig. 30. As pointed out by Gloor [261],
these interesting findings mean that the degradation procedure outlined by
Simon et al. [256, 257] is of more general applicability, since it can take
place with isoprenyl side chains of different length and different degree of
unsaturation, even if there is no hydroxy group available in the side chain
from the beginning.

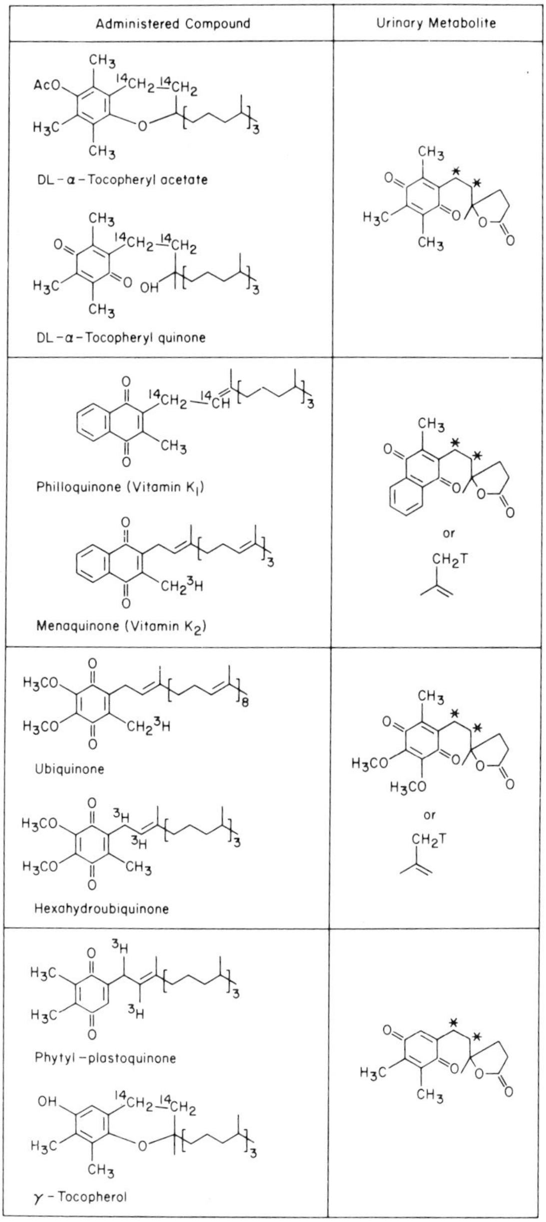

FIG. 30 Comparison of the metabolic products of tocopherol and other isoprenyl-containing substances. Notice the general applicability of the degradation procedure outlined by Simon et al. [256, 257].

VI. EXCRETION

A. Excretion in Urine, Feces, and Skin

Under physiological conditions, urinary excretion of vitamin E is in the form of Simon's metabolites. This represents a normal pathway, but its contribution seems to be quantitatively unimportant, since only 1% of the administered dose is excreted in the urine. Fecal elimination is undoubtedly a major route of excretion and varies widely, ranging from 10 to 75% of the administered dose depending upon the biological preparation used; as well as the analytical method employed. As discussed in Sec. VI.B., only small amounts of administered vitamin E are excreted in the bile. Therefore, tocopherol excreted in the feces arises from several sources, including: (1) incomplete absorption, (2) secretion from the intestinal mucosal cells back into the lumen, (3) desquamation of intestinal epithelial cells, and (4) biliary excretion. Vitamin E is not secreted in the pancreatic juice or other intestinal secretions. As previously discussed, significant amounts of tocopherol are deposited in the skin [179], suggesting that the skin plays a major role in the distribution and metabolism of vitamin E.

B. Biliary Excretion

Very little information exists on the biliary excretion of vitamin E or its metabolites. Schmandke and Proll [152] reported that rat bile contained 0.4-1.3 μg/ml tocopherol. Following intravenous administration of 5 mg dl-α-tocopherol, maximum excretion in the bile occurred on the second day. After 96 hr, 2.4% of the administered dose was excreted. It is not surprising to find tocopherol in bile, since other highly insoluble substances such as cholesterol and lecithin are present in bile in appreciable concentrations. These lipid molecules are normally kept in aqueous solution by virtue of incorporation into mixed micelles with the bile salts. In studies with lymph- and bile duct-cannulated rats, administered labeled tocopherol, MacMahon et al. [262] reported that up to 8% of the radioactivity was excreted in the bile during the 24 hr after intraduodenal administration. In opposition to the report of Schmandke and Proll [152] however, the studies of MacMahon et al. [262] demonstrated that less than 2% of the chromatographed radioactivity had the mobility of authentic α-tocopherol; most of the radioactivity remained at the origin, and no further characterization of the excretory product was done.

Studies on the quantitative biliary excretion of radioactivity were carried out in our laboratory in bile-cannulated rats after the intragastric administration of tritium-labeled tocopheryl acetate (TA) or tocopheryl nicotinate (TN). The esters of tocopherol were given in an emulsion containing proteins, carbohydrates, triolein, and saline. In these animals, the excretion rate of bile salts and lecithin was not changed. This was

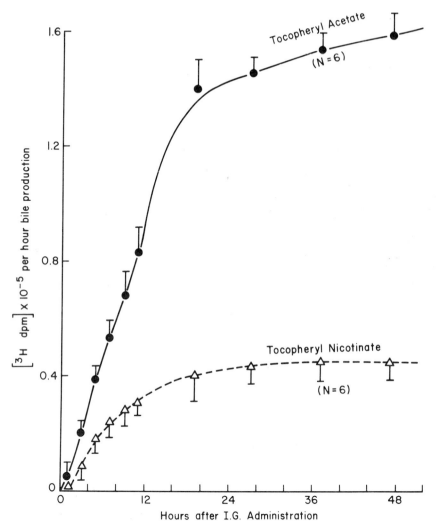

FIG. 31   Biliary excretion of total radioactivity (in the form of an unidentified metabolite) in rats administered labeled tocopherol esters. The animals were kept under steady state conditions of bile flow. Experimental conditions were otherwise the same as described in Figs. 3 and 4.

accomplished by the intraduodenal infusion of bile from rat donors. Although equimolar amounts were given, the biliary excretion of total radioactivity was significantly higher in the group receiving TA rather than TN (Fig. 31). Similar relative amounts of radioactivity appeared in

the bile of rats given free ^{3}H- or ^{14}C-labeled tocopherol (I.G.) and also
after the intravenous administration of the unesterified vitamin E, suggesting that the biliary excretion of vitamin E metabolic products is a normal,
physiologically significant event and not the expression of a detoxification
phenomenon which is only activated when high doses of the vitamin are
administered. In an effort to further delineate the nature of the biliary
radioactivity, the bile from rats given [^{14}C] tocopherol was pooled and
lyophilized. Concentration and fractionation of vitamin E metabolites were
achieved by extraction of the dry residue with chloroform/methanol and
subsequent thin-layer chromatographic separation. Authentic tocopherol,
tocopheryl-p-quinone, Simon's metabolites of tocopherol and tocopheryl-
glucuronide were used as standards. No unchanged TA or free tocopherol
was excreted in the bile of these rats, which received rather low doses
(1-2 mg) of the vitamin. The portion of radioactivity in the bile extract
behaving on TLC as tocopheryl-p-quinone or Simon's metabolites was
relatively small. However, most of the radioactivity in the bile extracts
cochromatographed with compounds more hydrophilic than TA, free tocopherol, tocopheryl-p-quinone, and the Simon's metabolites. The bulk of the
radioactivity was chromatographically similar to, and slightly more hydrophilic than the glucuronide of tocopherol. For further characterization of
the hydrophilic material, the corresponding chromatographic fractions
were incubated with β-glucuronidase/sulfatase. The chromatographic
behavior of the resulting product indicated that, in fact, one portion of the
vitamin E metabolite(s) must have been a substance bound to glucuronic
acid or sulfuric acid. After deconjugation, the metabolite was slightly
more polar than Simon's metabolite, but less polar than a synthetic glucuronide of tocopherol. This vitamin E metabolite has not previously been
identified in mammalian tissues. Although additional work is necessary
for the final elucidation of the structure of the bile metabolite, the described studies yielded evidence for the physiological occurrence of conjugated metabolites of vitamin E excreted in the bile of rats.

VII. OVERALL METABOLISM OF VITAMIN E

Vitamin E occurs in nature as a free alcohol, but it is usually administered
as an ester. In mammals, about 90% of the absorbed dose appears in the
lymph as a free vitamin, indicating that hydrolysis takes place either in the
intestinal lumen or at the mucosal cell. Mueller et al. [263] recently
demonstrated that duodenal esterase is the principal hydrolytic enzyme for
tocopherol esters. This suggests that, in the intestine, it is necessary to
solubilize the ester prior to hydrolysis. It was also shown that natural
bile salts, but not synthetic solubilizers, are important cofactors for the
reaction; there appears to be a specific interaction between cofactor and
enzyme. Thus, the poor hydrolysis of intravenously administered vitamin
E esters, in spite of abundant esterases throughout the body, may be due

TABLE 9   Chick Liver Tocopherol Levels 24 hr After a Single Oral Dosage with Esters of Tocopherol

Chemical structure	Tocopheryl-	Dosage (U)	Percent of liver tocopherol	
			Free	Ester
R-O-C(=O)-CH₃	Acetate	4	100.0	0.0
		8	100.0	0.0
		16	100.0	0.0
R-O-C(=O)-(pyridine ring)	Nicotinate	4	20.2	79.8
		8	27.7	72.3
		16	25.0	75.0
R-O-C(=O)-(pyridine ring)·H₂SO₄	Nicotinyl sulfate	4	67.0	33.0
		8	27.3	72.7
		16	34.0	66.0
R-O-C(=O)-(pyridine ring)·HCl	Nicotinyl hydrochloride	4	29.2	70.8
		8	25.6	76.4
		16	29.6	69.4
R-O-C(=O)-CH=CH-(phenyl ring)	Cinnamate	4	0.0	100.0
		8	1.7	98.3
		16	14.3	85.7
R-O-C(=O)-(phenyl ring)-NH₂	p-Aminobenzoate	4	36.3	63.7
		8	31.0	69.0
		16	0.0	0.0

Source: From Bunnell et al., unpublished observations.

to lack of suitable cofactors or adequate solubilization. In the intestine of birds, this hydrolytic mechanism is inefficient, for reasons that are not yet understood. Although tocopheryl acetate is extensively hydrolyzed, other esters of vitamin E may be absorbed as such (Table 9) [264]. Once absorbed, tocopherol is distributed throughout the body.

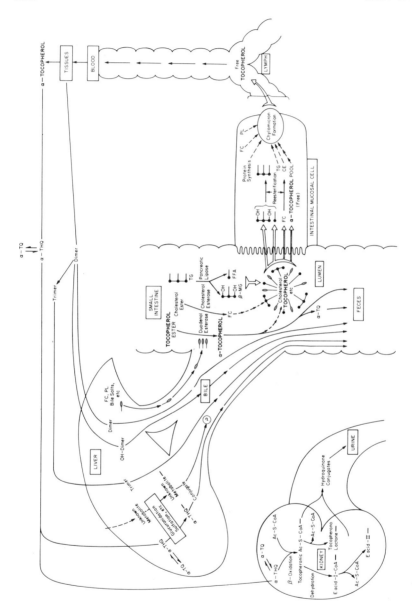

FIG. 32   A schematic representation of the general overview of the metabolism of vitamin E. This drawing is based on current available information.

An overview of the general metabolism of vitamin E, based on currently available information, is depicted in Fig. 32. No esters appear to
be formed in tissues. In the hypothetical scheme proposed by Simon et al.
[256,257], the chroman ring is hydrolyzed to α-tocopheryl quinone, which
is reduced to hydroquinone (TQ and THQ may normally exist in equilibrium), and at the same time, the terminal methyl group in the side chain is
oxidized. The resulting carboxylate is shortened, probably by β-oxidation,
giving rise to tocopheronic acid. Next, a nucleophilic attack by the hydroxy group in the side chain on the carbonyl carbon gives tocopheronolactone, releasing CoA in the process. Simon's proposal is supported by the
facts that TQ is formed in animal tissues and the administration of TQ
results in the urinary excretion of higher amounts of tocopheronolactone
than those observed after dosage with free tocopherol [154,265]. Draper
and Csallany [222] argue that the urinary excretory products are minor
metabolites of α-tocopherol since, under normal conditions, the rate of
quinone formation from α-tocopherol is limited, and most of it is eliminated with the stools. The amount of TQ in tissues, however, may depend
upon the experimental conditions employed. When large amounts of PUFA

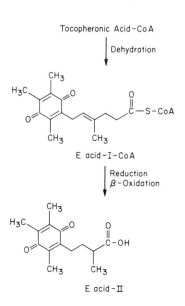

FIG. 33   The two new urinary excretion products of tocopherol reported
by Watanabe et al. [266].

are fed, large amounts of TQ are detected in the adipose tissue. Recently, Watanabe et al. [266] found two new urinary metabolites of vitamin E and proposed that the metabolic pathway proceeds somewhat differently (see Fig. 33). In this scheme, tocopheronic acid formed by β-oxidation is in part converted to tocopheronolactone and in part dehydrated so that an unsaturated, methylated CoA derivative is formed. By β-oxidation, and simultaneous reduction, a two-carbon unit is removed. These metabolites may be converted to their respective hydroquinones and excreted as conjugates. Also excreted as conjugates are the recently discovered biliary vitamin E metabolites. The final structure of these has not been yet completely elucidated, but it is possible that they may exist under physiological conditions. Dimers and trimers have been found in the liver. Urinary and biliary metabolites are excreted as either mono- or di-conjugates of glucuronic acid or sulfuric acid, or both.

VIII. SUMMARY

1. α-Tocopherol is transported in the lymph in the lipoproteins (LP), especially chylomicrons. The vitamin is distributed through the LP molecule; vitamin E exchanges less readily than cholesterol.

2. Tocopherol in plasma is also associated with lipoproteins, but there does not appear to be a specific lipoprotein carrier.

3. There is a rapid exchange of plasma tocopherol and erythrocyte tocopherol. All of the vitamin in the red blood cell is localized in the membrane.

4. α-Tocopherol is taken up by all tissues of the body. It is concentrated in the membrane-containing structures of the cell such as the mitochondria, microsomes, nucleus, and plasma membrane.

5. When either tocopheryl acetate or tocopheryl nicotinate is administered i.v., these compounds accumulate in the RES. It is not known whether the RES participates in the physiologic handling of orally administered vitamin E.

6. When a vitamin E-deficient diet is fed, plasma and liver levels of vitamin E decline rapidly. In the liver and several other tissues, there is a rapidly mobilized pool and a component which is retained for long periods. Depletion of tocopherol from adipose and muscle tissue is very slow and not bioavailable for practical purposes.

7. γ-Tocopherol is absorbed readily and deposited in tissues in a manner similar to α-tocopherol, but depletion rates from tissue are extremely rapid.

8. After administration of labeled tocopherol, almost all of the label is found in tissues as unchanged tocopherol. However, there is also some evidence for the existence in tissues of metabolites such as tocopheryl

quinone, tocopheryl hydroquinone, and dimers, trimers, and more-polar metabolites.

9. The major route of excretion is fecal elimination, which ranges from 10 to 75% of the dose administered. Usually less than 1% is excreted in the urine largely as tocopheronic acid or tocopheronic lactone (Simon's metabolites). A certain portion of tocopherol is excreted in the bile as an unidentified metabolite. It is not known whether vitamin E (or its metabolites) undergoes an enterohepatic circulation.

10. The metabolism of vitamin E is similar to that of other isoprenyl-containing compounds.

REFERENCES

1. K. E. Mason (ed.), Vitamin E, Ann. N.Y. Acad. Sci. 52:63 (1949).
2. K. E. Mason, in The Vitamins. Edited by W. H. Sebrell, Jr., and R. S. Harris, New York, Academic Press, 1954.
3. O. Wiss, R. H. Bunnell, and U. Gloor, Vit. Horm. 20:441 (1962).
4. O. A. Roels, Nutr. Rev. 25:33 (1967).
5. H. H. Draper, The tocopherols in "fat-soluble vitamins", in International Encyclopedia of Food and Nutrition, Vol. 9. Edited by R. A. Morton, 1970, p. 333.
6. N. Shimazono and Y. Takagi (eds.), International Symposium on Vitamin E, Hakone, Japan, Sept. 8-9, 1970. Tokyo, Kyoritsu Shuppan Co., 1972.
7. H. E. Gallo-Torres, Vitamin E in animal nutrition: Report of a Congress held at Hindsgavl Castle, Denmark, Sept. 8-11, 1971, Int. J. Vit. Nutr. Res. 42:312 (1972).
8. P. P. Nair and H. J. Kayden (eds.), International conference on vitamin E and its role in cellular metabolism, Ann. N.Y. Acad. Sci. 203:1 (1972).
9. J. Moustgaard and J. Hyldgaard-Jensen (eds.), Vitamin E in animal nutrition. Proceedings of a symposium of N.J.F., Sept. 8-11, 1971, Acta Agric. Scand. (Suppl.) 19 (1973).
10. M. K. Horwitt (ed.), Vitamin E: Biochemistry, nutritional requirements and clinical studies. International symposium held at Minneapolis, Minn., Sept. 27-28, 1973, Amer. J. Clin. Nutr. 9:939; 10:1105 (1974).
11. Congress Report, Fat soluble vitamins group meeting, University of Leeds, Apr. 4-5, 1975, Int. J. Vit. Nutr. Res. 46:205 (1976).
12. M. Boquillon, H. Carlier, and J. Clement, Digestion 10:255 (1974).
13. R. Blomstrand and L. Forsgren, Int. Z. Vit. Forschung 38:328 (1968).
14. L. K. Bjornson and H. E. Gallo-Torres, Fed. Proc. 34:913 (1975).

15. L. K. Bjornson, C. Gniewkowski, and H. J. Kayden, J. Lipid Res. 16:39 (1975).
16. M. L. Quaife and P. L. Harris, J. Biol. Chem. 156:499 (1944).
17. I. S. Wechsler, G. G. Mayer, and H. Sobotka, Proc. Soc. Exp. Biol. Med. 47:152 (1941); 53:170 (1943).
18. A. S. Minot and H. E. Frank, Amer. J. Dis. Child. 67:371 (1944).
19. C. Engel, Ann. N.Y. Acad. Sci. 52:292 (1949).
20. E. F. Week, F. J. Sevigne, and M. E. Ellis, J. Nutr. 46:353 (1952).
21. G. Klatskin and D. W. Molander, J. Clin. Invest. 31:159 (1952).
22. H. Rosenkrantz, A. T. Milhorat, and M. Farber, Metabolism 2:556 (1953).
23. J. Pomeranze and R. J. Lucarello, J. Lab. Clin. Med. 42:700 (1956).
24. W. R. H. Duncan, G. A. Garton, I. McDonald, and W. Smith, Br. J. Nutr. 14:371 (1960).
25. S. Krishnamurthy and J. G. Bieri, J. Lipid Res. 4:330 (1963).
26. F. Weber, U. Gloor, J. Würsch, and O. Wiss, Biochem. Biophys. Res. Commun. 14:189 (1964).
27. U. Gloor, J. Würsch, U. Schwieter, and O. Wiss, Helv. Chim. Acta 49:2303 (1966).
28. M. S. Losowsky and P. J. Leonard, Gut 8:539 (1967).
29. J. Kelleher and M. S. Losowsky, Br. J. Nutr. 24:1033 (1970).
30. I. R. Peake and J. G. Bieri, J. Nutr. 101:1615 (1971).
31. M. F. Sorrell, O. Frank, A. D. Thompson, H. Aquino, and H. Baker, Nutr. Rep. Int. 3:143 (1971).
32. J. T. Harries and D. P. R. Mueller, Gut 12:579 (1971).
33. T. Davies, J. Kelleher, C. L. Smith, B. E. Walker, and M. S. Losowsky, J. Lab. Clin. Med. 79:824 (1972).
34. M. S. Losowsky, B. E. Walker, and J. Kelleher, Nutrition in steatorrhea, in Malabsorption and Clinical Practice. Edinburgh, Churchill Livingstone, 1974, pp. 56-57.
35. M. A. Gassull, L. M. Blendis, D. J. A. Jenkins, A. R. Leeds, S. Hishon, and G. L. Metz, Int. J. Vit. Nutr. Res. 46:211 (1976).
36. M. K. Horwitt, Amer. J. Clin. Nutr. 29:569 (1976).
37. M. L. Quaife and P. L. Harris, Ind. Eng. Chem. Anal. Ed. 18:707 (1946).
38. M. Farber, A. T. Milhorat, and H. Rosenkrantz, Proc. Soc. Exp. Biol. Med. 79:225 (1952).
39. S. R. Ames and P. L. Harris, Anal. Chem. 28:874 (1956).
40. F. Bro-Rasmussen and W. Hjarde, Acta Chem. Scand. 11:34 (1957).
41. F. Bro-Rasmussen and W. Hjarde, Acta Chem. Scand. 11:44 (1957).
42. L. D. Matterson and M. W. Dicks, Feedstuffs, Dec. 24 (1960).
43. H. H. Draper, The tocopherols in "fat-soluble vitamins," in International Encyclopedia of Food and Nutrition, Vol. 9. Edited by R. A. Morton, 1970, p. 378.

44. P. W. R. Eggitt and L. D. Ward, J. Sci. Food Agric. 6:329 (1955).
45. E. E. Edwin, A. T. Diplock, J. Bunyan, and J. Green, Biochem. J. 75:450 (1960).
46. J. G. Bieri, C. J. Pollard, I. Prange, and H. Dam, Acta Chem. Scand. 15:783 (1961).
47. R. S. Harris and J. G. Wool (eds.), Vitam. Horm. 20:373 (1962).
48. M. Kofler, P. F. Sommer, H. R. Bollinger, B. Schmidli, and M. Vecchi, Vit. Horm. 20:407 (1962).
49. P. W. Wilson, E. Kodicek, and V. H. Booth, Biochem. J. 84:524 (1962).
50. J. G. Bieri and E. L. Andrews, Iowa State J. Sci. 38:3 (1963).
51. R. A. Dilley and F. L. Crane, Anal. Biochem. 5:531 (1963).
52. C. K. Chow, H. H. Draper, and A. S. Csallany, Anal. Biochem. 32:81 (1969).
53. H. J. Kayden, C. K. Chow, and L. K. Bjornson, J. Lipid Res. 14:533 (1973).
54. E. C. McCormick, D. G. Cornwell, and J. B. Brown, J. Lipid Res. 1:221 (1960).
55. P. R. Pelkonen, Acta Med. Scand. (Suppl.) 399:174 (1963).
56. H. J. Kayden and R. S. Silber, Trans. Assoc. Amer. Physicians 78:334 (1965).
57. H. Baker, O. Frank, S. Feingold, and C. M. Leevy, Nature (London) 215:84 (1967).
58. R. H. M. Rubinstein, A. A. Dietz, and R. Srinavasan, Clin. Chim. Acta 23:1 (1969).
59. T. Davies, J. Kelleher, and M. S. Losowsky, Clin. Chim. Acta 24:431 (1969).
60. I. R. Peake, H. G. Windmueller, and J. G. Bieri, Biochim. Biophys. Acta 260:679 (1972).
61. G. Brubacher, H. B. Stahelin, and J. P. Vuilleumier, Int. J. Vit. Nutr. Res. 44:521 (1974).
62. L. Aftergood, A. R. Alexander, and R. B. Alfin-Slater, Nutr. Rep. Intern. 11:295 (1975).
63. C. K. Chow, Amer. J. Clin. Nutr. 28:756 (1975).
64. O. V. Rajaram, P. Fatterparker, and A. Sreenivassan, Biochem. Biophys. Res. Commun. 52:459 (1973); C. L. Catignani, Biochem. Biophys. Res. Commun. 67:66 (1975).
65. Y. Takahashi, K. Uruno, and S. Kimura, J. Nutr. Sci. Vitaminol. 23:201 (1977); R. N. Patnaik and P. P. Nair, Arch. Biochem. Biophys. 178:333 (1977).
66. L. K. Bjornson, H. J. Kayden, E. Miller, and A. N. Moshell, J. Lipid Res. 17:343 (1976).
67. D. P. R. Mueller and J. T. Harries, Biochem. J. 112:28P (1969).

68. R. S. Overman, J. N. McNelly, M. E. Todd, and I. S. Wright, Amer. J. Clin. Nutr. 2:168 (1954).

69. R. W. Hillman, Amer. J. Clin. Nutr. 5:597 (1957).

70. T. E. Rousseau, Jr., M. W. Dicks, R. Teichman, C. F. Helmboldt, E. L. Bacon, R. M. Prouty, K. L. Dolge, H. D. Eaton, E. L. Jungherr, and G. Beall, J. Animal Sci. 16:612 (1957).

71. R. B. Goldbloom, Can. Med. Assoc. J. 82:1114 (1960).

72. F. Weber, U. Gloor, J. Würsch, and O. Wiss, Biochem. Biophys. Res. Commun. 14:186 (1964).

73. J. G. Bieri and E. L. Prival, Proc. Soc. Exp. Biol. Med. 120:554 (1965).

74. S. Dayton, S. Hashimoto, D. Rosenblum, and M. L. Pearce, J. Lab. Clin. Med. 65:739 (1965).

75. M. J. Bennett and B. F. Medawadowski, Amer. J. Clin. Nutr. 20:415 (1967).

76. W. L. Marusich, G. Ackerman, W. C. Reese, and J. C. Bauernfeind, J. Animal Sci. 27:58 (1968).

77. J. Kelleher and M. S. Losowsky, Biochem. J. 110:20P (1968).

78. H. Larsson and K. Heger, Pharmacol. Clin. 1:72 (1968).

79. H. Grimes and P. J. Leonard, Biochem. J. 115:15P (1969).

80. P. Weiss and J. R. Bianchine, Amer. J. Med. Sci. 258:275 (1969).

81. W. J. Pudelkiewicz and N. Mary, J. Nutr. 97:303 (1969).

82. H. F. Hintz, D. E. Hogue, and E. F. Walker, Jr., Proc. Soc. Exp. Biol. Med. 131:447 (1969).

83. K. C. Hayes, J. E. Rousseau, Jr., and D. M. Hegsted, J. Amer. Vet. Med. Assoc. 157:64 (1970).

84. M. T. MacMahon and G. Neale, Clin. Sci. 38:197 (1970).

85. K. Hoppner, W. E. J. Phillips, and T. K. Murray, Can. J. Physiol. Pharmacol. 48:321 (1970).

86. R. K. H. Poukka and J. G. Bieri, Lipids 5:757 (1970).

87. T. Fujii, H. Shimizu, and I. Eda, J. Vitaminol. 18:84 (1972).

88. I. Gontzea and N. Nicolau, Nutr. Rep. Intern. 5:225 (1972).

89. P. J. Leonard, E. Doyle, and W. Harrington, Amer. J. Clin. Nutr. 25:480 (1972).

90. G. Goransson, A. Norden, and B. Akesson, Scand. J. Gastroenterol. 8:21 (1973).

91. J. S. Lewis, A. K. Pian, M. T. Baer, P. B. Acosta, and G. A. Emerson, Amer. J. Clin. Nutr. 26:136 (1973).

92. S. Gross and D. K. Melhorn, J. Pediatr. 85:753 (1974).

93. F. X. Roth and M. Kirchgessner, Int. J. Vit. Nutr. Res. 45:333 (1975).

94. P. M. Farrell and J. G. Bieri, Amer. J. Clin. Nutr. 28:1381 (1975).

95. W. R. McWhirter, Acta Pediatr. Scand. 64:446 (1975).

96. A. Malm, W. G. Pond, E. F. Walker, Jr., M. Homan, A. Aydin, and D. Kirtland, J. Animal Sci. 42:393 (1976).

97. W. J. Darby, M. E. Ferguson, R. H. Furman, J. M. Lemley, C. T. Ball, and G. R. Meneely, Ann. N.Y. Acad. Sci. 52:328 (1949).

98. J. V. Straumfjord and M. L. Quaife, Proc. Soc. Exp. Biol. Med. 61:369 (1964).

99. J. Varangot, Compt. Rend. Acad. Sci. 214:691 (1942).

100. H. H. Gordon, H. M. Nitowsky, J. T. Tildon, and S. Levin, Pediatrics 21:673 (1958).

101. S. W. Wright, L. J. Filer, and K. F. Mason, Pediatrics 7:386 (1951).

102. H. M. Nitowsky, M. Cornblath, and H. H. Gordon, Amer. J. Dis. Child. 92:164 (1956).

103. R. B. Goldbloom and D. Cameron, Pediatrics 32:36 (1963).

104. F. A. Oski and L. A. Barness, J. Pediatr. 70:211 (1967).

105. J. B. MacKenzie, Pediatrics 13:346 (1954).

106. J. H. Ritchie, B. Fish, V. McMasters, and M. Grossman, N. Engl. J. Med. 279:1185 (1968).

107. R. Beckman, Die bedeutung des vitamin E in der padiätrie, in Vitamin A, E, and K. Edited by F. H. Von Kress and K. U. Blum, New York, Schattauer, 1969, p. 361-373.

108. A. Minkowski, E. Swierczewski, C. Chanez-Bel, and C. Gibelin, E'tudes Neo-Natales 7:81 (1958).

109. M. K. Horwitt and P. Bailey, Arch. Neurol. Psychiatr. 1:312 (1959).

110. J. Lehmann, M. W. Marshall, H. T. Slover, and J. M. Iacono, J. Nutr. 107:1006 (1977).

111. S. Postel, J. Clin. Invest. 35:1345 (1956).

112. V. McMasters, T. Howard, L. W. Kinsell, J. Van Der Veen, and H. S. Olcott, Amer. J. Clin. Nutr. 20:622 (1967).

113. R. Pelkonen, Acta Med. Scand. 174 (Suppl. 399):1 (1963).

114. R. M. H. Kater, W. J. Unterecker, C. Y. Kim, and C. S. Davidson, Amer. J. Clin. Nutr. 23:913 (1970).

115. M. K. Horwitt, A. L. Hall, J. A. Whitaker, and R. E. Olson, Fed. Proc. 28:758 (1969).

116. H. J. Binder, D. C. Herting, V. Hurst, S. C. Finch, and H. M. Spiro, New Engl. J. Med. 273:1289 (1965).

117. E. Cheraskin and W. M. Ringsdorf, Jr., Nutr. Rep. Int. 2:107 (1970).

118. V. E. Anisimov and B. S. Berezovski, Kazanskii Med. J. 5:27 (1960).

119. I. N. Iacovleva, Sovet. Med. 26:26 (1963).

120. R. H. Moorman, Jr., H. E. Snyder, C. D. Snyder, and W. A. Grosjean, Arch. Surg. 67:137 (1963).

121. I. P. Nikitin, Vop. Pitan 21:22 (1962).

122. A. H. Ratcliffe, Lancet 2:1128 (1949).

123. W. E. Shute and E. V. Shute, Alpha-tocopherol in Cardiovascular Disease, Toronto, Ryerson Press, 1954.

124. N. V. Sirnina and V. P. Stronkovskii, Therap. Arch. 33:26 (1961).
125. E. Szirmai and G. Ruecker, Z. Ges. Int. Med. 15:222 (1960).
126. V. Bohlau, Arzneim-Forsch. (Drug Res.) 21:674 (1971).
127. C. K. Donegan, A. L. Messer, E. S. Orgain, and J. M. Ruffin, Amer. J. Med. Sci. 217:294 (1949).
128. L. A. Gervasoni and A. Vannotti, Schweiz. Med. Wschr. 24:708 (1956).
129. M. Hamilton, G. M. Wilson, P. Armitage, and J. T. Boyd, Lancet 1:367 (1953).
130. M. Hamilton, G. M. Wilson, P. Armitage, and J. T. Boyd, Lancet 1:743 (1954).
131. R. Silber, R. Winter, and H. J. Kayden, J. Clin. Invest. 48:2089 (1969).
132. H. J. Kayden and L. Bjornson, Ann. N.Y. Acad. Sci. 203:127 (1972).
133. F. C. Jager and U. M. T. Houtsmuller, Nutr. Metab. 12:3 (1970).
134. J. G. Bieri and R. K. H. Poukka, Int. J. Vit. Nutr. Res. 40:344 (1970).
135. M. A. Chadd and A. J. Fraser, Int. J. Vit. Nutr. Res. 40:604 (1970).
136. F. Hruba, Vulterinova, V. Novakova, and Z. Placer, Int. J. Vit. Nutr. Res. 41:521 (1971).
137. Q. F. Ankong, D. Fisher, W. Tampion, and J. A. Lucy, Biochem. J. 136:147 (1973).
138. A. T. Diplock and J. A. Lucy, FEBS Lett. 29:205 (1973).
139. M. L. Quaife and M. Y. Dju, J. Biol. Chem. 180:263 (1949).
140. M. Y. Dju, K. E. Mason, and L. J. Filer, Jr., Etudes Neo-Natales 1:49 (1952).
141. K. E. Mason, M. Y. Dju, and L. J. Filer, Jr., Fed. Proc. 11:449 (1952).
142. M. Y. Dju, K. E. Mason, and L. J. Filer, Jr., Amer. J. Clin. Nutr. 6:50 (1958).
143. M. Y. Dju, L. J. Filer, Jr., and K. E. Mason, Amer. J. Clin. Nutr. 6:61 (1958).
144. J. G. Bieri and R. Poukka Evarts, Amer. J. Clin. Nutr. 28:717 (1975).
145. B. A. Underwood, H. Siegel, M. Dolinski, and R. C. Weisell, Amer. J. Clin. Nutr. 23:1314 (1970).
146. M. Mino, H. Nishino, T. Yamaguchi, and M. Hayashi, J. Nutr. Sci. Vitaminol. 23:63 (1977).
147. J. Sternberg and E. Pascoe-Dawson, Can. Med. Assoc. J. 80:266 (1959).
148. A. P. Grifo, Jr., H. D. Eaton, J. E. Rousseau, Jr., and L. A. Moore, J. Animal Sci. 18:232 (1959).
149. R. T. Chatterton, Jr., D. G. Hazzard, H. D. Eaton, B. A. Dehority, and A. P. Grifo, Jr., J. Dairy Sci. 44:1061 (1961).

150. E. E. Edwin, A. T. Diplock, J. Bunyan, and J. Green, Biochem. J. 79 (1961).
151. M. V. Zaehringer, C. A. Rickard, and W. P. Lehrer, Jr., J. Animal Sci. 22:592 (1963).
152. H. Schmandke and J. Proll, Int. Z. Vitaminf. 34:312 (1964).
153. A. Mellors and M. McC. Barnes, Br. J. Nutr. 20:69 (1966).
154. U. Gloor and O. Wiss, Helv. Chim. Acta 49:2590 (1966).
155. J. Kelleher, T. Davies, and M. S. Losowsky, Biochem. J. 114:74P (1969).
156. M. Hidiroglou, K. J. Jenkins, J. R. Lessard, and E. Borowsky, Can. J. Physiol. Pharmacol. 48:751 (1970).
157. C. K. Pearson and M. McC. Barnes, Br. J. Nutr. 24:581 (1970).
158. R. Poukka Evarts and J. G. Bieri, Lipids 5:757 (1970).
159. H. E. Gallo-Torres, Lipids 5:379 (1970).
160. H. E. Gallo-Torres, Int. J. Vit. Nutr. Res. 40:505 (1970).
161. H. E. Gallo-Torres, O. N. Miller, J. G. Hamilton, and C. Tratnyek, Lipids 6:318 (1971).
162. H. E. Gallo-Torres, F. Weber, and O. Wiss, Int. J. Vit. Nutr. Res. 41:504 (1971).
163. I. R. Peake and J. G. Bieri, Fed. Proc. 32:639 (1973).
164. H. E. Gallo-Torres, Acta Agric. Scand. (Suppl.) 19:97 (1973).
165. R. Poukka Evarts and J. G. Bieri, Lipids 9:860 (1974).
166. H. Kobayashi, C. Kanno, K. Yamauchi, and T. Tsugo, Bioch. Biophys. Acta 380:282 (1975).
167. F. R. Engelhardt, Can. J. Physiol. Pharmacol. 55:601 (1977).
168. G. B. J. Glass, Routes for absorption, in Introduction to Gastro-intestinal Physiology. Englewood Cliffs, N.J., Prentice-Hall, 1968, p. 146.
169. P. R. Holt, Medium chain triglycerides: Their absorption, metabolism and clinical applications, in Progress in Gastroenterology, Vol. I. Edited by G. B. J. Glass, New York, Grune and Stratton, 1968, p. 277.
170. H. E. Gallo-Torres, J. Ludorf, and M. Brin, Int. J. Vit. Nutr. Res., 48:240 (1978).
171. H. Fisher and H. Kaunitz, Proc. Soc. Exp. Biol. Med. 120:175 (1965).
172. Y. I. Takahashi and B. A. Underwood, Lipids 9:855 (1974).
173. P. Tantibhedhyangkul and S. A. Hashim, Bull. N.Y. Acad. Sci. 47:17 (1971).
174. J. G. Bieri, Ann. N.Y. Acad. Sci. 203:181 (1972).
175. L. J. Machlin and J. Keating, unpublished observations (1978).
176. L. W. Marusich, E. De Ritter, E. F. Ogrinz, J. Keating, M. Mitrovic, and R. H. Bunnell, Poul. Sci. 54:831 (1975).
177. V. Mc Masters, J. K. Lewis, L. W. Kinsell, J. Van der Veen, and H. S. Olcott, Amer. J. Clin. Nutr. 17:357 (1965).

178. H. E. Gallo-Torres and O. N. Miller, Int. J. Vit. Nutr. Res. 41:339 (1971).

179. T. Shiratori, Life Sci. 14:929 (1974).

180. C. Caravaggi, M. W. Gibbons, and E. Wright, N.Z. J. Agr. Res. 11:313 (1968).

181. H. H. Tikriti, Diss. Abtr. Int. 31:1717-B (1970).

182. H. L. Newmark, W. Pool, J. C. Bauernfeind, and E. De Ritter, J. Pharm. Sci. 64:655 (1975).

183. J. C. Bauernfeind, H. Newmark, and M. Brin, Amer. J. Clin. Nutr. 27:234 (1974).

184. E. Bonetti and F. Novello, Int. J. Vit. Nutr. Res. 46:244 (1976).

185. E. Bonetti, F. De Stefano, and F. Stirpe, J. Nutr. 90:387 (1966).

186. M. G. Spratt and C. C. Krantzig, J. Reticuloendother. Soc. 10:319 (1971).

187. M. Frigg and H. E. Gallo-Torres, Int. J. Vit. Nutr. Res. 47:145 (1977).

188. H. Eckert, in Autoradiography of Diffusable Substances. Edited by L. J. Roth and W. E. Stumpf, New York, Academic, 1969, p. 321.

189. S. E. Bjorkman, Acta Med. Scand. (Suppl. 191) (1947).

190. F. M. McCormick and M. Krashgarian, Amer. J. Clin. Pathol. 43:332 (1965).

191. L. A. Walkers, J. Lab. Clin. Med. 36:404 (1950).

192. R. J. Stenger, M. Petrelli, A. Segel, J. N. Williamson, and E. A. Johnson, Amer. J. Pathol. 57:689 (1969).

193. D. C. Bird and J. N. Sheagren, Proc. Soc. Exp. Biol. Med. 133:34 (1970).

194. H. H. Draper and A. S. Csallany, Proc. Soc. Exp. Biol. Med. 99:739 (1958).

195. R. H. Bunnell, E. De Ritter, and S. H. Rubin, Amer. J. Clin. Nutr. 28:706 (1975).

196. L. A. Witting, E. M. Harmon, and M. K. Horwitt, Proc. Soc. Exp. Biol. Med. 120:718 (1965).

197. L. J. Machlin, J. Keating, J. Nelson, M. Brin, R. Filipski, and O. N. Miller, J. Nutr. 109:105 (1979).

198. P. R. Cheeke and L. R. Shull, Nutr. Reports Int. 6:93 (1972).

199. W. Boguth, Vit. Horm. 27:1 (1970).

200. M. S. Blois, Nature (London) 181:1199 (1958).

201. W. A. Skinner and P. Alaupovic, J. Org. Chem. 28:2854 (1963).

202. W. Boguth and S. Blahser, in Vitamin A, E, and K. Edited by H. F. von Kress and K. U. Blum, Stuttgart, Schattauer, 1969, p. 235.

203. R. Repges and M. Sernetz, Ber. Bunsenges. Phys. Chem. 73:264 (1969).

204. W. A. Skinner and R. M. Parkhurst, J. Org. Chem. 29:3601 (1964).

205. W. Boguth and R. Hackel, Int. Z. Vitaminforsch. 38:169 (1964).

206. W. Durckheimer and L. A. Cohen, Biochem. Biophys. Res. Commun. 9:262 (1962).
207. C. T. Goodhue and H. A. Risley, Biochemistry 4:854 (1965).
208. C. R. Seward, G. Vaughan Mitchell, L. C. Argett, and E. L. Hove, Lipids 4:629 (1969).
209. A. S. Csallany, H. H. Draper, and S. N. Shah, Biochim. Biophys. Acta 59:527 (1962).
210. A. S. Csallany and H. H. Draper, J. Biol. Chem. 100:335 (1963).
211. D. R. Nelan and C. D. Robeson, J. Amer. Chem. Soc. 84:2963 (1962).
212. B. S. Strauch, H. M. Fales, R. C. Pittman, and J. Avigan, J. Nutr. 97:194 (1969).
213. A. S. Csallany, Int. J. Vit. Nutr. Res. 41:376 (1971).
214. R. A. Dilley and F. L. Crane, Biochim. Biophys. Acta 75:141 (1963).
215. J. V. Scudi and R. P. Buhs, J. Biol. Chem 149:549 (1943).
216. L. R. Hines and H. A. Mattill, J. Biol. Chem. 149:549 (1943).
217. R. A. Morton and W. E. J. Phillips, Biochem. J. 73:427 (1959).
218. A. T. Diplok, J. Green, E. E. Edwin, and J. Bunyan, Biochem. J. 76:563 (1960).
219. A. S. Csallany, H. H. Draper, and S. N. Shah, Arch Biochem. Biophys. 98:142 (1962).
220. F. Weber and O. Wiss, Helv. Physiol. Pharmacol. Acta 21:131 (1963).
221. P. S. Plack and J. G. Bieri, Biochim. Biophys. Acta 84:729 (1964).
222. H. H. Draper and A. S. Csallany, Fed. Proc. 28:1690 (1969).
223. W. A. Skinner, M. Leaffer, J. Johansson, and C. Mitoma, Experientia 26:502 (1970).
224. S. A. Aristarkhova, Ye. B. Burlakova, and N. G. Khrapova, Biophysics (Eng. transl.) 19:703 (1974).
225. H. Shimasaki and O. S. Privett, Arch. Biochem. Biophys. 169:506 (1975).
226. A. L. Tappel, Vit. Horm. 20:493 (1962).
227. L. A. Witting, Lipids 2:109 (1967).
228. J. Green, A. T. Diplock, J. Bunyan, D. McHale, and I. R. Muthy, Br. J. Nutr. 21:69 (1967).
229. S. Krishnamurthy and J. G. Bieri, J. Lipid Res. 4:330 (1963).
230. F. Weber, H. Weiser, and O. Wiss, Z. Ernahrungsw. 4:245 (1964).
231. A. S. Csallany, M. Chiu, and H. H. Draper, Fed. Proc. 28:757 (1969).
232. C. Golumbic and H. A. Matill, J. Biol. Chem. 134:535 (1940).
233. A. Issidorides and H. A. Matill, J. Biol. Chem. 188:313 (1951).
234. C. K. Chow, H. H. Draper, A. S. Csallany, and M. Chiu, Lipids 2:390 (1967).

235. J. Proll and H. Schmandke, Int. Z. Vitaminforsch. 39:304 (1969).
236. J. Bunyan, D. McHale, and J. Green, Br. J. Nutr. 17:391 (1963).
237. J. B. Mackenzie, H. Rosenkrantz, S. Ulick, and A. T. Milhorat, J. Biol. Chem. 183:655 (1950).
238. W. T. West and K. E. Mason, Amer. J. Physiol. Med. 34:223 (1955).
239. J. B. Mackenzie and C. G. Mackenzie, J. Nutr. 67:223 (1959).
240. J. B. Mackenzie and C. G. Mackenzie, J. Nutr. 72:322 (1960).
241. S. I. Mauer and K. E. Mason, J. Nutr. 105:491 (1975).
242. J. Bunyan, J. Green, A. T. Diplock, and E. E. Edwin, Biochim. Biophys. Acta 49:420 (1961).
243. M. D. Henniger and F. L. Crane, Bioc1im. Biophys. Acta 75:144 (1963).
244. W. A. Skinner and R. M. Parkhurst, J. Org. Chem. 31:1248 (1966).
245. W. A. Skinner and R. M. Parkhurst, Lipids 6:240 (1971).
246. J. L. Nilsson, J. O. Branstad, and H. Sievertsson, Acta Pharm. Suecica 5:509 (1968).
247. M. Komoda and I. Harada, J. Amer. Oil Chem. Soc. 47:249 (1970).
248. H. W. Gardner, K. Eskins, G. W. Grams, and G. E. Inglett, Lipids 7:324 (1972).
249. W. L. Porter, L. A. Levasseur, and A. S. Henick, Lipids 6:1 (1971).
250. W. L. Porter, A. S. Henick, and L. A. Levasseur, Lipids 8:31 (1973).
251. H. H. Draper, A. S. Csallany, and S. N. Shah, Biochim. Biophys. Acta 59:527 (1962).
252. A. S. Csallany and H. H. Draper, Arch. Biochem. Biophys. 100:335 (1963).
253. P. Alaupovic, B. C. Johnson, Q. Crider, H. N. Bhagavan, and B. J. Johnson, Amer. J. Clin. Nutr. 9:76 (1961).
254. P. Schudel, H. Mayer, J. Metzger, R. Reugg, and O. Isler, Helv. Chim. Acta 46:636 (1963).
255. H. A. Lloyds, E. A. Sokoloski, B. S. Strauch, and H. M. Fales, Chem. Commun. D. No. 6, 1934 (1969).
256. E. J. Simon, C. S. Gross, and A. T. Milhorat, J. Biol. Chem. 221:797 (1956).
257. E. J. Simon, A. Eisengart, L. Sundheim, and A. T. Milhorat, J. Biol. Chem. 221:807 (1956).
258. J. Green, E. E. Edwin, A. T. Diplock, and J. Bunyan, Biochim. Biophys. Acta 49:417 (1961).
259. H. Schmandke and G. Schmidt, Int. Z. Vitaminforsh. 38:75 (1968).
260. M. Uchiyama, M. Ito, and K. Fukuzaroa, J. Vitaminol. 16:225 (1970).
261. U. Gloor et al., unpublished observations.

262. M. T. MacMahon, G. Neale, and G. R. Thompson, Eur. J. Clin. Invest. 1:288 (1971).
263. D. P. R. Mueller, J. A. Manning, P. M. Mathias, and J. T. Harries, Int. J. Vit. Nutr. Res. 46:207 (1976).
264. R. H. Bunnell, unpublished observations.
265. O. Wiss and U. Gloor, Vit. Horm. 24:575 (1966).
266. M. Watanabe, M. Toyoda, I. Imada, and H. Morimoto, Chem. Pharm. Bull. 22:176 (1974).

Part 5C/ Biogenesis

HAROLD H. DRAPER

University of Guelph
Guelph, Ontario, Canada

Biosynthesis of the tocochromanols of the vitamin E group shares contain features in common with that of the structurally related plastochromanols and that of the more distantly related naphthoquinones of the vitamin K group, as well as the benzoquinones of the ubiquinone (coenzyme Q) series. Tocopherols are synthesized by higher plants and algae, but their presence in yeasts and fungi is disputed. They appear to be absent in bacteria. α-Tocopherol is the main form of vitamin E in algae and in the leaves of higher plants, where it is located mainly in the chloroplasts. γ-Tocopherol predominates in some seed oils (notably corn and soybean) and is present in the leaves of some plants. β- and δ-tocopherols are generally minor forms. The unsaturated derivatives of α- and β-tocopherol, i.e., α- and β-tocotrienol, are prevalent in some cereal grains, notably wheat, oats, and barley. The endosperm fraction of corn and wheat contains the bulk of the tocotrienols, whereas the germ contains most of the α-tocopherol [1].

Reviews on the biosynthesis of vitamin E have been published by Threlfall [2] and by Janiszowska and Pennock [3]. Studies on the incorporation of specifically labeled precursors into the unsaponifiable lipids of corn plants, chiefly by Threlfall and coworkers, demonstrated that shikimic acid is incorporated into the aromatic nuclei of tocopherols and plastochromanols and into the p-benzoquinone nuclei of tocopheryl quinones and plastoquinones. p-Hydroxyphenylpyruvate is a key intermediate in this process. Additional studies showed that, in higher plants, shikimate is also a precursor of the p-benzoquinone nucleus of the ubiquinones and the naphthoquinone nucleus of the K vitamins. The shikmic acid pathway is present in plants, algae, and bacteria, but is lacking in animals. The nucleus of ubiquinones synthesized in animal tissues is derived from the aromatic amino acids phenylalanine and tyrosine.

The pathway of tocotrienol biosynthesis from homogentisate suggested by these studies is outlined in Fig. 1. The steps between homogentisate and δ-tocotrienol are still obscure. Isotope experiments have shown that the 8-methyl group of the tocopherols and plastochromanols and their corresponding quinones can be derived from the β-carbon of p-hydroxyphenylpyruvate (the α-carbon of homogentisate). However, attempts to detect toluquinol (the decarbozylation product of homogentisate) or some similar intermediate have been unsuccessful. It has been proposed that a concerted reaction occurs involving simultaneous polyprenylation and nonoxidative decarboxylation of homogentisate, giving rise to a tetraprenyl methyl-quinol, which subsequently undergoes cyclization to form δ-tocotrienol (Fig. 1). In support of this view, synthesis of polyprenyltoluquinols from homogentisate and polyprenylpyrophosphates in particulate fractions of Euglena and sugar beet leaves has been reported by Thomas and Threlfall [4]. Radioactivity from mevalonic acid-2-[14C] has been found in the prenyl portions of α- and γ-tocopherol, α-tocopheryl quinone, plasto-quinone, phylloquinone, and β-carotene. The isoprene units are trans, and hydrogen is incorporated sterospecifically.

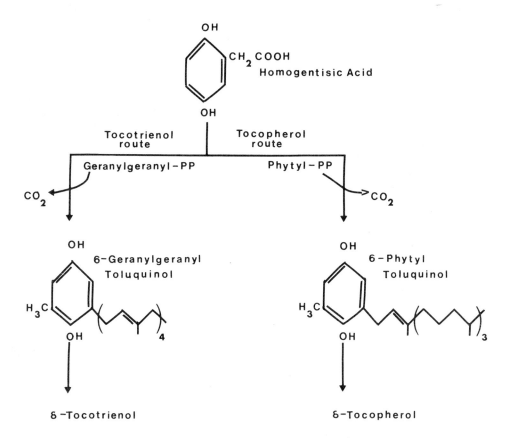

FIG. 1 Proposed pathways for the biosynthesis of δ-tocotrienol and δ-tocopherol. (From Refs. 2 and 3.)

It was originally proposed that δ-tocotrienol is the parent compound for the biosynthesis of all other naturally occurring tocotrienols as well as the tocopherols [2]. There was support for this conclusion from both isotopic and biogenetic studies. Analysis of seeds at various stages of germination has revealed changes in the distribution of vitamin E isomers indicative of successive methylations of the aromatic nucleus followed by hydrogenation of the polyprenyl side chain. For example, in germinating wheat seeds (which contain α- and β-tocotrienol and the corresponding tocopherols), the tocotrienols disappear by the time the plant is a few centimeters high and β-tocopherol disappears during the second month of growth [5]. Beyond this stage the plant resembles grasses in containing only α-tocopherol. The tocotrienols reappear in the ripening heads. Analogous changes involving other isomers of vitamin E have observed in germinating peas, corn, and barley; in each case, the changes indicate that interconversion of tocotrienols occurs by methyl additions to the nucleus and that the tocopherols are formed by subsequent hydrogenation of the tocotrienol side chains (Fig. 2).

Hall and Laidman [6] concluded that methylation of β- and γ-tocopherol to form α-tocopherol is not an important reaction in germinating seeds. Nevertheless, there is evidence that γ-tocopherol is converted to α-tocopherol in the leaves of several plant species. The aforementioned observations on wheat seedlings [5] are compatible with a similar conversion of β-tocopherol; however, studies with radioactive compounds indicate that this is not an important pathway [7]. The study of these conversions is complicated by evidence that α-tocopherol is localized in chloroplasts whereas the other tocopherols are located in extrachloroplastic organelles [8]. This distribution pattern raises the possibility that there is more than one site of biosynthesis. Whether the alternate route of α-tocopherol biosynthesis through β- and α-tocotrienol is a significant pathway is also unclear.

The remaining nuclear methyl groups of α-, β- and γ-tocotrienols and the corresponding tocopherols are derived from the S-methyl group of methionine. Experiments utilizing [^{3}H]NADPH indicated that this compound serves as a source of hydrogen for the conversion of tocotrienols to the analogous tocopherols [9].

More recent studies by Pennock and associates [3] have provided strong evidence for an alternate "tocopherol route" for the biosynthesis of α-tocopherol. The key distinction between this route and the "tocotrienol route" is that a phytyl (rather than a geranylgeranyl) side chain is added to the 6-position of homogentisic acid to form a phytyltoluquinol which cyclizes to yield δ-tocopherol directly (Fig. 1). According to this scheme, α-tocopherol is synthesized from δ-tocopherol via two successive methylation reactions with γ-tocopherol as intermediate. Conversion of [^{3}H]δ-tocopherol (8-methyl tocol) to [^{3}H]γ-tocopherol and [^{3}H]α-tocopherol by Hevea brasiliensis and Phaseolus vulgaris leaves was demonstrated

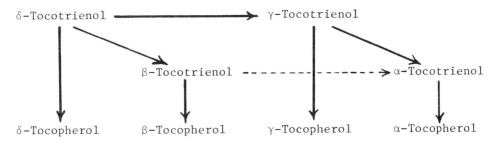

FIG. 2 Synthesis of non-δ-tocotrienols and tocopherols via the tocotrienol route. (From Ref. 2.)

and, in addition, P. vulgaris was found to methylate the 5- and 7-methyl tocols. This finding raised still further possibilities for the biosynthesis of α-tocopherol from isomeric intermediates of 6-phytyltoluquinol (Fig. 1), and evidence was obtained for conversion of the 5-phytyl as well as the 6-phytyl derivative by P. vulgaris. These possibilities are discussed in detail by Janiszowska and Pennock [3], along with evidence that there are at least two distinct sites of synthesis, one for α-tocopherol in the chloroplasts and another for non-α-tocopherols in extrachloroplastic organelles.

REFERENCES

1. G. W. Grams, C. W. Blessin, and G. E. Inglett, J. Amer. Oil Chem. Soc. 47:337 (1970).
2. O. R. Threlfall, Vit. Horm. 29:153 (1971).
3. W. Janiszowska and J. F. Pennock, Vit. Horm. 34:77 (1976).
4. G. Thomas and D. R. Threlfall, Biochem. J. 142:437 (1974).
5. J. Green, J. Sci. Food Agric. 9:801 (1958).
6. G. S. Hall and D. L. Laidman, Biochem. J. 108:475 (1968).
7. K. M. Botham, I. R. Peake, and J. F. Pennock, Biochem. J. 124:22P (1971).
8. R. P. Newton and J. F. Pennock, Biochem. J. 124:21P (1971).
9. A. R. Welburn, Phytochemistry 9:743 (1970).

Part 5D/ Nutrient Interrelationships

HAROLD H. DRAPER
University of Guelph
Guelph, Ontario, Canada

I.	Introduction	272
II.	Polyunsaturated Fatty Acids	274
III.	Selenium	276
IV.	Amino Acids	279
V.	Antioxidants	280
VI.	Iron	282
VII.	Other Vitamins	283
	A. Vitamin A	283
	B. Vitamin C	284
	C. Choline	284
VIII.	Quinones	285
	References	285

I. INTRODUCTION

The dietary requirement for vitamin E is influenced by other components of the diet to such an extent that it cannot be intelligibly defined except in relation to the intake of other nutrients. Because of variations in the composition of the free-choice human diet, arising from individual dietary habits and the peculiarities of national food supplies, the vitamin E requirement of humans, expressed in terms of a minimum daily intake, may vary by a factor of at least two. This variation complicates the problem of setting a recommended dietary allowance which can be confidently applied to the whole population. Studies on laboratory animals have shown that manipulation of the diet can result in vitamin E requirements which vary by at least one order of magnitude. Even in domestic farm animals fed standardized commercial rations the requirement may be influenced by fluctuations in the concentration of selenium and other indigenous constituents.

In 1968, the U.S. National Academy of Sciences issued a recommended dietary allowance (RDA) for adult males of 30 IU of vitamin E activity per day (equivalent to 20 mg of natural RRR-α-tocopherol) [1]. Since surveys showed that many diets provided less than this amount of vitamin E, the 1968 recommendation implied that a substantial portion of the population was at risk. On the other hand, assessment of plasma vitamin E levels in several segments of the U.S. population provided consistent evidence of adequate status.

The 1968 RDA was based in part on an estimate of the vitamin E requirement of experimental subjects fed diets high in polyunsaturated fatty acids (PUFA) [2]; and in part on the amount of vitamin E estimated to be available in the food supply [3]. Reassessment of the normal range of PUFA intakes and of the vitamin E content of U.S. diets as consumed led, in 1974, to a revised recommendation for adult males of 15 IU (10 mg RRR-α-tocopherol [4]. While evidence derived from experiments on human subjects implies that this recommendation contains "little, if any, safety factor" [5], diet surveys indicate that there are significant numbers of individuals in apparently adequate vitamin E status who consume less. Analysis of typical U.S. daily diets as consumed have yielded estimates averaging 7.4 and 9.0 mg α-tocopherol [6, 7]. A composite Canadian diet was estimated to contain 7 mg α-tocopherol or not more than 13 IU if allowance is made for a 20% contribution from other isomers [8]. English, Dominican Republic, and Japanese diets contain somewhat lower amounts [8]. It is apparent, therefore, that many diets provide less than the current RDA of 15 IU of vitamin E activity. However, despite a lack of epidemiological evidence of inadequate vitamin E status in any population, marked variations in individual eating habits may justify this recommendation as a standard of reference. There remains an unexplained discrepancy between the estimate of the vitamin E requirement based on epidermiological and dietary evidence and that derived from human experiments by Horwitt [5], who considers that 15 IU is at the lower end of a range of requirements extending to 45 IU/day.

The vitamin E requirements of domestic and laboratory animals have been reviewed by Blaxter [9], Horwitt [10], and Draper [11]. The requirement is markedly influenced by the PUFA content of the diet, to a lesser extent by the selenium content, and to a still smaller extent by the concentration of sulfur amino acids. The influence of dietary PUFA is vividly illustrated by the results of a study on calves conducted by Blaxter [9], who concluded that addition of cod-liver oil to the diet raised the vitamin E requirement about 100-fold, and by the observation of Bieri and coworkers [12] that chickens could be raised to maturity with a vitamin E-dificient diet by minimizing the intake of polyenoic fatty acids. In contrast to human diets, many practical rations for livestock may lead to a deficiency state unless augmented with vitamin E or a suitable substitute. The main vitamin E deficiency diseases of farm animals are white muscle disease (nutritional muscular dystrophy) of calves, lambs, and swine, and encephalomalacia of chicks.

Information on the vitamin E requirements of most laboratory and domestic animals is given in publications of the U.S. National Academy of Sciences. Under conditions of adequate selenium and normal fatty acid intake the vitamin E requirement of growing chicks and poults appears to be about 10 IU/kg of ration. In the absence of definitive information on the requirements of growing swine, a similar recommendation has been tentatively adopted for this species. The requirements of other farm species are still poorly defined.

II. POLYUNSATURATED FATTY ACIDS (PUFA)

As for animals, the primary determinant of the vitamin E requirements of humans appears to be the concentration of PUFA in the tissues [13]. Over protracted periods of time, the PUFA content of tissue lipids approaches equilibrium with that of the diet, and, hence, the vitamin E requirements can be related to the composition of dietary fatty acids in the habitual diet. Since the consumption of polyunsaturated oils in many industrialized countries has increased in recent years, it follows that the vitamin E requirement also has increased.

The possibility that vitamin E deficiency may be induced by consuming a diet high in PUFA is buffered by a positive correlation between the total vitamin E and PUFA content of edible oils and fats. This phylogenetic relationship is evident across a broad range of plant species and extends to different varieties of the same species (e.g., corn). Conceivably, a sudden marked reduction in vitamin E intake following a prolonged period of high PUFA consumption could result in an inadequate concentration of vitamin E in the tissues to prevent peroxidation of accumulated polyenoic fatty acids. However, a radical change in vitamin E intake is unlikely to occur unless it is prescribed for clinical reasons. Furthermore, most of the commercial plant oils consumed in the mixed diet of developed countries are subjected to partial hydrogenation, which has the effect of increasing the vitamin E/PUFA ratio.

Attempts to define the vitamin E requirement of humans in terms of a necessary ratio to dietary PUFA have failed to yield an accepted value. An analysis of published results on the vitamin E requirement of experimental animals and human subjects fed diets varying in vitamin E and PUFA content led to a proposed requirement of 0.6 mg α-tocopherol per gram of PUFA consumed [3]. This value coincided with the average ratio for the U.S. diet calculated from foods available for consumption in 1961. According to this criterion, most raw edible plant oils, which are generally regarded as good sources of vitamin E activity, would lead to depletion of vitamin E in the tissues because they are relatively higher in PUFA than α-tocopherol, whereas animal fats, despite their lower content of vitamin E, would sustain tissue vitamin E levels because of their low PUFA content.

Subsequent experimentation with animals and human subjects generally failed to support a need for an E/PUFA ratio as high as 0.6. Formulas with a ratio of 0.4 have been found to sustain a normal concentration of plasma vitamin in children [14]. A similar ratio has been found to be adequate for students consuming cafeteria meals [15], and this value evidently is characteristic of the current U.S. mixed diet [7]. The estimated contribution of isomers other than α-tocopherol to total vitamin E activity would raise this value to approximately 0.5. Analysis of a composite diet representative of the daily per capita consumption of foods in Canada yielded an α-tocopherol/PUFA ratio of 0.52 [8]. Some investigators have concluded that a ratio as low as 0.18 is sufficient to maintain normal plasma vitamin E levels in infants [16]; however, it is common practice to fortify infant formulas containing vegetable oils with vitamin E, especially those for premature babies, who generally exhibit lower plasma levels than term infants. Eskimo adults and children consuming diets rich in highly unsaturated marine oils have been observed to be in normal vitamin E status [17]. A longitudinal study on rats revealed no adverse effects on vitamin E status of feeding processed vegetable oils over two generations [18]. Weanling rats fed diets containing raw corn or soybean oil, which have E/PUFA ratios of about 0.1 and 0.2, respectively, were found to have greater concentrations of α-tocopherol in the blood and liver than rats fed the same amounts of lard or beef tallow [19]. These and other observations suggest that the relationship between the vitamin E requirement and PUFA intake may not be linear. Jager [20] concluded that, in normal animals in which the membrane systems are "saturated" with essential fatty acids, dietary linoleic acid has little effect on the vitamin E requirement except at very high intakes. A fixed dietary E/PUFA ratio, therefore, need not exist. He also found that saturated fats were poorer sources of "net" vitamin E activity than polyunsaturated vegetable oils. The vitamin E/PUFA relationship is further complicated by evidence that the intestinal absorption of vitamin E may be reduced by a high intake of linoleic acid [21].

The difficulties inherent in attempts to define the adequacy of human diets in terms of a vitamin E/PUFA ratio have been pointed out by Thompson and associates [8]. The fatty acid composition of foods is extremely variable owing to the wide variety of plant oils used in processing and to marked differences in the degree of hydrogenation. Many "vegetable oils" are not identified on food labels. Moreover, vitamin E status is dependent primarily on the composition of foods consumed over a previous period of months, or even years, rather than on current intake [13]. Isomers of vitamin E other than α-tocopherol make a significant, but variable, contribution to total biological activity. In the latest compilation of recommended dietary allowances for the U.S. population this contribution has been estimated at 20% [4]. The non-α-tocopherol isomer of primary significance is γ-tocopherol, which exceeds α-tocopherol in the mixed diet, but exhibits only about 10% as much biological activity [22]. On the basis of these various considerations, Thompson et al. [8] concluded that the vitamin E/PUFA ratio is impractical and is not a useful indication of the adequacy of foods and diets.

III. SELENIUM

Following the discovery that selenium, as well as vitamin E, was effective in the prevention of nutritional necrotic liver degeneration in rats fed a Torula yeast diet [23], this element was also reported to be effective in the prevention of several field diseases of farm animals, which previously had been attributed to vitamin E deficiency. These diseases included nutritional muscular dystrophy in ruminants, exudative diathesis in chicks, necrotic liver degeneration in swine, and myopathy of the heart and gizzard in poults. The epidemiology of these conditions appears to be affected by a low selenium concentration in the soil in some geographical areas, and, hence, to an insufficient uptake of selenium by plants to meet the nutritional requirements of animals. However, none of these diseases has been shown to be the result of selenium deficiency specifically, and all of them are apparently prevented by adequate amounts of vitamin E alone. A recent investigation of the causes of white muscle disease in lambs has led to the conclusion that vitamin E deficiency is the primary etiological factor in this condition [24].

For more than a decade, the nutritional and metabolic interrelationships between vitamin E and selenium, and indeed the status of selenium as an essential nutrient, remained ambiguous and contentious. While selenium was reported to be useful in the prevention of several diseases of livestock, there was no unequivocal demonstration that this element was essential under conditions of adequate vitamin E nutriture. Selenium administration was potentially more economical as a prophylactic measure but field cases of so-called "selenium-vitamin E deficiency" also responded to therapeutic amounts of vitamin E alone. The effectiveness of selenium appeared to be attributable to some "sparing" effect on the vitamin E requirement. The classical experimental diseases produced by feeding a vitamin E-deficient diet (such as muscular dystrophy in the rabbit and resorption gestation in the rat) were found not to be prevented by selenium administration. On the contrary, the experimental syndromes produced by feeding a diet low in both selenium and vitamin E (necrotic liver degeneration in the rat and exudative diathesis in the chick) were prevented by vitamin E. Hence, for some years the status of selenium as an essential nutrient remained tenuous.

The uncertain nutritional status of selenium was clarified by the experiments of Thompson and Scott [25] who demonstrated that when the diet of chicks is exceptionally low in selenium (< 0.005 ppm), vitamin E no longer substitutes for this element. Under these conditions a new nutritional syndrome, pancreatic fibrosis, was observed. This disease cannot be prevented by vitamin E even when the associated decrease in vitamin E absorption caused by reduced secretion of pancreatic lipases is circumvented by administration of bile salts to sustain a normal concentration of the vitamin in the blood plasma. An experimental syndrome in rats characterized by growth inhibition, reproductive failure, and hairlessness also appears to be specifically attributable to selenium deficiency [26]. Hence, the essentiality of selenium in nutrition has been firmly established.

While these studies clarified the dietary significance of selenium, the biochemical interrelationship between this element and vitamin E remained a mystery until the experiments of Rotruck and coworkers [27] demonstrated that selenium is a component of the enzyme, glutathione peroxidase. This discovery provided a rationale for the dietary interrelationships among selenium, vitamin E, and PUFA, since it implied that all three nutrients affect the metabolism of lipid-free radicals and peroxides in the tissues.

Glutathione peroxidase (glutathione/H_2O_2 oxidoreductase, EC 1.11.1.9) catalyzes the reduction of hydroperoxides of fatty acids (ROOH) and other compounds to their corresponding alcohols (ROH). It is nonspecific with respect to substrate, but has a specific requirement for glutathione as hydrogen donor:

$$ROOH + 2GSH \rightarrow ROH + GSSG + H_2O$$

Reduced glutathione (GSH) is regenerated through the action of glutathione reductase:

$$GSSG + NADPH + H^+ \rightarrow 2GSH + NADP$$

Glutathione peroxidase is a selenoprotein (mol wt 88,000) containing four atoms of selenium per mole of protein. Its primary role in metabolism appears to be the reduction of unsaturated fatty acid hydroperoxides to their hydroxy acid analogs, thereby preventing lipid-free radical chain reactions, which otherwise cause peroxidative damage to proteins, phospholipids, nucleic acid, and other macromolecules. The development of exudates in chicks is correlated with the level of glutathione peroxidase in the blood plasma, and this enzyme has been postulated to constitute the prime protective mechanism against peroxidation of unsaturated lipids in the capillary membrane [28]. A low concentration of glutathione peroxidase in brain tissue may explain the failure of selenium to prevent encephalomalacia [29]. Tissues exposed to oxygen (lung and red blood cells) are rich in this enzyme.

Vitamin E is now postulated to exert its antioxidant effect by preventing the formation of acyl hydroperoxides; however, there is still little direct

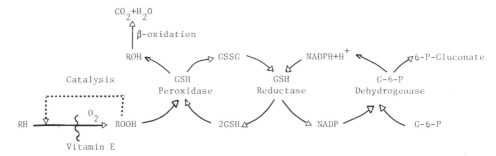

FIG. 1   Proposed involvement of vitamin E and selenium in lipid peroxidation. (From Chow et al., Ref. 32.)

experimental evidence as to its exact mechanism of action. Dimorphecolic acid, the reduction product of 9-hydroperoxy trans, trans-linoleic acid, is a naturally occurring constituent of mustard seed oils. When fed to animals it is deposited in the adipose tissues, but not in the liver where it is rapidly oxidized to CO_2 and H_2O [30]. There is little information relative to the significance for membrane function of hydroxy acids generated by reduction of hydroperoxides in situ, but it is of interest that hydroxy fatty acid esters of sterols have been reported to occur in atherosclerotic plaques [31].

A scheme of the proposed involvement of vitamin E and selenium in lipid peroxidation, taken from Chow and coworkers [32], is shown in Fig. 1.

Some aspects of the vitamin E-selenium relationship are still not entirely resolved. Since simple selenium deficiency does not result in muscular dystrophy, the effectiveness of this element in preventing myopathies in farm animals is evidently due to some mitigation of metabolic requirements for vitamin E. The most plausible explanation is that less vitamin E is required for the prevention of peroxidative damage to muscle cells when there is a normal complement of gluthathione peroxidase available for the decomposition of fatty acid hydroperoxides. Alternatively, it is possible that the efficiency of vitamin E absorption is impaired by pancreatic dysfunction caused by selenium deficiency; however, pancreatic lesions have not been found in farm mammals or poultry fed practical rations. Evidently, feeds grown on selenium-deficient soils contain sufficient selenium to prevent degeneration of the pancreas, but insufficient selenium to prevent exudates when the intake of vitamin E is also low. White muscle disease in ruminants, as it occurs under typical field conditions, is probably a consequence of low intakes of both selenium and vitamin E. Under conditions of mild vitamin E inadequacy selenium supplementation may suffice; otherwise, a vitamin E supplement may be required.

Muscle dystrophy also may occur in the presence of adequate selenium as a result of simple vitamin E deficiency. This is the case with the myopathies of mink and cats fed diets based on fish.

Selenium is ineffective in the prevention of encephalomalacia in chicks, resorption gestation in rats, and muscular dystrophy in rabbits. Exudative diathesis presents an unusual case, since the lesions are completely prevented by either vitamin E or selenium alone [25]. Necrotic liver degeneration may be similar in this respect. Hence, the occurrence of these two diseases signifies a diet low in both nutrients. Hoekstra [29] has postulated that selenium-specific diseases, such as pancreatic fibrosis, are the result of damage to cell components by H_2O_2, which is a substrate for glutathione peroxidases. However, Cantor and associates [33] found no relationship between glutathione peroxidase activity and the prevention of this disease. There is evidence for the existence of other selenoproteins in the tissues and for functions of selenium that are not associated with the action of this enzyme. Herrman and McConnell [34] have detected a novel selenium-containing protein in rat serum. Diplock [35] has obtained evidence for the presence of selenium (in the form of selenide) in nonheme iron proteins of microsomes, and has postulated that vitamin E and synthetic antioxidants function in maintaining these proteins in the reduced state. The situation has been further complicated by the discovery of a selenium-independent glutathione peroxidase [36].

IV. AMINO ACIDS

The amount of vitamin E required for the prevention of some deficiency diseases is modified by the intake of sulfur amino acids. This effect is most evident in the case of necrotic liver degeneration, which is prevented by vitamin E, cystine, or selenium [23]. Induction of muscular dystrophy in chicks requires a vitamin E-deficient diet containing a low concentration of S-amino acids, a low level of synthetic antioxidant to prevent encephalomalacia, and enough selenium to prevent exudates. A vitamin E-sparing effect of methionine and/or cystine has also been observed with respect to other deficiency states.

An apparent explanation of the role of S-amino acids was provided by the finding that reduced glutathione (a tripeptide containing cysteine) is specifically required in the glutathione peroxidase reaction. However, this explanation has been disputed by Hull and Scott [37] who found that the reduced glutathione content of dystrophic chick muscle was twice normal, and that glutathione peroxidase activity also was increased. This observation indicates that muscle degeneration is not precluded by the presence of normal concentrations of glutathione and glutathione peroxidase and is in agreement with the fact that dystrophy occurs in rabbits fed a vitamin E-deficient diet which is adequate in cystine and selenium.

While the partial activity of sulfur amino acids in vitamin E deficiency diseases is still not completely understood, it presumably derives from the reducing properties of the sulfhydryl forms of these compounds or their metabolic products. Sulfur compounds have been shown to act synergistically with chain-breaking antioxidants in the inhibition of peroxidation. The variable activity of sulfur amino acids and selenium, with respect to the prevention of different lesions of vitamin E deficiency, indicates that the protective mechanisms against lipid peroxidation in vivo are not identical at all sites.

Bunce and Hess [38] recently have described a novel interrelationship between vitamin E and tryptophan in the prevention of lenticular opacities in young rats. Simultaneous restriction of both nutrients (but not of either alone) in the maternal diet led to a high incidence of opacities in the progeny. The biochemical explanation of this relationship is unknown.

V. ANTIOXIDANTS

The lipid-antioxidant properties of α-tocopherol were demonstrated shortly after its structure was elucidated. These properties were shown to extend to in vivo systems by Moore [39], who found that vitamin E conserved vitamin A and carotene stores in rat tissues. The possibility that synthetic reducing substances might have a similar effect was confirmed by Dam, who showed that methylene blue was partially active in the prevention of resorption gestation in vitamin E-deficient rats [40].

A need for inexpensive stabilizers of unsaturated lipids in foods and feeds stimulated research on a number of synthetic fat-soluble antioxidants. The synthetic rubber antioxidant N,N^1-diphenyl-p-phenylenediamine (DPPD) was found not only to prevent the oxidation of β-carotene in feeds but also to be effective in the prevention of encephalomalacia in chicks [41]. Subsequently it came into widespread use in poultry rations for these purposes. Although this compound had been shown to be well tolerated by growing rats and chicks at concentrations of 0.5-1.0% in the diet, later studies revealed that it had an adverse effect on reproduction in female rats at levels used in poultry feeds (approximately 0.025%), and consequently it was withdrawn from commercial feed use. In small concentrations, however, DPPD has been found to be the most effective synthetic substitute for vitamin E in the prevention and treatment of deficiency diseases in experimental animals.

The synthetic compounds butylated hydroxyanisole (BHA) and butylated hydroxytoluene (BHT), which are in widespread use as food and feed antioxidants, have little biological activity as vitamin E substitutes [42]. Ethoxyquin resembles DPPD in its ability to replace vitamin E for the prevention of encephalomalacia and muscular dystrophy in chicks, and in the high concentrations necessary to prevent exudates [43]. Alkyl derivatives of p-phenylenediamine are less toxic to pregnant female rats than DPPD, but also are less effective in the prevention of resorption gestation [44].

The demonstrated ability of some synthetic antioxidants to prevent vitamin E deficiency diseases led to studies designed to determine what proportion of the vitamin E requirement is attributable to its antioxidant role in vivo, and what proportion, if any, is attributable to other possible functions. In experiments on the efficacy of DPPD in the prevention and remission of resorption gestation in vitamin E-deficient female rats, this antioxidant (when fed at a dietary concentration of 0.01% or less) was found to have curative as well as prophylactic activity. This finding indicated that its activity was not due to conservation of vitamin E stores but to direct substitution for the vitamin in metabolic processes. Difficulties inherent in devising experimental diets completely free of vitamin E made it uncertain, however, whether reproduction was sustained by traces of the vitamin in such diet ingredients as casein, glucose monohydrate, and essential fatty acid preparations. Further refinement of the experimental diets, including the substitution of synthetic amino acids for protein, ether-extracted sucrose for glucose monohydrate, and use of essential fatty acids recovered from crystallized derivatives, showed that DPPD administration to sterile female rats still resulted in restoration of fertility [42]. Under these experimental conditions, DPPD was found to be at least as active as vitamin E itself, whereas ethoxyquin was inexplicably inactive. Analogous experiments with vitamin E-deficient rabbits showed that dystrophic animals given DPPD underwent remission of gross symptoms, creatinuria, and hypercholesterolemia while fed an amino acid diet devoid of vitamin E [45].

These nutritional experiments on the two classical deficiency diseases, resorption gestation and muscular dystrophy, indicated that the function of vitamin E in animals is entirely associated with its antioxidant properties. This view is supported by several other lines of evidence. The dietary requirement for vitamin E is determined largely by the concentration of pro-oxidants (mainly PUFAs) in the tissue [13]. Studies on the metabolism of $[^{14}C]\alpha$-tocopherol in animals indicated that this compound undergoes limited conversion to oxidation products (α-tocopheryl quinone, dimers, and a trimer) which are analogous to the products formed under controlled autoxidation conditions in unsaturated oils [46]. The varied symptoms of vitamin E deficiency can be rationalized in terms of peroxidative attack on membrane phospholipids, proteins, and other macromolecules in different tissues [47].

Criticisms of the antioxidant theory of vitamin E function generally center on the inability of some synthetic antioxidants to substitute completely for vitamin E with respect to the prevention of certain deficiency symptoms, and on the paucity of direct experimental evidence for the formation of lipid peroxides in vivo [48, 49]. These objections have, to a considerable degree, been abated by recent discoveries. Some antioxidant refractory symptoms have been shown to be due to a primary deficiency of selenium, for which synthetic compounds generally are weak substitutes. The formation of lipofuscin pigments in the adipose tissues of vitamin E-deficient animals can be explained only in terms of peroxidative processes [50]. Direct evidence for peroxidation of PUFAs in vivo recently has been furnished by the observation that vitamin E-deficient animals expire increased quantities of ethane, a product evidently derived from the peroxidation of ω-3 fatty acids [51]. The failure of lipid peroxides to accumulate in the tissues of vitamin E-deficient animals can be explained by the presence of glutathione peroxidase.

The inability of some synthetic lipid antioxidants to substitute for vitamin E may be due to inefficient absorption, transport, translocation at cell boundaries, or binding to active sites. For example, whereas vitamin E is concentrated in the mitochondrial and microsomal membranes of liver cells, DPPD is apparently passively distributed in cell lipids [52]. Some synthetic antioxidants which are generally classified as "biologically inactive" (BHA, propyl gallante) are effective in preventing symptoms of vitamin E deficiency when fed in high concentrations [53]. Considering the gross structural dissimilarities of the compounds involved, it is remarkable that any synthetic antioxidants are capable of substituting for vitamin E in vivo.

VI. IRON

From a study on low birth-weight infants (in whom plasma vitamin E levels are characteristically low), Williams and coworkers [54] concluded that iron administration may lead to the development of vitamin E deficiency anemia. Hemolytic anemia, characterized by a low hemoglobin value, a high reticulocyte count, and morphological changes in the erythrocytes, has been associated with low plasma vitamin E levels in some premature babies. This condition was observed to be induced by feeding a formula containing a high concentration of linoleic acid (32% of total fatty acids) along with iron (12-13 mg/liter). Infants fed the high PUFA formula had lower serum vitamin E levels than those fed a formula containing less linoleic acid (12%), and their erythrocytes were more susceptible to H_2O_2-induced hemolysis in vitro. Interestingly, however, iron administration did not affect the serum level of vitamin E.

Dallam [55], in a similar study on preterm infants, concluded that iron doses of > 3 mg/kg body weight should be avoided because of the possible development of vitamin E deficiency, especially during the first 3 months of life. Even large doses of vitamin E did not raise serum vitamin E levels or prevent H_2O_2-induced erythrocyte hemolysis in vitro in some infants. He recommended administration of 5-25 IU of a water-soluble form of vitamin E per day during the first 3 months. Thereafter, the deficiency was observed to be self-limiting. Similar effects of administering excessive iron to premature infants have been observed by Melhorn and Gross [56].

Hemolysis in mice can be induced by giving an acute iron-dextran load [57]. Susceptibility to hemolysis was increased by vitamin E deficiency and administration of the vitamin before the load was protective. There is "limited evidence" that deaths may occur following iron administration to baby pigs born of sows deficient in vitamin E [58].

These adverse effects of iron on vitamin E status appear to be due to catalysis of peroxidation of polyunsaturated fatty acids in erythrocytes and possibly in other membranes. In thalassemia major and other severe forms of congenital hemolytic anemia, iron overload is associated with peroxidation of erythrocyte lipids and reduced serum vitamin E levels [59]. Parenchymal iron deposits are decreased by treatment with iron-chelating agents and the symptoms of peroxidation with therapeutic doses of vitamin E. A drug-nutrient interaction in thalassemia patients is suggested by the finding that the response to the chelating compound desferrioxamine is blocked by vitamin E in iron-overloaded animals [59].

VII. OTHER VITAMINS

A. Vitamin A

The interrelationship between vitamins A and E has been extensively investigated since it was first reported by Moore [39] that vitamin E reduced the rate of vitamin A depletion in rat liver. This relationship is usually explained in terms of the general lipid-antioxidant role of vitamin E, which has been extended to include vitamin A as a "co-oxidizable" substrate. This view was supported by the findings of Dam and coworkers [60], as well as several other investigators. However, Green et al. [61] were unable to find an association between lipid peroxidation, vitamin E status, and vitamin A depletion of rat or chick tissues, and they concluded that the relationship between the two vitamins in vivo was not attributable to an antioxidant function of vitamin E.

It appears that the vitamin E-vitamin A relationship in vivo, as has been suggested for the vitamin E/PUFA ratio [20], is conspicuous only within prescribed concentrations of vitamin A in the tissues. Further experiments by Green and associates [62] indicated that vitamin E increased the retention of high levels of vitamin A in the liver, albeit by a mechanism which they concluded did not involve an antioxidant mechanism. High levels of dietary vitamin A increase the vitamin E requirement [63] and some of the effects

of vitamin A toxicity can be counteracted by vitamin E administration [64].
Since alleviation of vitamin A toxicity by vitamin E occurred in spite of
higher concentrations of vitamin A in the tissues, the protective effect of
vitamin E evidently was not due to a reduction in vitamin A absorption or
deposition, but to amelioration of the biochemical pathology which occurs
at reactive sites [64]. In a long-term study on rats, liver vitamin A storage was increased by vitamin E, but the effect of feeding 25, 000 IU/kg diet
was the same as that of feeding 25 IU/kg [65]. However, megadoses of
vitamin E have been reported to increase absorption and catabolism of a
large does of vitamin A in children without affecting retention [66].

The interactions between vitamin A and vitamin E have been reviewed
by Berger [67]. This relationship does not appear to be of major nutritional significance within the range of normal vitamin A intakes.

B. Vitamin C

Under different conditions, ascorbic acid may act either as an inhibitor or
as a catalyst of lipid peroxidation. Vitamin C exhibits mild pseudovitamin E activity in animals under some conditions, such as in vitamin E-
selenium deficiency in ducks [68], but increases liver thiobarbituric acid
formation and erythrocyte hemolysis in rats [69]. When added to tissue
preparations in vitro, it may either decrease or increase the formation of
lipid peroxides, depending upon the presence of other compounds.

The mechanisms of lipid peroxide formation in animal tissues have
been extensively studied by Wills [70]. Catalysis of PUFA peroxidation by
liver mitochondria and microsomes at pH 7.4 is inhibited by ascorbic acid,
whereas it is enhanced in the supernate. These contrasting results have
been attributed to an inhibitory role of ascorbic acid in hemoprotein-
catalyzed peroxidation and a stimulatory effect on catalysis by nonheme
iron. Ascorbic acid releases iron from ferritin and activates the catalysis
of lipoxidation by either ferrous or ferric ions [70].

Addition of ascorbic acid to adrenal cells from vitamin E-deficient rats
increases thiobarbituric acid formation and inhibits adrenocorticotropic
hormone-induced steroidogenesis [71]. Since steroid synthesis was restored by cyclic adenosine 5'monophosphate (AMP) but not by adrenocorticotropic hormone (ACTH), it was concluded that binding of ACTH to
the cells was disrupted by ascorbic acid-catalyzed peroxidation of membrane lipids. Administration of vitamin E to the animals 16 hr prior to
preparation of the cells abolished the ascorbic acid effect.

C. Choline

Wilson and coworkers [72, 73] observed medial hepatic arteriosclerosis,
preventable by feeding BHA or BHT, in choline-deficient rats. Spratt and

Kratzing [74] reported phagocytosis, in addition to fat accumulation, in the liver of choline-deficient rats; phagocytic activity was increased by replacing saturated with polyunsaturated dietary fat and was prevented with vitamin E. These studies indicate that some of the lesions of choline deficiency are attributable to concomitant effects of lipid peroxidation.

VIII. QUINONES

Conflicting data have been reported relative to the effect of vitamin E deficiency on coenzyme Q (ubiquinone) concentrations in the tissues and on the effect of coenzyme Q administration on vitamin E-deficient animals. Coenzyme Q (CoQ) concentration in the liver varies substantially with diet but has not consistently been found to be influenced by vitamin E [75-77]. However, reduced CoQ_{10} levels have been found in more severely affected tissues including the heart and skeletal muscle of dystrophic rabbits [78]. Moreover, administration of CoQ_{10} or one of its derivatives (hexahydro CoQ_4 or CoQ_7) has been observed to prevent or cure a number of manifestations of vitamin E deficiency including resorption gestation in rats and muscular dystrophy in rabbits, along with their associated enzyme dyscrasias [78].

There are several possible explanations of the response of vitamin E-deficient animals to CoQ compounds. It may be due to the restoration of CoQ concentrations at enzyme sites in the respiratory chain of affected tissues. Loss of CoQ_{10} may occur as a result of epoxidation of this quinone under conditions of antioxidant deficiency [79]. Disruption of mitochondrial membranes in vitamin E deficiency may cause a reduced rate of CoQ synthesis. Another possibility is that reduction of CoQ compounds to their hydroquinones may add to the available lipid-antioxidant activity in the tissues. Tocopheryl hydroquinone is an active form of vitamin E if given in frequent doses to compensate for its rapid turnover rate [80]. Large doses of α-tocopheryl quinone also induce remission of symptoms of muscular dystrophy [80]. From a study of the metabolism of [^{14}C] d-α-tocopheryl-p-quinone, Chow and coworkers [81] postulated that when large doses of this compound are administered, reduction to the hydroquinone proceeds faster than conjugation of the latter with glucuronic acid, resulting in an effective antioxidant titer of the reduced compound. A similar explanation may apply to the pseudovitamin E activity of CoQ compounds.

REFERENCES

1. Food and Nutrition Board, Recommended Dietary Allowances (7th ed). Washington, D.C., U. S. Natl. Acad. Sci. Publ. 1694 (1968).

2. M. K. Horwitt, B. Century, and A. A. Zeman, Amer. J. Clin. Nutr. 12:99 (1963).

3. P. L. Harris and N. D. Embree, Amer. J. Clin. Nutr. 13:385 (1963).

4. Food and Nutrition Board, Recommended Dietary Allowances (8th ed.). Washington, D.C., U.S. Natl. Acad. Sci. Publ. 2216 (1974).

5. M. K. Horwitt, Amer. J. Clin. Nutr. 27:1182 (1974).

6. R. H. Bunnell, J. Keating, A. Quaresimo, and G. K. Parman, Amer. J. Clin. Nutr. 17:1 (1965).

7. J. G. Bieri and R. P. Evarts, J. Amer. Diet. Assoc. 62:147 (1973).

8. J. N. Thompson, J. L. Beare-Rogers, P. Erdody, and D. C. Smith, Amer. J. Clin. Nutr. 26:1349 (1973).

9. K. L. Blaxter, Vit. Horm. 20:633 (1962).

10. M. K. Horwitt, Borden Rev. Nutr. Res. 22:1 (1961).

11. H. H. Draper, in International Encyclopedia of Food and Nutrition, Vol. 9. Edited by R. A. Morton, 1970, p. 373.

12. J. G. Bieri, G. M. Briggs, C. J. Pollard, and M. R. Spivey Fox, J. Nutr. 70:47 (1960).

13. L. A. Witting, Amer. J. Clin. Nutr. 27:952 (1974).

14. J. S. Lewis, A. K. Pian, M. T. Baer, P. B. Acosta, and G. A. Emerson, Amer. J. Clin. Nutr. 26:136 (1973).

15. L. A. Witting and L. Lee, Amer. J. Clin. Nutr. 28:571 (1975).

16. S. A. Hashim and R. H. Asfour, Amer. J. Clin. Nutr. 21:7 (1968).

17. C. K. Wei Wo and H. H. Draper, Amer. J. Clin. Nutr. 28:808 (1975).

18. R. Alfin-Slater, P. Wells, and L. Aftargood, J. Amer. Oil Chem. Soc. 50:479 (1973).

19. H. H. Draper, unpublished results.

20. J. C. Jager, Linoleic acid intake and vitamin E requirement. Vlaardingen, The Netherlands, Unilever Research, 1973.

21. H. E. Gallo-Torres, Acta Agric. Scand. (Suppl.) 19:97 (1973).

22. J. G. Bieri and R. P. Evarts, J. Nutr. 104:850 (1974).

23. K. Schwarz and C. M. Foltz, J. Amer. Chem. Soc. 79:3292 (1957).

24. P. D. Whanger, P. H. Weswig, J. A. Schmitz, and J. E. Oldfield, J. Nutr. 107:1298 (1977).

25. J. N. Thompson and M. L. Scott, J. Nutr. 97:355 (1969).

26. K. E. McCoy and P. H. Weswig, J. Nutr. 98:383 (1969).

27. J. T. Rotruck, A. L. Pope, H. E. Ganther, A. B. Swanson, D. G. Hafernan, and W. G. Hoekstra, Science 179:588 (1973).

28. T. Noguchi, A. H. Cantor, and M. L. Scott, J. Nutr. 103:1502 (1973).

29. W. G. Hoekstra, Fed. Proc. 34:2083 (1975).

30. R. J. Reber and H. H. Draper, Lipids 6:983 (1970).

31. C. J. W. Brooks, G. Steel, J. D. Gilbert, and W. A. Harland, Atherosclerosis 13:223 (1971).

32. C. K. Chow, K. Reddy, and A. L. Tappel, J. Nutr. 103:618 (1973).

33. A. H. Cantor, M. L. Langevin, T. Noguchi, and M. L. Scott, J. Nutr. 105:106 (1975).
34. J. L. Herrman and K. P. McConnell, Fed. Proc. 34:925 (1975).
35. A. T. Diplock, Proc. Nutr. Soc. 33:315 (1974).
36. R. A. Lawrence and R. F. Burk, Fed. Proc. 35:578 (1976).
37. S. J. Hull and M. L. Scott, J. Nutr. 106:181 (1976).
38. G. E. Bunce and J. L. Hess, J. Nutr. 106:222 (1976).
39. T. Moore, Biochem. J. 34:1321 (1940).
40. H. Dam, Pharmacol. Rev. 1:9 (1957).
41. E. P. Singsen, R. H. Bunnell, L. D. Matterson, A. Kozeff, and E. L. Jungherr, Poult. Sci. 34:262 (1955).
42. H. H. Draper, J. G. Bergan, Mei Chiu, A. Saari Csallany, and A. V. Boaro, J. Nutr. 84:395 (1964).
43. G. F. Combs, Jr. and M. L. Scott, J. Nutr. 104:1297 (1974).
44. H. H. Draper and B. C. Johnson, J. Agric. Food Chem. 6:920 (1958).
45. A. Saari Csallany and H. H. Draper, Arch. Biochem. Biophys. 92:462 (1961).
46. H. H. Draper and A. Saari Csallany, Fed. Proc. 28:1690 (1969).
47. A. L. Tappel, Vit. Horm. 20:493 (1962).
48. J. Green and J. Bunyan, Nutr. Abstr. Rev. 39:321 (1969).
49. J. Glavind, Acta Agric. Scand. (Suppl.) 19 (1973).
50. K. S. Chio, V. Reiss, B. Fletcher, and A. L. Tappel, Science 166:1535 (1969).
51. D. G. Hafernan and W. G. Hoekstra, J. Nutr. 107:666 (1977).
52. A. Saari Csallany and H. H. Draper, Proc. Soc. Exp. Biol. Med. 104:739 (1960).
53. L. J. Machlin, J. Amer. Oil Chemists Soc. 40:368 (1963).
54. M. L. Williams, R. J. Shott, P. L. O'Neal, and F. A. Oski, N. Eng. J. Med. 292:887 (1975).
55. P. R. Dallam, J. Pediatr. 85:742 (1974).
56. D. K. Melhorn and S. Gross, J. Pediatr. 79:569 (1971).
57. K. A. Smith and C. E. Mengel, J. Lab. Clin. Med. 72:505 (1968).
58. Anonymous, in Nutrient Requirements of Swine. Washington, D.C., U.S. National Academy of Sciences, 1973.
59. C. Hershko and E. A. Rachmilewitz, Proc. Soc. Exp. Biol. Med. 152:249 (1976).
60. H. Dam, I. Prange, and E. Sondergaard, Acta Pharmacol. 8:1 (1952).
61. J. Green, I. R. Muthy, A. T. Diplock, J. Bunyan, M. A. Cawthorne, and E. A. Murrell, Br. J. Nutr. 21:845 (1967).
62. M. A. Cawthorne, J. Bunyan, A. T. Diplock, E. A. Murrell, and J. Green, Br. J. Nutr. 22:133 (1968).
63. W. J. Pudelkiewicz, L. Webster, and L. D. Matterson, J. Nutr. 84:113 (1964).

64. M. Y. Jenkins and G. V. Mitchell, J. Nutr. 105:1600 (1975).

65. N. Y. J. Yang and I. D. Desai, J. Nutr. 107:1418 (1977).

66. J. A. Kusin, V. Reddy, and B. Sivakumar, Amer. J. Clin. Nutr. 27:774 (1974).

67. S. Berger, Bibl. Nutr. Diet. 15 (No. 15):85 (1969).

68. E. T. Moran, Jr., H. C. Carlson, R. G. Brown, P. R. Sweeney, J. C. George, and D. W. Stanley, Poultry Sci. 54:266 (1975).

69. L. H. Chen and K. J. Barnes, Nutr. Rep. Intern. 14:699 (1976).

70. E. D. Willis, Biochem. J. 99:667 (1966).

71. A. E. Kitabchi, A. H. Nathans, and C. L. Mitchell, J. Biol. Chem. 248:835 (1973).

72. R. B. Wilson, N. S. Kula, P. M. Newberne, and M. W. Conner, Exp. Biol. Pathol. 18:357 (1973).

73. R. B. Wilson, P. M. Newberne, and N. S. Kula, Exp. Biol. Pathol. 21:118 (1974).

74. M. G. Spratt and C. C. Kratzing, Res. J. Reticuloendothel. Soc. 10:319 (1971).

75. R. A. Morton and W. E. J. Phillips, Biochem. J. 73:416 (1959).

76. A. T. Diplock, E. E. Edwin, J. Bunyan, and J. Green, J. Nutr. 15:425 (1961).

77. D. J. Lee, Mei Chiu, and H. H. Draper, Nature (London) 204:288 (1965).

78. K. Folkers, Amer. J. Clin. Nutr. 27:1026 (1974).

79. D. Jones, D. J. Scholler, and K. Folkers, Int. J. Vit. Nutr. Res. 41:215 (1971).

80. J. B. Mackenzie and C. G. Mackenzie, J. Nutr. 72:322 (1960).

81. C. K. Chow, H. H. Draper, A. S. Csallany, and Mei Chiu, Lipids 2:390 (1967).

Part 5E/ Biochemical Function

Section 1 Vitamin E: Its role as a biologic free radical scavenger
and its relationship to the microsomal mixed-function oxidase system

PAUL B. McCAY* AND M. MARGARET KING*
Oklahoma Medical Research Foundation
Oklahoma City, Oklahoma

I.	Introduction	289
II.	The Antioxidant Role of Vitamin E	291
	A. Free Radical Reactions	291
	B. Tocopherol as an Antioxidant	292
	C. Endogenous Sources of Free Radicals	296
	D. Free Radicals Formed from Exogenous Compounds	303
III.	Vitamin E and the Drug-Metabolizing System	306
	A. Introduction	306
	B. Influence of Vitamin E on Hemoprotein Synthesis	307
	C. Drug Metabolism	309
IV.	Conclusion	311
	References	312

I. INTRODUCTION

While the vitamin E requirement in animals in many respects seems to be met by structurally unrelated compounds possessing antioxidant properties, it is not certain that the latter compounds do so by actually substituting for a α-tocopherol, or whether they act by preventing oxidative loss of very small quantities of the vitamin that may already be present in the animal's tissues. The weight of evidence at the current time supports the concept that nontocopherol antioxidants can substitute for vitamin E, but that their effectiveness may be influenced by their particular chemical structure. However, a certain fraction of α-tocopherol might be required for a cellular function unrelated to its lipid antioxidant properties. Arguments for the latter case have been outlined in detail by Green and coworkers [1-3]. Clearly, the vitamin has some unusual effects on certain animals that cannot be related to its antioxidant property in any obvious way. For example,

---

*Additional present affiliation: University of Oklahoma Health Sciences Center, Oklahoma City, Oklahoma.

administration of additional α-tocopherol to normal chicks causes a significant reticulocytosis [4]. The authors suggest that the maturation of reticulocytes to erythrocytes involves reduction in the amount of total lipid present and that if peroxidation were somehow involved in the reduction of total lipid, antioxidants might retard maturation and promote reticulocytosis. Ethoxyquin (2, 2, 4-trimethyl-6-ethoxy-1, 2-dihydroquinoline), another very effective antioxidant, causes the same effect. Another unusual effect associated with α-tocopherol is its influence on the growth, phenotypes, and reproduction of the rotifer, Asplachna seiboldi. When this fresh-water metazoan is grown in a medium lacking α-tocopherol, these organisms multiply by parthenogenetic reproduction of females, with the body walls of the females incompletely developed. When α-tocopherol is added to the growth medium (other tocopherols are not effective), female body development is completed and the females can produce oocytes, which undergo meiosis to produce haploid eggs that develop into males. Male rotifers can then fertilize haploid eggs to produce females [5]. This highly specific function of α-tocopherol is not readily apparent from the antioxidant standpoint. In addition, α-tocopherol appears able to function as an ionophore for potassium and rubidium ions in mitochondria but not for sodium and lithium ions [6]. Furthermore, Kawai et al. have shown that α-tocopherol and its quinone are rather specific inhibitors of the Na^+-K^+ATPase of brain microsomes and that these substances give half-maximum inhibition at physiological blood levels of α-tocopherol (about 3×10^{-5} M). Similar effects were seen on the Ca^{2+}-activated ATPase of muscle [7].

There is no question, however, that the tocopherols possess reasonably good antioxidant properties and could function as free radical scavengers in vivo if radicals were to arise, particularly in intracellular membranous organelles where most of the vitamin is distributed. The localization of relatively large amounts of the highly unsaturated fatty acids in these membranes makes them highly vulnerable to lipid peroxidation. Lipid peroxidation occurs readily in mitochondria and microsomes in vitro under various conditions. Nonenzymic autoxidative lipid peroxidation in these organelles probably does not occur to any significant extent in vivo, primarily because steady state intracellular oxygen tension levels in most tissues are relatively low. On the other hand, if free radical formation is associated with the activity of certain types of enzymes, the possibilities for initiating peroxidative attacks on unsaturated membrane lipids would be considerably enhanced, particularly if a free radical-generating system were membrane-bound. This might present a particular hazard for membranous organelles because of the considerably greater solubility of oxygen in the lipid phase as compared to the aqueous phase of the cell. Studies in our laboratory and others over a period of several years have demonstrated that several oxidoreductase systems in liver promote lipid peroxidation in mitochondria, microsomes, and lysosomes via free radicals produced during the catalytic activity of these enzymes, and under circumstances which apparently would exist in vivo. Hence, the ongoing requirement for a free radical scavenger to prevent radical-mediated alteration of biological membranes would become clear if lipid peroxidation were promoted in vivo via certain types of enzyme-generated free radical reactions. This raises the question: does lipid peroxidation actually occur in the intact animal? Various types of evidence indicate that it does. The formation of ceroid pigments in antioxidant-deficient animals appears to be the result of a reaction of products of lipid peroxidation with protein to form products which are apparently metabolically inert. Such products normally accumulate slowly in certain tissues of animals (including humans), particularly in heart muscle and brain [8-10]. Other investigators have observed conjugated dienes in the lipid fractions of ceroid pigments, suggesting that a peroxidative process was involved.

Some hepatotoxic compounds appear to exert their damage on liver via lipid peroxidation. We have recently obtained direct evidence using isolated hepatocytes indicating that lipid peroxidation does occur as an ongoing process in isolated liver cells from normal rats and that it is induced by phenobarbital [11]. In this article we shall attempt to evaluate (1) the existing information concerning the biological role of antioxidants, particularly α-tocopherol, as free radical scavengers, and the relationship of such a function to membrane integrity; (2) the influence of tocopherol on a particular membrane function, namely, microsomal drug metabolism.

II. THE ANTIOXIDANT ROLE OF VITAMIN E

A. Free Radical Reactions

Free radicals in biological systems can be formed through cleavage of covalent bonds in organic compounds resulting in bond splitting, in which each fragment retains one electron of the original bonding pair:

```
      H   H   H   H   H
      |   |   |   |   |
  R — C = C — C — C = C — R'
              |       |
              H       H

              |
              |
              ▼

      H   H   H   H   H
      |   |   |   |   |
  R — C = C — C — C = C — R'  + H·
              |
              H
```

Such bond splitting is classified as homolytic and always gives rise to a pair of radicals. Radicals can also be produced from the capture of an electron by a molecule:

$$O_2 + e^- \longrightarrow O_2^-$$

In this example, the capture of an electron by molecular oxygen produces the superoxide anion radical, i.e., the free radical has a net negative charge because of the additional electron in its possession. Electron capture by molecular oxygen is known to occur by its interaction with flavin oxidoreductase systems [129].

Homolytic cleavage occurs more readily in compounds with certain types of bonds and is related to the dissociation energy of that bond [130]. Many free radicals produced by homolytic cleavage are very reactive compounds and have extremely short half-lives in solution. Some, however, are relatively stable (monodehydroascorbate, for example) and, due to their paramagnetic properties, can be detected and even determined quantitatively by electron spin resonance (ESR) spectroscopy. In cases where the radicals which are formed exist too briefly for such detection, the recently developed technique of spin trapping may be employed. In this procedure, the radical reacts with the spin trapping compound and produces an adduct which is a more stable radical and may be analyzed by the ESR method [131]. The characteristics of the spectrum provide information concerning the nature of the original radical [132].

Free radicals can initiate the formation of additional free radicals by reacting with polyunsaturated fatty acids, as illustrated in Fig. 1. Such fatty acids contain methylene groups from which the hydrogen atoms are easily abstracted by radicals. The fatty acid radical formed can react spontaneously with oxygen to form a fatty acid peroxy radical. This radical may propagate the peroxidation of an additional fatty acid by abstracting a hydrogen atom to form a hydroperoxide and a new fatty acid radical. In this way, a chain reaction may occur which can oxidize many fatty acid molecules as a result of the initial formation of a single fatty acid radical.

Malondialdehyde is a product of fatty acid peroxidation and, although it is not formed in amounts equivalent to the number of molecules oxidized, the relationship between the amount of malondialdehyde formed and the extent of fatty acid oxidized is a stoichiometric one within limits [25]. A possible mechanism by which malondialdehyde may be formed from a peroxidized fatty acid is shown in Fig. 2. Malondialdehyde can be determined easily and its analysis is often used as an indicator of the extent of peroxidation, but it cannot be used for determination of fatty acid peroxides per se, even though it has sometimes been employed in that sense.

B. Tocopherol as an Antioxidant

As pointed out a number of years ago by Dam, the principal role of vitamin E as an antioxidant must be to neutralize free radicals which could initiate

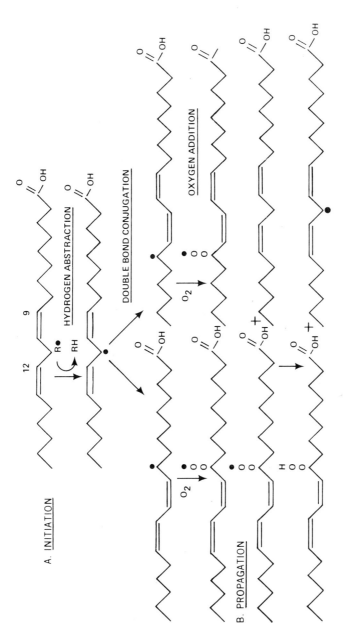

FIG. 1. Sequence of reactions involved in the initiation and propagation of free radical–mediated lipid peroxidation. (From Dahle et al., Ref. 142.)

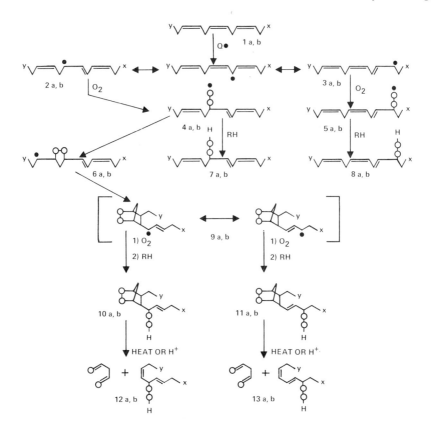

FIG. 2 Mechanism for conversion of methyl-linolenate to conjugated
hydroperoxides and prostaglandin-like endoperoxides, and the further
conversion of these prostaglandin-line endoperoxides to form the thiobarbituric acid-reactive material, i.e., malondialdehyde. Double bonds are
shown in their thermodynamically preferred *trans* form. a: x =
$(CH_2)_6CO_2CH_3$, y = CH_3; b: x = CH_3, y = $(CH_2)_6CO_2CH_3$; Q·: = Free
radical initiator; RH = Unsaturated fatty acid containing 1,4-pentadiene
portion. (From Pryor and Stanley, Lipids 11[5]:371, 1976; and Pryor
et al., J. Org. Chem. 40[24]:3616, 1975.)

a chain reaction, particularly in highly unsaturated lipids, resulting in the
formation of peroxides and products of their subsequent degradation [12].
The quenching of a free radical by vitamin E results in the formation of a
tocopherol semiquinone radical which rapidly degrades to other products
[13]. Since the free radical process involved in the oxidation of

unsaturated lipids entails both initiation and propagation, substances which can interfere with either of the parameters would inhibit the process and, as a group, would be called antioxidants. Antioxidants, however, may exert their action in different ways. Some substances, which are not antioxidants, inhibit lipid peroxidation by binding catalytic agents required for initiation. For example, ethylene diamine tetraacetate (EDTA) inhibits lipid peroxidation in various types of systems by chelating metal ions (iron) which may be involved. Mn^{2+} also inhibits lipid peroxidation, presumably by catalyzing the removal of superoxide anion from the system [43].

Other compounds prevent autocatalytic free radical reactions such as lipid peroxidation by reacting with the initial free radicals formed in the peroxidative process to yield products which are either unreactive or which degrade to nonradical products. An example of this type of free radical scavenger is α-tocopherol, which can donate a phenolic hydrogen atom to a free radical, thereby resolving the unpaired electron of the radical and oxidizing the tocopherol to its quinone form:

α-TOCOPHEROL

This reaction would effectively terminate a chain reaction that might have been propagated by the radical. The initial peroxide may be formed by the reaction of singlet oxygen ($^1O_2$) generated by photochemical processes and possibly enzymic activities [133, 134]. Because the lipids which are most susceptible to lipid peroxidation are located in the membranes of various subcellular organelles and form nonaqueous compartments within the cells, a fat-soluble antioxidant which terminates free radical reactions of unsaturated lipids may be required for membrane stability. α-Tocopherol can fill this requirement quite adequately and has the added advantage of being nontoxic at required levels. The latter property, in conjunction with the widespread occurrence of α-tocopherol in plants, may have been operating in the natural selection process, which culminated in its evolution as a vitamin for animals. Although other tocopherols have antioxidant properties, α-tocopherol has been demonstrated to be the most effective of the naturally occurring tocopherols in preventing biological deficiency symptoms and is the most abundant of the tocopherols which accumulate in animal tissues [135]. The most critical need for α-tocopherol by animals appears to be during the period of fetal development and during the rapid growth phase of newborn animals.

The question of whether or not vitamin E serves solely as a biological antioxidant peculiarly suited to the biological structures existing in cells has been under consideration for many years [14]. The disagreement on this point arises from studies which indicated that vitamin E could be replaced in the diet of rats by other antioxidants which were structurally unrelated to the tocopherols [15]. In these studies, rats were bred and maintained for at least two succeeding generations on synthetic diets containing antioxidant, but essentially no vitamin E. The argument has been advanced that the synthetic antioxidant functioned to protect exceedingly small amounts of vitamin E in purified diets from oxidative destruction and could have been sufficient to meet some specific requirement unrelated to its antioxidant properties.

Various specific functions for tocopherol have been proposed including a regulatory action at the genetic level [16]. However, in no case has a clearly defined regulatory function for this vitamin been elucidated and, at present, it appears that nearly all effects of vitamin E deficiency in animals could be explained on the basis of its antioxidant properties.

The variable capacity of different antioxidants to replace vitamin E in animals [17] may result from their differences in absorption, distribution, and metabolism. Since animal cell membranes are rich in polyunsaturated fatty acids, these structures could be expected to be most susceptible to oxidative attack in an antioxidant deficiency. Membrane alterations may be responsible for most of the effects observed as a result of vitamin E deficiency. Synthetic or substitute antioxidants might not orient themselves in membranes to provide the same efficiency of radical scavenging as α-tocopherol. Although this question has not been fully resolved at the present time, there is considerable evidence to suggest that at least part of the function of this vitamin is to protect the organization of cell membrane lipids from the disorganizing effect of free radical-mediated reactions initiated by the activity of certain enzyme systems.

C. Endogenous Sources of Free Radicals

The requirement for vitamin E is governed in large part by the amount of polyunsaturated fatty acids present in the diet, particularly in young animals [18]. In these animals, rapid growth may cause homeostatic mechanisms associated with maintaining the integrity of membranous structures to function at the limit of their capacity. It is also possible that in rapidly developing animals fed diets limited in vitamin E, the intake of tocopherol may not be adequate to provide a sufficient rate of deposition in newly formed membranes to prevent free radical-initiated peroxidative changes when diets are rich in polyunsaturated fats. Diets rich in polyunsaturated fats are known to enhance the content of such fatty acids in biolõgical membranes. Thus, young human infants which were fed a formula enriched with polyunsaturated fatty acids developed hemolytic anemia. The anemia was prevented by elevating the level of vitamin E supplementation [19]. The relationship between the polyunsaturated fatty acid content of animal diets, the tissue level of unsaturation, and the requirement for vitamin E has been thoroughly reviewed by Witting [20].

In 1963, Hochstein and Ernster and their colleagues observed that an iron-dependent formation of malondialdehyde occurred during the oxidation of reduced nicotinamide adenine dinucleolide phosphate (NADPH) by rat liver microsomes [21-23]. In 1968, May and McCay demonstrated that the oxidation of NADPH by liver microsomes in the presence of a low concentration of iron resulted in the oxidative destruction of significant amounts of polyunsaturated fatty acids in the microsomal membranes [24], and that there was a stoichiometric relationship between the amounts of NADPH oxidized, malondialdehyde formed, oxygen consumed, and polyunsaturated fatty acids lost [25]. The results indicated that the enzyme activity promoted a peroxidative attack on the unsaturated lipids of the microsomes and that the peroxidative process was not autocatalytic but required continuous enzyme activity to promote the process. Inhibition of the enzyme activity or depletion of the substrate (NADPH) resulted in immediate cessation of the peroxidative attack. The time of onset of the attack on the membrane lipids was a function of the dietary level of vitamin E fed to the animal. The higher the level of the vitamin being supplemented in the diet, the longer the catalytic activity of the enzyme system could be tolerated by the microsomal membrane before the attack on the polyunsaturated fatty acids began [26].

During oxidation of NADPH, superoxide anion (O_2^-) [27] and H_2O_2 [28] are produced. According to the studies of Haber and Weiss [29], these two factors can react to form the highly reactive hydroxyl radical:

$$[H_2O_2 + O_2^- \rightarrow HO\cdot + OH^- + O_2]$$

This reaction appears to be facilitated by Fe^{3+}. The superoxide anion radical itself is essentially unreactive with unsaturated lipids or with highly effective free radical scavengers. This is based on the observation that ethoxyquin, diphenyl-p-phenylenediamine, hydroquinone, ethanol, benzoate, mannitol, and α-tocopherol, did not interfere with the reduction of cytochrome c by the xanthine-xanthine oxidase system [27]. Since superoxide is the mediator of cytochrome c reduction in this system, significant

scavenging of O_2^- by these agents should have inhibited cytochrome c
reduction. However, Nishikimi and Machlin [33] have reported that
6-hydroxy-2, 5, 7, 8-tetramethylchroman-2-carboxylic acid (a reasonably
water-soluble tocopherol model compound) is oxidized by the xanthine-
xanthine oxidase system. This oxidation may have occurred via reaction
of the model compound with O_2^-. However, the xanthine-xanthine oxidase
system also produced H_2O_2 and, hence, has the potential for producing
hydroxyl radicals during the reaction. It is possible, therefore, that the
oxidation of the compound may have occurred via reaction with OH. If
that were the case, then the model compound would not be expected to
affect cytochrome c reduction by the enzyme system, and as mentioned
above, it does not. It is possible that the xanthine oxidase systems employed in both studies may have produced a sufficient flux of O_2^- to reduce
cytochrome c at a maximum rate and promote the oxidation of the tocopherol model compound as well, and the problem merits further study.

The capacity of O_2^- to reduce H_2O_2 with the resulting formation of
hydroxyl radicals makes O_2^- a potentially dangerous factor in living cells
which are also producing H_2O_2. Investigations with perfused livers indicate that the endoplasmic reticulum may not contribute very much to the
total perfusable H_2O_2 produced by liver cells [30]. However, if H_2O_2 can
readily penetrate membrane structures (as its solubility in ether and
ability to cross the plasma membrane suggest), then all sources of H_2O_2
in the cell may have the potential for initiating free radical-mediated lipid
peroxidation upon entering a membrane containing enzyme systems which
produce O_2^-. This would make the glutathione-peroxidase system particularly important in preventing free radical initiation in membranes since it
is a very effective scavenger of H_2O_2 (K_m of 1.0 μm according to Flohe
and Brand [31]), while catalase would be far less efficient at the low levels
of H_2O_2 occurring in intact cells since its K_m is reported by Ogura to be
1.1 M [32].

Glutathione peroxidase activity appears to be composed of two enzymic
components, at least one of which contains selenium as an essential constituent [136]. The selenium-containing component catalyzes the reduction
of both H_2O_2 and organic peroxides while the other component appears to
reduce only organic peroxides. Thus, a selenium deficiency resulting in
lowered total glutathione peroxidase activity might be expected to result in
tissue damage due to an inability of cells to eliminate low concentrations of
H_2O_2 generated by various enzymic activities. Catalase is an ineffective
scavenger of H_2O_2 at low concentrations [137]. In the rat, a combined
deficiency of selenium and fat-soluble antioxidant results in liver necrosis
[140]. Lowered glutathione peroxidase activity may allow elevated levels
of H_2O_2 to exist in the cell and the deficiency of fat-soluble free radical
scavengers (such as α-tocopherol) would not quench radical-mediated
attacks on unsaturated lipids in the membranes resulting from the interaction of H_2O_2 with O_2^-. Further support for the importance of the

glutathione peroxidase system in preventing initiation of free radical-mediated reactions comes from the work of Sies and Summer [34] who demonstrated that damage to isolated liver cells to which hydroperoxides have been added does not occur until the cellular NADPH is oxidized to the maximum extent with subsequent depletion of reduced glutathione.

Our studies indicate that glutathione peroxidase activity does not reduce lipid peroxides in biological membranes to lipid alcohols. Rather, it appears that the system prevents lipid peroxidation by removing H_2O_2 before it can react with superoxide anions to form hydroxyl radicals [66] (see Fig. 3). The catalytic activity of superoxide dismutase is highly effective in maintaining O_2^- (now known to be formed by a number of oxido-reductase systems) at low levels [35, 36]. Nevertheless, it appears that the presence of superoxide dismutase, catalase, and glutathione peroxidase is not always sufficient to protect against hydroxy radical-induced damage by enzymes that generate O_2^- and H_2O_2, and which are embedded in the hydrophobic matrix of membranes (as the NADPH-oxidase system of liver microsomes appears to be). Oxygen is approximately eight times more soluble in the lipid phase of cells than it is in the aqueous phase [128]. Hence, any enzyme system capable of generating O_2^- and H_2O_2 during its catalytic activity in the hydrophobic matrix will have adequate O_2 available to do so under aerobic conditions. Furthermore, H_2O_2

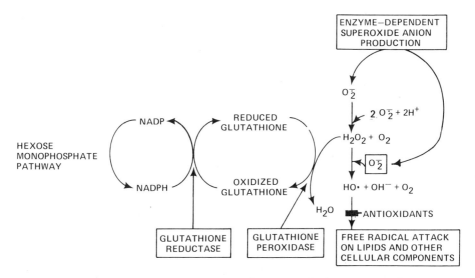

FIG. 3 Diagrammatic representation of events which appear to be involved in enzyme-catalyzed lipid peroxidation and its control.

might be expected to remain in the nonaqueous phase sufficiently long in
some cases to permit reaction with O_2^-, thereby forming a hydroxyl radical
in the immediate vicinity of polyunsaturated fatty acids from which it could
promptly abstract a hydrogen to form a fatty acid radical ($R^{\cdot}$). Since none
of the soluble enzymes which control H_2O_2 and O_2^- levels in the cytosol
could be expected to have a direct participation in the events occurring
within the nonaqueous phase of the membrane, the presence of lipid-
soluble free radical scavengers such as vitamin E would be necessary to
quench $HO^{\cdot}$ and/or $R^{\cdot}$ (lipid) radicals. Otherwise, the reaction of $R^{\cdot}$ with
O_2 to form $ROO^{\cdot}$ and subsequent radical-mediated reactions involving
other unsaturated lipids would disrupt the hydrophobic nature of the membrane interior, resulting in membrane fragmentation (a feature often seen
in electron micrographs of tissues affected by vitamin E-deficiency) [37-
39]. A representation scheme of our concept of the sequence of events
which seems to fit the known information about NADPH oxidase-catalyzed
microsomal lipid peroxidation is shown in Fig. 4. In further support of
this concept are the studies of Vos et al. [122], who demonstrated that
mitochondria and microsomes isolated from vitamin E-deficient ducks
contained less arachidonic acid than those from control animals. Studies
by Hogberg et al. have shown that NADPH-dependent lipid peroxidation in
microsomal membranes results in membrane alterations accompanied by
loss of certain membrane-bound enzyme activities, some at an early time,
some occurring only after extensive lipid alterations occurred [40].

The sequence of events leading to enzyme-catalyzed lipid peroxidation
in biological membranes as represented in Fig. 4 is supported by the following observations:

1. Addition of superoxide dismutase to microsomal membranes
    undergoing lipid peroxidation due to NADPH oxidase activity does
    not inhibit the attack on the lipids, but addition of superoxide
    dismutase to a solubilized and purified NADPH-cytochrome P_{450}
    reductase system does protect other membrane structures (such
    as lysosomes) from peroxidative attack during the catalytic
    activity of the reductase [27].

2. Fat-soluble antioxidants, such as α-tocopherol, administered in
    vivo protect biological membranes from the effects of membrane-
    bound NADPH oxidase activity while water-soluble scavengers do
    not (McCay et al., unpublished observations).

3. Since neither tocopherol, other antioxidants, nor polyunsaturated
    fatty acids appear to react at measurable rates with O_2^- in vitro,
    some other radical species must be responsible for the rapid
    attack on the lipids [27].

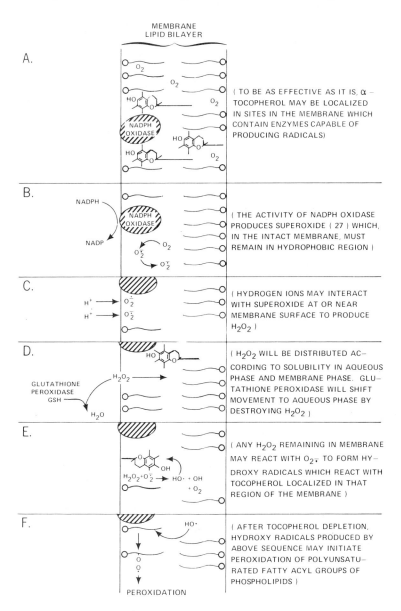

FIG. 4   Sequence of events indicated to occur in the liver microsomal membrane during NADPH-oxidase activity leading to a peroxidative attack on unsaturated membrane lipids.

4. If the radical species responsible for the oxidative attack is the hydroxyl radical, it must be formed in the immediate vicinity of the polyunsaturated fatty acid chain because of the extreme reactivity of this radical. Diffusion of this radical from a reaction of O_2^- and H_2O_2 in the cytosol into the membrane to attack an unsaturated fatty acid in the membrane interior would not be likely to occur under these conditions.

5. ESR studies with spin-trapping compounds have provided direct evidence for the formation of carbon-centered radicals by microsomes oxidizing NADPH and may represent lipid radicals $(R\cdot)$ [41].

6. Loss of polyunsaturated fatty acids has been shown to occur in membranes of subcellular organelles mitochondria and microsomes of vitamin E-deficient animals (see discussion by Molenaar et al. in Chap. 4.G).

7. Vitamin E is consumed in microsomal membranes during enzymic reactions known to generate radicals before an attack begins on the unsaturated lipids [42].

Interestingly, a low concentration of iron is required for a significant rate of lipid peroxidation by enzyme-catalyzed systems. Our studies indicate that the role of Fe^{3+} in these systems is to enhance the formation of hydroxyl radicals via the following reactions [43]:

$$O_2^{\cdot -} + O_2^{\cdot -} + 2H^+ \rightarrow H_2O_2 + O_2$$

$$O_2^{\cdot -} + Fe^{3+} \rightarrow O_2 + Fe^{2+}$$

$$Fe^{2+} + H_2O_2 \rightarrow Fe^{3+} + HO\cdot + OH^-$$

The last reaction is a Fenton-type system which is known to be a fast reaction capable of hydroxylating organic compounds [44].

In summary, the studies are compatible with the concept that α-tocopherol functions as a free radical scavenger in membranes. This does not exclude the possibility, however, that it may exert other highly specific functions. One reason for considering that α-tocopherol may have another specific function is the fact that while structurally unrelated antioxidants can substitute for α-tocopherol in the animal diet reasonably well, examples of inability to provide full protection exist. However, this could be due to toxicity of the antioxidant or to an inability of the synthetic antioxidant to localize into membrane structure in the same manner as

α-tocopherol at sites of high vulnerability to radical attack. This would result in inefficient scavenging of radicals with chronic membrane perturbations that eventually affect cullular activities. An example of such alterations is the loss of cytochrome P_{450} from microsomal membranes which have been subjected to lipid peroxidation [77, 78].

D. Free Radicals Formed from Exogenous Compounds

Free radical sources other than those produced by endogenous metabolic processes may also result in alteration of cellular constituents and cause dysfunction or cell death. One example is carbon tetrachloride, a hepatotoxic compound which is believed to exert its damaging effects on the liver during its metabolism. Reviews of the hepatotoxicity of this compound, its relationship to lipid peroxidation, and the association of the metabolism of CCl_4 with the peroxidation process, are available [45-48], as well as descriptions of the morphological events associated with CCl_4-mediated injury of liver tissue [49, 50]. This discussion concerns the protective action of antioxidants (including α-tocopherol) against the toxicity of carbon tetrachloride and the possible mechanisms of the injury and protection.

About 10 years ago, it was shown almost simultaneously by three different laboratories that the toxic action of CCl_4 on the liver was associated with its metabolism by the endoplasmic reticulum of that tissue [48, 51, 52]. The metabolism of CCl_4 by liver microsomes was also shown to be associated with lipid peroxidation of homogenates and subcellular fractions of rat liver [51, 53-55]. These studies led to a general investigation of the effects of antioxidants on carbon tetrachloride toxicity, especially in view of a much earlier observation by Hove [56] that dietary α-tocopherol protected rats against the toxicity of CCl_4. It was soon determined that various antioxidant compounds provided substantial protection against CCl_4-induced necrosis [48, 51, 54, 57]. Meldolesi demonstrated that pretreatment of Sprague-Dawley rats with α-tocopherol (125 mg/kg in corn oil, i.p.) before administering CCl_4 (2.5 ml/kg, diluted 1:2 in paraffin) resulted in almost uniform reduction of the degree of severity of lesions observed [58] and concluded that the studies were consistent with the hypothesis that peroxidation of the structural lipids was a major mechanism in CCl_4 liver damage as proposed by Goshal and Recknagel [59], Slater [51], and others. Alpers et al. demonstrated that either α-tocopherol or N, N'-diphenyl-p-phenylenediamine (both administered i.p.) prevented fatty liver and necrosis by CCl_4, but did not prevent inhibition of protein synthesis in liver slices or by polyribosomes resulting from CCl_4 treatment [60], suggesting that the protein synthesis defect was not a consequence of lipid peroxidation. In fact, they could not produce any diminution of [^{14}C] L-leucine incorporation by liver microsomes exposed to peroxidizing conditions in vitro [60]. Other antioxidants were also found to be effective in protecting liver against damage by CCl_4. Dianzani and Ugazio reported that propyl gallate and reduced glutathione prevented fatty infiltration of the liver of animals following CCl_4 poisoning [61]. Benedetti et al. studied the effect of α-tocopherol on CCl_4 toxicity in the rat and observed that the microsomal concentration of α-tocopherol was strictly correlated to both a decrease in peroxidation of microsomes (as measured by conjugated diene content) and decrease liver triglyceride accumulation [62].

Perhaps the most convincing information which supports the lipid peroxidation theory of CCl_4-induced liver necrosis is the observation that conjugated dienes are present in microsomal lipids from these animals and the evidence indicating that CCl_4 is metabolized in vitro via homolytic cleavage, which results in free radical production (bond dissociation energy = 68 kcal/mole) [63].

$$Cl - \underset{\underset{\textstyle Cl}{|}}{\overset{\overset{\textstyle Cl}{|}}{C}} - Cl \xrightarrow[\text{SYSTEM}]{\substack{\text{MICROSOMAL} \\ \text{ENZYME}}} Cl - \underset{\underset{\textstyle Cl}{|}}{\overset{\overset{\textstyle Cl}{|}}{C}} \cdot\ +\ Cl\cdot$$

Haloalkane radicals of this type would easily abstract methylene hydrogen atoms from polyunsaturated fatty acyl groups of membrane phospholipids. The lipid radical would then react spontaneously with molecular oxygen to form a hydroperoxyl radical which could then initiate further free radical reactions. The enzymes of the drug-metabolizing system are located in the membrane of the endoplasmic reticulum of the liver. It would appear likely, therefore, that if the metabolism of carbon tetrachloride involved homolytic cleavage, lipid peroxidation might result unless adequate radical-scavenging compounds were present in the membrane. Interestingly, the effectiveness of haloalkane compounds such as chloroform, carbon tetrachloride, and bromotrichloromethane in promoting lipid peroxidation in microsomal membranes during their metablism by these particles increases in accordance with decreasing halide bond dissociation energy of the compound [63].

Peroxidized polyunsaturated fatty acid groups contain conjugated diene structures resulting from double bond migration, as a consequence of a free radical attack. A significant increase in conjugated dienes is observed in rat liver microsomal lipid 24 hr after administration of carbon tetrachloride. This increase in conjugated dienes at 24 hr occurs only to a small extent in animals protected with antioxidants [63]. The onset of the double bond shift actually begins within a few minutes after administration of CCl_4 [64].

Recently, Diaz Gomez et al. [138] have concluded that the lipid peroxidation is not a causal factor in CCl_4-induced liver injury. They based this conclusion on the lack of correlation between the irreversible membrane binding of ^{14}C from $[^{14}C]Cl_4$ with conjugated diene content of the mouse liver lipids. In the rat, a correlation can be found. Since the mouse is more susceptible to the necrogenic action of CCl_4 than the rat, these authors concluded that lipid peroxidation (as indicated by conjugated diene content) was not correlated with the necrotic effect of CCl_4 nor with the binding of ^{14}C from $[^{14}C]Cl_4$ to the microsomal membrane. The binding of ^{14}C apparently occurs through metabolic formation of $[^{14}C]Cl_3\cdot$ and $Cl\cdot$ radicals which then react with lipids and proteins [71]. We have recently obtained direct evidence employing the ESR technique with a spin-trapping agent [72] for the formation of free radicals by liver microsomes metabolizing CCl_4. However, studies in our laboratory indicate that peroxidized portions of the endoplasmic reticulum detach from that membrane and, as a result, the lipids containing the conjugated dienes would be lost during isolation of the microsomal fraction and could account for the results of Diaz Gomez et al. above. Our studies indicate that lipid peroxidation in the endoplasmic reticulum does, indeed, appear to be correlated with the necrotic effect of CCl_4 and was verified by determination of the total content of the various polyunsaturated fatty acids present in the microsomal fraction after CCl_4 exposure [11]. The mouse shows considerable total loss of these fatty acids, exceeding that observed in rat microsomes [65]. The results also correlated well with malondialdehyde formation by mouse microsomes [65]. Similar results were obtained using isolated rat hepatocytes with which we demonstrated that CCl_4 results in loss of a significant fraction of the microsomal lipids and proteins in a very short time [11]. These results are consistent with reports of the loss of drug-metabolizing functions in microsomal membranes of CCl_4-treated rats [67].

It seems quite possible, therefore, that the protective action of α-tocopherol and other antioxidants on the hepatotoxic action of CCl_4 occurs in part through the scavenging, either of $CCl_3\cdot$ and $Cl\cdot$ radicals or of lipid radicals which result from the attack of the CCl_4-derived radicals. Several workers have reported that polyunsaturated fatty acids decrease in the microsomal membranes after CCl_4 poisoning [68-70]. On the other hand, there is also evidence that antioxidants delay the entry of CCl_4 into the liver [61], which would further contribute to a protective action.

Antioxidants, including α-tocopherol, have been shown to inhibit carcinogenesis by various compounds [73, 74], and it seems worthwhile to consider that the protective effect may result from an interference with a free radical-mediated step in the activation of the carcinogen. Floyd et al. have shown that a lipid hydroperoxide (linoleic acid hydroperoxide) in the presence of methemoglobin or hematin, activates the carcinogen, N-hydroxy-N-acetyl-2-aminofluorene (N-OH-AAF), to 2-nitrosofluorene and N-acetoxy-N-acetyl-2-aminofluorene, the latter being considerably more carcinogenic than N-OH-AAF [139]. Of particular interest is the fact that malondialdehyde (a product of lipid peroxidation) has been shown to be both a tumor initiator [75] and a mutagenic compound [79]. In addition, elevated levels of polyunsaturated fat in animal diets enhances their susceptibility to carcinogen-induced tumor formation [76]. Possibly, some of the effects of antioxidants on chemical carcinogenesis may be exerted through the effect of the antioxidants on the drug-metabolizing system. The following section considers the interaction of antioxidants with that system.

III. VITAMIN E AND THE DRUG-METABOLIZING SYSTEM

A. Introduction

The metabolism of lipids, steroids, various drugs, carcinogens, and numerous other xenobiotics is catalyzed in liver via an electron transport pathway associated with the endoplasmic reticular membrane. The system requires NADPH and O_2, and has been designated a mixed-function oxidase system [80]. In purified, reconstituted systems, NADPH-cytochrome P_{450} reductase, cytochrome P_{450}, and phospholipid are required for activity [81,82]. Each molecule of substrate acted upon requires one molecule of oxygen, with one atom of oxygen adding to the substrate, and the other being reduced to form H_2O. The terminal hemoprotein of this microsomal electron transport system has recently been shown to be a family of closely related hemoproteins known as cytochromes P_{450} [83,84] which act as terminal oxidases for a considerable variety of oxidative reactions [85-89]. It is of great interest that this family of heme proteins is induced by many different compounds, and that different forms of P_{450} are produced when animals are exposed to one type of compound as compared to another [90,91]. As a result, a compound may be metabolized in different ways, depending on the types and amounts of these cytochromes that are present [92].

The significance of the term P_{450} lies in the ability of the reduced form of these hemoproteins to react with carbon monoxide, yielding complexes which absorb strongly at 450 or 448 nm, and which can be used to quantitate the hemoproteins [90,93]. In the scheme of electron flow, NADPH is oxidized by the flavoprotein NADPH-cytochrome P_{450} reductase, with transfer of an electron from the reduced flavoprotein to the oxidized form(s) of cytochrome P_{450} to which the substrate to be oxidized has been bound (Fig. 5). The mechanism of mixed-function oxidations is not well understood, particularly the form of oxygen which interacts with the substrate. It has been clearly demonstrated that rats which are deficient in vitamin E have decreased microsomal drug-metabolizing functions [31,50, 95,96,121]. However, the cause of the decreased function of this system is not known. The activity cannot be restored by the direct addition of

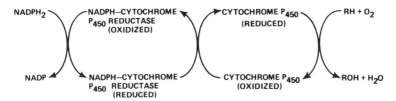

FIG. 5   Metabolic reactions known to occur during the activity of the mixed-function oxidase system in liver microsomes.

α-tocopherol to the microsomal system. In this discussion, we shall deal with the effects of vitamin E sufficiency and deficiency on the functioning of the microsomal mixed-function oxidase system. This may bring into clearer focus the possible action of vitamin E on the mixed-function oxidase system and how it may relate to microsomal fatty acids, hemoproteins, flavoproteins, and the ability of certain synthetic antioxidants to mimic many in vivo effects of this vitamin.

B.   Influence of Vitamin E on Hemoprotein Synthesis

A deficiency of vitamin E produces a great variety of species-specific syndromes including encephalomalacia, exudative diathesis, fetal resorption, defective spermatogenesis, degeneration of skeletal and cardiac muscle, and anemia. The development of a nutritional anemia has been demonstrated in vitamin E-deficient monkeys [97-99], and it was postulated that the locus of vitamin E influence was in the biosynthesis of heme and heme proteins [98, 99]. If vitamin E does influence heme synthesis or the biosynthesis of heme proteins, then the effect of a deficiency of α-tocopherol on microsomal drug metabolism might be expected when the content of the cytochrome P_{450} in the endoplasmic reticulum is diminished. This would be anticipated to occur at an early stage of deficiency since this heme protein or family of heme proteins has a rather rapid turnover. Other investigators have also suggested the possible involvement of vitamin E with heme synthesis [102-104]. Since cytochrome P_{450} turns over rapidly in liver it could be expected to reflect any restriction in heme synthesis rather quickly.

Nair and coworkers have reported that vitamin E functions in the regulation of heme biosynthesis presumably by controlling the mechanisms of induction and repression of the two key enzymes, δ-aminolevulinic acid synthetase (δ-ALA synthetase) in bone marrow, and δ-aminolevulinic acid dehydratase (δ-ALA dehydratase) in liver [101, 105-107]. The biosynthesis of heme (Fig. 6) is common to all aerobic cells and begins with the

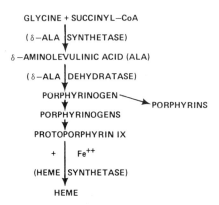

FIG. 6   Pathway for the biosynthesis of heme.

intramitochondrial condensation of glycine and succinyl CoA to form
δ-aminolevulinic acid (ALA). This first step is catalyzed by δ-ALA synthetase. The second step is the condensation of two molecules of amino-
levulinic acid to form porphobilinogen (PBG) and is catalyzed by δ-ALA
dehydratase, a soluble cytosolic enzyme. As catalysts of the first two
essential steps in the heme synthetic pathway, these two enzymes, either
individually or in combination, are rate determining. The terminal step is
catalyzed by the enzyme heme synthetase. This involves the incorporation
of ferrous iron into protoporphyrin IX, and occurs intramitochondrially.
Once synthesized, the heme is conjugated with apoproteins to function in a
great many cellular activities.

If a deficiency of vitamin E results in decreased synthesis of heme, a
change in the levels and/or activities of δ-ALA synthetase or δ-ALA
dehydratase might be observed. It would also follow that the amounts of
hepatic heme and hemoproteins would decrease, reflecting the levels of
available heme. More recent evidence indicates that a vitamin E deficiency
has little effect, if any, on the level of heme-containing proteins, at least
in the liver [95, 108, 109]. Carpenter [108] found that quantitative determinations of cytochrome P_{450} content of liver microsomes in control and
vitamin E-deficient rats showed no difference in amounts of P_{450}. Diplock
[109] investigated cytochrome constituents in the microsome and showed
that their biosynthesis was unimpaired, even if a selenium deficiency also
accompanied the vitamin E deficiency.

It has also been suggested that the toxicity of iron described in vitamin
E deficiency [110, 111] may be the result of a limited production of protoporphyrin IX, a pathway that is available for the uptake of iron if the
heme synthetic pathway is functioning normally [106]. Inorganic iron which

is not utilized properly may promote peroxidative processes in tissues in the same way that it does in the in vitro systems described earlier. This likelihood is enhanced by the fact that iron toxicity is known to be prevented by tocopherol and other antioxidants [111]. Since synthetic antioxidants given at the same time as iron afford protection to anemic animals being given iron therapy, it does not seem likely that a specific function for vitamin E in protoporphyrin IX biosynthesis exists [112].

Bartlett et al. [141] investigated the influence of vitamin E on lead toxicity in the rabbit. Lead inhibits several enzymes in the heme synthesis pathway, especially δ-ALA dehydratase [113-115]. Moreover, vitamin E was found to diminish the anemia and coproporphinuria in lead-poisoned rats [117]. Bartlett and coworkers investigated the effect of tocopherol on the inhibition of δ-ALA dehydratase and δ-ALA synthetase by lead [141]. They found that vitamin E did not prevent a decrease of δ-ALA dehydratase activity in rabbits fed diets containing lead, nor did it have any stimulatory effect on δ-ALA dehydratase in rabbits fed no lead. They concluded that there was no experimental evidence for a defect in either δ-ALA synthetase or δ-ALA dehydratase in vitamin E-deficient rabbits.

Recently Horn et al. [95] have examined the role of vitamin E in the regulation of liver heme proteins and report no differences in amounts of cytochromes P_{450} or P_{448}, or in catalase levels between control and tocopherol-deficient rats. Further evidence for a lack of correlation between tocopherol intake and hemoprotein synthesis was seen in a concurrent induction of cytochrome P_{448} levels of both control and deficient animals during a 4-day period of treatment with 3-methylcholanthrene.

The evidence available at the present time indicates that there is no direct effect of vitamin E on heme synthesis, at least in the liver. It may still be true that heme synthesis is altered in bone marrow during vitamin E deficiency, especially in view of the anemia which develops in several types of animals deprived of tocopherol, and in view of the work of Porter and Fitch in which a decrease in δ-ALA synthetase activity was found in bone marrow deterioration caused by a peroxidative alteration of erythroid cells, and may suggest an antioxidant function for vitamin E in this respect.

C. Drug Metabolism

Several investigators, Carpenter [108, 118, 119], Diplock [120], and Giasuddin et al. [121], have performed careful studies on the demethylation of the antipyretic drug, aminopyrine. These investigators all concurred that over a wide range of substrate concentrations, the demethylation of aminopyrine by the mixed-function oxidase system is depressed in liver microsomal fractions from rats deprived of vitamin E. It was found that in vitro addition of antioxidants such as ethoxyquin and/or exogenous α-tocopherol [120, 121] to either the homogenate or to the assay medium had no significant effect on the decreased enzyme activity. This suggested that the effect of vitamin E deficiency was probably not due to an increased rate of in vitro peroxidation of the membrane polyunsaturated lipids. This does not, however, eliminate the possibility that peroxidative damage to the endoplasmic reticulum may have already occurred in vivo as a result of tocopherol deficiency.

Horn et al. [95] observed that even though the concentrations of heme proteins did not differ in vitamin E-sufficient and vitamin E-deficient rats, there was a significant decrease in the activities of the drug-metabolizing enzymes as measured in vitro by ethylmorphine demethylation or of benzo(α)pyrene hydroxylation, and that sleeping times following treatment with pentobarbital or zoxazolamine did not differ between vitamin E-deficient and vitamin E-supplemented rats. In this study it was also shown that vitamin E deficiency had no effect upon the inducing abilities of benzo(α)pyrene-hydroxylase by 3-methylcholanthrene and that no difference in the time course of induction between control and deficient groups could be demonstrated.

A more complete study of this phenomenon was done with reaction kinetics of the overall demethylase system. In this approach there were some differences in results among the investigators. Carpenter reported that the V_{max} values were reduced by one-half for both aminopyrine and codeine demethylation but observed no change in K_m values, suggesting that the microsomal content of hydroxylase in the microsomes of the control animals is greater than in vitamin E-deficient ones [108]. Diplock obtained similar results for codeine demethylation but opposite results for aminopyrine. He observed a threefold increase in the K_m for aminopyrine and no change in the apparent V_{max} values in normal and vitamin E-deficient rats [120]. Again, the in vitro addition of α-tocopherol or ethoxyquin was without effect on the K_m values obtained with liver microsomes from E-deficient rats. From this information, Diplock concludes that this decrease in drug metabolism caused by vitamin E deficiency is probably not due to in vivo lipid peroxidation. However, this conclusion is based upon an in vitro addition to the assay system, and it does not seem likely that a subsequent addition of an antioxidant to the system can rectify membrane changes which might have already occurred in vivo, especially peroxidative-type reactions.

Carpenter [108] investigated the effects of the in vivo administration of the antioxidant N,N'-diphenyl-ρ-phenylenediamine (DPPD) upon microsomal demethylation reactions. Microsomal lipid peroxidation was completely inhibited in microsomes from animals which had received DPPD in their diet. However, no differences were observed in the demethylation of either codeine or aminopyrine between antioxidant-deficient and control animals. It was assumed that the DPPD was incorporated into the microsomes since lipid peroxidation was inhibited but that it could not function in the same manner as vitamin E in microsomal hydroxylation reactions.

It has been suggested that α-tocopherol is required as a structural component of the endoplasmic reticulum and possesses configurational properties which make it ideal for stabilizing membranes containing polyunsaturated fatty acids [123]. In this model, two interactions are proposed between methyl groups of the phytyl chain of α-tocopherol and the cis-double bonds of the fatty acid. Under normal circumstances, some of the arachidonate residues may be associated with cholesterol, and according to Lucy's theory [123], a 1:1 ratio of vitamin E to polyunsaturated fatty acid in membranes is not required, but membranes containing high levels of polyunsaturated fatty acids will require higher levels of vitamin E for structural stability. Without sufficient amounts of vitamin E, the arrangement of the hydrocarbon regions of membranes will become disordered. This disorder may facilitate the oxidative destruction of polyunsaturated fatty acids. Rowe and Wills have demonstrated that both polyunsaturated fatty acids and vitamin E are essential in the diet for maximal activity of oxidative drug metabolism [124]. Neither vitamin E nor polyunsaturated fat given alone is as effective as a combination of both factors. They found that a delicate balance between these two dietary factors was required for maximal activity.

In summary, the effects of vitamin E deficiency on drug metabolism are still unexplained. It must be determined whether or not the reported effects exist in the intact animal or intact liver cell and whether or not it is a general effect of vitamin E deficiency among different species. Assuming that such differences in drug-metabolizing parameters do exist in vivo between vitamin E-deficient and vitamin E-sufficient animals, the relationship between such an effect and the variety of deficiency disorders observed among different species seems baffling. A deficiency of vitamin E may initiate a cascade of events which may perturb a number of cell parameters, of which only one may be sufficiently deranged to interfere with the expression of the cell's function. Reconstruction of such a chain of events to unequivocally identify the initial consequence of vitamin E lack may lie some distance in the future.

IV. CONCLUSION

The evidence supporting the hypothesis that animals require dietary antioxidants to minimize extraneous free radical-mediated membrane damage promoted by endogenous enzyme activity is reasonably convincing. The hypothesis can explain most of the effects of vitamin E deficiency including the initially confusing relationship between selenium and α-tocopherol in dietary liver necrosis. In this disorder, either vitamin E or dietary selenium can prevent liver necrosis [125]. Since selenite itself does not possess antioxidant properties [126], it appears likely that it exerts its protective action in this liver disorder by providing an essential component in the enzyme glutathione peroxidase [127], in particular, the form of the enzyme which catalyzes the destruction of H_2O_2 [136]. This selenoenzyme would eliminate accumulation of H_2O_2 and apparently interrupt the sequence of events leading to generation of hydroxyl and lipid-free radicals. Vitamin E supplementation in lieu of selenium may provide a sufficient edge of scavenging capacity to protect the liver cell membranes from free radical attack and prevent membrane damage and necrosis even at low levels of the form of glutathione peroxidase which acts on hydrogen peroxide.

It is not unlikely that subtle radical-mediated perturbations of membrane structure might alter receptor sites, transport functions, and membrane-bound enzyme activities which could produce serious consequences in some tissues, yet leave other organs which are less dependent on those parameters seemingly unaffected. If the systems perturbed to the greatest extent are species specific, the variety and severity of tocopherol deficiency symptoms observed among different animals would be explained.

REFERENCES

1. J. Green, A. T. Diplock, J. Bunyan, D. McHale, and I. R. Muthy, Br. J. Nutr. 21:69-101 (1967).
2. J. Bunyan, A. T. Diplock, and J. Green, Br. J. Nutr. 21:217-224 (1967).
3. A. T. Diplock, J. Bunyan, D. McHale, and J. Green, Br. J. Nutr. 21:103-114 (1967).
4. B. E. March, V. Coates, and J. Biely, Science 164:1398-1400 (1969).
5. J. J. Gilbert, Amer. J. Clin. Nutr. 27:1005-1016 (1974).
6. J. B. Chappell and A. R. Crafts, Biochem. J. 95:393-402 (1965).
7. K. Kawai, M. Nakao, T. Nakao, and G. Katsui, Amer. J. Clin. Nutr. 27:987-994 (1974).
8. G. Siebert, P. P. Diezel, K. John, E. Krug, A. Schmitt, E. Grunberger, and A. Bottke, Histochimie 3:17-25 (1962).
9. A. N. Siakotos, I. Watanabe, A. Saito, and S. Fleischer, Biochem. Med. 4:361-375 (1970).
10. R. D. Taubold, A. N. Siakotos, and E. G. Perkins, Lipids 10:383-390 (1975).
11. C. C. Weddle, K. R. Hornbrook, and P. B. McCay, J. Biol. Chem. 251:4973-4978 (1976).
12. H. Dam, Pharmacol. Rev. 25:1-16 (1957).
13. L. Michaelis and S. H. Wollman, Science 109:313-314 (1949).
14. H. A. Mattill, Ann. Rev. Biochem. 16:177-192 (1947).
15. H. H. Draper and A. S. Csallany, Proc. Soc. Exp. Biol. Med. 99:739-742 (1958).
16. R. E. Olson, Science 145:926-928 (1964).

17. S. Krishnamurthy and J. G. Bieri, J. Nutr. 77:245-252 (1962).
18. M. K. Horwitt, in International Symposium on Vitamin E. Edited by N. Shimazono and Y. Togaki. Tokyo, Kyoritsu Shuppan Co. Ltd., 1972, pp. 45-62.
19. H. Hassan, S. A. Hashim, T. B. Van Itallie, and W. H. Sebrell, Amer. J. Clin. Nutr. 19:147-157 (1966).
20. L. A. Witting, Amer. J. Clin. Nutr. 27:952-959 (1974).
21. P. Hochstein and L. Ernster, Biochem. Biophys. Res. Commun. 12:388-394 (1963).
22. P. Hochstein, K. Nordenbrand, and L. Ernster, Biochem. Biophys. Res. Commun. 14:323-328 (1964).
23. R. Nilsson, S. Orrenius, and L. Ernster, Biochem. Biophys. Res. Commun. 17:303-309 (1964).
24. H. E. May and P. B. McCay, J. Biol. Chem. 243:2288-2295 (1968).
25. H. E. May and P. B. McCay, J. Biol. Chem. 243:2296-2305 (1968).
26. P. B. McCay, J. L. Poyer, P. M. Pfeifer, H. E. May, and J. M. Gilliam, Lipids 6:297-306 (1971).
27. K-L. Fong, P. B. McCay, J. L. Poyer, B. B. Keele, and H. Misra, J. Biol. Chem. 248:7792-7797 (1973).
28. A. G. Hildebrandt, M. Speck, and I. Roots, Biochem. Biophys. Res. Commun. 54:968-975 (1973).
29. F. Haber and J. Weiss, Proc. R. Soc. Edinburgh Sec. A. 147:332-351 (1934).
30. N. Oshino, D. Jamieson, and C. Chance, Biochem. J. 146:53-65 (1975).
31. L. Flohe and L. Brand, Biochim. Biophys. Acta 191:541-549 (1969).
32. Y. Ogura, Arch. Biochem. Biophys. 57:288-300 (1955).
33. M. Nishikimi and L. J. Machlin, Arch. Biochem. Biophys. 170:684-689 (1975).
34. H. Sies and K-H. Summer, Eur. J. Biochem. 57:503-512 (1975).
35. J. M. McCord and I. Fridovich, J. Biol. Chem. 244:6049-6055 (1969).
36. C. Beauchamp and I. Fridovich, J. Biol. Chem. 245:4641-4646 (1970).
37. I. Molenaar, F. A. Hommes, W. G. Braams, and H. A. Polman, Proc. Natl. Acad. Sci. 61:982-988 (1968).
38. I. Molenaar, J. Vos, F. C. Jager, and F. A. Hommes, Nutr. Metab. 12:358-370 (1970).
39. J. F. Van Vleet, B. V. Hall, and J. Simon, Amer. J. Pathol. 52:1067-1079 (1968).
40. J. Hogberg, A. Bergstrand, and S. V. Jakobsson, Eur. J. Biochem. 37:51-59 (1973).
41. P. B. McCay, J. L. Poyer, R. A. Floyd, K-L. Fong, and E. K. Lai, Fed. Proc. 35:1421 (1976).
42. P. B. McCay, P. M. Pfeifer, and W. H. Stipe, Ann. N.Y. Acad. Sci. 203:62-73 (1972).

43. K-L. Fong, P. B. McCay, J. L. Poyer, H. P. Misra, and B. B. Keele, Chem.-Biol. Interact., in press.
44. Hj. Staudinger, B. Kerekjarto, V. Ullrich, and Z. Zubrzycki, in Oxidases and Related Redox Systems. Edited by T. E. King, H. S. Mason, and M. Morrison, New York, Wiley, 1965, pp. 815-837.
45. R. O. Recknagel and A. K. Goshal, Lab. Invest. 15:132-148 (1966).
46. R. O. Recknagel, Pharmacol. Rev. 19:145-208 (1967).
47. T. F. Slater, in Free Radical Mechanisms in Tissue Injury. Edited by T. F. Slater, London, Pion, Ltd., 1972, pp. 91-170.
48. R. O. Recknagel and E. A. Glende, Jr., CRC Critical Reviews in Technology, November 1973, 263-297.
49. C. T. Ashworth, F. J. Luibel, E. Sanders, and N. Arnold, Arch. Pathol. 75:212-225 (1963).
50. E. S. Reynolds and H. J. Ree, Lab. Invest. 25:269-278 (1971).
51. T. F. Slater, Nature (London) 209:36-40 (1966).
52. E. A. Smuckler, Lab. Invest. 15:157-164 (1966).
53. C. Comporti, C. Saccocci, and M. U. Dianzani, Enzymologia 29:186-203 (1965).
54. N. R. Di Luzio and F. Costales, Exp. Mol. Pathol. 4:141-154 (1965).
55. A. K. Goshal and R. O. Recknagel, Life Sci. 4:2195-2209 (1965).
56. E. L. Hove, Arch. Biochem. 17:467-473 (1948).
57. C. H. Gallagher, Austr. J. Exp. Med. 40:241-254 (1962).
58. J. Meldolesi, Exp. Mol. Pathol. 9:141-147 (1968).
59. A. K. Goshal and R. O. Recknagel, Life Sci. 4:2195-2209 (1965).
60. D. H. Alpers, M. Solin, and K. J. Isselbacher, Mol. Pharmacol. 4:566-573 (1968).
61. M. U. Dianzani and G. Ugazio, Chem.-Biol. Interact. 6:67-79 (1973).
62. A. Benedetti, M. Ferrali, E. Chieli, and M. Comporti, Chem.-Biol. Interact. 9:117-134 (1974).
63. R. O. Recknagel, E. A. Glende, G. Ugazio, R. R. Koch, and S. Srinivasan, Isr. J. Med. Sci. 10:301-311 (1974).
64. K. S. Rao and R. O. Recknagel, Exp. Mol. Pathol. 9:271-278 (1968).
65. K. R. Hornbrook, J. L. Poyer, and P. B. McCay, The Pharmacologist, 18(2):246, 1976.
66. P. B. McCay, D. D. Gibson, K-L. Fong, and K. R. Hornbrook, Biochim. Biophys. Acta 431:459-468 (1976).
67. D. Sgoutas, Metabolism 16:382-291 (1967).
68. E. A. Glende, Jr., Biochem. Pharmacol. 21:1-7 (1972).
69. M. G. Horning, M. J. Earle, and H. M. Maling, Biochim. Biophys. Acta 56:177-180 (1962).
70. M. Comporti, E. Burdino, and G. Ugazio, Ital. J. Biochem. 20:156-165 (1971).
71. M. C. Villarruel and J. A. Castro, Research communication, Chem. Pathol. Pharmacol. 10:105-116 (1975).

72. P. B. McCay, R. A. Floyd, E. K. Lai, J. L. Poyer, and K-L. Fong, Biophys. J. 16:66a (1976).
73. S. L. Haber and R. W. Wissler, Proc. Soc. Exp. Biol. Med. 111:774-775 (1962).
74. L. W. Wattenberg, J. Natl. Cancer Inst. 48:1425-1430 (1972).
75. R. S. Shamberger, T. L. Andreone, and C. E. Willis, J. Natl. Cancer Inst. 53:1771-1773 (1974).
76. E. B. Gammal, K. K. Carroll, and E. R. Plunkett, Cancer Res. 27:1737-1742 (1967).
77. W. Levin, A. Y. H. Lu, M. Jacobson, R. Kuntzman, J. L. Poyer, and P. B. McCay, Arch. Biochem. Biophys. 158:842-852 (1973).
78. B. A. Schaerer, H. S. Marver, and U. A. Meyer, Biochim. Biophys. Acta 279:221-227 (1972).
79. F. N. Mukai and B. D. Goldstein, Science 191:868-869 (1976).
80. H. S. Mason, J. C. North, and M. Vanneste, Fed. Proc. 24:1172-1180 (1965).
81. A. Y. H. Lu, R. Kuntzman, S. West, M. Jacobson, and A. H. Conney, J. Biol. Chem. 247:1727-1734 (1972).
82. R. M. Kashnitz and M. G. Coon, Biochem. Pharmacol. 24:295-297 (1975).
83. A. H. Conney, W. Levin, M. Jacobson, R. Kuntzman, D. Y. Cooper, and O. Rosenthal, in Microsomes and Drug Oxidations. Edited by J. R. Gillette, A. H. Conney, G. J. Cosmides, R. W. Estabrook, J. R. Fouts, and G. J. Mannering, New York, Academic, 1969, pp. 279-295.
84. A. G. Hildebrandt and R. W. Estabrook, in Microsomes and Drug Oxidations. Edited by J. R. Gillette, A. H. Conney, G. J. Cosmides, R. W. Estabrook, J. R. Fouts, and G. J. Mannering, New York, Academic, 1969, pp. 331-343.
85. A. H. Conney, Pharmacol. Rev. 19:317-366 (1967).
86. J. R. Gillette, D. C. Davis, and H. A. Sasame, Ann. Rev. Pharmacol. 12:57-84 (1972).
87. R. Kuntzman, Annu. Rev. Pharmacol. 9:228-245 (1969).
88. P. E. Thomas, A. Y. H. Lu, D. Ryan, S. B. West, J. Kawalek, and W. Levin, J. Biol. Chem. 251:1385-1391 (1976).
89. G. J. Mannering, Metabolism 20:228-245 (1971).
90. A. P. Alvares, G. Schilling, W. Levin, and R. Kuntzman, Biochem. Biophys. Res. Commun. 29:521-526 (1967).
91. A. Y. H. Lu, R. Kuntzman, S. West, M. Jacobson, A. H. Conney, J. Biol. Chem. 247:1727-1734 (1972).
92. P. E. Thomas, A. Y. H. Lu, D. Ryan, S. B. West, J. Kawalek, and W. Levin, J. Biol. Chem. 251:1385-3191 (1976).
93. D. Ryan, A. Y. H. Lu, S. West, and W. Levin, J. Biol. Chem. 250:2157-2163 (1965).

94. D. A. Haugen, M. J. Coon, D. W. Nebert, J. Biol. Chem. 251:1817-1827 (1976).

95. L. R. Horn, L. J. Machlin, M. O. Barker, and M. Brin, Arch. Biochem. Biophys. 172:270-277 (1976).

96. J. C. Sosa-Lucero, F. A. de la Iglesia, G. Lumb, and G. Feuer, Rev. Can. Biol. 32:69-75 (1973) (Autumn Suppl.).

97. J. S. Dinning and P. L. Day, J. Exp. Med. 105:395-402 (1957).

98. F. S. Porter, C. D. Fitch, and J. S. Dinning, Blood 20:471-477 (1962).

99. F. S. Porter and C. D. Fitch, Scand. J. Hematol. 3:175-185 (1966).

100. D. K. Melhorn and S. Gross, J. Pediatr. 79:569-580 (1971).

101. P. P. Nair, E. Mezey, H. S. Murty, J. Quartner, and A. I. Mendeloff, Arch. Intern. Med. 128:411-415 (1971).

102. W. J. Darby, Vit. Horm. 26:685-704 (1968).

103. A. S. Majaj, J. S. Dinning, S. A. Azzam, and W. J. Darby, Amer. J. Nutr. 12:374-379 (1963).

104. J. A. Whitaker, E. G. Fort, S. Vimokesant, and J. S. Dinning, Amer. J. Clin. Nutr. 20:783-789 (1967).

105. H. S. Murty, P. I. Cassi, S. K. Brooks, and P. P. Nair, J. Biol. Chem. 245:5498-5504 (1970).

106. P. P. Nair, Ann. N.Y. Acad. Sci. 203:53-61 (1972).

107. P. P. Nair, H. S. Murty, P. I. Caasi, S. K. Brooks, and J. Quartner, J. Agr. Food. Chem. 20:476-480 (1972).

108. M. P. Carpenter, Ann. N.Y. Acad. Sci. 203:81-92 (1972).

109. A. T. Diplock, Amer. J. Clin. Nutr. 27:995-1004 (1974).

110. L. Goldberg and J. P. Smith, Amer. J. Pathol. 36:125-150 (1960).

111. G. Tollerz and N. Lannek, Nature (London) 201:846-847 (1964).

112. C. P. J. Caygill, A. T. Diplock, and E. H. Jeffery, Biochem. J. 136:851-858 (1973).

113. R. A. Goyer and B. C. Rhyne, Int. Rev. Exp. Pathol. 12:1-77 (1973).

114. R. L. C. Kao and R. M. Forbes, Proc. Soc. Exp. Biol. Med. 143:234-237 (1973).

115. S. Hernberg and J. Nikkanen, Prac. Lek. 24:77-83 (1972).

116. P. P. Nair, H. S. Murty, and N. R. Grossman, Biochim. Biophys. Acta 215:112-118 (1970).

117. R. de Rosa, Acta Vitaminol. 8:167-172 (1954).

118. M. P. Carpenter, Fed. Proc. 26:475 (1967).

119. M. P. Carpenter, Fed. Proc. 27:677 (1968).

120. A. T. Diplock, Vit. Horm. 32:445-461 (1974).

121. A. S. M. Giasuddin, C. P. J. Caygill, A. T. Diplock, and E. H. Jeffery, Biochem. J. 146:339-359 (1975).

122. J. Vos., I. Molenaar, M. Searle-van Leeuwen, and F. A. Hommes, Ann. N.Y. Acad. Sci. 203:74-80 (1972).

123. J. A. Lucy, Ann. N.Y. Acad. Sci. 203:4-11 (1972).
124. L. Rowe and E. D. Wills, Biochem. Pharmacol. 25:175-179 (1976).
125. T. Moore, Proc. Nutr. Soc. 21:179-185 (1962).
126. R. Caputto, P. B. McCay, and M. P. Carpenter, Amer. J. Clin. Nutr. 9:61-70 (1961).
127. J. T. Rotruck, A. L. Pope, H. E. Ganther, A. B. Swanson, D. G. Hafeman, and W. G. Hoekstra, Science 179:588-590 (1973).
128. H. B. Demopoulos, Fed. Proc. 32:1859-1861 (1973).
129. I. Fridovich, in Free Radicals in Biology, Vol. I. Edited by W. A. Pryor, New York, Academic, 1976, p. 239.
130. W. A. Pryor, in Introduction to Free Radical Chemistry, Englewood Cliffs, N.J., Prentice Hall, 1966, p. 9.
131. J. R. Harbour, V. Chow, and J. R. Bolton, Can. J. Chem. 52:3549 (1974).
132. E. G. Janzen, Acc. Chem. Res. 4:31 (1971).
133. M. M. King, E. K. Lai, and P. B. McCay, J. Biol. Chem. 250:6496-6502 (1975).
134. N. Nakano, T. Noguchi, K. Sugioka, H. Fukuyama, and M. Sato, J. Biol. Chem. 250:2402-2406 (1975).
135. F. D. Vassington, S. M. Reichard, and A. Nason, Vit. Horm. 18:43-87 (1960).
136. R. A. Lawrence and R. F. Burk, Biochem. Biophys. Res. Commun. 71:952-958 (19).
137. H. Misra, J. Biol. Chem. 249:2151-2155 (1974).
138. M. I. Diaz Gomez, C. R. de Castro, N. D'Acosta, O. M. de Fenos, E. C. de Ferreyra, and J. A. Castro, Toxicol. Appl. Pharmacol. 34:102-114 (1975).
139. R. A. Floyd, L. M. Soong, R. N. Walker, and M. Stuart, Cancer Res. 36:2761-2767 (1976).
140. J. Green, A. T. Diplock, J. Bunyan, I. R. Muthy, and D. McHale, Br. J. Nutr. 21:497-506 (1967).
141. R. S. Bartlett, J. E. Rousseau, Jr., H. I. Frier, and R. C. Hall, Jr., J. Nutr. 104:1637-1645 (1974).
142. L. K. Dahle, E. G. Hill, and R. T. Holman, Arch. Biochem. Biophys. 98:253-261 (1962).
143. W. A. Pryor and J. P. Stanley, J. Org. Chem. 40:3615-3617 (1975).
144. W. A. Pryor, J. P. Stanley, and E. Blair, Lipids 11:370-379 (1976).

Section 2   Role in nucleic acid and protein metabolism

GEORGE L. CATIGNANI*
National Institute of Arthritis,
Metabolism, and Digestive Diseases
National Institutes of Health
Bethesda, Maryland

   I. Introduction   318
  II. Nucleic Acid Metabolism   319
 III. Protein Metabolism   320
  IV. Enzyme Function   321
   V. Creatine Kinase   321
  VI. Xanthine Oxidase   324
       References   330

I. INTRODUCTION

One of the most frequently suggested hypotheses on the mode of action of
vitamin E is that it serves some specific, but thus far undefined, regulatory role [1-3]. Through the years, a number of proposals have been put
forth concerning such a role for vitamin E in nucleic acid and protein
metabolism [2-10]. Moreover, the number of publications describing
efforts to define a direct regulatory function for vitamin E is indeed large.
A variety of experimental approaches has been used, but from this wealth
of information no clearly defined regulatory role can yet be ascribed to
this vitamin.

In recent years, however, sufficient evidence has emerged to warrant
encouragement regarding the resolution of this dilemma. This includes
the work of Dinning and coworkers on nucleic acid metabolism [11] and
work from several laboratories on the effects of vitamin E deficiency on
general protein synthesis [3,9,10,12,13], specific enzymes [3,8,14,15],
and enzyme systems [6,16,17]. Although in vitro studies on the protein-
synthesizing machinery of deficient animals have failed to yield a unified

---

*Present affiliation: North Carolina State University, Raleigh, North
Carolina.

concept regarding the function of vitamin E in this process, it appears that the vitamin does indeed exert an influence on the synthesis of specific proteins as suggested by Green [2].

II. NUCLEIC ACID METABOLISM

Vitamin E deficiency produces significant alterations in the tissue content of nucleic acids [18,19]. Certain tissues accumulate RNA during vitamin E deficiency [18,19]. An increase in the specific activity of RNA from deficient animals, after administration of labeled nucleotide precursors [5,20, 21] without an increase in specific activity of the RNA using labeled preformed nucleotides [11,22], demonstrated that the rate of synthesis of RNA is not altered during deficiency. Since the nucleotide precursor pool size was unaffected, these results indicated that an increased rate of nucleotide synthesis de novo results in the increased specific activity of RNA from deficient animals, and suggest that the accumulation of RNA is due to a decrease in the rate of nucleic acid degradation.

Young and Dinning reported an approximately twofold increase in the DNA content of skeletal muscle from vitamin E-deficient rabbits. Subsequently, with the use both of labeled nucleotide precursors [5,20,21] and of preformed nucleotides [11,22], it was established that this increase resulted from a 20-fold increase in the rate of DNA synthesis, with a concomitant increase in the rate of de novo synthesis of nucleotides [11]. The rate of DNA synthesis in other rabbit tissues examined was not altered [11]. The increased DNA content of skeletal muscle and bone marrow [18] in the monkey likewise results from an increased rate of DNA synthesis [11].

Further study on DNA synthesis of monkey bone marrow revealed that the increased rate of synthesis and content was apparently the result of hyperplasia observed in the deficient marrow [23], and indicated an increase in erythropoiesis. Since vitamin E deficiency shortens erythrocyte survival [23,24] and results in morphologically abnormal erythroid precursors [23], an increase in erythropoiesis may represent an attempt to maintain a normal level of functional erythrocytes. Whether vitamin E serves only to protect and maintain normal erythroid precursor membranes, whether it has a more direct role in DNA metabolism, or, as Fitch has suggested [25], whether it exerts an influence over other erythrocyte components, remains obscure.

Various enzymes of nucleic acid metabolism have been examined during vitamin E deficiency. Dinesen and Konat [26] have reported that the activity of rat liver RNA polymerase I decreases approximately 30% after 47 days of deficiency. However, Bonetti et al. [13] found no significant difference in either RNA polymerase I or II as a result of vitamin E deficiency, and only a slight, but not significant, decrease in RNA polymerase II in nuclei from necrotic livers (diet deficient in vitamin E and selenium).

Vitamin E deficiency produces a marked increase in the activity of rabbit muscle RNase [27]. However, this observation seems inconsistent with the observation that there is an increased accumulation of RNA in the deficient muscle [19] without an increase in RNA synthesis. The increase in free RNase observed may not reflect the actual conditions in vivo, since the vitamin E-deficient lysosome would be more susceptible to release of hydrolytic enzymes during tissue preparation.

Detailed examination of the effects of vitamin E deficiency on different species of RNA are lacking, with the exception of reports on the content of ribosomal RNA and the extent to which tRNA is charged. Olson [3] has demonstrated a fourfold increase in the ribosomal content of vitamin E-deficient rabbit muscle. This observation is consistent with the increases in RNA content reported by Young and Dinning [19], considering that rRNA represents a large proportion of the total RNA content of the cell. Reiss and Tappel [12] have reported a decrease in the phenylalanine-accepting activity of tRNA from deficient animals. Using a soluble fraction and activating enzymes from the liver of chow-fed animals, and tRNA from control and deficient rat liver, a consistent 12% decrease in phenylalanine-charging activity was observed with deficient tRNA, as compared to controls.

III. PROTEIN METABOLISM

It is known that the rate of muscle protein synthesis in vivo is increased during vitamin E deficiency [20, 28, 29]. However, in vitro experiments designed to pinpoint an effect of vitamin E deficiency on protein synthesis have given rise to a variety of conflicting results. De Villers et al. [9] have reported that the incorporation of [^{14}C]phenylalanine into protein by polysomal preparations of dystrophic rabbit muscle is increased 27% when compared to control. Density gradient analysis of the polysomal material indicated that, compared with controls, the concentration of heavy polysomes and monosomes decreased during deficiency, while that of the light polysomes increased. The addition of poly U to the deficient polysome preparation restored the profile to that of controls. Simard and Srivastava [10], from the same laboratory, reported an increase in phenylalanine incorporation into protein of 355% and 64% at 3 and 4 weeks, respectively, by deficient polysomes, as compared to controls when poly U was added to the system in vitro. These results were interpreted as evidence, possibly, for a differential rate of synthesis of specific muscle proteins. They also led to the speculation that there may be insufficient mRNA in the deficient muscle.

In contrast, Olson [3] found no change either in rate of incorporation of phenylalanine into protein by polysomal preparations, with or without added poly U, or in the polysome profile in dystrophic muscle (deficient).

Olson [3] has shown by SDS-acrylamide gel analysis that there is a change in the proportion of certain myofibrillar proteins during vitamin E deficiency, in agreement with the suggestion of De Villers et al. [9] that there may be a change in the rate of synthesis of certain muscle proteins. However, at present, the reasons for the difference observed in the in vitro rates of amino acid incorporation and polysome profiles by these two groups remains obscure.

A similar discrepancy exists in results from experiments on protein synthesis by rat liver microsomes. Reiss and Tappel [12] have reported that vitamin E deficiency reduced by 40% the capacity of microsomes to incorporate phenylalanine into protein, while Bonetti et al. [13] were not able to find any significant difference in the rate of incorporation of leucine into protein by microsomal preparations from deficient and control animals.

Presently it is difficult to evaluate what role vitamin E may play in protein synthesis from examination by in vitro methods and it appears that the effect must await further experimentation.

IV. ENZYME FUNCTION

Vitamin E deficiency appears to influence a number of enzyme activities (Table 1). Changes observed during deficiency have been attributed to a variety of considerations, including loss of compartmentation, shift in isozymic pattern, and changes in food intake and levels of dietary constituents other than vitamin E. These considerations, however, fail to explain changes in activity for most of the enzymes listed. In many cases, the specific activity of these enzymes increases during deficiency and it was on this basis that Olson [7] postulated that the vitamin may serve as a corepressor for the synthesis of certain enzymes.

V. CREATINE KINASE

In search of support for this hypothesis, Olson and Carpenter [8] examined the effects of vitamin E deficiency on rabbit muscle and serum creatine kinase. Both activities were observed to increase significantly after 10 days of deficiency. By day 25, the muscle level had returned to normal, but the serum creatine kinase activity had increased approximately

TABLE 1   Reported Alterations in Enzymatic Activity Due to Vitamin E Deficiency

Enzyme	Reference	Enzyme	Reference
Acid phosphatase (M)[a] ↑ [b]	30, 31	Glutathione reductase ↑	45
Alanine aminotransferase ↑	30	Hyaluronidase (M) ↑	47
Aldolase ↑	32, 33	Hydroxyacyl Co A dehydrogenase (M) ↑	42
Aminopyrine demethylase (M) ↓	34, 35	Hydroxybutyrate dehydrogenase (M) ↑	46
cAMP phosphodiesterase ↑	36	Isocitric dehydrogenase (M) ↓	40
Aniline hydroxylase (M) ↓	34	Lactate dehydrogenase ↓	31, 39
Aryl sulphatase (M) ↑	27, 30	Lipoxygenase (M) ↑	48
Aspartate aminotransferase ↑	30, 37	Malate dehydrogenase (M) ↓	39
ATPase (Na$^+$, K$^+$) (M) ↑	39	Neuraminidase (M) ↑	48
Carbamyl phosphate synthetase (M) ↓	40	Nitroanisole-O-demethylase (M) ↑	26
Cathepsins (M) ↑	27, 41	5'Nucleotidase (M) ↓	38

Enzyme	Ref.	Enzyme	Ref.
Codeine demethylase (M) ↓	34	Ornithine-keto acid aminotransferase (M) ↑	40
Creatine kinase ↑	8	Ornithine transcarbamylase (M) ↓	40
Cytochrome oxidase (M) ↑	42	Phospholipase A (M) ↑	48
Dimethylaniline demethylase (M) ↓	43	Pyruvate kinase ↑	56
Dimethylaniline oxygenase (M) ↑	43	RNA polymerase I (M) ↓	26
DNase (M) ↑	44	RNase (M) ↑	27
Glucose-6-phosphate dehydrogenase ↑	31, 45	Serine dehydratase ↑	36
β-Galactosidase (M) ↑	27	Xanthine dehydrogenase ↑	14
β-Glucuronidase (M) ↑	30	Xanthine oxidase ↑	14, 49, 50
Glutathione peroxidase ↑	45		

[a] M indicates enzyme is localized in a membranous portion of the cell. Enzymes present in both soluble and membrane fractions are listed as localized in the portion of the cell assayed. See individual references.

[b] Arrows indicate direction of change (↑increase, ↓decrease) in enzyme activity during vitamin E deficiency.

180-fold. Refeeding vitamin E or injecting ethionine resulted in a return of the activity of the enzyme to near normal levels after 48 hr, an indication that vitamin E inhibited its synthesis. Furthermore, measurements of the half-life of purified creatine kinase administered intravenously revealed that the rate of degradation of the serum enzyme was similar in the normal, deficient, ethionine-treated and vitamin E-treated animals.

Subsequent experiments [3] demonstrated that vitamin E deficiency resulted in a doubling of the turnover rate of the muscle creatine kinase. If one assumes that muscle is the source of the serum enzyme, these results are consistent with the idea that there is an increased rate of synthesis of this enzyme sufficient to not only maintain normal muscle level, but also the elevated serum level seen during deficiency.

Purification and characterization of the enzyme from control and vitamin E-deficient muscle indicated that neither the size, shape, charge, or kinetic properties were altered as a result of deficiency.

Although these data can only implicate vitamin E indirectly, they virtually eliminate the possibility that the deficiency results in a catalytically altered enzyme and indicate that the observed increase in activity may represent a state of excessive synthesis of the enzyme which in turn could be repressed by vitamin E.

VI. XANTHINE OXIDASE

It has long been known that vitamin E deficiency produces a marked increase in liver xanthine oxidase activity in rabbits [49] and rats [50], the largest increase being manifest in rabbits, where activity may be 4- to 12-fold higher than in corresponding controls. A recent report has indicated that the assay of xanthine oxidase in freshly prepared supernatant fractions of tissue may not reflect the true enzymatic capacity for purine oxidation in vivo. It was found that xanthine oxidase activity in a freshly prepared supernatant fraction of rat liver was stimulated by the addition of NAD^+. After storage [52,53] or incubation of the supernatant fraction at $37°$ C for 1 hr [51], the xanthine oxidase activity increased while the stimulation by NAD^+ was lost. This observation led to the suggestion that in fresh preparations the enzyme exists mostly as a dehydrogenase, while subsequent storage results in a gradual conversion to the oxidase [51].

The relationship between xanthine oxidase and xanthine dehydrogenase activities has been further clarified [54]. The xanthine dehydrogenase of freshly prepared rat liver homogenates can be converted completely into xanthine oxidase activity (loss of stimulation by NAD^+) by treatment with reagents such as N-ethylmaleimide or p-hydroxymercuribenzoate. Eighty percent of xanthine oxidase can be reconverted to the NAD^+-dependent dehydrogenase by treatment with dithioerythritol. This indicated that both activities are present in the same enzyme; inactivation of some functionally important sulfhydryl group is necessary for loss of NAD^+ binding and concomitant activation of a functional group binding O_2.

While these treatments result in complete conversion of xanthine dehydrogenase to xanthine oxidase, the conversion during storage is time dependent and may require 6-8 days for completion [52, 53]. These data underscore the importance of assaying xanthine oxidase in the presence of NAD^+ if the true rate of xanthine oxidation is to be determined in freshly prepared tissue extracts. Accordingly, a study was undertaken of the effects of vitamin E deficiency on rabbit liver xanthine dehydrogenase activity [14]. The results demonstrated that xanthine dehydrogenase activity was converted to oxidase activity. When equal volumes of homogenates from control and vitamin E-deficient animals were mixed, the activity was found to be additive (Table 2), and addition of serum from control or deficient animals to homogenates from each of these animals did not affect the enzymatic activity. These results indicated that the change in activity of xanthine dehydrogenase was not due to the loss of an inhibitor or in the presence of an activator, and led to the suggestion that vitamin E may influence the rate of synthesis of this enzyme.

This hypothesis was tested by immunochemical titration of the quantity of xanthine oxidase protein from liver cytosol of control and vitamin E-deficient animals [15]. An antiserum produced against a preparation of rabbit liver xanthine oxidase purified to homogeneity [55] was used to quantitate the amounts of enzyme protein present in normal and vitamin E-deficient liver [15].

Since conversion of xanthine dehydrogenase to xanthine oxidase occurred upon storage, incubation at 37°C, and following various preparative treatments, the data reported on the immunological experiments are for the fully converted preparations. This eliminated the necessity to produce antisera to both forms of the enzyme in the event that they were immunologically different, and assured antibody specificity toward the oxidase form of the enzyme in immunochemically titrated cytosols.

Results of immunochemical titrations of xanthine oxidase from control and vitamin E-deficient rabbit liver cytosol (105,000 $\underline{g}$ fraction) are shown in Table 3. Equivalence points represent the volume of each cytosol from which a constant amount of antibody will remove all measurable xanthine oxidase activity.

It can be seen that the amount of immunochemically reactive xanthine oxidase parallels the increase in enzyme activity observed in the deficient cytosols. To determine if increases in activity were due to a proportional increase in enzyme protein, the immunochemical data were plotted on an activity basis (Fig. 1). As illustrated, all points fall essentially on the same line, thus demonstrating not only that the increase in activity of xanthine oxidase during vitamin E deficiency is due solely to increased

TABLE 2 Liver Xanthine Oxidase and Xanthine Dehydrogenase Activities from Control and Vitamin E-Deficient Rabbits and the Influence of Storage and Pre-Incubation with Buffer

Livers	Experimental conditions	Xanthine oxidase		Xanthine dehydrogenase			
				Methylene blue		NAD$^+$	
		Exp. 1	Exp. 2	Exp. 1	Exp. 2	Exp. 1	Exp. 2
Control	Assayed immediately	0	0.075	0	1.92	0	1.025
Control	24 hr storage at 4°C	0	0.20	0	1.16	0	1.0
Control	1 hr preincubation of homogenate at 37°C	0	1.0	0	0.50	0	0.20
E deficient	Assayed immediately	0.90	0.40	15.6	4.0	8.5	2.50
E deficient	24 hr storage at 4°C	2.0	0.60	6.0	1.40	5.2	1.80
E deficient	1 hr preincubation of homogenate at 37°C	8.60	2.90	3.90	0.85	1.2	1.50
Mixture	1 hr preincubation, equal parts control and E-deficient liver homogenates	4.10	1.80	1.80	0.70	0.50	0.80

TABLE 3   Comparison of the Xanthine Oxidase Activity with the Amounts of Xanthine Oxidase Protein Present in Liver Cytosol from Control and Vitamin E-Deficient Rabbits by Immunochemical Titration with Specific Antibody

	Enzyme activity X 10^2a	Activity as % of control	Point of equivalence (ml)	Relative amounts of immunoreactive material as % of control
Experiment I				
Control	4.18	100	0.475	100
Deficient	16.7	400	0.115	410
Experiment II				
Control	3.69	100	0.520	100
Deficient	24.6	660	0.080	650
Deficient	33.2	900	0.060	830

a Enzyme activities are expressed as micromoles uric acid formed per minute per gram of wet weight of liver.

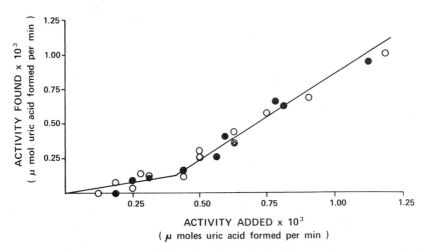

FIG. 1   Immunochemical behavior of liver xanthine oxidase from control and vitamin E-deficient rabbits.

TABLE 4 Incorporation of [^{14}C]Leucine into Liver Cytosol Proteins and Xanthine Oxidase

Source of cytosol	Activity X 10^2 [a]	Total cytosol proteins (cpm/g of liver X 10^{-3})	Immunoprecipitable proteins (enzyme) (cpm/g of liver)	Immunoprecipitable proteins (% of control)	Specific activity of acid-soluble leucine (cpm/ μmole X 10^{-3})
Control	3.69	216	14	100	18
Deficient	24.6	203	50	357	11
Deficient	33.2	220	115	821	10

[a] Enzyme activities are expressed as micromoles of uric acid found per minute per gram of wet weight of liver.

accumulation of additional enzyme, but also that the enzyme from the deficient animals is immunologically indistinguishable from the enzyme of control animals. To study the role of synthesis in the accumulation of this enzyme, the rate of incorporation of [^{14}C]leucine into both total and immunoreactive protein was determined. The results of these experiments are shown in Table 4. Vitamin E deficiency did not alter the incorporation of label into total soluble protein compared with controls. The immuno-precipitable material, however, contained significantly higher amounts of radioactivity. It should also be noted that the specific activity of the acid-soluble leucine decreased approximately 40% in the deficient animals.

These results demonstrate an elevated rate of synthesis of xanthine oxidase during vitamin E deficiency. A dilution of the specific activity of leucine by 40% indicated an increase in the rate of general protein synthesis in the deficient liver, since there was equal incorporation into total protein in deficient and control animals. The fact that the rate of [^{14}C]leucine incorporation into xanthine oxidase increased by several-fold substantiates the hypothesis that the rate of synthesis of this enzyme is selectively increased during deficiency. While it is yet undetermined what role degra-dation may play in the accumulation of xanthine oxidase during vitamin E deficiency, the data certainly suggest that a large part of this accumulation is due to an increase in the de novo synthesis of this enzyme. Further-more, since the enzyme which accumulates during deficiency is catalytical-ly and antigentically indistinguishable from that of controls, the rate of transcription of mRNA for this enzyme may be altered during deficiency. Although it would be a bit premature to say that vitamin E regulated gene transcription, the fact that deficiency affects the rates of synthesis of only certain proteins suggests this and opens an interesting avenue for continued research efforts.

One of the most useful initial approaches directed at testing such a hypothesis for a given compound involves the identification and function of specific soluble binding (receptors). This line of investigation is presently being pursued for tocopherol. Recent studies from this laboratory [57] have demonstrated that when the 105,000 g supernatant of rat liver is incubated in the presence of [^{3}H]tocopherol, a protein capable of binding tocopherol can be detected both by sucrose density gradient centrifugation and by gel filtration. The protein has an apparent molecular weight of 31,000 and exhibits a high affinity (detectable at a tocopherol concentration 20 nM) and specificity for α-tocopherol. Whether this binding protein exhibits characteristics analogous to other binding proteins (receptors) in mediating cellular events is presently under investigation and may provide the means necessary for determining the action of vitamin E at the mole-cular level.

ACKNOWLEDGMENT

The author wishes to acknowledge the Division of Nutrition, Department of Biochemistry, Vanderbilt University, with which he was affiliated while gathering the data describing the effects of vitamin E on xanthine oxidase.

REFERENCES

1. R. H. Wasserman and A. N. Taylor, Ann. Rev. Biochem. 41:179-202 (1972).
2. J. Green, in The Fat Soluble Vitamin. Edited by H. F. DeLuca and J. W. Suttie, Madison, The University of Wisconsin Press, 1970, Chap. 19.
3. R. E. Olson, Amer. J. Clin. Nutr. 27:1117-1129 (1974).
4. K. E. Mason, Vit. Horm. 2:107-153 (1944).
5. J. S. Dinning, J. Biol. Chem. 212:735-739 (1975).
6. M. P. Carpenter, Ann. N.Y. Acad. Sci. 203:81-92 (1972).
7. R. E. Olson, Can. J. Biochem. 43:1565-1573 (1965).
8. R. E. Olson and P. C. Carpenter, Adv. Enzyme Regulation 5:325-333 (1967).
9. A. De Villers, P. Simard, and V. Srivastava, Can. J. Biochem. 51:450-459 (1973).
10. P. Simard and V. Srivastava, J. Nutr. 104:521-531 (1974).
11. J. S. Dinning, Vit. Horm. 20:511-519 (1962).
12. U. Reiss and A. L. Tappel, Biochim. Biophys. Acta 312:608-615 (1973).
13. E. Bonetti, A. Abbondanza, E. Della Corte, F. Novello, and F. Stirpe, J. Nutr. 105:364-371 (1975).
14. G. L. Catignani and J. S. Dinning, J. Nutr. 101:1327-1330 (1971).
15. G. L. Catignani, F. Chytil, and W. J. Darby, Proc. Natl. Acad. Sci., USA 71:1966-1968 (1974).
16. M. P. Carpenter and C. N. Howard, Amer. J. Clin. Nutr. 27:966-979 (1974).
17. A. T. Diplock, Amer. J. Clin. Nutr. 27:995-1004 (1974).
18. J. S. Dinning and P. L. Day, J. Nutr. 63:393-397 (1957).
19. J. M. Young and J. S. Dinning, J. Biol. Chem. 193:748-747 (1951).
20. J. S. Dinning, J. T. Sime, and P. L. Day, J. Biol. Chem. 217:205-211 (1955).
21. J. S. Dinning, J. T. Sime, and P. L. Day, J. Biol. Chem. 222:215-217 (1956).
22. J. S. Dinning, J. T. Sime, and P. L. Day, Biochim. Biophys. Acta 21:383-384 (1956).

23. F. S. Porter, C. D. Fitch, and J. S. Dinning, Blood 20:471-477 (1962).
24. H. N. Marvin, J. S. Dinning, and P. L. Day, Proc. Soc. Exp. Biol. Med. 105:473-475 (1960).
25. C. D. Fitch, Ann. N.Y. Acad. Sci. 203:172-176 (1972).
26. B. Dinesen and G. Konat, Envir. Physiol. 1:110-118 (1971).
27. H. Zalkin, A. L. Tappel, K. A. Caldwell, S. Shibko, I. D. Desai, and T. A. Holliday, J. Biol. Chem. 237:2678-2682 (1962).
28. J. F. Diehl, Arch. Biochem. Biophys. 87:339-340 (1960).
29. I. M. Weinstock, Ann. N.Y. Acad. Sci. 138:199-212 (1966).
30. B. Eschraghi, I. Elmadfa, and W. Feldheim, Internat. Z. Vit. Ern. Forsc. 44:32-45 (1973).
31. A. A. Pokrovsky, T. A. Orlova, and K. A. Korovnikov, Voprosy Pitaniia 32:17-22 (1973).
32. R. J. Helmsen and A. A. White, Proc. Soc. Exp. Biol. Med. 136:785-789 (1971).
33. R. Beckmann and E. Buddecke, Klin. Wochenschr. 34:818-819 (1956).
34. M. P. Carpenter and C. N. Howard, Amer. J. Clin. Nutr. 27:966-979 (1974).
35. A. S. M. Giasuddin, C. P. J. Caygill, A. T. Diplock, and E. H. Jeffery, Biochem. J. 146:339-350 (1975).
36. J. Schroeder, Biochim. Biophys. Acta 343:173-181 (1974).
37. M. A. Barber, D. H. Basinski, and H. A. Mattill, J. Biol. Chem. 181:17-21 (1949).
38. E. A. Machado, E. A. Porta, W. S. Hartroft, and F. Hamilton, Lab. Invest. 24:13-20 (1971).
39. M. Fedelesova, P. V. Sulakhe, J. C. Yates, and N. S. Dhalla, Can. J. Physiol. Pharmacol. 49:909-918 (1971).
40. K. Shimbayashi and S. Shoya, Agr. Biol. Chem. 35:983-988 (1971).
41. I. M. Weinstock, S. Epstein, and A. T. Milhorat, Proc. Soc. Exp. Biol. Med. 99:272-276 (1958).
42. K. Bernhard and R. Markstein, Helv. Chim. Acta 55:519-526 (1972).
43. E. Arrhenius, Cancer Res. 28:264-273 (1968).
44. I. M. Weinstock and M. Lukacs, Proc. Soc. Exp. Biol. Med. 115:716-718 (1974).
45. C. K. Chow, K. Reddy, and A. L. Tappel, J. Nutr. 103:618-624 (1973).
46. I. Elmadfa and W. Feldheim, Internatl. Z. Vit. Ern. Forsc. 43:165-173 (1973).
47. E. A. Irving, Nature (London) 183:398 (1959).
48. A. A. Linchevskaya, A. M. Saburova, and Y. A. Epshtein, Tsitologiia 13:911-914 (1971).
49. J. S. Dinning, J. Biol. Chem. 202:213-215 (1953).

50. R. E. Olson and J. S. Dinning, Ann. N.Y. Acad. Sci. 57:889-894
    (1954).
51. F. Stirpe and E. Della Corte, J. Biol. Chem. 244:3855-3863 (1969).
52. E. Della Corte and F. Stirpe, Biochem. J. 108:349-351 (1968).
53. D. G. R. Blair and B. D. McLennan, Can. J. Biochem. 46:1047-1056
    (1968).
54. E. Della Corte and F. Stirpe, Biochem. J. 126:739-745 (1972).
55. G. L. Catignani, F. Chytil, and W. J. Darby, Biochim. Biophys.
    Acta 377:34-41 (1975).
56. C. K. Chow, J. Nutr. 105:1221-1224 (1975).
57. G. L. Catignani, Biochem. Biophys. Res. Commun. 67:66-72 (1975).

Section 3   The role of vitamin E in mitochondrial metabolism

LAURENCE M. CORWIN
Boston University School of Medicine
Boston, Massachusetts

I.   Introduction   332
      Location of α -Tocopherol in Mitochondrial
      Preparations and Other Parts of the Cell   333
III. Antioxidant Theory   334
IV.   Metabolic Effects of Tocopherol   335
V.   Oxidative Phosphorylation   341
VI.   Interactions between Antioxidant and Biochemical
      Theories   342
VII. Experiments with Cells in Culture   343
VIII. Conclusions   344
      References   345

I. INTRODUCTION

Studies of the role of vitamin E in intermediary metabolism have been
many and varied. Biochemical effects have been found which could be
attributable to almost all of the cellular organelles and structures. This
review will only cover functions associated with the mitochondria, some
of which may be influenced by other parts of the cell. No attempt has

been made to make this a complete literature survey. Instead, a presentation of the biochemical theories of tocopherol function is provided with the view towards the possibility of the confluence of these theories with the antioxidant theory, a subject which has been the subject of much controversy in the past.

II. LOCATION OF α-TOCOPHEROL IN MITOCHONDRIAL PREPARATIONS AND OTHER PARTS OF THE CELL

Before it was possible to make any sort of assertions concerning the metabolic role of α-tocopherol, it was considered essential to show that the vitamin was located where it could exert its effects. An early and persistant theory of tocopherol function was that it was either a part of the electron transport chain or somehow associated with its function. The rationale behind the approach to the problem was first to demonstrate its presence by measuring it after isolating the various cellular fractions. Secondly, the vitamin was removed either by creating a dietary deficiency or by extracting the vitamin with organic solvents such as isooctane. If the extraction decreased enzyme activity, which could then be restored by tocopherol addition, it was assumed that tocopherol was involved in that enzyme reaction and in that location in the cell.

Nason and Lehman implicated vitamin E as a possible cofactor for NAD and succinate-cytochrome c reductases of rat skeletal muscle and bovine heart muscle using such an approach [1-3]. The enzymatic activity was completely lost following isooctane extraction and could be completely restored by addition of tocopherol or even more effectively by addition of the lipid residue extracted by isooctane. These results were confirmed by Morrison et al. [4,5] using isooctane-extracted succinate-cytochrome c reductase from pig heart. The nontocopherol lipid active in restoring activity to cytochrome c reductases was found to be a mixed triglyceride with stearate, palmitate, and oleate components [6]. It was subsequently shown that the crude lipid residue extracted by isooctane contained tocopherol and, presumably, tocopherol quinone [7]. By repeated extractions and "aging" for 1 week with daily freezing and thawing, it was found that materials which could reactivate cytochrome c reductase after one isooctane extraction could no longer do so.

The interpretation of the restorative properties of tocopherol on isooctane-extracted preparations was clouded considerably when Pollard and Bieri [8,9] and Igo et al. [10] demonstrated that isooctane was toxic to the enzymatic preparations previously described. Simple expedients, such as freeze-drying isooctane-extracted preparations, centrifuging at high speeds, followed by reconstitution of the pellet in water, or simple dilution of the enzymes, restored most of the activity. Pollard and Bieri [11] have also observed the aging effect in creating a rather specific tocopherol requirement for restoration of NAD-cytochrome c reductase of digitonin-treated chick heart muscle preparation. However, since similar specificity was observed in reversing the inhibition by dibenzoyl peroxide, they concluded that the aging effect was due to the accumulation of peroxides in the preparations.

Bouman and Slater [12] were able to demonstrate the presence of α-tocopherol in a Keilin-Hartree heart muscle preparation. The amount they isolated, mostly in the form of the quinone, was about 2 μmol/g protein compared with 10 μmol found by Donaldson and Nason [13]. Similarly, Crane et al. [14] found tocopherol and an unknown quinone in beef heart mitochondria. This quinone was later demonstrated to be coenzyme Q (Q275) when extracted by isooctane from the electron transport particle (ETP) of beef heart mitochondria [15]. Coenzyme Q was effective in restoring succinoxidase activity to isooctane-extracted ETP, especially when added with phospholipid.

More recent work has solidified the existence of tocopherol in bovine heart mitochrondria [16]. The concentration ranged from 0.05 to 0.44 μmol tocopherol per gram of protein and appears independent of cytochrome oxidase activity in the same samples. The vitamin was found in all the enzymatically active lipoprotein complexes of the electron transport system, but no direct quantitative relationship with the enzymatic activities was observed. It was demonstrated that only the inner mitochondrial membranes contained tocopherol. The nuclear fraction contained tocopherol, but the supernatant after centrifugation of the mitochondria contained very little. Experiments with [3H]tocopherol have shown that it is bound to a specific lipoprotein found in the cell sap [17]. It was suggested that this lipoprotein is involved in the intracellular transport and distribution of the vitamin.

There has been some criticism of many of the experiments purporting to assess the quantity of tocopherol in tissues. Edwin et al. [18] remind us that tocopherol is quite unstable and that assay methods that do not take this into account are seriously in error. Furthermore, there are many other reducing substances in tissues which can interfere with tocopherol assays that do not involve separation of tocopherol from such interference by methods such as paper chromatography.

III. ANTIOXIDANT THEORY

The extraction of tocopherol from cell fractions has not led to the discovery of its function. However, it is still possible that tocopherol affects cellular oxidative metabolism. The most prevalent hypothesis to explain the function of vitamin E in preventing disease relates to its ability to act as an antioxidant [19]. There has been much evidence to support this notion [20-23]. It has been shown that antioxidants are able to replace vitamin E in the diet, and thus prevent sterility [18] and necrotic liver degradation [24]. One function of tocopherol in vitro is to maintain the oxidation of α-ketoglutarate and succinate by rat liver homogenates [25, 26]. The prevention of oxidative decline could also be duplicated by N, N'-diphenyl-p-phenylenediamine (DPPD), menadione, methylene blue, and a tocopherol metabolite, 2-(3-hydroxy-3-methyl-5-carboxy)-pentyl-3, 5, 6-trimethyl-benzoquinone [27]. These agents are quite potent in vitro, with DPPD having the greatest activity. Nevertheless, it has been shown that in this in vitro system, tocopherol can be added in quantities sufficient to prevent the decline of α-ketoglutarate oxidation, but not enough to prevent peroxide formation [28]. In this system, at least, it has been possible to distinguish between a metabolic effect and its ability to prevent peroxide formation.

There is other evidence that tocopherol does not prevent the auto-oxidation of unsaturated lipids in vivo [29, 30]. For example, Siakotos et al. [31] have shown that in Batten's disease, a disorder of lipid peroxidation, the illness progresses in spite of an ample supply of tocopherol in the blood stream. Despite these indications that tocopherol may not act as an in vivo antioxidant, the lack of correlation between in vivo peroxide formation and the tocopherol status of the animal does not preclude some sort of antioxidant function.

METABOLIC EFFECTS OF TOCOPHEROL

The more definitive way of researching the role of a vitamin such as tocopherol is a comparison of enzymatic activities of animals deficient in or supplemented with the vitamin, as compared to such techniques as solvent extraction. The effect of tocopherol-deficiency on tissue oxidation has been the subject of many early studies. Accompanying the muscular dystrophy produced by deprivation of vitamin E, an excessive rate of respiration from skeletal muscle has been repeatedly demonstrated (Table 1). [32, 34]. The rate of oxygen uptake of rabbit skeletal muscle has been muscle strips increased even before symptoms of muscular dystrophy were noted [35]. This rate increased as the deficiency disease progressed. The respiratory quotient and the rate of glycolysis was unchanged; however, Morgulis and Jacobi suggested that the increased oxygen consumption might be due to higher ATPase activities in these tissues [36], but they were unable to demonstate any difference in ATPase activity by either muscle or liver homogenates during early or late stages of the vitamin deficiency [37]. In fact, there is evidence that vitamin E deficiency uncouples phosphorylation in muscle homogenates during aerobic and anaerobic glycolysis and lowers ATPase activity [38]. Weinstock et al. [39] demonstrated an

TABLE 1   Effect of Vitamin E-Deficiency on Oxidation

Preparation	Animal	Substrate or enzyme	Oxidation[a]	Reference
Muscle strips	Rabbit	Endogenous	Increase	32, 34
Liver homogenate	Rabbit	Krebs cycle	Increase	39
Muscle	Rabbit	Cytochrome c reductase and cytochrome oxidase	Increase	41
Muscle	Hamster	Succinate	Increase	32, 42
Muscle	Hamster	Sucinnate	No change	43
Liver and muscle	Rabbit	Succinate	Decrease	44
Muscle	Rabbit	Succinate	No change	45
Muscle	Rabbit	α-Ketoglutarate	Decrease	46
Liver slice	Rat	Endogenous	Decrease	48
Liver homogenate	Rat	α-Ketoglutarate and succinate	Decrease	25, 26

[a] Represents the change produced by a vitamin E deficiency compared with vitamin E-supplemented controls.

increase in oxidation of Krebs cycle intermediates by washed rabbit liver homogenates deficient in vitamin E. Except for citrate oxidation, which was unaffected, the increase was enhanced by the presence of ATP [40]. They too were unable to demonstrate a difference in Mg-ATPase activity. Addition of tocopherol or tocopherol succinate in vitro did not eliminate the effect of the in vivo deficiency. Cytochrome c reductase activity became elevated in rabbit muscle homogenates in late stages of the deficiency, but was unaffected after 2 weeks [41]. Cytochrome oxidase was relatively unaffected. Houchin and Mattill [32, 42] reported a several-fold increase in succinoxidase activity by hamster dystrophic muscle. However, Basinski and Hummel could show no difference in succinoxidase activity of hamster muscle homogenates [43]. On the other hand, Shirley et al. [44] reported an increase in succinoxidase activity of heart and skeletal muscle and liver from vitamin E-fed animals, thus completing the state of confusion. Jacobi et al. [45] not only could not detect a difference in succinoxidase of muscle homogenates from rabbits with incipient muscular dystrophy but found no differences in malic and lactic dehydrogenases, fumarase, cytochrome oxidase, and ATPase activities. A decrease in activity of the Krebs cycle enzymes, α-ketoglutarate and isocitrate dehydrogenases, was found in dystrophic muscle of rabbits in terminal stages [46]. Other studies from muscle preparations of animals in terminal stages of disease found increases in cytochrome oxidase and cytochrome reductase [41].

Some concern over the use of tissues from terminal animals seems justified, i.e., see Ref. 47. Damaged tissue could conceivably result either in an increase of apparent activity due to a breakdown of barriers between substrate and enzyme, or a decrease in activity due to cell destruction by lysozomal enzymes. In both cases, the enzymatic alterations would occur as a secondary event to tissue breakdown by other causes, such as toxic effects by organic peroxides. If tocopherol is in fact involved as a necessary component of oxidative mechanisms, the tissue damage in tocopherol deficiency should result from a prior breakdown in oxidative metabolism. Thus, enzymatic studies should be made either on undamaged tissue, during a latent phase of the disease, or both. Chernick et al. [48] described a phenomenon called respiratory decline in liver slices obtained from rats on a diet deficient in vitamin E and selenium. The rats were in a latent phase of the disease, 1-2 weeks prior to the onset of liver necrosis. Respiratory decline was described as the inability to maintain the endogenous oxidation of the liver slices over a period of 2 hr. This decline was found to be preventable by dietary tocopherol and also by injection of tocopherol intraportally 10-30 min before extirpation of the liver [49]. The effect of intraportal injection of tocopherol precludes an effect of the vitamin on prior tissue damage. Respiratory decline could be reproduced in liver homogenates [25, 26]. The oxidation of α-ketoglutarate and succinate declined about 60-70% over 90 min using tocopherol-deficient homogenates; this was completely preventable by tocopherol added either in the diet or to the homogenate. Selenium was ineffective, but DPPD, menadione, methylene blue, and α-tocopherol metabolite were effective in vitro. As mentioned previously, a protective effect of tocopherol can be observed at levels which do not inhibit peroxide formation [28]. Furthermore, tocopherol does not appear to be altered during incubation with the homogenate, indicating that it is effective without having to act through a metabolite [50]. No evidence of a tocopherol dimer was obtained, which Durckheimer and Cohen have shown to be a product of tocopherol with free radicals [51]. Draper et al. [52] have found this dimer in tocopherol-deficient liver. An important observation is that respiratory decline could be observed in liver homogenates from animals which were fed selenium but not tocopherol [26]. Since these animals were not destined to come down with liver necrosis, the decline probably represents the loss of a specific function of tocopherol. Apparently, this decline is not enough to cause damage to the liver unless selenium is also absent. Whether the requirement for a selenium deficiency is related to glutathione peroxidase is speculative at this stage.

A more detailed analysis of the phenomenon of respiratory decline has revealed thst the phenomenon is complex and superficially appears to involve more than one mechanism. It was first necessary to discover if the effect of tocopherol in preventing respiratory decline involved in the cytochrome chain. Nason et al. [53] demonstrated that digitonin inhibited NADH and succinatc cytochrone c reductases of bovine heart muscle. Inhibition was rather specifically prevented by α-, β, γ-, or δ-tocopherols, and the restored activity was sensitive to antimycin A. Dilution of the digitonin-treated enzyme preparation restored activity without further addition. This was attributed to dissociation of the digitonin. Corwin and Schwarz [54] also sought for the location of tocopherol action in the electron transport scheme to account for the progressive loss of ability to oxidize succinate and α-ketoglutarate. Cytochrome oxidase activity declined only about 15% in a 90-min period in E-deficient homogenates, not enough to account for the decline of Krebs cycle acid oxidation. Tocopherol did not prevent antimycin A inhibition of substrate oxidation even at limiting antimycin A concentrations. This was contrary to the competitive inhibition between antimycin A and tocopherol reported by Nason and Lehman in the digitonin-treated NADH-cytochrome c reductase from rat skeletal muscle [3]. In fact, the more recent results by Nason et al. [53] also indicate that tocopherol restores antimycin A-sensitive enzyme activity. When it was found that sulfhydryl protective agents such as glutathione (GSH) and British anti-Lewisite (2,3-dimercaptopropanol), would prevent respiratory decline, it was suspected that tocopherol may involve protection of sulfhydryl groups of dehydrogenases [54]. This was supported by the finding that tocopherol could prevent the decline produced in α-ketoglutarate oxidation by the dithiol inhibitors: arsenite and Cd^{2+} ions. Similarly, it could also prevent inhibition of glutamate and β-hydroxybutyrate oxidation by the monothiol inhibitor, p-hydroxymercuribenzoate. It was also demonstrated that tocopherol maintained the reduced status of cell sulfhydryl groups. Tocopherol was not acting as a reducing agent, since it was only effective when present at the beginning of the incubation. It was concluded that tocopherol must be sterically situated to mask dehydrogenase sulfhydryl groups in order to protect them from sulfhydryl inhibitors.

An interesting aspect of respiratory decline in rat liver homogenates is the requirement of the microsomal fraction for the decline to occur [55]. By differential centrifugation one can obtain mitochondrial, microsomal, and cytosol (microsomal supernatant) cell fractions. The combination of mitochondria and cytosol will oxidize substrates such as α-ketoglutarate, β-hydroxybutyrate, and glutamate. Even if these cell fractions were obtained from vitamin E-deficient rat liver homogenates, very little decline was observed [54,55]. Readdition of the microsomal fraction reinstated decline in deficient preparations. One can substitute sulfhydryl inhibitors such as Cd^{2+}, arsenite, and pHMB for the microsomes, and also produce a decline in E-deficient mitochondrial plus cytosol preparations, which are correctable by tocopherol. Grove et al. [56] studied this microsomal inhibitor in detail and have found it to be inactivated by boiling and bound to microsomal membranes. They suggested that the inhibitor was protein in nature. Grove and Johnson [57] later provided evidence that the addition of increased NAD to E-deficient rat liver homogenates delayed the onset of respiratory decline. They therefore implicated microsomal NADase as the cause of microsomal-induced decline. However, these authors pointed out that the presence of the cytosol can prevent respiratory decline in the presence of E-supplemented microsomes even though the NAD concentration was low. The possibility that metal ions might be involved in microsome-induced decline was given support by the finding that EDTA and diethyl-dithiocarbamate, effective metal-chelating agents, prevented the decline [58]. Thus, it remains possible that respiratory decline associated with vitamin E-deficient rat liver homogenates is due in part to metal ion inhibition of sulfhydryl groups, which can be prevented by the masking of these groups by tocopherol. In the case of α-ketoglutarate oxidation, the sulfhydryl connection has been made even stronger by the observation of Schwarz [59] that lipoyl dehydrogenase activity also declines in E-deficient homogenates. This enzyme is involved in the oxidation of the dithiol groups of lipoic acid which were reduced by α-ketoglutarate and other α-keto acids.

$$\alpha\text{-ketoglutarate} \xrightarrow{\alpha\text{KGDH, TPP, CoA}} \text{succinyl CoA}$$

$$\text{lipoic} \left\langle \begin{matrix} S \\ | \\ S \end{matrix} \right. \qquad \text{lipoic} \left\langle \begin{matrix} SH \\ \\ SH \end{matrix} \right. \tag{1}$$

$$\text{lipoyl dehydrogenase}$$

$$\text{NADH} + \text{H}^+ \longleftarrow \text{NAD}$$

At this point, it is worth while to put the phenomenon of respiratory decline in perspective. The very real effect of tocopherol in preventing decline may in fact just be a result of the presence of tocopherol in proximity to enzyme sulfhydryl groups. However, since the oxidation process starts out normally enough with E-deficient, but selenium-supplemented homogenates, from livers which are not destined to become diseased, it appears likely that respiratory decline is at best an in vitro symptom of an unstable condition in the tissue. Apparently more damage must aggravate this condition, before overt clinical symptoms appear. Nevertheless, the linkage of tocopherol with sulfhydryl groups does indicate an important potential role in metabolism. Ideally, one would like to find that a deficiency of the vitamin would result in a metabolic lesion which would not require a period of in vitro incubation before it can be seen. Thus, respiratory decline and peroxide formation which require incubation in vitro of the E-deficient homogenate seem to be secondary phenomena. The question is whether or not a primary role for tocopherol can be found which will result in a metabolic defect that is immediately observable in fresh tissue preparations.

An attempt to discover a more direct role was begun with a survey of the oxidation of Krebs cycle acids by liver mitochondria from rats whose diets were deficient or supplemented with vitamin E [60]. Only succinate oxidation was decreased by the vitamin E deficiency and this could be seen in initial oxidation measurements. This could be reversed by intraportal tocopherol injection 30 min before liver extirpation, but was unaffected by dietary selenite. This biochemical lesion was seen only in the presence of NAD, indicating that some reaction further along the Krebs cycle was necessary in order to see the effect, since succinate oxidation itself does not require NAD. Unlike the more generalized effect of E deficiency in homogenates, the mitochondrial phenomenon seems much more specific. The cause of the decline of succinate oxidation in mitochondria was thought to be due to an accumulation of oxaloacetic acid (OAA). Compounds known to cause the removal of OAA, such as Mn, Al, and Mg ions, acetyl CoA, and ATP were all effective in preventing the inhibition of succinate oxidation in the presence of NAD and in the absence of vitamin E. OAA is a well-known competitive inhibitor of succinate oxidation and would, of course, be formed from malate in the presence of NAD

$$\text{Succinate} \rightarrow \text{fumarate} \xrightarrow{\text{H}_2\text{O}} \text{malate} \xrightarrow{\text{NAD}} \text{oxaloacetate} \qquad (2)$$

Corwin [61] subsequently demonstrated an increase in OAA accumulation in E-deficient mitochondria, but showed that this was not due to a difference in the removal of OAA. Tocopherol, therefore, must then prevent the synthesis of OAA from malate. Since it was found that tocopherol stimulated the NAD-linked reduction of acetoacetate by succinate

Succinate ⟶ fumarate

FAD_s ⇌ $\text{FAD}_\text{s} \cdot \text{H}_2$

$\text{FAD}_\text{NAD} \cdot \text{H}_2$ ⇌ FAD_NAD

NAD ⇌ NADH

β-hydroxybutyrate ⟵ acetoacetate $\qquad (3)$

it was concluded that tocopherol therefore increased oxidation by decreasing the amount of available NAD. Chance and Hagihara [62] have shown
that a reduction of up to 30% of mitochondrial NAD will maintain uninhibited
succinate oxidation. They also proved that addition of a phosphate (P_i)
acceptor causes a rapid oxidation of NADH to NAD, nearly to the 100%
level, allowing a rapid conversion of malate to OAA. The addition of P_i
acceptor increased succinate oxidation in the E-deficient mitochondria and
increased the decline in the E-supplemented mitochondria, probably due to
the reoxidation of NADH [61]. Carabello and Bird [63] have confirmed
these observations in E-deficient and E-supplemented guinea pig liver
mitochondria, and have shown that succinate control of -hydroxybutyrate
oxidation to acetoacetate is enhanced by tocopherol. Since this enhancement was removed by P_i acceptor, they also concluded that tocopherol
controls the energy-dependent succinate control of NAD-linked oxidations.
As this control involves reverse electron transport, tocopherol must be
involved in the accumulation of energy to push this thermodynamically difficult reaction. One must again ask the question if this is the role of
tocopherol or whether it is just another manifestation of a more generalized
function of the vitamin. Since sulfhydryl groups are required for oxidative
phosphorylation and tocopherol protects sulfhydryl groups, the sulfhydryl
connection begins to have more appeal as a primary site for tocopherol
function.

V. OXIDATIVE PHOSPHORYLATION

There have been other reports that tocopherol may affect oxidative phosphorylation. It was found that methyllinoleate hydroperoxide decreased the
P:O ratio during -hydroxybutyrate and succinate oxidation [64]. In addition, mitochondrial ATPase was inhibited. Tocopherol prevented inhibition
by the peroxide. The significance of such a finding is not clear with regard
to tocopherol function in vivo. Such peroxides are not known to exist in
E-deficient mitochondria. Furthermore, one cannot be certain if this
effect is an uncoupling phenomenon of a nonspecific enzyme inhibition.
Nevertheless, it does leave open the possibility that tocopherol may prevent a peroxidative attack on the groups required for oxidative phosphorylation such as vicinal dithiols.
    Carbello et al. [65] have obtained more direct evidence for an effect of
tocoperol on the P:O ratio. They reported in an abstract that phosphorylation during citrate oxidation by E-deficient guinea pig liver mitochondria
was 22% lower than controls. This could be prevented by intraportal
tocopherol injection prior to sacrifice. N,N'-diphenyl-p-phenylenediamine

did not substitute for tocopherol. Since tocopherol did not affect phosphorylation associated with ascorbate oxidation, it was assumed that only phosphorylation stemming from the early part of the respiratory chain was affected, a result which is consistent with the site I phosphorylation effect found by Corwin [61].

VI. INTERACTIONS BETWEEN ANTIOXIDANT AND BIOCHEMICAL THEORIES

An interesting paper presenting another viewpoint concerning the role of vitamin E in electron transport is that of McCay et al. [66]. They studied the effect of NADPH oxidation on electron transport in mitochondria (Mt) and microsomes (Mc) from vitamin E-deficient or E-supplemented animals. NADPH-dependent oxidation by Mt and Mc resulted in increased malondialdehyde formation which could be prevented by dietary vitamin E. They concluded, therefore, that NADPH oxidation involves the formation of a free radical which, in the absence of vitamin E, results in the peroxidation of polyunsaturated fatty acids associated with the electron transport system. This treatment essentially destroyed further oxidation by E-deficient mitochondria such as that of α-ketoglutarate and succinate. Mitochondria from animals fed 50 mg/kg vitamin E were protected against such loss of oxidation. Diets containing 25 mg/kg vitamin E afforded some protection but much less than with 50 mg/kg. These observations do not seem to be exclusively related to oxidation of NADPH. In experiments with the metabolism of Krebs cycle intermediates, Corwin [67] has shown that the production of malondialdehyde by E-deficient rat liver homogenates is greatly affected by what is being oxidized. For example, although suc-cinate does not increase malondialdehyde formation over controls, α-ketoglutarate oxidation does to some extent, and this production is enhanced by ADP, ATP, and AMP. The oxidation of pyruvate plus malate produced up to three times that of the unsupplemented control homogenates. Tocopherol prevented malondialdehyde formation under all these conditions. Electron transport inhibitors such as cyanide, antimycin A, and amytal prevented the increase of malondialdehyde formation produced by α-ketoglutarate over that of the control homogenate without substrate. Similarly glutathione was quite effective in inhibiting substrate-induced peroxidation. Dietary and in vitro addition of tocopherol prevented all malondialdehyde formation even in the control homogenate. Interestingly, malondialdehyde formation associated with α-ketoglutarate oxidation by mitochondria was very low, only about 7% of that seen with the whole homogenate. Stimulation of production was slight when microsomes were added to the mitochondria, but tripled by the addition of the microsomal supernatant fraction. All three fractions added together restored complete malondialdehyde formation seen with the homogenate.

Thus, although malondialdehyde production varies a great deal depending on the substrate involved, there can be no doubt that there is a substrate-dependent production of peroxides when tocopherol is absent from cell-free preparations. One possible explanation for such results may be that polyunsaturated fatty acids associated with the electron transport chain may act as electron acceptors and form peroxides. Tocopherol must prevent this metabolic electron transfer to PUFA and prevent damage to the electron transport system. One might even speculate that tocopherol could be involved in a catalytic role of electron transfer. Since the tocopherol concentration is at about the level of the cytochromes in the inner membranes of the mitochondria [16] and only 1/50 of the arachidonic acid concentration, it obviously cannot be used as an electron sink during routine mitochondrial oxidation. It must be able to retransfer electrons or else be used up by forming dimers and other metabolites. At this point, however, no evidence of an electron acceptor for reduced tocopherol has been obtained, so such a hypothesis is speculative.

However, an interesting new theory by Diplock and Lucy [68] now indicates that tocopherol can exist in close proximity to PUFA in cellular membranes. By model building, they have shown that the C-4 and C-8 methyl groups of tocopherol's phytol side chain fit tightly into the pockets provided by cis double bonds of arachidonic acid. Thus, membrane fluidity created by a large amount of membrane PUFA should be decreased by such an interaction, much in the same way as cholesterol does in membranes. Since mitochondrial membranes are known to contain more PUFA than other membranes, they should be affected by such an interaction. Unlike cholesterol, however, tocopherol has the additional advantage of the semiquinone chromanol ring to participate in redox functions associated with the sulfur or selenium of membrane proteins.

VII. EXPERIMENTS WITH CELLS IN CULTURE

A rather good way to obtain evidence for the Diplock-Lucy hypothesis would be to demonstrate the effectiveness of the vitamin on whole cells in vitro. Most cell culture media do not contain tocopherol, but are nevertheless able to support the growth of many different kinds of cells. Corwin and Humphrey [69] have hypothesized that this may be due to the fact that glucose is the major carbon source in these media. In bacteria, glucose represses Krebs cycle enzymes, and animal cells growing in glucose-containing media do not seem to require the entire Krebs cycle, i.e., succinic dehydrogenase is greatly decreased in cultured cells. This makes them comparatively insensitive to malonate, compared to their parent tissue [70]. When Chinese hamster cells are forced to utilize the Krebs cycle by substituting pyruvate for glucose as a carbon source, the cells require tocopherol for optimal growth and then become sensitive to malonate, a Krebs cycle inhibitor [69].

It has also been shown that tocopherol is required for the decarboxylation of 1-[^{14}C]pyruvate in these cells. Thus, it appears that tocopherol is
involved in mitochondrial function in these cells, and under conditions
which require such functions for growth, tocopherol becomes a growth
factor.

To supply more direct evidence for the membrane hypothesis mentioned above, another approach was taken involving a study of the interaction of PUFA and tocopherol on growth and the membrane-regulated uptake
of 2-deoxyglucose (DOG) [71]. Chinese hamster fibroblasts growing in
lipid-depleted media are inhibited by arachidonic and linoleic acids. This
growth inhibition is relieved by tocopherol. An endothelial cell line,
BALB/c3T3 mouse cells, is stimulated by tocopherol both in growth and
DOG uptake. Further experiments have shown that such an interaction of
tocopherol with oleic acid does not alter DOG uptake, which is consistent
with the Diplock-Lucy theory. Oleic acid with only one double bond does
not permit close interaction with the tocopherol-phytol side chain as does
arachidonic acid. These experiments show a plasma membrane function
for tocopherol, although the differing results with the different types of
cells indicate that other membrane factors influence the direction in which
the cell will respond to its presence. It also seems clear from the many
different kinds of data presented earlier, that tocopherol probably also acts
at the mitochondrial membrane and at other cell organelles as well.

VIII. CONCLUSIONS

Through the years tocopherol has been found to be associated with many
deficiency diseases and many metabolic disorders. The first hypothesis
which tried to link together so many effects of a vitamin E deficiency into a
unified whole was the antioxidant theory. Although reflecting a valid property of the vitamin, too many difficulties in explaining in vivo findings such
as the lack of demonstration of peroxides in deficient animals, has made
alternative hypotheses necessary. Tocopherol has been found to affect
several mitochondrial and microsomal functions, many of them relating to
the ability to oxidize. In mitochondria, the effect of vitamin E seems to
involve the early part of the electron transport chain, perhaps close to the
dehydrogenases themselves. In this regard, it has been shown that tocopherol is involved with sulfhydryl groups of the dehydrogenases. It has been
shown that in a tocopherol deficiency, oxidation of substrates produces
peroxides in vitro and thus it appears possible that PUFA associated with
the electron transport particle may become peroxidized locally and cause
damage to oxidative systems. Since tocopherol has been shown to be
capable of interacting closely with PUFA in a structural way by means of
its side chain, the vitamin may be properly situated so that its seminquinone

chromanol ring can serve a redox function to protect sulfur and selenium proteins and, speculatively, perhaps to transfer single electrons.

REFERENCES

1. A. Nason and I. R. Lehman, Science 122:19 (1955).
2. I. R. Lehman and A. Nason, J. Biol. Chem. 222:497 (1956).
3. A. Nason and I. R. Lehman, J. Biol. Chem. 222:511 (1956).
4. M. Morrison, R. Crawford, and E. Stotz, Biochim. Biophys. Acta. 22:579 (1956).
5. G. V. Marinetti, J. Erbland, M. Morrison, and E. Stotz, J. Amer. Chem. Soc. 80:402 (19).
6. K. O. Donaldson, A. Nason, I. R. Lehman, and A. Nickon, J. Biol. Chem. 233:566-571 (1958).
7. K. O. Donaldson, A. Nason, and R. H. Garret, J. Biol. Chem. 233:572-579 (1958).
8. C. J. Pollard and J. G. Bieri, Biochim. Biophys. Acta 30:658-659 (1958).
9. C. J. Pollard and J. G. Bieri, J. Biol. Chem. 234:1907-1911 (1959).
10. R. P. Igo, B. Mackler, and D. J. Hanahan, J. Biol. Chem. 234:1312-1314 (1959).
11. C. J. Pollard and J. Bieri, J. Biol. Chem. 235:1178 (1960).
12. J. Bouman and E. C. Slater, Biochim. Biophys. Acta 26:624-633 (1957).
13. K. O. Donaldson and A. Nason, Proc. Natl. Acad. Sci. 43:364 (1957).
14. F. L. Crane, Y. Hatefi, R. L. Lester, and C. Widmer, Biochim. Biophys. Acta 25:220 (1957).
15. F. L. Crane, C. Widmer, R. G. Lester, and Y. Hatefi, Biochim. Biophys. Acta 31:476-489 (1959).
16. M. M. Oliveira, W. B. Weglicki, A. Nason, and P. P. Nair, Biochim. Biophys. Acta 180:98-113 (1969).
17. O. V. Rajaram, P. Fatterpaker, and A. Sreenivasan, Biochim. Biophys. Acta 52:459-465 (1973).
18. E. E. Edwin, A. T. Diplock, J. Bunyan, and J. Green, Biochem. J. 75:450 (1960).
19. A. L. Tappel, Vitam. Horms. 20:493 (1962).
20. H. Dam, Pharmacol. Rev. 9:1 (1957).
21. P. L. Harris and K. E. Mason, Intern. Congr. Vit. E., Third Congr., Venice, Italy, 1955, pp. 1-25.
22. H. A. Mattill, Nutr. Revs. 10:225 (1952).
23. E. L. Hove, Amer. J. Clin. Nutr. 3:328 (1955).
24. K. Schwarz, Proc. Soc. Exp. Biol. Med. 99:20 (1958).
25. L. M. Corwin and K. Schwarz, Nature (London) 186:1048 (1960).

26. L. M. Corwin and K. Schwarz, J. Biol. Chem. 235:3387 (1960).
27. K. Schwarz, W. Mertz, and E. J. Simon, Biochim. Biophys. Acta 32:484-491 (1959).
28. L. M. Corwin, Arch. Biochem. Biophys. 97:51-58 (1962).
29. J. Green, A. T. Diplock, J. Bunyan, D. McHale, and I. R. Muthy, Br. J. Nutr. 21:69 (1967).
30. A. T. Diplock, M. A. Cawthorne, E. A. Munell, J. Green, and J. Bunyan, Br. Nutr. 22:465 (1968).
31. A. N. Siakatos, N. Koppang, S. Youmans, and C. Bucana, Amer. J. Clin. Nutr. 27:1152-1157 (1974).
32. J. Victor, Amer. J. Physiol. 108:229 (1934).
33. O. B. Houchim and H. A. Mattill, J. Biol. Chem. 146:301 (1942).
34. J. P. Hummel and D. H. Basinski, J. Biol. Chem. 172:417 (1948).
35. J. P. Hummel and R. S. Melville, J. Biol. Chem. 191:391-394 (1951).
36. S. Morgulis and H. P. Jacobi, Q. Bull. Northwestern Univ. Med. School 20:92 (1946).
37. H. P. Jacobi, S. Rosenblatt, V. M. Wilder, and S. Morgulis, Arch. Biochem. Biophys. 27:19 (1950).
38. J. P. Hummel, J. Biol. Chem. 172:421 (1948).
39. I. M. Weinstock, I. Shoichet, and A. T. Milhorat, Fed. Proc. 13:482 (1954).
40. I. M. Weinstock, Amer. J. Phys. Med. 34:320-324 (1955).
41. J. R. Allen, B. A. Sullivan, and H. L. Dobson, Arch. Biochem. Biophys. 86:6-9 (1960).
42. O. B. Houchin and H. A. Mattill, J. Biol. Chem. 146:309-312 (1942).
43. D. H. Basinski and J. P. Hummel, J. Biol. Chem. 167:339-343 (1947).
44. R. L. Shirley, T. F. Easly, and G. K. Davis, Abst. 129th Meeting Amer. Chem. Soc., Texas, 1956, p. 29.
45. H. P. Jacobi, S. Rosenblatt, V. M. Wilder, and S. Morgulis, Arch. Biochem. 27:19-21 (1950).
46. H. Rosenkrantz, Fed. Proc. 17:299 (1958).
47. F. D. Vasington, S. M. Reichard, and A. Nason, Vit. Horm. 18:43-87 (1960).
48. S. S. Chernick, J. G. Moe, G. P. Rodman, and K. Schwarz, J. Biol. Chem. 217:829 (1955).
49. G. P. Rodman, S. S. Chernick, and K. Schwarz, J. Biol. Chem. 221:231 (1956).
50. C. R. Seward and L. M. Corwin, Arch. Biochem. Biophys. 101:71-74 (1963).
51. W. Durckheimer and L. A. Cohen, Biochem. Biophys. Res. Commun. 9:262 (1962).

52. H. H. Draper, A. S. Csallany, and S. N. Shah, Biochim. Biophys. Acta 59:529 (1962).
53. A. Nason, R. H. Garrett, P. P. Nair, F. D. Vasington, and T. C. Detweiler, Biochem. Biophys. Res. Commun. 14:220-226 (1964).
54. L. M. Corwin and K. Schwarz, Arch. Biochem. Biophys. 100:385-392 (1963).
55. L. M. Corwin, Fed. Proc. 20:145 (1961).
56. J. A. Grove, R. M. Johnson, and J. H. Cline, J. Biol. Chem. 241:5564 (1966).
57. J. A. Grove and R. M. Johnson, J. Biol. Chem. 242:1623 (1967).
58. K. Schwarz, Vit. Horm. 20:463 (1962).
59. K. Schwarz, Fed. Proc. 24:58 (1965).
60. L. M. Corwin and K. Schwarz, J. Biol. Chem. 234:191 (1959).
61. L. M. Corwin, J. Biol. Chem. 240:34 (1965).
62. B. Chance and B. Hagihara, J. Biol. Chem. 237:3540 (1962).
63. F. B. Carabello and J. W. C. Bird, Biochem. Biophys. Res. Commun. 34:92 (1969).
64. H. Naito, B. Johnson, and B. C. Johnson, Proc. Soc. Exp. Biol. Med. 122:545 (1966).
65. T. Carabello, F. Lien, C. Canes, and J. Bird, Fed. Proc. 30:639 (1971) abstract.
66. P. B. McCay, P. M. Pfeifer, and W. H. Stipe, Ann. N.Y. Acad. Sci. 203:62 (1972).
67. L. M. Corwin, Arch. Biochem. Biophys. 97:51 (1962).
68. A. T. Diplock and J. Lucy, FEBS Lett. 29:205 (1973).
69. L. M. Corwin and L. P. Humphrey, Proc. Soc. Exp. Biol. Med. 141:609 (1972).
70. G. S. Turner, Nature (London) 193:164 (1962).
71. L. P. Humphrey and L. M. Corwin, Fed. Proc. 33:671 (1974).

Part 5F/ Hormonal Status in Vitamin E Deficiency

ABBAS E. KITABCHI
*University of Tennessee Center
for the Health Sciences
and Veterans Administration Hospital
Memphis, Tennessee*

I.	Introduction	348
II.	Gonadal Function	349
III.	Hormone-Mediated Glucose Oxidation and Lipolysis in Isolated Fat Cells	352
IV.	Adrenal Function	353
V.	Prostaglandins	364
VI.	Thyroid Function	367
VII.	Effects on Physiology of Rotifers	369
VIII.	Summary and Prospects	369
	References	370

I. INTRODUCTION

In regard to the role of tocopherol and hormonal function, it suffices to note that the chemical name of vitamin E, i.e., tocopherol, taken from the Greek "tokos" meaning childbirth, "phero" meaning to bear or to bring forth, and "ol" designating oil solubility—thus, the "oil of fertility"—has implied an important function of this vitamin in reproduction, fertility, and possibly hormonal alteration.

The lack of convincing evidence for a specific role of vitamin E in direct hormonal action has been due in part to our failure to understand the mechanism of hormone action at the cellular level. Recent knowledge regarding the interaction of the hormone receptor complex, availability of extremely sensitive methods for determination of hormones in blood by radioimmunoassay, as well as the emergence of newer hormones such as prostaglandins, with a wide variety of actions in numerous tissues, has permitted inquiry into the interrelation of this vitamin with various hormones. Nevertheless, because of the limitations of the studies on this subject, the present review has concentrated, of necessity, on contemporary work which is in progress on prostaglandins as well as on steroid hormones.

In addition to these works, a brief review in the field of gonadal function and vitamin E has been included as this has been the cornerstone of vitamin E research.

II. GONADAL FUNCTION

The relationship of vitamin E to gonadal function had been admirably reviewed up to 1939 by Mason [1]. The salient points of these studies which still hold true are briefly mentioned below. As early as 1919, it was shown that rats fed purified diets in addition to amounts of vitamins A, B, C, and D failed to reproduce, which suggested gonadal injury [2]. The factor responsible for this was not designated until later when the evidence leading to vitamin E as a distinct entity was reported by Evans, Mason, and others [3-5]. The early description of testicular degeneration in rats has been summarized in the review by Mason [1]. It is important to note that the earlier findings regarding histological changes associated with inhibition of spermatogenic activity consisted of extensive nuclear chromolysis of spermatids and secondary spermocytes which coalescend to form numerous giant cells of all sizes, followed by varying degrees of nuclear and cytoplasmic degeneration in the primary spermatocyte and spermatogonia.

It is also important to point out that although these changes after testicular degeneration have been observed, investigators essentially agree that interstitial cells showed no significant alterations. Furthermore, it was clearly established before 1930 that the histological injury which appeared in testicular tissue in the rat was a degenerative process which could not be reversed by additional tocopherol.

In spite of these severe changes in the germinal epithelium, the "accessory sex glands" (i.e., prostate, seminal vesicle, etc.) are unaffected by vitamin E deficiency. Although some progressive atrophy of accessory sex glands had been noted, it was attributed to the retarded growth and constitutional inferiority of E-deficient rats after prolonged maintenance on the experimental diets.

These findings suggest that the germ cells are not essential to production of male sex hormones and that their synthesis is apparently unimpaired by E deficiency. Apparently, interstitial tissue represents the source of sex hormones and lack of vitamin E induces no grave disturbance of gonad-hypophyseal relationships in the male.

In the female E-deficient rats, estrus, ovulation, and implantation processes are normal, and no structural changes occur in the ovary or uterus. Pregnancies, however, are terminated by resorption of the fetus in utero. Although the mechanism is not clear, it would appear that, on the seventh day of gestation, a significant retardation of fetal development occurs with rarefaction of fetal tissues, especially those of mesodermal origin, which suggests a possible suppression of hematopoietic development in the yolk sac, allantois, fetal placenta, liver, and blood vascular system of the fetus and fetal membrane. It is of interest that the maternal placenta shows no significant deviation from normal but the early fetal placenta is retarded in its differentiation and in its invasion of the maternal decidua. This results in the thwarting of the establishment of a normal vascular connection between the mother and fetus. The consequent asphyxia and starvation result in fetal death between the tenth and thirteenth day of gestation with coagulation necrosis of fetal tissue which is rapidly resorbed [1].

Although in the 1930s it was postulated that gonadotropic hormones of the hypophysis may play an important role in reversing the vitamin E effect on reproduction, such observations have not been based on unequivocal results. In fact, large bodies of evidence in the early part of 1930 suggested that the sterility of the female E-deficient rat did not respond to treatment with follicular hormone, corpus luteum extract, or anterior pituitary extract, and that gonadotropic hormones were ineffective in repairing testicular injury in male deficient rats.

Thus, it appears that estrus, ovulation, and implantation in the female rats, as well as hormonal control of the accessory sex glands in the male, are unaffected by E deficiency. Furthermore, the data available at the time indicated that, if impaired gonadal-hypophyseal relationships existed in the E-deficient animals, it should be regarded as the result rather than the cause of the reproductive abnormalities characteristic of the sterility of vitamin E deficiency.

Although this statement is true in particular for rats, other studies on the reproductive organs of vitamin E-deficient animals in other species do not show these characteristic results, i.e., studies in dairy cattle fail to demonstrate any lack of productivity, but the mothers do show some mortality or morbidity just before and after delivery [6].

Testicular degeneration after vitamin E deficiency has been reported not only in rats but also in monkeys, dogs, rabbits, guinea pigs, and mice. The histopathological changes, however, have not been described in detail and their response to vitamin E has not been reported. Studies on vitamin E-deficient hamsters by Mason and Mauer [7] showed that daily oral supplementation of d-α-tocopherol to these animals which had changes in the germinal epithelium and impaired spermatogenesis resulted in repair of the germinal epithelium and reappearance of spermatoza in ducts of the epididymus. The testicular injury in these animals, and especially the repairability of the germinal epithelium after vitamin E therapy, was in striking contrast to the irreversible testicular injury characteristically seen in vitamin E-deficient rats.

Thus, it would appear that, in the early part of the work on vitamin E deficiency, there was no direct evidence that the androgen status of the animals on a vitamin E-deficient diet was impaired and the injury was entirely limited to the germinal cells. Since that time, however, additional indirect evidence has confirmed the work of Mason and others. Thus, neither Lutwak-Mann [8] nor Carpenter [9] observed a hypertrophy of the accessory sex glands in vitamin E-deficient rats. Griesbach et al. [10] found an increase in the weights of the accessory sex glands in the vitamin E-deficient rat, and histological evidence that the pituitary showed some increase in the number of foccile-stimulating hormone (FSH) cells and in the population of undeveloped luteinizing hormone (LH) cells.

Since the function of the accessory sex glands is also an indication of the androgen status of animals, Carpenter studied the content of fructose and/or citrate in the accessory sex glands of E-deficient rats [9]. No differences were found in either the weight of the glands or fructose and/or citrate content of the dorsal prostate, ventral prostate, coagulating glands, or seminal vesicles in the tocopherol-deficient rats as compared to the supplemented controls, in rats from 1 week postweaning to adults. Both the weights of the glands and the amount of fructose and citrate were found to increase markedly at 6 weeks of age. No fructose and only trace amounts of citrate were detectable before 6 weeks. Rats fed vitamin E-deficient diets for 7-12 months had increased seminal vesicle weight, but the total amount of citrate per gland was not changed.

The rate of production of fructose also was studied by investigating the biosynthetic pathway of fructose through the glucose-sorbital pathway. No reduction in aldose and ketose reductase in either coagulating gland or the dorsal lateral prostate was observed in glands from vitamin E-deficient rats compared with control animals. Thus, it appears that indirect measurement of androgen status of rats does not indicate differences between the vitamin E-deficient and control animals.

Direct measurement of androgenic hormone levels in the blood of E-deficient and control rats have been made by Carpenter and Kling using radioimmunoassay procedures [11]. They have measured testosterone and dihydrotestosterone during vitamin E deficiency in the sera of rats ranging in age from 4 weeks to 10 months. These studies show that blood testosterone concentration progressively increased from 0.37 ng/ml in the immature rat (4 weeks old) to an average of 1.44 ng/ml in animals 4 months and older. Corresponding levels of dihydrotestosterone were 0.18 ng/ml and 0.45 ng/ml, respectively. Both androgens increased during the transition from prepubertal to adult rat in a parallel manner in the experimental, vitamin E-deficient rat. However, the levels of both hormones dropped significantly (P < 0.01) in deficient rats between 13 and 16 weeks of age: testosterone 1.06 ng/ml and dihydrotestosterone 0.19 ng/ml (Table 1).

Although there were statistically significant differences in the levels of testosterone in the sera of vitamin E-deficient rats after the testes began to degenerate, the above workers point out that the absolute values fall within the normal range for adult rats. Additionally, these animals do not

TABLE 1   Serum Androgen Levels [a, b]

Animal	Testosterone (ng/dl)	Dihydrotestosterone (ng/dl)
Control		
Immature (10)	36.50 ± 6.74	18.41 ± 3.10
Adult (7) ′	143.89 ± 8.64	44.80 ± 3.69
Experimental		
Immature (12)	31.97 ± 6.56	17.70 ± 2.23
Adult	105.68 ± 8.13 [c]	18.58 ± 1.30 [c]

[a] Numbers in parentheses indicate the numbers of animals. Immature rats were 4-5 weeks old, adult rats were 4-10 months old. Control rats were fed a tocopherol-supplemented diet. Experimental rats were fed a tocopherol-deficient diet.
[b] Data courtesy of M. P. Carpenter.
[c] $p < 0.01$ compared with the adult control group.

appear to be androgen deficient, i.e., the accessory sex glands do not atrophy and appear to function normally.

III.   HORMONE-MEDIATED GLUCOSE OXIDATION AND LIPOLYSIS IN ISOLATED FAT CELLS

Although lipid peroxidation as tested by the thiobarbituric acid (TBA) test has now been shown to be present in most tissues of vitamin E-deficient rats [12] in the studies conducted by Dr. Lavis in our laboratories, this phenomenon could not be correlated with the state of vitamin E deficiency in isolated fat cells from epididymal fat pads of adult rats [13]. In spite of the fact that tocopherol could not be detected in any significant amount in this tissue, significant lipid peroxidation could not be measured in these preparations. This finding may be partially explained by the characteristic fatty acid pattern of the tissue, which consists mainly of saturated fatty acids, in contradistinction to the highly unsaturated fatty acid content of the adrenal, which is a highly peroxidizable tissue [14].

    Additional metabolic studies on the isolated fat cells of vitamin E-deficient rats showed that the rate of glucose oxidation in CO_2 in response to ACTH or epinephrine was not significantly different in the vitamin E-deficient and vitamin E-supplemented rats [13]. Thus, it would appear that the metabolic apparatus of hormonally sensitive fat tissue is not adversely affected by the lack of vitamin E either through the insulin-mediated glucose oxidation or ACTH-induced lipolysis.

Since the major site of action of these two hormones on the fat cell is believed to be on the plasma membrane [15], one may presume that the above study indirectly supports the thesis that the fat cell membrane in vitamin E deficiency is not impaired in response to lipolytic and antilipolytic hormones.

Similar lack of correlation between lipid peroxidation and the state of vitamin E deficiency was also noted in our laboratory in cardiac muscle, where the intact perfused heart showed no difference in CO_2, phosphorylated respiration, or nonmitochondrial oxygenation in the vitamin E-deficient or vitamin E-supplemented group [16]. Homogenates of this tissue, however, did show a significantly higher lipid peroxidation may be an entirely artifactual and in vitro phenomenon as a result of antioxidant deficiency, and that it may not be the prevailing reaction in vivo. Nevertheless, there is no doubt that this phenomenon does exist in certain tissues and is the index of vitamin E deficiency states in certain experimental animals.

IV. ADRENAL FUNCTION

That the TBA phenomenon may not be directly related to the state of vitamin E deficiency was more clearly established when the adrenal was tested for its ability to synthesize corticosterone. Similar to our findings in isolated perfused rat heart, the quartered gland of vitamin E-deficient rats showed no higher TBA index than the control group, but contrary to our findings in the perfused heart and isolated fat cells of vitamin E-deficient rats, the quartered adrenal glands of these rats produced significantly lower corticosterone than the E-sufficient controls [17]. These studies on the heart and adrenal tissues are demonstrated in Table 2.

Because of the unique metabolic status of the adrenal gland, i.e., high concentrations of tocopherol, ascorbic acid, and highly unsaturated fatty acids, and because of our preliminary work on the inhibited synthesis of corticosterone in a vitamin E deficiency, we were encouraged to further investigate the relationship of steroidogenesis to vitamin E lack and lipid peroxidation.

Our first attempt was to investigate the nature of lipid peroxidation. In a series of studies, we undertook a comparative study of the TBA index in numerous endocrine and nonendocrine tissues and evaluated the relative lipid peroxidizability of various tissues as tested by the TBA index in both E-deficient and E-sufficient controls [14].

TABLE 2 Adrenal and Myocardial Status of Vitamin E-Deficient and
-Sufficient Rats

	Adrenal[a]		Heart[c]	
	Corticosterone ($\mu g/10$ mg/hr)	TBA Index (OD 530 nm)	qO_2 (ml O_2/min/g)	OD 530 nm
E-Sufficient	2.380 ± 0.29	0.01	0.155 ± 0.02	0.000
E-Deficient	1.360 ± 0.26	0.00	0.148 ± 0.01	0.001

[a] Data Taken from Kitabchi [17].
[b] Data taken from Kitabchi et al. [16].

These studies, which are demonstrated in Table 3 for the E-deficient
rats and control, showed that adrenal contains the highest TBA index
compared to the next most peroxidizable tissue—liver, i.e., the adrenal
had 10 times more TBA index per milligram of tissue than liver of the
E-deficient group. There was no special pattern which we could discern
in other endocrine organs, such as testes, pancreas, etc. Furthermore,
this phenomenon was related to the extent of vitamin E deficiency in rats,
i.e., whereas vitamin E deficiency caused a prompt rise in TBA index in
the liver which reached a plateau within a few days of tocopherol deprivation, the adrenal did not reach its maximal response until the fifth to
seventh week of deprivation (Figs. 1 and 2). Additional biochemical
investigations demonstrated that the TBA-reaching material in the adrenal
was indeed malonaldehyde [14], similar to our earlier findings in the liver
[18]. In an attempt to explain the high rate of lipid peroxidation in this
tissue, the fatty acid profiles of adrenals were compared in the two groups.
But, the percentage of arachidonic acid as well as other highly unsaturated
fatty acids in the vitamin E-deficient and control groups was similar [14].
Thus, greater concentrations of unsaturated fatty acids were not demonstrated and did not explain the greater rate of lipid peroxidation in the
adrenals of E-deficient rats. Additional studies on the soluble and particulate fractions of adrenal homogenates revealed that in addition to the
rich source of unsaturated fatty acid in the particulate fraction of the
adrenal homogenate, the presence of high concentrations of ascorbate in
the soluble fraction could provide additional factors for the high lipid peroxidation in the vitamin E-deficient state. However, again the concentration of ascorbate in both groups was similar [14]. Thus, neither the high
concentrations of ascorbic acid nor the unsaturated fatty acids in adrenals,
individually or collectively, were capable of producing lipid peroxidation in
the presence of the high concentrations of tocopherol which prevailed in the

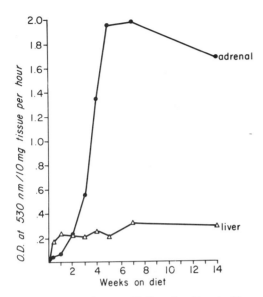

FIG. 1   Lipid peroxidation in vitro in liver and adrenal homogenates of vitamin E-deficient rats during various periods of vitamin deprivation. Each point represents the average of values from four rats. Incubation system is similar to that of Table 3. Reproduced with permission from The Journal of Biological Chemistry [14].

TABLE 3   Comparison of Lipid Peroxidation in Vitro in Various Tissues of Vitamin E-Deficient Rats and Their Controls[a]

Organ	Vitamin E deficient	Control
Adrenal	1.306	0.069
Liver	0.109	0.014
Heart	0.104	0.032
Brain	0.101	0.077
Testes	0.090	0.025
Kidney	0.062	0.045
Skeletal muscle	0.021	0.011
Pancreas	0.020	0.014
Epididymal fat	0.011	0.011

[a] Data taken from Kitabchi and Williams [14]. The incubation system was 10 mg whole homogenate in 1 ml phosphate buffer, 0.1 M, pH 7.35. Incubation was for 60 min at 37 °C in air.

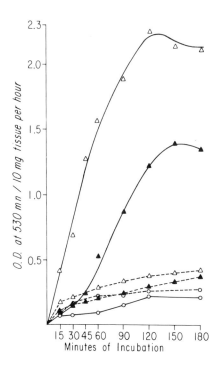

FIG. 2   The TBA chromogen formation in liver and adrenal homogenates
of vitamin E-deficient rats during various periods of vitamin E deprivation.
Each point represents the average value from four rats. Incubation system
is similar to Table 3 but at different periods of incubation. Adrenal:
△——△, 9 weeks; ▲——▲, 3 weeks; and o——o, 1 week. Liver:
△------△, 9 weeks; ▲-----▲, 3 weeks; and o-----o, 1 week. Reproduced
with permission from The Journal of Biological Chemistry [14].

normal adrenal homogenate. It thus appeared that, in the presence of high
ascorbate and unsaturated fatty acids, tocopherol deprivation in the adrenal
of vitamin E-deficient rats may have been responsible for high lipid peroxidation in vitro.

Having demonstrated a direct relationship between lipid peroxidation
(albeit a purely in vitro phenomenon) and of malonaldehyde and the time-
dependent vitamin E deprivation, we next proceeded to examine the phenomenon of lipid peroxidation and enzyme activity in the other membranous
structures of the adrenal. Both adrenal mitochondria and microsomes
are rich in hydroxylating enzymes, the enzymes responsible for steroidogenesis. As the amount of tissue is limited in the rat, we studied the

hydroxylase system of beef adrenal cortex. A 21-hydroxylase source was provided by the microsomes and 11-hydroxylase by the mitochondria. Addition of ascorbate produced high levels of peroxidation with concomitant inhibition of 11-β-hydroxylase and 21-hydroxylase in mitochondria [19] and microsomes [20], respectively. Addition of tocopherol in vitro prevented both lipid peroxidation and enzyme inhibition induced by ascorbate.

To determine if lipid peroxidation is associated with actual alteration of unsaturated lipid, the lipid profile of the 21-hydroxylase system in the microsome was analyzed. It was shown that lipid peroxidation and 21-hydroxylase inhibition in the microsomes were accompanied by diminution of arachidonic acid in the phospholipid moiety of the microsomal lipid [20].

Although all the above studies demonstrated interesting phenomenon which essentially provided definitive evidence for lipid peroxidation, malonaldehyde formation, alteration of unsaturated lipids and decrease in enzyme activity in vitro of two hydroxylase systems, the relationship of these phenomena to the in vivo state of the adrenal in vitamin E deficiency was not established.

Using a modified [21] method of Swallow and Sayers [22], we were able to demonstrate that the isolated adrenal cell system is particularly suitable to simulate in vivo conditions because these cells: (1) have intact cell membranes [23]; (2) are homogenous, consisting mainly of fasiculata cells [23]; and (3) produce corticosterone in response to physiological concentrations of ACTH [24]. Furthermore, although these cells at the beginning of the preparation are rich with ascorbate, by the end of the trypsin digestion procedure they have essentially lost all their ascorbate [25], and, therefore, the system could be enriched with any amount of exogenous ascorbate if one wished to investigate the role of this prooxidant in steroidogenesis. In collaboration with Mrs. Nathans, we were able to undertake a series of studies to investigate lipid peroxidation and steroidogenesis in vitamin E deficiency in response to ACTH and dibutyryl cyclic AMP (dcAMP) (the presumed second messenger analog for ACTH) with and without ascorbate.

Following are the salient points of our findings [26]:

1. ACTH- or dcAMP-induced steroidogenesis in vitamin E-deficient rats was lower than the control. There was no significant difference between lipid peroxidation in the two groups.

2. Addition of ascorbate inhibited ACTH-induced steroidogenesis with concomitant formation of lipid peroxide in the isolated adrenal cells of vitamin E-deficient rats but not in the control group (Fig. 3).

3. Addition of ascorbate did not affect dcAMP-induced steroidogenesis in either group but caused lipid peroxidation in the deficient group.

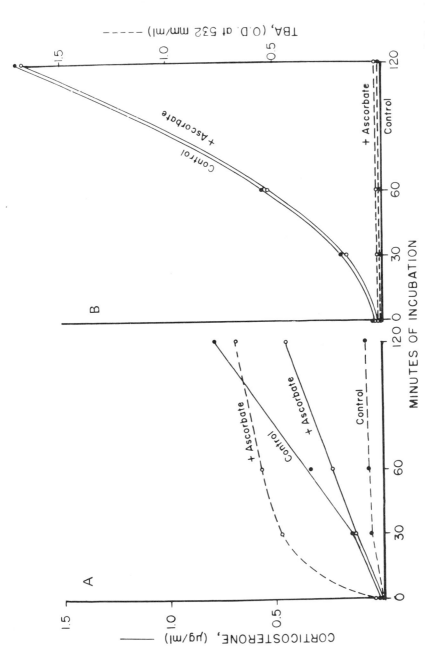

FIG. 3   Lipid peroxidation (TBA) and corticosterone formation in isolated adrenal cells of vitamin E-deficient (A) and vitamin E-sufficient (B) rats. Control tubes in each case contain 50 μU of ACTH per ml of incubation mixture, and steroidogenesis (o——o) or lipid peroxidation (o–––-o) is measured at different periods of incubation. Reproduced with permission from The Journal of Biological Chemistry [26].

4. Ascorbate produced lipid peroxidation with both steroid stimuli (ACTH or dcAMP). However, only the ACTH-induced steroidogenesis was inhibited by ascorbate.

5. The administration of tocopherol in vivo to the deficient rats 12 hr before killing them prevented the inhibition of ACTH-induced steroidogenesis by ascorbate.

6. The injection of another antioxidant, DPPD, however, did not reverse the ascorbate-inhibited steroidogenesis in the deficient group.

7. Increase in the concentration of ascorbate increased the half-maximum concentration of ACTH in the deficient group but not the control group (Fig. 4).

The fact that ascorbate inhibited ACTH-induced but not dcAMP-induced steroidogenesis, and tocopherol reversed this inhibition, suggested that the effect of tocopherol may be at the membrane site where ACTH is known to stimulate the release of the second messenger for steroidogenesis [19,26].

Our next attempt was to investigate the effect of vitamin E deficiency on adenylate cyclase, a membrane-bound enzyme. This system is particularly intriguing since it is shown to contain lipids, specifically phophatidylinositol. Since our isolated adrenal cell preparations are devoid of cAMP phosphodiesterase [27], formation of cAMP could be measured in the vitamin E-deficient and sufficient rats by prelabeling the ATP pool of isolated adrenal cells by [^{14}C]adenine and studying the conversion of [^{14}C]ATP to [^{14}C]cAMP with various concentrations of ACTH in the presence or absence of ascorbate. These studies demonstrated that ascorbate caused the inhibition of adenylate cyclase in the deficient group but not the control [28]. The inhibition was noted within 30 min but stayed the same for the remaining period of incubation up to 2 hr, whereas the formation of cAMP in the control tube (without ascorbate) or the vitamin E-supplemented cells showed time dependence (Fig. 5). Similar to our findings in the earlier studies with steroidogenesis, ascorbate-induced inhibition could be overcome with additional doses of ACTH (Fig. 6). These studies thus provide indirect evidence that the phenomenon may be related to membrane binding and receptor interaction with ascorbate and ACTH, which is consistent with the competitive inhibition kinetics that are exaggerated in the deficient group.

Of particular interest was the relationship of calcium to ascorbate-inhibited cAMP formation. Since our earlier studies on the isolated adrenal cells of normal rats that demonstrated that certain levels of calcium were necessary for optimum steroidogenesis and adenylate cyclase activity [29], the effect of various concentrations of calcium was investigated in the adrenal cells from vitamin E-deficient rats and controls.

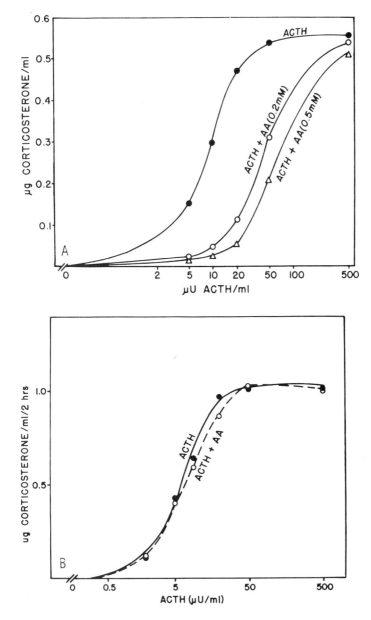

FIG. 4   Effect of ascorbic acid (AA) on the concentration response curve
of ACTH-induced steroidogenesis in isolated adrenal cells of vitamin E-
deficient (A) and vitamin E-supplemented rats (B). Reproduced with permission from The Journal of Biological Chemistry [26].

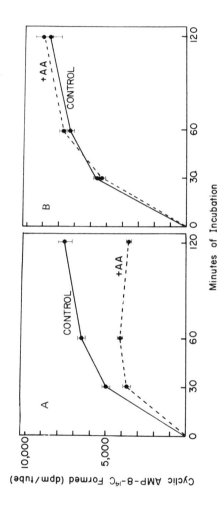

Minutes of Incubation

FIG. 5 Time course of cyclic [8-^{14}C]AMP formation in response to 500 μU of ACTH in the presence (+AA) or absence of 0.5 mM ascorbate in vitamin E-deficient (A) and vitamin E-supplemented (B) rats. The standard error of the mean is depicted for each point. Reproduced with permission from Biochimica et Biophysica Acta [28].

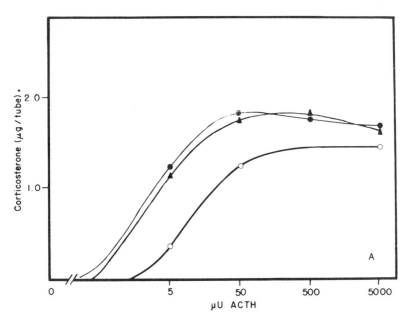

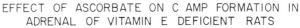

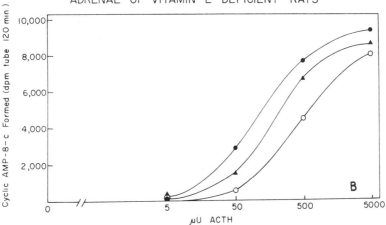

FIG. 6   Concentration response curve of ACTH-induced steroidogenesis (A) and cyclic [^{14}C]AMP formation (B) in isolated adrenal cells of vitamin E-deficient rats in the presence (○——○) or absence (●——●) of ascorbate (0.5 mM) or ascorbate (0.5 mM) plus -tocopherol, 144 μg/ml (▲——▲). The values reported are for 2 hr of incubation.   Reproduced with permission of Biochimica et Biophysica Acta [28].

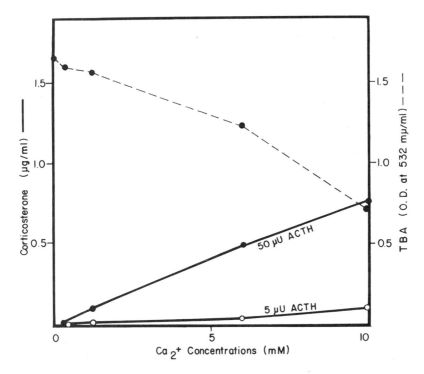

FIG. 7   Effect of varying concentrations of calcium on the inhibitory effect of ascorbate on steroidogenesis and its stimulatory effect on TBA formation in the isolated adrenal cells of vitamin E-deficient rats.

These results are depicted in Figs. 7-9. As can be seen in Fig. 7, inhibition of corticosterone production was reversed with an increasing concentration of calcium. This was accompanied by a concomitant decrease in lipid peroxidation. Figures 8 and 9 demonstrate the effect of various concentrations of calcium on the inhibitory effect of ascorbate on ACTH-induced steroidogenesis and cAMP formation in vitamin E-deficient adrenal cells, respectively. Thus, it would appear that in addition to the well-known effect of calcium in the hormone receptor complex, this cation may also provide an additional effect on the cell membrane where it may help stabilize membranes from vitamin E-deficient animals against oxidative stress.

It is interesting that in our studies, the nonspecific antioxidants had no effect on reversing the ascorbate-induced inhibition of steroidogenesis or adenylate cyclase [28]. It would appear that tocopherol has a specific role in preventing these inhibitory effects rather than acting as a nonspecific antioxidant.

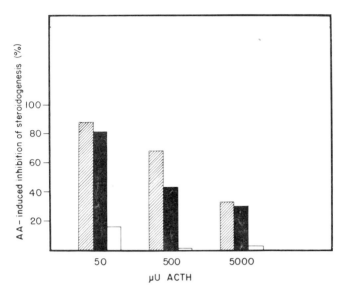

FIG. 8 Effect of calcium on the inhibitory action of ascorbate on ACTH-
induced steroidogenesis in isolated adrenal cells of vitamin E-deficient rats.
Hatched bar, 0.3 mM Ca^{2+}; solid bar, 1.2 mM Ca^{2+}; clear bar, 10 mM
Ca^{2+}.

The role of tocopherol in this case may, therefore, be more than a
mere antioxidant. Tocopherol may stabilize the adenylate cyclase membrane complex by providing optimal configuration for the phospholipid
moiety of the membrane.

For a more direct involvement of tocopherol in steroidogenesis, the
receptor studies by the isolated adrenal cell membrane with tocopherol
are essential. To determine the physiological role of tocopherol in
steroidogenesis, extensive studies in vivo on the status of the adrenals
are needed.

V. PROSTAGLANDINS

In addition to the above areas of hormonal studies and α-tocopherol in
vitamin E deficiency, α-tocopherol has been implicated for modulation of
prostaglandins in other hormonal systems and their metabolites, some of
which will be briefly described.

Studies by Carpenter et al. have shown that prostaglandins occur in
normal rat testes [30] and that they are synthesized by this tissue [31,32].
The primary species that are synthesized and released by this tissue are
prostaglandin E_2 and prostaglandin $F_{2\alpha}$.

Prostaglandins are rapidly synthesized and released after removal of a tissue and during homogenization, which makes the determination of "endogenous" values difficult to determine. To circumvent this problem, they have carefully standardized the conditions for the removal of tissue; to minimize prostaglandin synthesis and release, they perform homogenizations in the presence of a prostaglandin synthetase inhibitor, indomethacin. The term endogenous level refers to amounts of prostaglandins observed under these conditions. Extractions carried out without indomethacin or after tissue has been frozen and thawed, are a reflection of net synthesis, release, and turnover. Prostaglandin synthesis in testes from rats fed with vitamin E-deficient diets has been investigated by these procedures [33]. These studies are summarized in Tables 4-6.

These observations (Table 4) suggest that the levels of endogenous prostaglandins are higher in the testes of E-deficient rats than controls. Moreover, there is some suggestion of increased synthesis and release of prostaglandin in testes from E-deficient rats. This is particularly obvious when tissues are frozen and thawed (Table 6), a process which may expose more of the prostaglandin synthetase to the substrate.

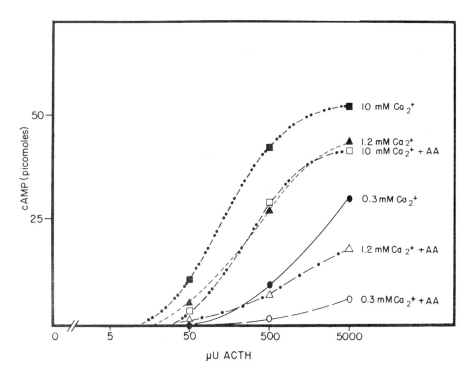

FIG. 9   Effect of calcium and ascorbate on ACTH-induced cAMP formation in isolated adrenal cells of vitamin-E deficient rats.

TABLE 4   Testicular "Endogenous" Prostaglandins [a,b]

| Age (wk) | Vitamin E sufficient | | Vitamin E deficient | |
	$PGF_{2\alpha}$ (ng/g, mean ± SE)	PGE_2	$PGF_{2\alpha}$ (ng/g, mean ± SE)	PGE_2
5-6	0.42 ± 0.05	2.77 ± 1.0	1.07 ± 0.16 [c]	2.06 ± 0.76
7-10	1.07 ± 0.12	–	1.46 ± 0.21	–
13-25	1.02 ± 0.30	3.79 ± 1.01	3.16 ± 0.50 [d]	3.77 ± 0.59
17-25 [e]			3.53 ± 0.56 [d]	6.32 ± 1.13

[a] Data courtesy of M. P. Carpenter.
[b] The term endogenous prostaglandin has been defined in the text.
[c] $P = < 0.02$.
[d] $P = < 0.01$.
[e] Degenerate testes.

Machlin et al. have studied the prostaglandin (PG) levels in the blood of rats in vitamin E deficiency by measuring serum prostaglandin in these animals by means of bioassay [34] as well as identification of these compounds by gas chromatography-mass spectrometry [35]. These studies showed that prostaglandin E_2 concentrations were increased as compared to the control rats. The concentration of tocopherol was inversely related to the serum concentration of PGE_2 (Fig. 10). These data may suggest that the conversion of endogenous concentrations of arachidonic acid into PGE_2 and $PGF_{2\alpha}$ may be inhibited by tocopherol through inhibition of the formation of endoperoxide intermediates by PGE_2 and $PGF_{2\alpha}$. An alternative theory advanced by the authors may be that tocopherol could be altering phospholipase activation. These findings may be important in the relationship of tocopherol deficiency and platelet aggregation.

Additional studies on the effect of vitamin E and prostaglandin were conducted by Anderson and Menzel [36]. These authors used isotonic contraction of rat fundus strip to assay "prostaglandin-like" activity present in the incubation of fundus homogenates carried out in the presence of glutathione, hydroquinone, and arachidonic acid. Prostaglandin-like activities were inhibited in tocopherol-treated animals but not after treatment with other antioxidants. These preliminary results may suggest a role for tocopherol in the modulation of prostaglandin metabolism or function.

VI. THYROID FUNCTION

Weiser et al. [37] have investigated the role of the thyroid in rats fed a diet deficient in tocopherol and quinone (T-Q). These authors have assayed the pituitary-thyroid system by measurement of follicle epithelial height and by interferometric determinations of the colloid density. From these studies, the authors concluded that diminished activity of pituitary-thyroid function results from long-term feeding of this diet. Substitution with tocopherol or quinone normalizes morphological changes but other antioxidants do not. Apparently, the site of action of tocopherol or quinone was not in the pituitary gland [37]. Unfortunately, no direct measurements of thyroid function, such as measurement of thyroid hormones or immunoassay of TSH or uptake of ^{131}I by the tissue was reported. It is difficult, therefore, to arrive at any direct conclusion on the status of the thyroid glands in these animals.

The relationships of thyroid status with serum tocopherol was studied by Bartuska [38] in a group of 20 hyperthyroid, 20 hypothyroid, and 30 euthyroid patients. These studies showed an inverse relationship between serum levels of tocopherol and thyroid activity, i.e., hyperthyroid patients had lower levels of tocopherol, whereas hypothyroid patients had higher levels of tocopherol than euthyroid patients. The significance of these findings to clinical states of patients, however, is not established.

TABLE 5   Testis Prostaglandins – Indocin Absent [a]

Animals [b]	$PGF_{2\alpha}$ (ng/g, mean ± SE)	PGE_2 (ng/g)
Immature		
Control (4) [d]	4.24 ± 1.13	8.31 ± 1.13
Experimental (3)	4.40 ± 1.32	7.88 ± 1.34
Adult		
Control (4)	8.25 ± 1.13	6.16 ± 0.22
Experimental (5)	15.72 ± 1.20 [c]	8.73 ± 0.02

[a] Data courtesy of M. P. Carpenter.
[b] Conditions similar to Table 1.
[c] Number of animals in parentheses.
[d] Significantly different from control $P = < 0.01$.

TABLE 6   Testicular and Prostaglandins – Frozen Tissue[a]

	Testes	
Animals[b]	PGF$_{2\alpha}$ (ng/g)	PGE$_2$
Immature		
Control	2.76	2.14
Experimental	17.60	13.50
Adult		
Control	5.15	1.77
Experimental	89.00	40.40

[a] Data courtesy of M. P. Carpenter.
[b] Conditions similar to Table 1. Immature animals were 4 weeks old; adult animals were 19 weeks old.

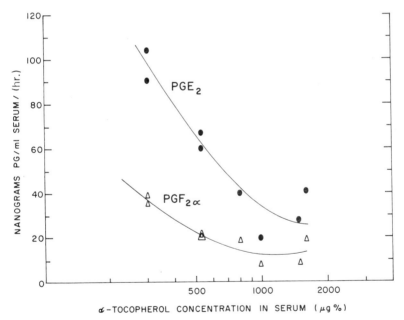

FIG. 10   Relationship of α-tocopherol concentration to PGE$_2$ and PGF$_{2\alpha}$ accumulations in rat serum. Three week old rats were maintained on diet containing 0, 10, 40 or 200 mg. dl α-tocopherol acetate per kg of diet for 7 weeks. The blood was removed by abdominal aorta puncture and was allowed to stand for one hour at 37° before preparation of serum. Each point represents a serum sample pooled from four rats. Recoveries of PGF$_{2\alpha}$-9-^{3}H added to serum: lipid extraction, 100%; silicic acid column chromatography, 87%; and silica gel TLC plates, 35% [35].

VII. EFFECTS ON PHYSIOLOGY OF ROTIFERS

The effect of tocopherol on the growth of fresh water rotifer, Asplanchna sieboldi was studied by Gilbert [39]. These studies showed that addition of α-tocopherol to the medium stimulated growth of these animals which did not occur with other antioxidants. The effect seemed to be specific and brings an increase in body size rather than an increase in rate of growth. Tocopherol also caused the normally parthenogenic females to have an altered phenotype and produce male offsprings. Although this effect has only been noted in lower invertebrates, nevertheless it is a novel effect which may implicate a role for tocopherol in genetic regulation. Additional studies, on mitotic activity, etc., are needed to evaluate a possible role of tocopherol in this regulation.

VIII. SUMMARY AND PROSPECTS

That α-tocopherol has an important role in the maintenance of the germinal epithelium in many species is well established, but similar action in the testosterone-producing cells of the testes has not been demonstrated. Preliminary work from one laboratory [9], however, suggests that diminution of testosterone and dihydrotestosterone in vitamin E-deficient rats occurs, but these values are still within normal limits and furthermore, the diminution is not accompanied by functional alteration of accessory sex glands.

Other work that has failed to show a direct effect of tocopherol on hormonal modulation has been the studies on the isolated fat cells of rats on deficient and control diets. These studies have demonstrated that insulin-mediated glucose metabolism or ACTH-induced lipolysis in fat cells from E-deficient rats is not significantly different from that in tissue of control animals.

It has been observed that release of PGE_2 and PGF_2 from platelets was inversely related to the vitamin E status of rats. Release of PG from rat testicular tissue was also higher in tissue from E-deficient animals. It has been suggested that tocopherol could inhibit PG synthesis either by preventing endoperoxide synthesis or altering phospholipase activity. Further studies are needed to prove such a hypothesis and to determine the physiological significance of these findings. Other studies in testicular tissue suggest that tocopherol may modulate synthesis or turnover of prostaglandin in this tissue.

In adrenal tissue, tocopherol appears to have two distinct functions. One is its stimulating effect on the steroid hydroxylase systems of subcellular organelles. In the hydroxylase system of mitochondria and microsome of beef adrenal tissue, tocopherol reverses ascrobate-induced inhibition. This inhibition is correlated with lipid peroxidation. This effect of tocopherol, however, is not specific since other antioxidants will also reverse the ascorbate-induced inhibition of hydroxylase. The second function of tocopherol which is noted in the isolated adrenal cell with intact membranes is more specific in that the ascorbate-inhibited, ACTH-induced steroidogenesis is reversed with tocopherol but not with other antioxidants. Furthermore, the effect is not related to lipid peroxidation. In the latter system, tocopherol appears to be involved in modulation of the membrane-bound ACTH-stimulated enzyme, adenylate cyclase.

In light of the above work, as well as the studies from other laboratories, it is suggested that one function of tocopherol in hormone action may be as a stabilizer of the phospholipid moiety of adenylate cyclase in the membrane. Much additional work, however, is needed with the isolated membrane preparation to substantiate this hypothesis.

Addendum: Since the submission of this review the author has had the opportunity to examine the adenylate cyclase (AC) activity in the adrenal cell membrane of vitamin E-deficient and -sufficient rats. These studies demonstrated inhibited AC activity in the deficient group which was further exaggerated by the addition of ascorbate [40]. Of interest is also our recent finding that a specific tocopherol binding site is present in the membrane of adrenal cells [41].

ACKNOWLEDGMENTS

The studies of the author referred to in this review have been in part supported by Research Grants AM 13102, AM 15509, AM 19717, Training Grant AM 05497, and General Clinical Research Grant RR 00211 from the National Institutes of Health and VA Projects 4966-01 and 4966-02.

The author is grateful to Drs. M. P. Carpenter, L. Machlin, and K. Mason for providing some of their original and unpublished works for this review. Appreciation is also expressed to the above individuals for their review of this manuscript prior to publication.

REFERENCES

1. K. E. Mason, Sex and Internal Secretion, 2:1149, 1939.
2. T. B. Osborne and L. B. Mendel, J. Biol. Chem. 38:223, 1919.
3. H. M. Evans and G. G. Burr, Proc. Natl. Acad. Sci. U.S.A. 11:334, 1925.
4. K. E. Mason, J. Exp. Zool. 45:159, 1926.
5. H. A. Mattil, JAMA 110:1831, 1938.
6. T. W. Gullickson, Ann. N.Y. Acad. Sci. 52:256, 1949.
7. K. E. Mason and S. Mauer, J. Nutr. 105:484, 1975.
8. C. Lutwak-Mann, Vit. Horm. 16:35, 1958.
9. M. P. Carpenter, personal communication.
10. W. E. Griesbach, M. E. Bell, and M. Livingston, Endocrinology 60:729, 1957.
11. M. P. Carpenter and R. O. Kling, manuscript in preparation.
12. J. G. Bieri and A. A. Anderson, Arch. Biochem. Biophys. 90:105, 1960.

13. V. R. Lavis, A. E. Kitabchi, and R. H. Williams, J. Biol. Chem. 244:4382, 1969.
14. A. E. Kitabchi and R. H. Williams, J. Biol. Chem. 243:3248, 1968.
15. A. E. Kitabchi, Otolaryngol. Clin. N.A. 8:335, 1975.
16. A. E. Kitabchi, D. R. Challonder, and R. H. Williams, Proc. Soc. Exp. Biol. Med. 127:647, 1968.
17. A. E. Kitabchi, Nature (London) 203:4945, 1964.
18. A. E. Kitabchi, P. B. McCay, M. P. Carpenter, R. E. Trucco, and R. Caputto, J. Biol. Chem. 235:1591, 1960.
19. A. E. Kitabchi, Ann. N.Y. Acad. Sci. 203:123, 1972.
20. A. E. Kitabchi, Steroids 10:567, 1967.
21. A. E. Kitabchi and R. K. Sharma, Endocrinology 88:1109, 1971.
22. R. L. Swallow and G. Sayers, Proc. Soc. Expl. Biol. Med. 131:1, 1969.
23. R. K. Sharma, K. Hashimoto, and A. E. Kitabchi, Endocrinology 91:994, 1972.
24. A. E. Kitabchi, R. K. Sharma, and W. H. West, Horm. Metab. Res. 3:133, 1971.
25. A. E. Kitabchi and W. H. West, Ann. N.Y. Acad. Sci. 258:422, 1975.
26. A. E. Kitabchi, A. H. Nathans, and C. L. Kitchell, J. Biol. Chem. 248:835, 1973.
27. A. E. Kitabchi, D. B. Wilson, and R. K. Sharma, Biochem. Biophys. Res. Commun. 44:898, 1971.
28. A. H. Nathans and A. E. Kitabchi, Biochim. Biophys. Acta 399:244, 1975.
29. F. Bowyer and A. E. Kitabchi, Biochem. Biophys. Res. Commun. 57:100, 1974.
30. M. P. Carpenter, Lipids 9:397, 1974.
31. P. W. Weidenbach and M. P. Carpenter, Fed. Proc. 33:1425, 1974.
32. M. P. Carpenter and L. M. Manning, Fed. Proc. 34:2575, 1975.
33. M. P. Carpenter, manuscript in preparation.
34. L. J. Machlin et al., Fed. Proc. 34:3923, 1975.
35. W. C. Hope, C. Dalton, L. J. Machlin, R. J. Filipski, and F. M. Vane, Prostaglandins 10:557, 1975.
36. W. G. Anderson and D. B. Menzel, Fed. Proc. 34:3919, 1975.
37. H. Weiser, V. Acterrath, and W. Boguth, Acta Agricul. Scand. Suppl. 19:208, 1973.
38. D. G. Bartuska, Program of 55th Meeting of the Endocrine Society, Chicago, Illinois, June 1973, Abstr. 294.
39. J. J. Gilbert, Amer. J. Clin. Nutr. 27:1005, 1974.
40. A. E. Kitabchi, A. Nathans, J. A. Barker, L. Kitchell, and B. W. Watson, In: de Duve C., Hayaishi, O., ed., Tocopherol, Oxygen, and Biomembranes. Amsterdam: Elsevier/North Holland Biomedical Press, 1:201-219, 1978.
41. A. E. Kitabchi, J. A. Barker, and M. Anderson, Program of 6th International Endocrine Society, Melbourne, Australia, February 1980.

Part 5G/ Role in Function and Ultrastructure
of Cellular Membranes

IZAÄK MOLENNAAR, CAESAR E. HULSTAERT, AND
MACHIEL J. HARDONK
University of Groningen
Groningen, The Netherlands

I.	Introduction	372
II.	Role of the Membrane in Cellular Metabolism	373
III.	Structure and Composition of Membranes	374
IV.	Membranes in Relation to Vitamin E	376
	A. Membrane Phospholipids	376
	B. Membrane Fragility	380
	C. Membrane Permeability	381
	D. Membrane Proteins	382
	E. Membrane Recognition	384
V.	Hypothesis	384
	References	387

I. INTRODUCTION

In this part we shall try to link the first half of this monograph, in which the tocopherol molecule and its role in metabolism have been discussed, to the second part, in which the reader will learn what happens to cells and tissues if that molecule is missing in animal and humans. That this link could be found at the membrane level of cellular organization does not seem to be too much of a speculation. All cells are enveloped by cell membranes (also called plasma membranes) and contain cell organelles as mitochondria, rough and smooth endoplasmic reticulum, Golgi complexes, lysosomes, etc., all having the membrane as a general, common structure (Fig. 1). Moreover, membranes are of utmost importance for cellular life. It has become clear that the function of all cell organelles is not only dependent on the molecules in their "soluble" interior but also on their constituting membranes. Finally, although membranes differ largely in their chemical composition, they all contain lipid, which is nature's solvent for tocopherol. Thus it seems warranted to examine whether cellular membranes contain the clue for cellular pathology in vitamin E deficiency.

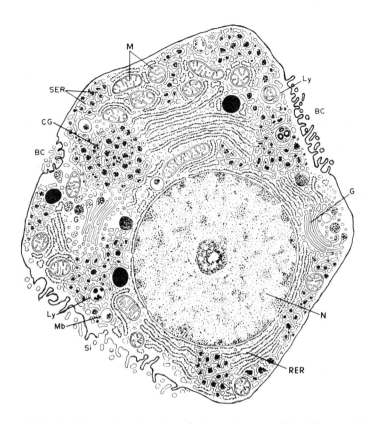

FIG. 1   Schematic drawing of a hepatocyte. BC, bile canaliculus; CG, cisternal granule; G, Golgi complex; Ly, lysosome; M, mitochondrion; Mb, microbody; N, nucleus; RER, rough endoplasmic reticulum; SER, smooth endoplasmic reticulum; Si, sinusoid. All these organelles have cellular membranes as general common structure. (From Ref. 1 with permission.)

In this way we may better understand the function of vitamin E in the healthy organism.

II. ROLE OF THE MEMBRANE IN CELLULAR METABOLISM

Biological membranes are indispensable for cellular life. In the first place, they divide tissues into cells and cells into organelles leading to many different compartments. This determines the difference between biochemistry in a test tube and in vivo; some compartments might even be too small for mass-action laws to apply directly [2]. The membrane as a compartmentalizing structure not only brings together molecules taking part in metabolic reactions but also regulates the concentrations of ions and molecules within the compartment by its permeability properties. Thus, each compartment* has its own micromilieu, particularly determined and controlled by specific properties of its enveloping membrane. One example is the lysosome, whose membrane, packing the hydrolytic enzymes, determines some of the most important features of the organelle and its function [3]. Inside the lysosome a pH of 5 is maintained [4] by the strongly acidic glycolipid component [5] and acidic lipoproteins [6] of the membrane.

Secondly, the membrane provides possibilities for a spatial distribution of certain molecules. They can either form an integral part of the membrane or interact with its surface, depending on their physicochemical properties. This offers the opportunity for a specific organization of macromolecular complexes in the membrane [7]. In these complexes a new dimension of cellular control may be represented—one in which the effects mediated by the interaction of a specific metabolite with one protein may be transmitted via heterologous protein interaction to other proteins (e.g., enzymes) in a cluster arrangement [8]. These complexes may be associated through interactions with nonprotein matrix structures that have the possibility to bring about conformational changes [9]. Indeed, it has been found that profound differences exist between the properties of membrane-bound and extracted enzymes [10]. Some of these properties are: inhibitor sensitivity, pH optimum, K_M, redox potential, cold lability, and substrate specificity. To perform enzymatic function the enzyme protein must possess the correct conformation for activity. Variations in the activity of many enzymes, caused by modification or loss of lipid may be due to changes in the association between lipid and enzyme molecule, resulting in a change of the spatial folding of the enzyme. The lipid requirement may be rather nonspecific; the availability of the hydrophobic part of the lipids appears to be the most important factor. But examples also exist of a much higher degree of specificity for lipid requirement, suggesting that both polar and nonpolar parts of the lipid molecule may influence the enzymatic conformation [10].

III. STRUCTURE AND COMPOSITION OF MEMBRANES

Membranes are composed mainly of lipids and proteins. How these molecules are thought to be assembled is described in membrane models. These models are hypothetical visualizations of the molecular anatomy of

*It should be mentioned that this definition of "compartment" is not necessarily identical with that used in some of the biochemical literature.

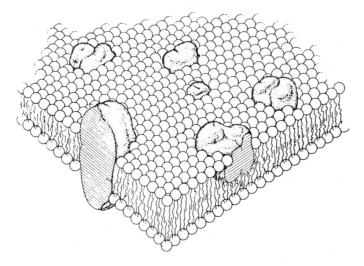

FIG. 2   The fluid mosaic membrane model; schematic three-dimensional and cross-sectional view. The solid bodies with stippled surfaces represent the globular integral proteins, embedded with their nonpolar surface in the phospholipid matrix. Peripheral proteins and glycoproteins are not depicted. (From Ref. 12, with permission.)

the membrane. The oldest in the Danielli-Davson model or laminar bilayer model in which the lipids are sandwiched between outer protein layers held to the lipid by electrostatic bonding [11].

Since its presentation in 1935, new models have been brought forward. In the newest, the fluid model of Singer and Nicolson, the organization of lipids and proteins has developed into a structural configuration of minimum free energy and thus is consistent with the restrictions imposed by thermodynamics [12]. The proteins belonging to the membrane in a narrow sense ("integral" proteins) are a heterogenous set of globular molecules, each arranged in an amphipathic structure, i.e., with the ionic and highly polar groups protruding from the membrane into the aqueous phase and the nonpolar groups largely buried in the hydrophobic interior of the membrane (Fig. 2). These globular molecules are partially embedded in a matrix of phospholipids, the latter being organized mainly as a discontinuous fluid bilayer although a small fraction of the lipid may interact specifically with the membrane proteins. Formally therefore, the fluid mosaic structure is analogous to a two-dimensionally oriented solution of integral proteins (or lipoproteins) in the viscous phospholipid bilayer solvent [12]. Although it has been claimed [7] that most integral proteins are much less mobile than

is assumed in the fluid mosaic model, the model is of great value for
membrane research.

Although the chemical composition of different kinds of membranes
varies considerably, it is possible on the basis of lipid characteristics
(e.g., the degree of saturation) to divide all cellular membranes into two
main groups [13]:

1. Plasma membranes, lysosomal membranes, and membranes of
   the Golgi complex, containing a large proportion of saturated and
   monounsaturated fatty acids, cholesterol, and sphingomyelin

2. Mitochondrial membranes and membranes of the endoplasmic
   recticulum, containing a high content of polyunsaturated fatty acids
   but less sphingomyelin

Finally it should be mentioned that in various tissues nearly all
tocopherol seems to be located in the membranous subcellular fractions of
the cell (Table 1) [13a].

Apart from the integral proteins described above, the membrane contains "peripheral" proteins which are loosely bound to the membrane
surface. Many of the proteins of both groups consist of enzymes. It is
generally assumed that in a given tissue, nearly every type of cellular
membrane has a specific set of enzymes corresponding with its metabolic
capacities. These so-called marker enzymes can be used for classifying
membranes as has been very elegantly demonstrated [14,15].

Furthermore, membranes contain carbohydrates which are attached
to the proteins as well as to the lipids (glycoproteins, glycolipids) [16].
They are distributed asymmetrically and play an important role in the
functioning of cellular membranes with regard to the process of recognition.

IV. MEMBRANES IN RELATION TO VITAMIN E

In vitamin E deficiencies (Chaps. 4, 6, and 7), an increasing number of
observations point to the membrane as the cellular structure which is
primarily impaired. This literature has been extensively reviewed up to
1972 [13]. In this section, the relations between vitamin E and phospholipids, membrane fragility, permeability, and membrane proteins will be
discussed, as well as the possible effect of vitamin E on membrane
recognition.

A. Membrane Phospholipids

In the above-mentioned review [13] it was explained how morphological
observations led to a biochemical analysis of membranes. In brief,

TABLE 1 Tocopherol Content of Subcellular Fractions of Tissues [a]

Fraction	Liver	Heart	Lung	Liver	Heart	Lung
	(μg/mg protein)			(μg tocopherol per total fraction)		
Homogenate	0.04	0.12	0.14	104	58	99
Nuclear	0.03	0.25	0.18	34	28	24
Heavy mitochondrial	0.27	0.26	0.60	31	4	12
Light mitochondrial	0.12	0.29	0.26	19	4	13
Microsomal	0.08	0.37	0.56	18	9	12
Soluble	0.002	0.02	0.04	2	5	13

[a] From Taylor et al. [13a].

membranes on electron micrographs of osmiumtetroxide-fixed tissue are
normally visualized in positive contrast, i.e., as black lines. At high
magnification, these membranes, when sectioned perpendicular to their
surface, appear to be triple-layered: a central light zone bordered by two
dark zones. These zones can be interpreted as follows. In model experiments it has been established that osmiumtetroxide reacts stoichiometrically with the double bonds of fatty acyl chains [17]. During tissue fixation
with osmiumtetroxide, it is reasonably certain that this compound reacts
primarily with the lipid double bonds in the bilayer of the membrane. Subsequently the formed monoester anionic groups would migrate to the polar
parts of the membrane, resulting in the dark zones [17].

However, on electron micrographs of jejunal epithelial cells of two
patients suffering from vitamin E deficiency (secondary to an abetalipoproteinemia), no positive membrane contrast could be found in the mitochondrial and endoplasmic reticular membranes; the contrast was restored
by administration of vitamin E [18]. It was supposed that the loss of
positive membrane contrast resulted from a decrease of the content of unsaturated fatty acids in these membranes, caused by vitamin E deficiency.

To a lesser extent this loss of membrane contrast was also found in
jejunal epithelial cells and in liver parenchymal cells of vitamin E-deficient
ducklings. It appeared that the outer mitochondrial membrane lost more
contrast than the inner one [19]. It was attractive to suppose that this
differential loss of positive contrast visualized a critical difference in the
loss of double bonds caused by vitamin E deficiency [20]. This turned out
to be the case. The fatty acid analyses of outer and inner mitochondrial
membranes of livers of vitamin E-deficient ducklings showed a specific
loss of polyunsaturated fatty acids (Table 2) [13]. Of the mitochondrial
membranes, the outer membrane indeed showed a larger decrease in
arachidonic acid and in linoleic acid. The relative decreases in polyunsaturated fatty acids were found to be compensated by relative increases in
monounsaturated fatty acids. In vitamin E-deficient rats, similar alterations in the fatty acid composition of the liver homogenate fractions were
found (Table 2) [21]. The alterations in the rat liver fractions were more
pronounced than in the duckling liver fractions. Even the microsomes
demonstrated a loss of polyunsaturated fatty acids contrary to those of the
livers of vitamin E-deficient ducklings.

The above-mentioned results are suggestive of a functional link
between vitamin E and polyunsaturated fatty acids. The investigations of
McCay and associates [22,23] of a NADPH-dependent enzyme system in
microsomal and mitochondrial fractions of rat liver homogenates give an
indication how the changes in the fatty acid composition in vitamin E
deficiency could be brought about. During the first 3 min of an in vitro
incubation of microsomes or of mitochondria in the presence of NADPH
and Fe^{3+}, 90% of the α-tocopherol present in these fractions was
metabolized, and subsequently the polyunsaturated fatty acids were per-

TABLE 2 Fatty Acid Composition (Wt% of Total Fatty Acids) of Membranes from Livers of Control and Vitamin E-Deficient Ducklings and Rats [a]

Fatty acid	Inner mitochondrial membrane		Outer mitochondrial membrane		Microsomes		Supernatant [b]	
	C	D	C	D	C	D	C	D
Duckling liver [c]								
Total saturated	46.5	46.4	55.6	53.6	45.8	48.2		
C16:1ω7+C18:1ω9	22.8	28.8	23.8	28.6	23.2	22.1		
C18:2ω6	13.3	12.2	6.8	3.6	4.5	4.7		
C20:4ω6	13.3	7.6	9.4	3.3	16.9	14.7		
C22:6ω3	1.6	1.0	1.2	2.0	2.0	3.4		

Fatty acid	Mitochondria		Microsomes		Supernatant [b]	
	C	D	C	D	C	D
Rat liver [d]						
Total saturated	40.6	43.1	43.6	44.3	32.6	41.5
C16:1ω7+C18:1ω9	7.2	25.2	6.7	26.1	18.5	51.5
C18:2ω6	19.0	10.2	16.1	7.5	32.0	4.2
C20:4ω6	24.0	19.4	24.3	17.5	11.9	3.0
C22:6ω3	8.0	2.9	9.8	3.2	5.2	Trace

[a] C = control, D = vitamin E-deficient.
[b] 105,000 g.
[c] Molenaar, Vos, and Hommes (1972) [3].
[d] Fujita and Matsumoto (1974) [21].

oxidized. As the level of α-tocopherol in the diet increased, the peroxidation of polyunsaturated fatty acids decreased but was never completely suppressed. It must be noted, however, that this reaction probably proceeds at a much slower rate in vivo than in vitro. It was found by others that, in a period of 3 weeks, 93% of the radioactive α-tocopherol that had been present in the livers of rats and chickens was metabolized [24]. It was concluded that the function of vitamin E is to protect the polyunsaturated fatty acids in membranes with electron transport functions against the attack by free radicals generated by the reaction system [23].

It must be noted that the importance of vitamin E for the protection of mitochondrial and microsomal membranes was already stressed by Tappel [25, 26]. He considered the nonenzymatic peroxidation of polyunsaturated fatty acids by molecular oxygen as the only initiating damaging process that is inhibited by vitamin E. However, this hypothesis ignores the possibility that normal biochemical processes in the membrane are capable of initiating peroxidation [27, 28]. For example, peroxidation in vitamin E deficiency could be generated in the microsomal and mitochondrial membranes as a result of NADPH-dependent reactions as described by McCay and coworkers [22, 23]. It is possible, however, that in late stages of vitamin E deficiency peroxidation (according to Tappel) will take place, wherever oxygen is sufficiently available.

It seems plausible that a functional link between vitamin E and polyunsaturated fatty acids, as described above, would work through a structural link. On the basis of studies of molecular models it was jointly proposed by Lucy and Diplock [29, 30] that vitamin E forms a complex with phospholipids containing arachidonyl residues. The methyl groups at C-4 and C-8 of the phytyl chain of tocopherol would fit into pockets created by the cis double bonds of the fatty acid. In this way the packing of this acid in the membrane would be facilitated, resulting in a protection of the fatty acid against oxidative destruction; thus, the membrane would be stabilized. The chromanol ring of α-tocopherol and the polar groups of the phospholipid would both lie at the same end of the complex where they are thought to participate in polar interactions at the membrane surface. We think, however, that it remains to be seen whether the polyunsaturated fatty acyl chains are more protected against oxidative destruction by the closer packing of the carbon chains in the membrane than by the presence of the chromanol ring at the membrane surface.

B. Membrane Fragility

It was to be expected that membranes lacking vitamin E would be less stabile [29] and this indeed turned out to be the case. It was established that the erythrocyte membrane, proven to contain vitamin E [31], appeared to be less stabile in vitamin E-deficient rats [32,33], chickens [34], ducklings [35], and guinea pigs [36], as was shown by the hemolysis that occurred when their erythrocytes were incubated in the presence of dialuric acid. Further investigation of the influence of dialuric acid on the rat erythrocyte membrane and on micellar suspensions of this membrane showed that, in vitamin E deficiency, dialuric acid causes losses of polyunsaturated fatty acids, especially arachidonic acid and the 16-carbon plasmalogen [37]. It was also shown that in vitamin E deficiency hemolysis was accelerated when partially peroxidized cells were treated with phospholipase A and C. This suggests that peroxidation exposes both polar and nonpolar lipid sites. The latter experiments indicate how membranes could be gradually degraded in vitamin E deficiency.

There are also indications of an increased fragility of intracellular membranes. The rise in activity of lysosomal enzymes found in timescale studies on the development of muscular dystrophy in vitamin E-deficient rabbits [38] could be the result of lesions in the lysosomal membrane. Further, it appeared that mitochondrial inner and outer membrane of vitamin E-deficient ducklings were more fragmented than those of control ducklings when fractions of these membranes were negatively stained for electron microscopy [13,39]. In the healthy organism, the outer mitochondrial membrane does not contain α-tocopherol [40]; thus, it is not easy to understand why this membrane shows an increased fragility in vitamin E deficiency. Damage to the outer membrane can be thought to be inflicted by free radicals generated in the inner mitochondrial membrane, as the distance between the outer and the inner mitochondrial membrane is probably less than is commonly accepted [41], possibly not exceeding 3 nm which is the range of action of free radicals [42]. In the outer membrane, cholesterol is known to be present [43], possibly fulfilling a stabilizing function by forming a complex with the monounsaturated fatty acids [44]. If this membrane is attacked by free radicals, the presence of cholesterol can, however, lead to the formation of cholesterolhydroperoxides [45].

C. Membrane Permeability

According to the hypothesis by Lucy and Diplock [29,30], vitamin E in the membrane would reduce permeability and vitamin E deficiency would increase permeability. The studies of their group on the permeability of liposomes containing α-tocopherol [46] are in good agreement with their postulation. It appeared that α-tocopherol could reduce the permeability to glucose and chromate ions when the liposomes consisted of phospholipids containing arachidonic acid residues. This effect of tocopherol on permeability was larger, with the phospholipid having a higher content of arachidonic acid residues.

Also, the experiments of McCay and associates [22], who found a decrease of turbidity in a microsomal suspension concomitant with a peroxidation of polyunsaturated fatty acids following the metabolic breakdown of α-tocopherol, could be interpreted as an increase in the permeability of the microsomal membrane. In a different experimental system, other investigators found that liver mitochondria of vitamin E-deficient ducklings showed a decreased uptake of ammonium phosphate and of ammonium malate in the presence of phosphate [47]. The decreased incorporation of [^{14}C]cholesterol into androgens by testis homogenates, and into androgens and corticosterone by adrenal homogenates of vitamin E-deficient rats, could be also due to a decreased transport of precursors through the mitochondrial membranes, since the initial steps of steroidogenesis occur in mitochondria [48].

The above-mentioned data seem to be rather confusing, but one should realize that they are concerned with different experimental systems and are related to different transport systems. The tocopherol to arachidonate ratio is 1:50 in mitochrondria [13] and 1:500 in erythrocytes [30]. This suggests that a complex of tocopherol and arachidonate is not likely to play a role in the passive diffusion of molecules through cellular membranes. Rather, it would point to a specific localization of the tocopherol molecule in the membrane (to be discussed in Sec. V).

The decreased uptake of phosphate in mitochondria [47], as mentioned above, can be explained by a change in the translocation process. In the literature, two specific mechanisms are proposed for this process: the carrier mechanism and the fixed-pore mechanism [49]. According to the carrier mechanism, the entire transport protein with its binding site is rotated across the membrane; according to the fixed pore mechanism, a conformational change of the protein translocates the binding site across the membrane. The fatty acid composition in the direct vicinity of either carrier or pore mechanism will influence the translocation process. Vitamin E deficiency, proven to cause a decreased unsaturation in the mitochondrial membranes [13], would be expected to hamper the translocation process because of the increasing rigidity of the membrane adjacent to the transport mechanism. This argument could also be valid for the findings on the decreased steroidogenesis as mentioned above [48].

D. Membrane Proteins

As described earlier in this section, proteins besides lipids form an important constituent of cellular membranes, and therefore it would not be surprising if membrane-bound proteins, such as membrane-bound enzymes, are affected in vitamin E deficiency as well. However, until recently, relatively little attention has been paid to the investigation of

membrane-bound enzymes in vitamin E deficiency. It was found that succinate dehydrogenase activity was reduced in liver mitochondria of
vitamin E-deficient rats [50] and guinea pigs [51]. In vitamin E-deficient
rabbits the Na^+, K^+-dependent ATPase activity of the erythrocyte plasma
membrane was higher than in control rabbits [52]. Furthermore, a progressive decrease was found in the activity of Na^+, K^+-dependent ATPase in
the plasma membrane of liver parenchymal cells of vitamin E-deficient
rats [53].

In a histochemical investigation of 20 enzymes in vitamin E-deficient
duckling livers, five membrane-bound enzymes turned out to be stimulated:
5'-nucleotidase, glucose-6-phosphatase, isocitrate dehydrogenase ($NADP^+$),
tetrazolium reductase (NADH), and tetrazolium reductase (NADPH) [41].
Of these enzymes, 5'-nucleotidase and glucose-6-phosphatase appeared to
be stimulated most. Biochemically a stimulation of these two enzymes
could be demonstrated per milligram of protein, per milligram of phospholipid, per milligram of RNA, and per milligram of DNA. The increase per
milligram of DNA was largest (glucose-6-phosphatase, 46%; 5'-nucleotidase,
49%), whereas the increase per milligram of protein, phospholipid, and RNA
was only one-half the increase per milligram of DNA. Morphometrical
investigation of the liver parenchymal cells made it clear why this discrepancy occurred. The volume of the liver parenchymal cell in the
vitamin E-deficient ducklings had increased by 30% as was also found by
other investigators in vitamin E-deficient rats [54]. As this increase is
almost completely due to an increase of the volume of the cytoplasmic
compartment, the amount of protein, phospholipid, and RNA will have
increased per cell as well, thus masking the increase of the enzyme
activity. Further investigation on the nature of the increase of the enzyme
activity with digitonin preincubation made it likely that for both enzymes
the amount of enzyme molecules has increased in vitamin E deficiency [41].
This means that the balance between degradation and synthesis of membrane
proteins has been disturbed. We cannot decide which of the two is of primary importance.

The influence of vitamin E deficiency on membrane proteins was also
studied by a morphometrical analysis of membranes of liver parenchymal
cells, fixed according to a method to preserve as much as possible the
physiological conformation of the proteins [41]. With this method it is
possible to visualize protein particles in the membrane [55]. In vitamin E
deficiency the diameter of these protein particles in the outer mitochondrial
membrane was found to have decreased. The thickness of this membrane
had decreased as well, which is probably due to the smaller size of the
protein particles. This smaller size could be a reflection of conformational changes [9] brought about by free radicals generated in the inner
mitochondrial membrane, as explained before in relation to the increased
membrane fragility (Sec. IV.B).

E. Membrane Recognition

Lately it appeared that administration of high doses of vitamin E enhanced
the humoral immune response in chickens [56, 57] and in mice [58]. Also,
the in vitro administration of α-tocopherol to a suspension of mouse spleen
cells stimulated the antibody production to a large extent [59]. Although
the chain of processes involved in antibody production is rather extensive,
it is not unlikely that there is a direct effect of the vitamin on the plasma
membrane. Possibly, vitamin E affects the glycoprotein component which
is involved in the process of membrane recognition.

V. HYPOTHESIS

Considering the above-mentioned experimental results, we propose the
following hypothesis for the function of vitamin E. This hypothesis is
based on an assumed specific distribution of unsaturated fatty acyl chains
in the membrane. This assumption is based on the following arguments:
It has been suggested [60] that phospholipid molecules are not randomly
distributed throughout the membrane but that the phospholipids of interest
for a particular enzyme are localized in the immediate vicinity of this
enzyme. In this respect, it is of importance for our hypothesis that most
membrane-bound enzymes require unsaturated phospholipids for activity
[60]. This is apparent from investigations of mutants of bacteria that are
unable to synthesize unsaturated fatty acids [10, 60], from studies on the
reactivation of lipid-depleted membrane-bound enzymes by adding defined
phospholipids [10, 60, 61], and from studies on enzyme activity in membranes where endogenous phospholipids are substituted by defined exogenous
phospholipids [62].
     The integral proteins in the Singer-Nicolson model contain hydrophobic
groups on their intramembranous surface. Such a surface would be especially suited to accommodate the twisted chains of the unsaturated phospholipids, facilitating their packing in the membrane (Fig. 3). Such a location
of unsaturated fatty acyl chains adjacent to an integral protein may, however, endanger membrane integrity. This would be the case if such a
protein forms part of an electron transport system capable of generating
free radicals, such as the mixed-function oxidases [63]. The NADPH-
dependent enzyme system as studied by McCay and associates [22, 23]
probably forms part of this enzyme complex. To cope with the ever-
existing danger of peroxidation by free radicals, the unsaturated fatty acids
surrounding the mixed-function oxidases are protected by the redox function
of the chromanol ring of the tocopherol molecule (Fig. 3, protein II). The
phytyl chain of the tocopherol molecule forms a complex with the arachidonyl residue of the phospholipids [29, 30]. Thus, the chromanol ring is

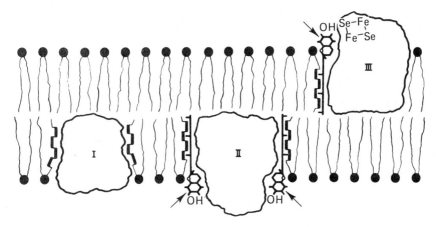

FIG. 3   Proposed localization of the tocopherol molecule (see arrows) in
the membrane.   I = integral protein; II = integral protein, forming part of
a mixed function oxidase; III = integral selenide-containing non-heme iron
protein.

anchored in the direct vicinity of the mixed-function oxidases. Because the
range of action of a free radical is about 3 nm [42], tocopherol molecules
are only needed directly adjacent to integral proteins that produce free
radicals. Unsaturated lipids at a greater distance are not expected to be
subject to free radical attack. The aforementioned location of tocopherol
could also explain the protection of the selenide, possibly forming part of
the active center of the nonheme iron protein (of the mixed-function oxidase
complex) as proposed by Diplock and Lucy [30,64] (Fig. 3, protein III).

The fact that more arachidonic acyl chains than tocopherol molecules
are present in most membranes can be explained because not all integral
proteins contain free-radical-producing systems. In this respect it is
interesting to note that it can be calculated that the inner mitochondrial
membrane, containing electron transport systems, contains 1 molecule of
tocopherol per 50 arachidonic acyl chains [13], whereas the plasma membrane of the erythrocyte without such systems contains 1 molecule of
tocopherol per 500 arachidonic acyl chains [30].

As explained above, the most important function of vitamin E is
believed to be the prevention of free radical attack of unsaturated fatty·
acids in the membrane and thus the prevention of lipid hydroperoxide
formation. Recently it has become evident that vitamin E is not the only
protective factor against peroxidative damage to membranes. In this
respect glutathione peroxidase, a seleno-enzyme, can be considered to
function as an extra defense system in the cytosol as it metabolizes H_2O_2

and lipid hydroperoxides [65]. This would explain why many vitamin E deficiency symptoms disappear when the concentration of selenium in the diet exceeds a critical value [66]. Indeed it was found that the activity of glutathione peroxidase increases with the concentration of selenium in the diet [65].

If the proposed hypothesis is valid, what are the molecular events that will take place in vitamin E deficiency? Free radical damage will lead to peroxidation of polyunsaturated fatty acids in the membrane, which is consistent with the changes found in the fatty acid composition [13, 21]. Once membrane-generated peroxidation has started, the opportunity for a nonenzymatic peroxidation [25, 26] can develop. In general this can be expected in the later stages of deficiency. One specific tissue, the adipose tissue, will be especially liable to nonenzymatic peroxidation, because nonstructural lipid in the form of droplets is present in the relatively large vacuoles of the adipose cells. Once peroxidation has started in the droplet it cannot be easily controlled, because membranes are only present at the outer circumference of these cells. Indeed, a high increase in the amount of lipid peroxides in vitamin E deficiency has been found in adipose tissue [67]. Furthermore, free radical damage may influence membrane proteins, permeability, and membrane-bound enzymes as has been discussed before (Sec. IV.C and D).

Can we, with the help of this combined working hypothesis, understand more of the pathology of vitamin E deficiency?

With the localization of the tocopherol molecule in mind it is clear that in a deficiency two factors contribute to the pathological symptoms. The first one relates to the molecular interactions in which the missing molecule normally takes part (i.e., the mixed-function oxidase). The second factor is the membrane whose function is influenced, due to the missing tocopherol molecule. This can be illustrated by experiments with mitochondria [47], in which the permeability disturbances for phosphate are explained as a change in the translocation process caused by changes in the membrane lipids (see Table 2). Thus it can be understood that vitamin E has an influence on oxidative phosphorylation, not directly as was earlier supposed [50], but because the membrane localization of the molecule affects the supply of phosphate ions for the continuation of the process. Also, the influence of vitamin E deficiency on the steroid metabolism [48] may not be direct, but can be interpreted in terms of an effect on membrane permeability because transport of precursors through mitochondrial membranes are initial steps in steroidogenesis.

The specific changes in membrane structure and function will be dependent upon the kind of membrane which is affected most. We think that this is probably the reason why in vitamin E deficiency there is such a large variety of macroscopical and microscopical lesions in different organs of the same animal and in the different species—not because of intricate molecular events but because tocopherol is located in all, or nearly all cellular membranes, all of which differ in composition and function, leading to unspecific or at least nonvitamin E-specific pathological manifestations. Organ pathology in vitamin E deficiency is probably partly determined by vitamin E aspects on the molecular level, but especially by the dysfunction of the affected membrane system. Whether a difference exists in the need for vitamin E between different membrane systems, or in terms of pathology, between the sensibility for vitamin E deficiency remains to be investigated. It is known that among the very susceptible tissues are testis, liver, and adrenal cortex. It is to be noted that the smooth endoplasmic reticulum is especially abundant in these tissues. Would the membranes of this cellular organelle represent the "heel of Achilles"? There is reason enough for this supposition: mixed-function oxidases are rather active in these tissues.

In conclusion, vitamin E has a most important function in the protection of the integrity of cellular membranes as the basic structural units of cells. By its membrane localization it helps to maintain compartmentalization and permeability, thus contributing importantly, but probably rather unspecifically to cellular metabolism. It guarantees that metabolic interrelations based upon and coupled with the membrane surface can be developed undisturbed. In our opinion, that is how vitamin E, through membranes, contributes to the functioning of cells.

REFERENCES

1. T. L. Lentz, Cell Fine Structure. Philadelphia, Saunders, 1971, p. 189.
2. R. A. Peters, Biochemical Lesions and Lethal Synthesis. Oxford, Pergamon, 1963, p. 212.
3. A. H. Gordon. In Lysosomes in Biology and Pathology. Edited by J. T. Dingle, Amsterdam, North-Holland, 1973, p. 87.
4. J. L. Mego, Biochem. J. 122:445 (1971).
5. A. J. Barrett and J. T. Dingle, Biochem. J. 105:20P (1967).
6. A. Goldstone, E. Szabo, and H. Koenig, Life Sci. (II) 9:607 (1970).
7. D. E. Green, S. Ji, and R. F. Brucker, Bioenergetics 4:527 (1972).
8. A. Ginsburg and R. Stadtman, Annu. Rev. Biochem. 39:429 (1970).
9. H. Baltscheffsky and M. Baltscheffsky, Annu. Rev. Biochem. 43:871 (1974).
10. R. Coleman, Biochim. Biophys. Acta 300:1 (1973).
11. J. F. Danielli and H. Davson, J. Cell. Comp. Physiol. 5:495 (1935).
12. S. J. Singer and G. L. Nicolson, Science 175:720 (1972).
13. I. Molenaar, J. Vos, and F. A. Hommes, Vit. Horm. 30:45 (1972).

13a. S. L. Taylor, M. P. Lamden, and A. L. Tappel, Lipids 7:530 (1976).

14. A. Beaufay, E. Amar-Costesec, E. Feytmans, D. Thinès-Sempoux, M. Wibo, M. Robbi, and J. Berthet, J. Cell Biol. 61:188 (1974).

15. D. H. de Heer, M. S. Olson, and R. N. Pinckard, J. Cell Biol. 60:460 (1974).

16. G. L. Nicolson, Int. Rev. Cytol. 39:89 (1974).

17. J. C. Riemersma. In Biological Techniques in Electron Microscopy. Edited by D. F. Parsons, New York, Academic, 1970, p. 75.

18. I. Molenaar, F. A. Hommes, W. G. Braams, and H. A. Polman, Proc. Natl. Acad. Sci. USA 61:982 (1968).

19. I. Molenaar, J. Vos, F. C. Jager, and F. A. Hommes, Nutr. Metab. 12:358 (1970).

20. J. Vos, I. Molenaar, M. Searle-van Leeuwen, and F. A. Hommes, Acta Agr. Scand. 19:192 (1973).

21. T. Fujita and K. Matsumoto, J. Pharm. Soc. Jap. 94:147 (1974).

22. P. B. McCay, J. L. Poyer, P. M. Pfeifer, H. E. May, and J. M. Gilliam, Lipids 6:297 (1971).

23. P. B. McCay, P. M. Pfeifer, and W. H. Stipe, Ann. N.Y. Acad. Sci. 203:62 (1972).

24. S. Krishnamurthy and J. G. Bieri, J. Lipid Res. 4:330 (1963).

25. A. L. Tappel, Vit. Horm. 20:493 (1962).

26. A. L. Tappel, Fed. Proc. 24:73 (1965).

27. U. Reiss and A. L. Tappel, Biochim. Biophys. Acta 312:608 (1973).

28. A. L. Tappel, Amer. J. Clin. Nutr. 27:960 (1974).

29. J. A. Lucy, Ann. N.Y. Acad. Sci. 203:4 (1972).

30. A. T. Diplock and J. A. Lucy, FEBS Lett. 29:205 (1973).

31. R. Silber, R. Winter, and H. J. Kayden, J. Clin. Invest. 48:2089 (1969).

32. C. S. Rose and P. György, Amer. J. Physiol. 168:414 (1952).

33. F. C. Jager, Nutr. Diet. 10:215 (1968).

34. F. Christensen, H. Dam, R. A. Gortner, and E. Søndergaard, Acta Phys. Scand. 35:215 (1956).

35. F. C. Jager and J. A. Verbeek-Raad, Int. J. Vit. Nutr. Res. 40:597 (1970).

36. I. Elmadfa and W. Feldheim, Int. J. Vit. Nutr. Res. 41:490 (1971).

37. M. O. Barker and M. Brin, Arch. Biochem. Biophys. 166:32 (1975).

38. J. Zalkin, A. L. Tappel, K. A. Caldwell, S. Shibko, I. D. Desai, and T. A. Holliday, J. Biol. Chem. 237:2678 (1962).

39. J. Vos, I. Molenaar, M. Searle-van Leeuwen, and F. A. Hommes, Ann. N.Y. Acad. Sci. 203:74 (1972).

40. M. M. Oliviera, W. B. Weglicki, A. Nason, and P. P. Nair, Biochim. Biophys. Acta 180:98 (1969).

41. C. E. Hulstaert, W. P. Gijzel, M. J. Hardonk, A. M. Kroon, and I. Molenaar, Lab. Invest. 33:176 (1975).

42. F. Hutchinson, Science 134:533 (1961).
43. C. Schnaitman, V. G. Erwin, and J. W. Greenawalt, J. Cell Biol. 32:719 (1967).
44. R. A. Demel, L. L. M. van Deenen, and B. A. Pethica, Biochim. Biophys. Acta 135:11 (1967).
45. A. A. Lamola, T. Yamane, and A. M. Trozzolo, Science 179:1133 (1973).
46. A. T. Diplock, J. A. Lucy, M. Verrinder, and A. Zieleniewski, FEBS Lett. 82:341 (1977).
47. F. A. Hommes, D. J. Mastebroek-Helder, and I. Molenaar, Nutr. Metabol. 19:263 (1975).
48. M. McC. Barnes and A. J. Smith, Int. J. Vit. Nutr. Res. 45:342 (1975).
49. S. J. Singer, Ann. Rev. Biochem. 43:805 (1974).
50. L. M. Corwin, J. Biol. Chem. 240:34 (1965).
51. F. Carabello and J. Bird, Biochem. Biophys. Res. Commun. 34:92 (1969).
52. R. N. Farias, T. F. R. Celis, A. L. Goldemberg, and R. E. Trucco, Arch. Biochem. Biophys. 116:34 (1966).
53. E. A. Machado, E. A. Porta, W. S. Hartroft, and F. Hamilton, Lab. Invest. 24:13 (1971).
54. U. N. Riede, C. Stitny, S. Althaus, and H. P. Rohr, Beitr. Pathol. 145:24 (1972).
55. F. S. Sjöstrand and L. Barajas, J. Ultrastruct. Res. 25:121 (1968).
56. R. P. Tengerdy, R. H. Heinzerling, and C. F. Nockels, Inf. Immunol. 5:987 (1972).
57. R. H. Heinzerling, C. F. Nockels, C. L. Quarles, and R. P. Tengerdy, Proc. Soc. Exp. Biol. Med. 146:279 (1974).
58. R. P. Tengerdy, R. H. Heinzerling, G. L. Brown, and M. M. Mathias, Int. Arch. Allergy Appl. Immunol. 44:221 (1973).
59. P. A. Campbell, H. R. Cooper, R. H. Heinzerling, and R. P. Tengerdy, Proc. Soc. Exp. Biol. Med. 146:465 (1974).
60. L. Rothfield and D. Romeo. In Molecular Biology. Edited by L. I. Rothfield, New York, Academic, 1971, p. 251.
61. C. Garland and C. F. Cori, Biochemistry 11:4712 (1972).
62. G. B. Warren, P. A. Toon, N. J. M. Birdsall, A. G. Lee, and J. C. Metcalfe, FEBS Lett. 41:122 (1974).
63. H. S. Mason, Ann. Rev. Biochem. 34:595 (1965).
64. A. T. Diplock, Vit. Horm. 32:445 (1974).
65. W. G. Hoekstra, Fed. Proc. 34:2083 (1975).
66. C. E. Hulstaert, I. Molenaar, J. J. M. de Goeij, C. Zegers, and P. L. van Pijpen, Nutr. Metabol. 20:91 (1976).
67. J. Glavind, F. Nannestad Hansen, and C. Sylvén, Int. J. Vit. Nutr. Res. 46:258 (1976).

6 ROLE OF VITAMIN E IN PLANTS, MICROBES, INVERTEBRATES, AND FISH

HAROLD H. DRAPER
University of Guelph
Guelph, Ontario, Canada

I.	Plants	391
II.	Microbes	392
III.	Invertebrates	393
IV.	Fish	394
	References	394

I. PLANTS

The discovery that ubiquinone (coenzyme Q) is involved in mitochondrial electron transport in animals suggested that tocoquinones might serve a similar function in photosynthetic electron transport and photophosphorylation in plants. Evidence was obtained for light-catalyzed nicotinamide adenine dinucleotide phosphate (NADP)-linked oxidation of α-tocopheryl hydroquinone in spinach chloroplasts [1], and it was suggested that the reduced and oxidized forms of α-tocopheryl quinone might serve as an electron pair in photosynthetic electron transport. However, it was subsequently demonstrated that the concentration of these compounds in chloroplasts was too low to support this function and that the primary polyprenylquinones in chloroplasts are plastoquinone and phylloquinone. Ubiquinone was found in the mitochondria, whereas the tocopherols were located in several cell fractions [2,3].

In three species of plants in which non-α-tocopherols are prevalent (French bean, brown seaweed, and tomato) Newton and Pennock [3] found that α-tocopherol was located in the chloroplasts whereas γ-tocopherol and δ-tocopherol were located in extrachloroplastic fractions of the cell. This compartmentalization of different isomers of vitamin E suggests several possibilities: non-α-isomers may traverse the chloroplast membrane and then undergo methylation to form α-tocopherol; all tocopherols may be synthesized in one location and subsequently dispersed to different locations within the cell (this would imply that they have different functions); or there may be separate sites of synthesis for α-tocopherol and the other isomers.

These findings are in agreement with the general observation that α-tocopherol is associated with plant tissue that contains chlorophyll, whereas the other tocopherols are present predominantly in nonchlorophyll-containing tissues such as vegetable oils, nuts, fruits, and cereal seeds. The association of α-tocopherol with chlorophyll suggests some as yet undefined role in photosynthesis. If this is the case, the function of α-tocopherol in plants must be different from that of the tocotrienols, which are confined mainly to cereal oils.

There is a strong correlation between the concentrations of vitamin E in plant oils and the concentration of polyunsaturated lipids. This relationship extends to different varieties of the same species, as illustrated in the correlation between the concentrations of α-linoleic acid and vitamin E (mainly γ-tocopherol) in corn oil [4]. The highest concentration of this vitamin reported in natural oils to date is that in latex lipids, which have been found to contain 8.0% vitamin E by weight [5]. Presumably this high concentration is related to the susceptibility of latex (a high molecular weight unsaturated isoprenoid polymer) to oxidation. The association between vitamin E and unsaturated lipids in plant oils indicates that the antioxidant properties of this vitamin are important in plant as well as animal tissues.

II. MICROBES

Green and coworkers [6] surveyed a range of microorganisms for vitamin E. These organisms included Escherichia coli, Streptococcus faecalis, Bacillus cereus, Streptococcus aureus, the nitrogen-fixing bacterium Rhizobium leguminosarum, three sulfur bacteria, and the protozoa Ochromanas malhamensis, Euglena gracilis, and Tetrahymena pyriformis. Vitamin E (as α-tocopherol) was found only in Ochromonas, Euglena, and to a very small extent in Chlorobium thiosulfatophilum. The concentration of α-tocopherol was found to be related to the amount of chlorophyll synthesized. Subsequent studies revealed that α-tocopherol is also present in many green, brown, red, and blue-green algae. γ-Tocopherol has been found in Euglena gracilis and β-tocopherol in the blue-green algae Anabaena variabilis [7]. Whereas α-tocopheryl quinone is present in many algae, the tocotrienols apparently do not occur in microorganisms.

III. INVERTEBRATES

Gilbert [8] has shown that the fresh water rotifer Asplanchna sieboldi has a specific requirement for RRR-α-tocopherol for maximal growth and adult body size and for sexual reproduction. When cultured in the absence of vitamin E this species multiplies by diploid parthenogenesis, producing only females with a saccate phenotype. When α-tocopherol is added to the medium, females with altered phenotypes are produced which give birth to male offspring and sexual reproduction is initiated. Much of the added vitamin E is deposited in the male offspring where it is most highly concentrated in the testes. Sexual reproduction is conducive to survival of the species because it leads to the production of a resting egg which is less vulnerable to environmental stresses.

The response of A. sieboldi to RRR-α-tocopherol is noteworthy in that it appears to be stereospecific and not duplicable by administration of synthetic antioxidants which are active as substitutes for vitamin E in higher animals. N-N'-diphenyl-phenylenediamine (DPPD), butylated hydroxytoluene (2,6-di-tertiary butyl 4-methylphenol) (BHT), and tocopheramines are inactive, and Ethoxyquin has a growth-depressing effect. The rotifier, which is related to the nematode worms, is the most primitive animal in which vitamin E has been observed to be biologically active. Its biochemical role is unknown, but the circumstances under which its activity is manifested clearly indicate an essential function in male reproduction.

In a study of the nutritional requirements of the snail Biomphalaria glabrata raised under axenic conditions, Vieira [9] observed that vitamin E was necessary for egg production. Although growth was unaffected, this may have been due to the presence of traces of vitamin E in the semi-purified basal diet.

Several insect species have been shown to have a dietary requirement for vitamin E. Meikle and McFarlane [10] observed that when male house crickets (Acheta domesticus L.) were grown on a purified diet lacking in vitamin E, they exhibited impaired spermatogenesis and sterility. The deficiency appeared to block the transformation of spermatids to spermatozoa but did not produce testicular atrophy and other histopathological changes as seen in the male rat. Females apparently were unaffected. House [11] found that vitamin E is necessary for maximal growth and for reproduction of the fly Agria affinis (Fallen). The effects of feeding a vitamin E-deficient diet were reminiscent of those observed in female rats, viz., mating and fertilization occurred normally but embryonic development was arrested.

The presence of two factors in wheat germ oil which are required for normal growth and development of several moths of the genus Ephestia, one replaceable by linoleic acid and the other with vitamin E, has been reported by Fraenkel and Blewett [12]. Chumakova [13] found that vitamin E was essential for reproduction of female beetles of the species C. montrousieri.

These studies indicate that vitamin E is required by representative species of Coleoptera, Orthoptera, and Diptera. While its biochemical role is unknown, there is strong evidence of a general involvement in insect reproduction.

IV. FISH

Vitamin E has been found to be an essential nutrient for several species of fish including Chinook salmon, brown trout, and channel catfish. Extensive studies, particularly by Watanabe [14], Andrews [15], and their collaborators, have shown that vitamin E-deficient fish exhibit many of the deficiency symptoms of birds and mammals: muscular dystrophy, exudative diathesis, anemia, ceroid deposition, and lesions of the pancreas. Exophthalmia, ascites, and depigmentation are additional features of the deficient state.

Most of these conditions can be prevented by Ethoxyquin or other synthetic antioxidants, indicating that vitamin E acts as a lipid antioxidant in fish as it does in higher animals. The observation that the efficacy of synthetic compounds in the prevention of some aspects of the deficiency is substantially lower than that of vitamin E raises the possibility that the vitamin may have additional functions. The current state of knowledge of the role of vitamin E in fish metabolism is therefore similar to that pertaining to its function in warm-blooded animals.

REFERENCES

1. R. A. Dilley and F. L. Crane, Biochim. Biophys. Acta 75:142 (1963).
2. F. L. Crane. In Biochemistry of Quinones. Edited by R. A. Morton, Academic Press, New York, p. 193, 1965.
3. R. P. Newton and J. F. Pennock, Phytochemistry 10:2323 (1971).
4. R. D. Levy, Ph.D. Thesis, University of Illinois, 1972.
5. P. J. Dunphy, K. J. Whittle, J. F. Pennock, and R. A. Morton, Nature (London) 207:521 (1965).
6. J. Green, S. A. Price, and L. Gare, Nature (London) 184:1339 (1959).
7. D. R. Threlfall, Vit. Horm. 29:153 (1971).
8. J. J. Gilbert, Amer. J. Clin. Nutr. 27:1005 (1974).
9. E. C. Vieria, Amer. J. Trop. Med. Hyg. 16:792 (1967).
10. J. E. S. Meikle and J. E. McFarlane, Can. J. Zool. 43:87 (1965).

11. H. L. House, J. Insect Physiol. 12:409 (1966).
12. G. Fraenkel and M. Blewett, J. Exp. Biol. 22:172 (1946).
13. B. M. Chumakova, Vop. Ekol. Kievsk. 8:133 (1962); Biol. Abstr. 45:44502 (1964).
14. T. Watanabe, T. Tsuchiya, and Y. Hashimoto, Bull. Jap. Soc. Sci. Fish 33:843 (1967).
15. T. Murai and J. W. Andrews, J. Nutr. 104:1416 (1974).

7 PATHOLOGY OF VITAMIN E DEFICIENCY

JAMES S. NELSON
Washington University
School of Medicine
St. Louis, Missouri

I.	Introduction	397
II.	Lesions of the Reproductive System	398
	A. Embryopathy	398
	B. Testicular Atrophy	399
III.	Myopathy	402
IV.	Lesions of the Central Nervous System	407
	A. Nutritional Encephalomalacia	407
	B. Localized Axonal Dystrophy	413
V.	Lesions of the Cardiovascular System	417
VI.	Hematopoietic Disorders	418
VII.	Hepatic Necrosis	419
VIII.	Lipopigment	420
IX.	Summary	422
	References	423

I. INTRODUCTION

Dietary deficiency of vitamin E or α-tocopherol and its homologues may be associated with disorders of the vertebrate reproductive system, skeletal muscle, nervous system, cardiovascular system, hematopoietic tissue,

The preparation of this chapter was supported in part by U.S. Public Health Service Grant NS 11277 from NINDS.

*Additional present affiliation: Institut für Neuropathologie, Freie Universitat Berlin, Berlin, West Germany.

and liver. Clinical sydromes associated with these disorders are of
importance chiefly in the field of veterinary medicine. In some instances,
structural lesions may occur without overt clinical or physiological
disturbances (e.g., accumulation of lipopigment).

Several aspects of the pathology of vitamin E deficiency have been
extensively studied by light microscopy. The reviews by Mason [1] and
Follis [2] provide valuable summaries of this work. In the last decade
modern methods of pathological investigation including electron microscopy
and histochemistry have been used to explore the pathology and pathogenesis of lesions associated with vitamin E deficiency. In this chapter the
more recent observations are included with the information derived from
conventional methods of pathological investigation. Current views concerning the pathological effects of vitamin E deficiency on the central
nervous system and skeletal muscle as well as details of the relationship
between vitamin E deficiency and anemia in the premature human infant are
presented. For the most part, descriptive morphological observations
have been emphasized. Where possible, pathogenetic mechanisms are discussed; however, surprisingly little is known about them. The lack of
information results in part because the role of vitamin E in animal metabolism has not been fully defined. Further, many pathogenetic studies
focus chiefly on attempts to establish or eliminate lipid peroxidation as the
principal mechanism responsible for the lesions. Clearly, more frequent
use of a modern, systematic, pathobiological approach to the pathology of
vitamin E deficiency is desirable.

II. LESIONS OF THE REPRODUCTIVE SYSTEM

A. Embryopathy

Fetal death and resorption associated with maternal vitamin E deficiency
was first observed and subsequently studied extensively in the rat by Evans
and colleagues [3]. The disorder has also been described in mice [4],
guinea pigs [5], and swine [6]. According to the work of Evans [3], the
earliest structural abnormalities appear on the eighth gestational day when
the embryonic ectodermal cavity fails to develop. Prior to this time no
physiological abnormalities involving ovulation or the estrus cycle are
present. Ceroid pigment is present within macrophages and the smooth
muscle cells of the uterus. In all other respects, the uterus and the
ovaries are structurally intact.

Subsequent to retarded development of ectodermal structures, the
ectoplacental and amniotic cavities fail to form. Other tissues in which
developmental processes are delayed or abnormal include the mesoderm,
blood islands, and liver. Death of the embryo is evident as early as the
thirteenth gestational day. Following death, the embryo is resorbed. In
addition to embryopathic lesions, placental abnormalities are also seen

which include limited development and inadequate invasion of the placenta by vessels of fetal origin. Evans [3] has attributed death of the fetus to insufficient supply and distribution of nutrients resulting from defective development of the yolk sac and allantois. An alternative vascular mechanism was proposed by Mason [7] who observed dilatation, congestion, and stasis affecting the superficial vascular channels, especially in the head, shoulder, and dorsal trunk regions of the embryo. In the later stages of the process larger and deeper vessels including those in the central nervous system may be involved. On the basis of these observations Mason [7] suggested that a functional or structural defect in the fetal blood vessels was the primary event leading to fetal death.

B. Testicular Atrophy

Irreversible degeneration of the germinal epithelium develops in rats fed an E-deficient diet continuously from the time of weaning [8]. Similar effects are found in the hamster [1] and guinea pig [9]. Testicular atrophy morphologically resembling the lesion of E deficiency has also been observed in rabbits [10], dogs [11], monkeys [1], and pigs [6]. The seminiferous tubules of the mouse are said to be remarkably resistant to the effects of vitamin E deficiency. In one study, however, marked atrophy of the germinal epithelium of the mouse testis was observed after a prolonged period of vitamin E deficiency which extended approximately 18 months [12]. The basis for the species variation in the threshold of the seminiferous tubule to injury induced by vitamin E deficiency is not known.

The histopathology of testicular atrophy in the rat associated with vitamin E deficiency has been studied by a number of investigators [1]. The reports of Mason [1, 7, 8] provide a comprehensive account of the progressive histopathological changes as well as an account of the response of the damaged testis to tocopherol therapy. The degenerative process may be divided into five stages. Initial alterations appear between 50 and 100 days after beginning the dietary regimen in rats fed an E-deficient diet continuously after weaning. The cell bodies of mature spermatoza undergo agglutination with disintegration of the nuclei. Subsequently, the nuclei of spermatids and secondary spermatocytes undergo disintegration. Many germinal epithelial cells are sloughed and then fuse to form large multi-nucleated cells. Those germinal epithelial cells which are not sloughed undergo degenerative changes. In the end stages of the process only the basement membranes of the seminiferous tubule lined by Sertoli cells remain (Figs. 1 and 2). Ceroid pigment is present within the Sertoli cells and in macrophages located between the tubules. Interstitial or Leydig cells are normal. The entire degenerative process is complete approximately 35–50 days after its inception. The seminiferous tubules are not affected simultaneously, so that various stages of the process can be observed in adjacent tubules. Mason's studies also demonstrate that by

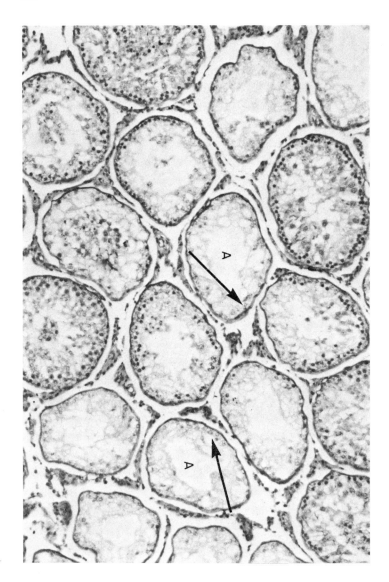

FIG. 1   Vitamin E-deficient rat testis, showing moderate to severe loss
of germinal epithelium in many seminiferous tubules (A) and relative
preservation of Sertoli cells and the basement membrane (arrows). Note
variation in extent of damage from tubule to tubule. X100, Trichrome.

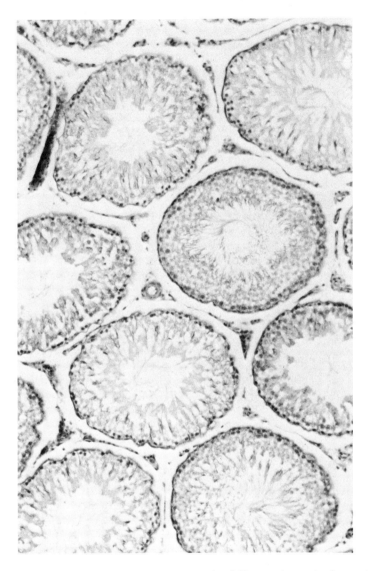

FIG. 2   Normal rat testis. Note the full complement of germinal epithelial cells. Compare tubular diameters in Figs. 1 and 2. X100, Trichrome.

the time light microscopic changes are evident irreversible damage to the germinal epithelium has already occurred. Such damage can be prevented only by administering vitamin E at least 10-15 days prior to the time at which histological lesions are first apparent. Treatment begun later than the 10-15 day period but before the onset of light microscopic changes results in the preservation of some, but not all, of the seminiferous tubules. The incomplete salvage of the testicular tubules is another manifestation of the asynchronous fashion in which the tubules are injured by vitamin E deficiency.

Testicular atrophy resulting from germinal epithelial injury also occurs in states of inanition or vitamin A deficiency. According to Mason [8] testicular damage resulting from vitamin E deficiency can be distinguished histopathologically from the lesions associated with inanition or vitamin A deficiency. Moreover, the germinal epithelial injury associated with these latter conditions is less severe than that induced by vitamin E deficiency and can be reversed by appropriate therapy even in the late stages of the disorders. These observations point to the existence of a relatively specific testicular injury resulting from vitamin E deficiency.

III. MYOPATHY

The first evidence of a muscular disorder in association with vitamin E deficiency is contained in studies reported by Evans and Burr in 1928 [14]. The offspring of E-deficient mother rats were observed to lose the righting reflex approximately 1 or 2 days before the weaning. The disability was progressive, leading eventually to paralysis and death. Less than 20% of the animals recovered; some of these were permanently paralyzed. Development of the disease was prevented by administration of substances rich in vitamin E.

The pathological basis of the weakness in suckling or weanling rats was not investigated until several years later when Lipshutz [15] examined material from the original study. He attributed the weakness and paralysis to widespread degenerative changes in the central nervous system. This work could not be confirmed in subsequent investigations. Extensive skeletal muscle necrosis, the lesion actually responsible for the weakness, was finally identified by Olcott [16] 10 years after the original report by Evans and Burr [14].

Shortly after the observations by Evans and Burr [14] but prior to the studies of Olcott [16], profound structural lesions in the skeletal muscles of experimentally malnourished rabbits and guinea pigs were noted by Goettsch and Pappenheimer [17]. The myopathy was called "nutritional muscular dystrophy." Although the disease was actually induced by feeding an E-deficient diet, its relationship to vitamin E deficiency was not recognized until several years later.

Acute or chronic necrotizing myopathy is now regarded as one of the most common manifestations of the vitamin E deficiency [1]. The histo-pathological changes may vary to some extent from species to species, in accordance with the methods used to induce the disorder, or as an expression of the rate at which the disease is evolving. In all cases, however, the basic process is a necrotizing myopathy (Figs. 3 and 4) [18]. Histologically there is marked random variation in the cross-sectional diameter of the muscle fibers. Occasional fibers contain internal nuclei. Necrosis and phagocytosis of individual muscle fibers are seen. Regenerative changes such as cytoplasmic basophilia and the formation of clusters of vesicular sarcolemmal nuclei frequently containing nucleoli may be present to some extent. The endomysial connective tissue is increased, particularly in areas where fibers have disappeared as a result of necrosis or atrophy. Acute or chronic inflammatory cells are found chiefly in relationship to necrotic muscle fibers. In the chronic stage of the myopathy there may be extensive focal replacement of muscle fibers by fat and fibrous tissue. The myopathic process affects virtually all of the skeletal muscles, includ-ing the diaphragm, in a symmetrical fashion. The extent and severity of the muscle lesions correlates well with the degree of weakness observed clinically.

The ultrastructural changes of the myopathy have been described in several species [19-21]. Alterations which antedate the onset of overt light microscopic lesions involve the mitochondria, the microcirculation, and fibroblasts. It is uncertain whether the ultrastructural damage directly causes or simply heralds the development of the widespread nectotizing myopathy. Similarly, increased lysosomal enzyme activities observed in the early stages of the process [22,23] could conceivably rep-resent an initiating event, or (as is more likely) reflect part of the non-specific response of skeletal muscle to injury.

The pathogenesis of the myopathy is incompletely understood. A number of studies clearly indicate that the disease results from a deficiency of vitamin E [24,25]. In some instances selenium deficiency may be asso-ciated with the myopathy [21]. Relatively little is known about the specific biological functions of selenium. Three enzyme-catalyzed reactions including glutathione peroxidase of erythrocytes are known to require a selenium-containing protein [26]. All are oxidation-reduction reactions. A fourth selenoprotein has been isolated from the heart and skeletal muscle of lambs. The biological function of the protein has not been defined; how-ever, its properties indicate that it may also be involved in an oxidation-reduction process [26]. Because the necrotizing myopathy is induced or strongly influenced by a deficiency of substances involved in oxidation reactions, lipid peroxidation has been suggested as a basic pathogenetic mechanism. This hypothesis is supported by studies demonstrating facilitated induction of the myopathy when the concentration of dietary polyunsaturated fatty acids is increased [27,28]. Conclusive evidence of

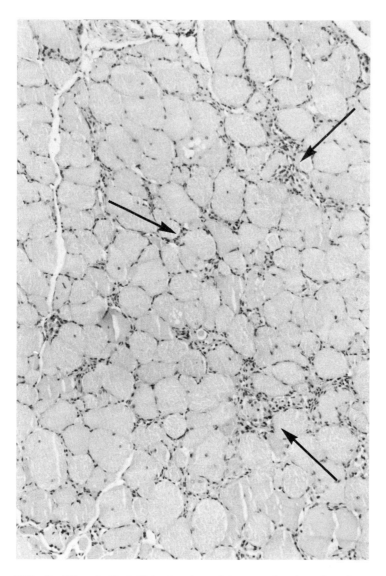

FIG. 3   Vitamin E-deficient rat quadriceps, showing chronic necrotizing myopathy (arrows).   X100, hematoxylin, and eosin.

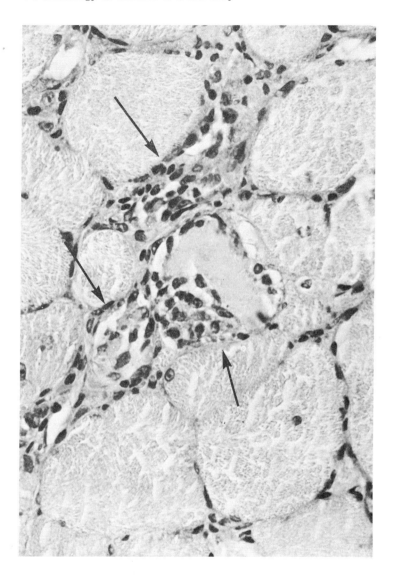

FIG. 4 Vitamin E-deficient rat quadriceps, showing necrosis and phagocytosis of individual muscle fibers (arrows). Note variability of intact muscle fibers, some of which contain internal sarcolemmal nuclei. X400, hematoxylin and eosin.

lipid peroxidation, however, in the affected skeletal muscles is not available. Further, in some species, antioxidants other than vitamin E have no effect on the progress of the myopathy.

The biochemical characteristics of the myopathy have been extensively studied. One of the most intriguing and still unexplained observations is the increased consumption of oxygen by E-deficient muscle [29-34]. The increase has been observed in association with well-developed histopathological changes and in the absence of such lesions [34]. Administration of vitamin E rapidly lowers the oxygen consumption to normal levels [31-33]. The evidence strongly suggests that the increased rate of oxygen consumption reflects an alteration in the E-deficient muscle fiber, rather than reactive changes in the muscle. The basis for the biochemical alteration is unknown. Conceivably, the increase in oxygen consumption could result from an uncoupling of oxidative phosphorylation secondary to damage affecting lipid-rich mitochondrial membranes.

Necrotizing myopathies histologically similar to the vitamin E deficiency disorder occur spontaneously in calves, sheep, swine, and horses [35, 36]. Form a pathogenetic standpoint these conditions are complex. Several factors have been implicated in their development including deficiencies of vitamin E and selenium, excessive amounts of dietary polyunsaturated fatty acids, the presence of legumes in the diet, and excessive muscular activity [36].

Throughout this discussion we have referred to the muscle disease associated with vitamin E-deficiency as a necrotizing myopathy rather than using the name suggested by Goettsch and Pappenheimer [17], nutritional muscular dystrophy. The latter term suggests that there may be a significant etiological relationship between the necrotizing myopathy of vitamin E deficiency and human muscular dystrophy. It is true that the pathological changes in both conditions are similar. The occurrence of these similarities, however, does not indicate that the two diseases are identical, only that similar mechanisms and similar structures are involved in their pathogenesis. The human muscular dystrophies are regarded as a distinct group of progressive, genetically determined, primary, degenerative myopathies in which muscle necrosis may sometimes be present [37]. The classification of a disease as a type of human muscular dystrophy is based on the concurrent use of a number of clinical and pathological characteristics, not simply the pathological changes alone. Since the clinicopathological characteristics of the human muscular dystrophies are clearly and sharply defined and because there is no obvious etiological relationship between the myopathy of vitamin E deficiency and human muscular dystrophy, it seems desirable to restrict the use of the term muscular dystrophy to the genetically determined human disorder and apply the term nutritionally induced necrotizing myopathy to the disorders resulting from tocopherol deficiency.

IV. LESIONS OF THE CENTRAL NERVOUS SYSTEM

A. Nutritional Encephalomalacia

Nutritional encephalomalacia (NE) is an acute central nervous system (CNS) disease of growing chicks with structurally organized but incompletely mature brains [38]. NE may be consistently produced by feeding chicks a diet deficient in tocopherol and other antioxidants and enriched with linoleic acid [39-43]. Spontaneous outbreaks of the disorder have been described in commercially bred chicks [44,45]. The clinical signs of NE in their usual order of development are ataxia of gait and stance, failure of righting reflexes, torsion of the neck and body, and eventually prostration and death. The rate at which the process evolves varies from a few hours to a few days.

The pathology of NE was described first by Wolf and Pappenheimer [46] who found edema and zones of acute parenchymal necrosis in the cerebellum and occasionally the cerebrum (Figs. 5 and 6). The necrosis was accompanied by microglial proliferation, phagocyte formation, capillary proliferation, and eventually, astrocytic and mesodermal organization of the lesions. The lesions were noted to be similar to infarcts caused by occlusive vascular disease. Hyalin thrombi were seen in small blood vessels, especially capillaries, but their significance with regard to the necrosis was discounted because of their inconstant relationship to the necrotic foci.

The pathogenesis of NE remains obscure. Tocopherol deficiency and inclusion of linoleic acid in the diet have been shown to be necessary prerequisites for the development of the disease [39-43]. The antioxidant activity of the tocopherols [47-52]; the arrest, reversibility, or prevention of the disease with synthetic antioxidants [53-57]; and the easy oxidizability of linoleic acid or its derivatives such as arachidonic acid suggest that NE may somehow be related to lipid peroxidation, for example, through accumulation of peroxides in toxic amounts or uncontrolled peroxidative alteration of membrane phospholipids containing unsaturated fatty acids. Direct evidence of peroxidation such as the demonstration of the products of peroxidation in the brains of affected chicks examined immediately after death is not available [58]. In one study, chicks given peroxides of linoleic acid developed acute neurological signs and died [59]. Pathological examination of these animals showed acute, nonspecific changes in the cerebellum. The relationship between this condition and NE has not been further clarified.

Progressive endothelial cell changes characterized by lysosomal activation selectively affecting the CNS microcirculation have been observed during the induction of NE, prior to the onset of neurological signs or the development of parenchymal necrosis [57,60,61]. The alterations include a progressive increase in the deposition of acid phosphatase reaction product

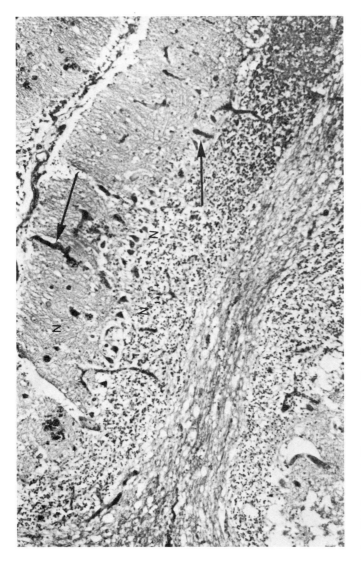

FIG. 5 Chick cerebellar cortex with vitamin E deficiency–nutritional encephalomalacia, showing necrosis of molecular, Purkinje, and granular layers with occasional hemorrhage (N). Note the darkly stained hyalin "thrombi" in a number of the distended capillaries (arrows). X100, Luxol fast blue–PAS.

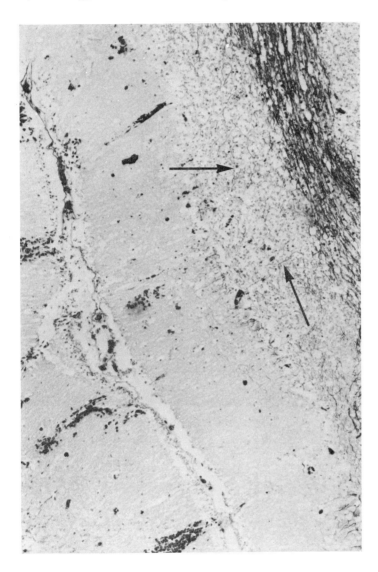

FIG. 6   Chick cerebellar cortex with vitamin E deficiency-nutritional encephalomalacia. This section, adjacent to the specimen in Fig. 5, was silver stained to demonstrate disintegration of axons and dendrites in the necrotic cortex (arrows). 100X, Sevier-Munger.

and an accumulation of yellow autofluorescent granules in and limited to
the endothelial cells of brain capillaries (Fig. 7). The alterations are not
seen in the heart, liver, kidney, spleen, or skeletal muscle. They are
absent when the diet is supplemented with α-tocopherol or promethazine.
The autofluorescent grangules are insoluble in alcohol and xylol and do not
stain with oil red "O" in frozen sections or with PAS and acid-fast techniques in paraffin sections [57, 60]. Similar vascular alterations develop
in tocopherol deficient rats when high levels of polyunsaturated fatty acids
are included in the tocopherol-deficient diet [62]. Lipid histochemical
studies suggest that the granules contain phospholipid [61]. The fluorescence of the granules is unaffected by immersion in dilute ammonium
sulfide or incubation in the Gomori acid phosphatase substrate solution.
Immersion of the sections in dilute ammonium sulfide after incubation in
the Gomori acid phosphatase substrate solution quenches the fluorescence.
Concomitant with the light microscopic accumulation of acid phosphatase
reaction product and autofluorescent granules, rounded, electron-dense
bodies accumulate within the endothelial cell cytoplasm of brain capillaries
(Fig. 8). The selective deposition of acid phosphatase reaction product in
these bodies (identifying their lysosomal character) has been demonstrated
by electron histochemistry [60].

The direct relationship of the capillary lysosomal alterations to the
development of the necrotic foci and edema is uncertain. Conceivably, the
changes may represent the initial stage of an endothelial injury leading
eventually to increased vascular permeability or endothelial necrosis and
thrombosis. This hypothesis is supported by a number of observations.
Increased vascular permeability to trypan blue associated with brain
necrosis occurs at or near the onset of overt neurological symptoms [63].
Quantitative changes in brain-water content are demonstrable shortly after
the onset of neurological symptoms characteristic of NE. The percent dry
weight of the lesion-containing cerebellum from chicks with neurological
symptoms is 20-25% less than the percent dry weight of normal chick
cerebellum or of the cerebellum from tocopherol-deficient chicks without
neurological symptoms [63]. This change reflects a substantial increase
in cerebellar water content apparently developing in conjunction with the
onset of neurological symptoms. Swelling and disintegration of cerebellar
endothelial cells have been reported in chicks with evidence of acute NE
including ataxia and gross cerebellar edema [64]. However, none of these
studies provide any direct evidence that overt vascular injury precedes
the development of parenchymal lesions. It is possible, for example, that
the changes in the capillaries as well as the parenchymal alterations are
components of a regional lesion produced by the same agent. A study in
which the temporal evolution of the vascular and parenchymal changes are

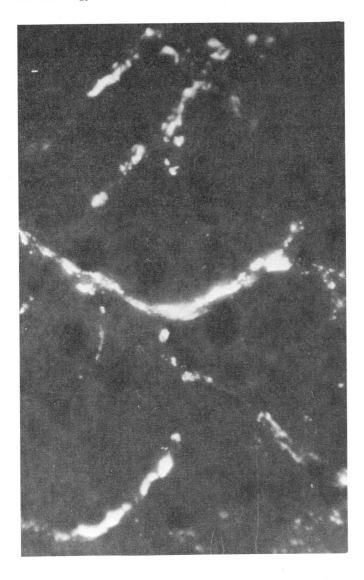

FIG. 7   Chick cerebellar cortex with vitamin E deficiency-prenecrotic
phase of nutritional encephalomalacia, showing accumulation of autofluorescent granules in capillary endothelium.   Unstained frozen section.
X400.

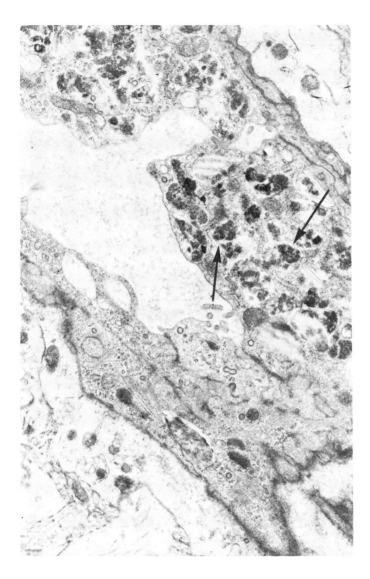

FIG. 8   Chick cerebellar cortex with vitamin E deficiency-prenecrotic phase of nutritional encephalomalacia, showing accumulation of electron-dense bodies (lysosomes) in capillary endothelial cytoplasm (arrows). X24,750.

carefully and systematically examined would aid in clarifying this point.

Some indirect evidence indicates that capillary damage is causally related to the development of the parenchymal lesions. The brain capillaries are selectively and constantly affected by the lysosomal abnormalities. These changes appear and in many cases progress in intensity prior to development of the necrotic lesions. The histological characteristics of necrotic parenchymal lesions resemble those of infarcts; their size and shape sometimes suggest that they occupy the territory supplied by small caliber vessels [57]. True thrombi are demonstrable in capillaries adjacent to the necrosis (Fig. 9). On the other hand, the lysosomal alterations are also seen in parts of the brain which are only occasional sites of necrosis in NE, e.g., the cerebrum [60]. Moreover, although every chick with NE shows the capillary changes, the necrotic lesions may occur at any stage in progression of the vascular reaction [60].

B. Localized Axonal Dystrophy

In contrast to the situation obtaining in chickens, definition of the neuropathological changes associated with vitamin E deficiency in mammals, particularly rats, has evolved slowly and with controversy. Ringsted [65] described a neurological syndrome consisting of ataxia, bilateral symmetrical muscle atrophy, and paralysis in adult rats maintained on a vitamin E-deficient diet for prolonged periods. Subsequently, Einarson and Ringsted [66] investigated the neuropathological basis of the syndrome. Lesions were found in the spinal cord, peripheral nerves, and skeletal muscles. The earliest alterations involved the dorsal roots and dorsal columns, especially the fasciculus gracilis. The process began at the lumbar level and gradually progressed rostrally sometimes as high as the lower cervical segments. Axons and myelin sheaths were lost in approximately equal numbers. These changes were accompanied by fibrillary astrocytosis and lipid phagocyte formation. Somewhat later, myopathic changes were evident in skeletal muscles. During the later stages of the process, degenerative changes in the anterior horns including the neuronal accumulation of lipofuscin or ceroid pigment and, possibly, nerve cell loss with mild astrocytosis were observed. Occasionally, degeneration of the corticospinal tracts was observed. The findings of Einarson and Ringsted [66] were supported by Monnier [67]. In contrast, Wolf and Pappenheimer [68] found no significant neuropathologic changes in rats maintained up to 365 days on an E-deficient diet. In a later publication [69], however, they noted the presence of lipopigment in CNS neurons of E-deficient rats and absence of the pigment in rats receiving protective doses of wheat germ oil

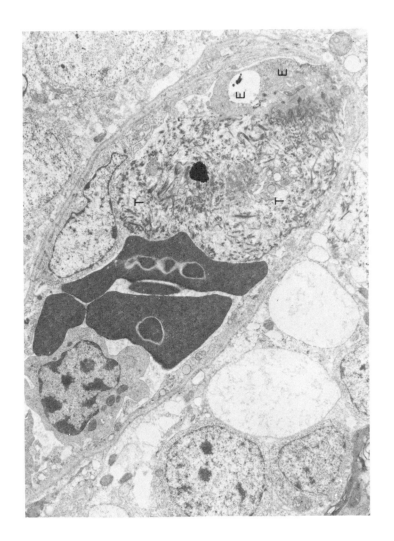

FIG. 9   Chick cerebellar cortex with vitamin E deficiency-necrotic phase of nutritional encephalomalacia. Capillary endothelial degeneration (E) and thrombosis (T).   X9000.

or tocopherol. The accumulation of lipopigment was not associated with nerve cell loss or neurological disturbances. The investigations of Wolf and Pappenheimer were stimulated in part by the growing use, in the late 1930s, of vitamin E as a treatment for amyotrophic lateral sclerosis and related motor neuron disorders. They provided early, substantial experimental evidence against an etiologic or pathogenetic relationship between tocopherol deficiency and amyotrophic lateral sclerosis. Later, in a critical review of his studies, Einarson [70] acknowledged that he had probably overemphasized the significance of the anterior horn cell alterations. He reaffirmed the occurrence of degeneration in the posterior columns of the spinal cord. It is this lesion, rather than the controversial and dubious anterior horn cell degeneration, that has been shown to be the characteristic neuropathological lesion in the E-deficient rat.

The regular occurrence of posterior column degeneration in rats maintained for prolonged periods on an E-deficient diet has been confirmed by several groups of investigators including Luttrell and Mason [71]; Malamud, Nelson, and Evans [72]; and Pentschew and Schwarz [73]. Pentschew and Schwarz [73] extended these observations. They noted the presence of swollen, dystrophic axons in the posterior columns, gracile and cuneate nuclei, the posterior horns, Clarke's column, the sensory nucleus of the fifth nerve and the nucleus of the tractus solitarius (Fig. 10).

Axonal changes in vitamin E deficiency are most numerous in the gracile and cuneate nuclei. The distal portions of the axons are most severely affected. With electron microscopy the axonal swelling has been shown to result from an accumulation of various cytoplasmic organelles including neurofilaments, mitochondria, and collections of electron-dense bodies descriptively identified as microbodies, or multivesicular or multigranular bodies [74-76].

The pathogenesis of the posterior column degeneration and its precise relationship to vitamin E are unknown. The severity of the lesions but not their incidence may be influenced by dietary lipids [71]. Histologically and topographically, similar lesions are found in humans with cystic fibrosis [77], congenital biliary atresia [78], and with advancing age [79, 80]. Conceivably, vitamin E deficiency could play a role in the development of the axonal changes in the first two conditions; both are known to be associated with disturbed absorption of fat-soluble vitamins and laboratory evidence of vitamin E deficiency. Axonal changes of a similar but not identical nature and with wider or different topographical distribution are seen in a number of human neurological disorders, including infantile neuroaxonal dystrophy [8] and Hallervorden-Spatz disease [82]. Vitamin E is without effect on the course or severity of infantile neuroaxonal dystrophy [83]. Similar axonal changes seen in the various experimental and naturally occurring conditions noted above probably represent the response of the axon to injuries of varying etiology and should not be regarded as specific indicators of a particular disease.

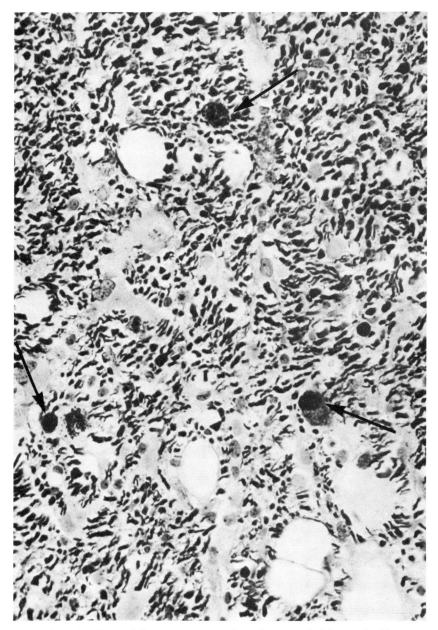

FIG. 10   Vitamin E-deficient rat spinal cord.   Rounded large darkly
stained axons are present in the posterior columns (arrows).   X400,
Sevier-Munger.

As noted previously, lysosomal changes have been observed in the cerebral capillaries of rats fed an E-deficient diet enriched with linoleic acid [62].

V. LESIONS OF THE CARDIOVASCULAR SYSTEM

The observations of Dam and Glavind and others have established that vitamin E protects chicks against a condition known as exudative diathesis [84-86]. In this disorder, plasma leaks from capillaries in the subcutaneous tissues, resulting in extensive accumulations of fluid which may have a green color. Adipose tissue, connective tissue, or muscle may be affected. Microscopically, in addition to the edema, small numbers of erythrocytes and leukocytes may be present.

Several lines of evidence suggest that lipid peroxidation is involved in the pathogenesis of the disorder. Exudative diathesis was one of the first instances in which vitamin E deficiency could be associated with peroxidation of fat in vivo [58]. The disease begins at approximately the time lipid peroxides are initially detected in subcutaneous fat [58]. Both vitamin E and selenium are completely effective in preventing development of the disease. Scott and his coworkers [87] have shown that vitamin E prevents development of the disease by interrupting the formation of peroxides from polyunsaturated fatty acids located within cell membranes. Selenium, as noted earlier, is an essential component of the glutathione peroxidase system responsible for the catalytic breakdown of peroxides [26]. Optimal function of this system facilitates destruction of fatty acid hydroperoxides before they cause serious membrane alterations.

A less well-defined relationship between vascular lesions and vitamin E is suggested by several experimental studies. Holman [88, 89] showed that a necrotizing arteritis in dogs induced by renal insufficiency and feeding of a high fat diet can be retarded or prevented by administration of vitamin E. The vascular damage associated with choline deficiency in rats can be decreased in severity by dietary supplementation with vitamin E [90].

Clinical or pathological evidence of myocardial disease in association with vitamin E deficiency has been observed in ruminants [91-95], swine [96, 97], rats [98], mice [99], and rabbits [100-102]. A necrotizing myopathy frequently accompanies the myocardial lesions. Occasionally, myocardial lesions are the dominant pathological abnormality. The gross form and distribution of the lesions may vary according to the species affected. Microscopically there is extensive necrosis of cardiac muscle fibers and moniliform calcification of myofibrils. The alterations resemble those seen in the necrotizing myopathy of skeletal muscle.

The cardiomyopathy of vitamin E deficiency in the pig has been studied extensively by Nafstad and coworkers [96, 97]. Swine fed a high fat diet deficient in vitamin E develop myocardial necrosis associated with fibrinoid necrosis of arteries. In some cases "mulberry heart disease" is observed. Ischemia caused by vascular insufficiency is thought to be responsible in part for the myocardial damage. The disease is prevented by dietary supplements of vitamin E.

Myocardial lesions similar to those of vitamin E deficiency may be seen in spontaneously occurring cardiomyopathies affecting cattle, sheep, pigs, and horses [35,36]. These diseases may at times respond to vitamin E or selenium. Primates exposed to E-deficiency regimens similar to those used to induce conspicuous heart disease in ruminants show no myocardial abnormalities [103].

VI. HEMATOPOIETIC DISORDERS

The increased susceptibility of erythrocytes from vitamin E-deficient birds and mammals to lysis in hydrogen peroxide or dialuric acid has been extensively documented [104-107]. In the absence of oxidant stress, E deficiency may not be associated with changes in the hematocrit, hemoglobin concentration, or erythrocyte count [108,109]. Anemia unrelated to apparent oxidant stress has been observed in E-deficient monkeys [103], pigs [110], and rats [111]. In the monkey, Fitch [103] has shown that anemia results from ineffective erythropoiesis. The disorder develops after 5-30 months of an E-deficient regimen. In addition to increased in vitro susceptibility to lysis by hydrogen peroxide, red cell survival is markedly reduced. In the bone marrow, morphological abnormalities are seen in the red blood cell precursors. The nuclear chromatin is homogeneously distributed and densely staining rather than clumped. The myeloid series and the megakaryocytes are normal. Similar bone marrow changes have been observed in anemic vitamin E-deficient pigs. Primate anemia responds dramatically to vitamin E therapy.

Vitamin E deficiency is associated with a mild normochromic normocytic anemia in the premature human infant [112,113]. The basis of the anemia is believed to be increased red cell hemolysis resulting from peroxidative damage to the erythrocyte membrane [113]. In addition to deficiency of vitamin E promoted in part by the limited capacity of the premature newborn to absorb fat-soluble vitamins, other factors such as iron or linoleic acid may play a role in development of the anemia [113]. Both of these latter substances are often contained in substantial concentrations in the dietary formulations given premature infants. In addition to anemia, an elevated reticulocyte count and thrombocytosis are frequently present. Acanthocytes may be seen in the peripheral blood smears. The anemia responds to administration of vitamin E; however, therapy is complicated by the fact that the premature newborn infant is capable of absorbing only small amounts of the vitamin. The limited intestinal absorptive capacity persists from birth to approximately 12 weeks of age.

Platelet aggregation is believed to be triggered by an endoperoxide formed during the synthesis of prostaglandin E_2 from arachidonic acid. Since vitamin E prevents the formation of the peroxides in adipose tissues, it is conceivable that it could inhibit peroxidation of arachidonate in platelets, thereby inhibiting platelet aggregation. Recent studies demonstrate that platelet aggregation and subsequently platelet counts are increased in rats fed a vitamin E-deficient diet [114].

VII. HEPATIC NECROSIS

Hepatic lesions chiefly at the histopathological level have been reported in a number of species [115-117]. For the most part, these lesions represent accumulation of lipofuscin or ceroid pigment. In mice [117], a form of fatty metamorphosis may occur.

More extensive and significant hepatic lesions occur in vitamin E-deficient rats. Spontaneous necrosis sometimes associated with hemorrhage develops in rats raised on diets low in vitamin E and sulfur-containing amino acids [118-120], or on diets containing high concentrations of certain types of yeast [121]. Necrosis develops approximately 2-3 weeks after initiation of the necrogenic dietary regimen. Prenecrotic changes are evident by light and electron microscopy. The studies of Hartroft and his colleagues [122, 123] indicate that regarding the genesis of the necrosis the most important of the prenecrotic changes is progressive degeneration of the hepatocellular plasma membranes facing the sinusoids. Although there is evidence of lipoperoxidation affecting the plasma membranes, the process is detected only late in the prenecrotic phase when other structure and enzyme histochemical changes are established. The initial foci of necrosis usually develop in the centrilobular zone (zone 3 of Rappaport's acinus). At a later stage other lobular zones are affected. Necrotic hepatocytes are replaced by inflammatory infiltrates composed chiefly of eosinophils, macrophages, and histiocytes. Initially, the Kupffer cells in necrotic areas are uninvolved. Eventually, however, ceroid pigment is present in Kupffer cells as well as in macrophages adjacent to the necrotic foci. Electron microscopic examination of the necrotic lesions discloses advanced degeneration of plasma membranes along the sinusoidal borders, erythrophagia in liver cells, and evidence of ceroid accumulation in Kupffer cells. Sinusoids adjacent to the necrotic foci are obstructed to varying degrees by masses of platelets, and occasionally, fibrin. Addition of vitamin E to the diet prevents development of the necrosis.

Since evidence of lipoperoxidation is demonstrable only late in the prenecrotic phase of the disorder after other changes are well established,

Hartroft et al. [123] have suggested that the membrane-stabilizing properties of vitamin E and selenium are unrelated to the antioxidant activities
of these substances. They further proposed that the decrease in sodium/
potassium-activated ATPase activity is a basic mechanism in the pathogenesis of the hepatic necrosis.

Acute centrilobular hepatic necrosis can be induced in otherwise
healthy rats by administration of carbon tetrachloride [124]. Treatment of
the rats with vitamin E prior to administration of carbon tetrachloride
prevents the development of liver necrosis and death. Other substances
which have antioxidant properties are also effective in this regard.

VIII. LIPOPIGMENT

The premature and/or excessive accumulation of lipopigment is one of the
most common cellular responses to injury linked to vitamin E deficiency.
The nomenclature of the lipopigments found in animal cells is variable
[125]. The material associated with vitamin E deficiency has been referred
to as lipofuscin, ceroid [126], or simply the lipopigment of vitamin E
deficiency (Fig. 11). Other types of lipopigments include wear and tear
pigment, lipochrome pigment, and age pigment. The physical, biochemical, and histochemical characteristics of these pigments, including the
lipopigment of vitamin E deficiency, are similar. It is not known whether
the same mechanisms are involved in the production of these pigments;
however, their closely related physical and chemical characteristics suggest that they originate from similar cellular materials [127].

The physical and histochemical characteristics of the lipopigments
include insolubility in xylol, autofluorescence, and positive staining in
paraffin sections with oil red "O" or sudanophilic dyes, and with PAS. In
some classifications, lipofuscin and ceroid are regarded as related but
distinct pigments. Part of this distinction is based on the fact that ceroid
is characteristically positive in acid-fast stains, while lipofuscin usually
is not [125]. At the ultrastructural level the morphology of both substances is similar; however, granules of ceroid exhibit greater morphological variability than lipofuscin bodies [127]. A number of experimental
studies indicate that ceroid and lipofuscin are not altogether different substances but represent different stages in the formation of a lipopigment
[128-131]. Using an experimental model, Hartroft [129,130] demonstrated
that the lipopigments formed initially (termed interceroids or preceroids)
were sudanophilic and insoluble in 95% alcohol, but soluble in xylol. As
the lesion evolved histologically, the substances became insoluble in xylol
and developed autofluorescence and PAS positivity. The latest stage in
the evolution of the pigment appeared to be the development of acid-fast,
positive staining characteristics. Larger amounts of ceroid were formed

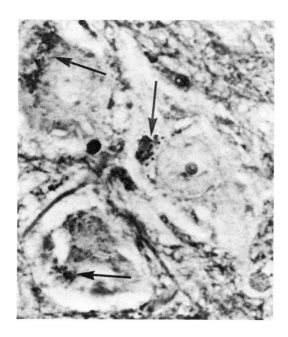

FIG. 11   Vitamin E-deficient rat spinal cord.   Lipopigment granules in cytoplasm of neurons in anterior horn (arrows).   X250, Luxol fast blue-PAS.

when the lipid precursors contained substantial amounts of polyunsaturated fatty acids.

The formation of lipopigment in connection with vitamin E deficiency has been observed in a number of animal species and in several different types of cells including smooth muscle [132], cardiac muscle [132], skeletal muscle [132], neurons [133-137], macrophages, and hepatocytes [1,138].   Lipid peroxidation has been implicated in the pathogenesis of lipopigment [139,140].   In the absence of an effective antioxidant such as tocopherol, the development and accumulation of intracellular free radicals and peroxides (normally limited processes) are greatly enhanced [141]. Lipid membranes containing highly reactive unsaturated fatty acids are particularly prone to peroxidation.   The excess free radicals and peroxides resulting from accelerated lipid peroxidation react with adjacent lipid membranes or other cellular components, thus producing peroxidative damage followed by accumulation of substances such as malonaldehyde, and eventually lipopigment.   The intracellular formation of lipopigment, even in substantial quantities, does not by itself appear to compromise cellular function. Furthermore, disturbances in cell physiology cannot be readily correlated with the formation of the pigment. The accumulation of the lipopigment may be regarded as evidence of a state of intracellular injury in which the degree of damage is balanced by a repair process so that overt physiological disorders are not apparent.

In humans and in some animals a group of hereditary nervous system disorders have been identified which are characterized clinically by progressive dementia, blindness, and movement disorders, and pathologically by the accumulation of large amounts of lipopigments in neurons in various parts of the central and peripheral nervous systems. The lipopigments have the histochemical characteristics of the lipofuscins or ceroids. They are often distinguishable, however, from the usual type of lipopigment encountered, e.g., during aging, by ultrastructural examination. Furthermore, the degree of intracellular accumulation is sufficient to produce obvious morphological enlargement of the cell body. In the later stages of the disease process frank and indisputable nerve loss with reactive astrocytosis is evident. The diseases are known by a variety of eponymic designations including Spielmeyer-Vogt-Batten disease. Other terms include late or juvenile onset amaurotic family idiocy. Zeman [142] has generically termed these disorders the neuronal ceroid lipofuscinoses.

The pathogenesis of these diseases is unknown, but disturbances in intracellular peroxidation have been suggested as a basic mechanism. Evidence of peroxidase deficiency has been observed in some cases, leading to the speculation that peroxides formed in the course of naturally occurring biochemical processes in these cases may accumulate within cells and cause membrane damage [143].

In some instances treatment of neuronal ceroid lipofuscinosis with antioxidants including vitamin E has been attempted. The results of the treatment are difficult to evaluate. Failure of patients to recover neurological function could be the result of irreversible damage rather than lack of therapeutic response. Consequently, the effect of antioxidant treatment may be best judged by its effect on the progress of the disease. The neuronal ceroid lipofuscinoses are slowly progressive so that therapy must be extended over a number of years to determine whether any change in the rate of progression has occurred.

IX. SUMMARY

Deficiency of vitamin E is associated with structural evidence of cellular injury in a number of tissues. The mechanisms involved in the pathogenesis of these injuries are largely unknown. Studies on the cerebral microcirculation [60-62], liver [122, 123], and gastrointestinal epithelium [144] from E-deficient animals indicate that the important initial damage involves membranes of cells or subcellular organelles. Identification and characterization of the cellular injury by modern pathological techniques will lead eventually to precise identification of all the processes associated with cellular injury in vitamin E deficiency and will contribute to our understanding of the normal functions of vitamin E.

REFERENCES

1. K. E. Mason. In The Vitamins. Edited by W. H. Sebrell and R. S. Harris, Vol. 3, Part VII, New York, Academic, 1954, pp. 514-562.
2. R. H. Follis, Jr., Deficiency Disease, Springfield, Ill., Charles C. Thomas, 1958, pp. 159-170, 383-384.
3. H. M. Evans, G. O. Burr, and T. Althausen, Memoirs of the University of California, Vol. 8, 1927, pp. 1-23.
4. W. L. Bryan and K. E. Mason, Amer. J. Physiol. 131:263 (1940).
5. A. M. Pappenheimer and M. Goettsch, Proc. Soc. Exp. Biol. Med. 47:268 (1941).
6. F. B. Adamstone, J. L. Krider, and M. F. James, Ann. N.Y. Acad. Sci. 62:260 (1949).
7. K. E. Mason, Yale J. Biol. Med. 14:605 (1942).
8. K. E. Mason, Amer. J. Anat. 52:153 (1933).
9. A. M. Pappenheimer and C. Schogoleff, Amer. J. Pathol. 20:239 (1944).
10. M. L. Chevral and M. Cormier, C. R. Acad. Sci. 226:1854 (1948).
11. K. M. Brinkhous and E. D. Warner, Amer. J. Pathol. 17:81 (1941).
12. Z. Menschik, M. K. Munk, T. Rogalski, O. Rymaszewski, and T. J. Szczesniak, Ann. N.Y. Acad. Sci. 52:94 (1949).
13. H. Kaunitz, A. M. Pappenheimer, and C. Schogoleff, Amer. J. Pathol. 20:247 (1944).
14. H. M. Evans and G. O. Burr, J. Biol. Chem. 76:273 (1928).
15. M. D. Lipshutz, Rev. Neurol. 65:221 (1936).
16. H. S. Olcott, J. Nutr. 15:221 (1938).
17. M. Goettsch and A. M. Pappenheimer, J. Exp. Med. 54:145 (1931).
18. B. Q. Banker. In Neuromuscular Disorders, Vol. 38, New York, Res. Publ. Assoc. Nerv. Ment. Dis., 1961, pp. 197-233.
19. E. L. Howes, H. M. Price, and J. M. Blumberg, Amer. J. Pathol. 45:599 (1964).
20. J. F. Van Vleet, B. V. Ball, and J. Simon, Amer. J. Pathol. 52:1067 (1968).
21. P. R. Sweeney, J. G. Buchanan-Smith, F. de Mille, J. R. Pettit, and E. T. Moran, Amer. J. Pathol. 68:493 (1972).
22. H. Zalin, A. L. Tappel, K. A. Caldwell, S. Shibko, I. D. Desai, T. A. Holliday, J. Biol. Chem. 237:2678 (1962).

23. I. D. Desai, C. C. Calvert, M. L. Scott, and A. L. Tappel, Proc. Soc. Exp. Biol. Med. 115:462 (1964).

24. A. M. Pappenheimer, Physiol. Rev. 23:37 (1943).

25. A. M. Pappenheimer, On Certain Aspects of Vitamin E Deficiency. Springfield, Ill., Charles C. Thomas, 1948.

26. T. C. Stadtman, Science 183:915 (1974).

27. L. A. Witting and M. K. Horwitt, J. Nutr. 82:19 (1964).

28. L. A. Witting and M. K. Horwitt, J. Nutr. 84:351 (1964).

29. J. Victor, Amer. J. Physiol. 108:229 (1934).

30. L. L. Madsen, J. Nutr. 11:471 (1936).

31. I. Friedman and H. A. Mattill, Amer. J. Physiol. 131:595 (1940).

32. O. B. Houchin, Fed. Proc. 1:117 (1942).

33. O. B. Houchin and H. A. Mattill, Proc. Soc. Exp. Biol. Med. 50:216 (1942).

34. H. Kaunitz and A. M. Pappenheimer, Amer. J. Physiol. 138:328 (1943).

35. W. J. Hadlow. In Comparative Neuropathology. Edited by J. R. M. Innes and L. Z. Saunders, New York, Academic, 1962, pp. 147-243.

36. W. J. Hadlow. In The Striated Muscle. Edited by C. M. Pearson and F. K. Mostofi, Baltimore, Williams and Wilkins, 1973, pp. 364-409.

37. J. N. Walton and D. Gardner-Medwin. In Disorders of Voluntary Muscle. Edited by J. N. Walton, Edinburgh, Churchill Livingstone, 1974, pp. 561-613.

38. A. M. Pappenheimer and M. Goettsch, J. Exp. Med. 53:11 (1931).

39. H. Dam, J. Nutr. 27:193 (1944).

40. H. Dam, J. Nutr. 28:297 (1944).

41. H. Dam, G. K. Nielsen, I. Prange, and E. Sondergaard, Nature (London) 182:802 (1958).

42. L. J. Machlin and R. S. Gordon, Proc. Soc. Exp. Biol. Med. 103:659 (1960).

43. M. G. Kokatnur, S. Okui, F. A. Kummerow, and H. M. Scott, Proc. Soc. Exp. Biol. Med. 104:170 (160).

44. E. Jungherr, Science 84:559 (1936).

45. E. Jungherr, Ann. N.Y. Acad. Sci. 52:104 (1949).

46. A. Wolf and A. M. Pappenheimer, J. Exp. Med. 54:399 (1931).

47. H. S. Olcott and H. A. Matill, J. Amer. Chem. Soc. 58:1627 (1936).

48. C. Golumbic, J. Amer. Chem. Soc. 63:1142 (1941).

49. R. H. Barnes, W. O. Lundberg, H. T. Hanson, and G. O. Burr, J. Biol. Chem. 149:313 (1943).

50. H. Dam and H. Granados, Acta Physiol. Scand. 10:162 (1945).

51. H. A. Mattill, Ann. Rev. Biochem. 16:177 (1947).

52. A. L. Tappel, Fed. Proc. 24:73 (1965).

53. H. Dam, I. Kruse, I. Prange, and E. Sondergaard, Acta Physiol. Scand. 22:299 (1951).

54. E. P. Singsen, R. H. Bunnell, L. D. Matterson, A. Kozeff, and E. L. Jungherr, Poultry Sci. 34:262 (1955).
55. L. J. Machlin, R. S. Gordon, K. H. Meisky, J. Nutr. 67:333 (1959).
56. E. L. Jungherr, E. P. Singsen, and L. D. Matterson, Lab. Invest. 5:120 (1956).
57. J. S. Nelson, V. W. Fischer, and P. A. Young, J. Neuropathol. Exp. Neurol. 31:317 (1972).
58. H. Dam, Pharmacol. Rev. 9:1 (1957).
59. H. Tsuchiyama, T. Nishida, and F. A. Kummerow, Arch. Pathol. 74:208 (1962).
60. V. W. Fischer and J. S. Nelson, J. Neuropathol. Exp. Neurol. 32:474 (1973).
61. V. W. Fischer and J. S. Nelson, Acta Neuropathol (Berl.) 29:65 (1974).
62. J. S. Nelson, L. J. Machlin, and R. Filipski, Fed. Proc. 33:671 (1974).
63. J. S. Nelson, unpublished observations.
64. W. A. Yu, M. C. Yu, and P. A. Young, Exp. Mol. Pathol. 21:289 (1974).
65. A. Ringsted, Biochem. J. 29:788 (1935).
66. L. Einarson and A. Ringsted, Effect of Chronic Vitamin E Deficiency on the Nervous System and Skeletal Musculature in Adult Rats. London, Oxford Univ. Press, 1938.
67. M. Monnier, Presse Med. 49:1272 (1941).
68. A. Wolf and A. M. Pappenheimer, Arch. Neurol. Psychiat. 48:538 (1942).
69. A. Wolf and A. M. Pappenheimer, J. Neuropathol. Exp. Neurol. 4:402 (1945).
70. L. Einarson, Acta Psychiat. Neurol. Scand. Suppl. 78 (1952).
71. C. M. Luttrell and K. E. Mason, Ann. N.Y. Acad. Sci. 52:113 (1949).
72. N. Malamud, M. M. Nelson, and H. M. Evans, Ann. N.Y. Acad. Sci. 52:135 (1949).
73. A. Pentschew and K. Schwarz, Acta Neuropathol. 1:313 (1962).
74. P. Lampert, J. M. Blumberg, and A. Pentschew, J. Neuropathol. Exp. Neurol. 23:60 (1964).
75. P. Lampert and A. Pentschew, Acta neuropathol. 4:158 (1964).
76. S. S. Schochet, Acta Neuropathol. Suppl. 5:54 (1971).
77. J. H. Sung, J. Neuropathol. Exp. Neurol. 23:567 (1964).
78. J. H. Sung and E. M. Stadlan, J. Neuropathol. Exp. Neurol. 25:341 (1966).
79. J. H. Sung., Proc. 5th Int. Congress Neuropathol. Amsterdam, Excerpta Medica Foundation, 1966, pp. 478-480.
80. W. Brannon, W. McCormick, and P. Lampert, Acta Neuropathol. 9:1 (1967).

81. D. Cowen and E. V. Olmstead, J. Neuropathol. Exp. Neurol. 22:175 (1963).

82. E. C. Dooling, W. C. Schoene, and E. P. Richardson, Arch. Neurol. 30:70 (1974).

83. P. R. Huttenlocker and F. H. Gilles, Neurology 17:1174 (1967).

84. H. Dam and J. Glavind, Nature (London) 142:1077 (1938).

85. H. Dam and J. Glavind, Nature (London) 143:810 (1939).

86. H. R. Bird and T. G. Culton, Proc. Soc. Exp. Biol. Med. 44:543 (1940).

87. M. L. Scott, T. Noguchi, and G. F. Combs, Vit. Horm. 32:429 (1974).

88. R. L. Holman, Proc. Soc. Exp. Biol. Med. 66:307 (1947).

89. R. L. Holman, Southern Med. J. 42:108 (1949).

90. P. M. Newberne, M. R. Bresnahan, and N. S. Kula, J. Nutr. 97:219 (1969).

91. T. W. Gullickson and C. E. Calverley, Science 104:312 (1946).

92. T. W. Gullickson, Ann. N.Y. Acad. Sci. 52:256 (1949).

93. A. M. Macdonald, K. L. Blaxter, P. S. Watts, and W. A. Wood, Br. J. Nutr. 6:164 (1952).

94. O. H. Muth, J. Amer. Vet. Med. Assoc. 126:355 (1955).

95. E. D. Andrews, W. J. Hartley, and A. B. Grant, N.Z. Vet. J. 16:3 (1968).

96. I. Nafstad and S. Tollersreed, Acta Vet. Scand. 11:152 (1970).

97. I. Nafstad, Vet. Pathol. 8:239 (1971).

98. G. J. Martin and F. B. Faust, Exp. Med. Surg. 5:405 (1947).

99. F. I. Dessau, L. Lipchuck, and S. Klein, Proc. Soc. Exp. Biol. Med. 87:522 (1954).

100. O. B. Houchin and P. W. Smith, Amer. J. Physiol. 141:242 (1944).

101. A. J. Gatz and O. B. Houchin, Anat. Record. 110:249 (1951).

102. J. H. Bragdon and H. D. Levine, Amer. J. Pathol. 25:265 (1951).

103. C. D. Fitch, Vit. Horm. 26:501 (1968).

104. V. W. Fischer, J. S. Nelson, and P. A. Young, Poultry Sci. 49:443 (1970).

105. P. Gyorgy and C. S. Rose, Science 108:716 (1948).

106. P. Gyorgy and C. S. Rose, Ann. N.Y. Acad. Sci. 52:231 (1949).

107. L. R. Horn, M. O. Barker, G. Reed, and M. Brin, J. Nutr. 104:192 (1974).

108. C. E. Mengel, Ann. N.Y. Acad. Sci. 203:163 (1972).

109. C. D. Fitch, Ann. N.Y. Acad. Sci. 203:172 (1972).

110. I. Nafstad, Pathol. Vet. 2:277 (1965).

111. L. R. Machlin, R. Filipski, J. Nelson, L. Horn, and M. Brin, submitted for publication, J. Nutr.

112. J. H. Ritchie, M. B. Fish, V. McMasters, and M. Grossman, N. Engl. J. Med. 279:1185 (1968).

113. P. R. Dallman, J. Pediatr. 85:742 (1974).
114. L. J. Machlin, R. Filipski, A. L. Willis, D. C. Kuhn, and M. Brin, Proc. Soc. Exp. Biol. Med. 149:275 (1975).
115. F. B. Adamstone, Arch. Pathol. 31:613 (1941).
116. H. Popper, P. Gyorgy, and H. Goldblatt, Arch. Pathol. 37:161 (1944).
117. Z. Menschik and T. J. Szczesniak, Anat. Record 103:349 (1949).
118. P. Gyorgy and H. Goldblatt, J. Exp. Med. 89:245 (1949).
119. E. L. Hove, D. H. Copeland, and W. D. Salmon, J. Nutr. 39:397 (1949).
120. K. Schwarz, Ann. N.Y. Acad. Sci. 52:225 (1949).
121. O. Lindan and H. P. Himsworth, Br. J. Exp. Pathol. 31:651 (1950).
122. E. A. Porta, F. A. de la Iglesia, and W. S. Hartroft, Lab. Invest. 18:283 (1968).
123. E. A. Machado, E. A. Porta, W. S. Hartroft, and F. Hamilton, Lab. Invest. 24:13 (1971).
124. C. H. Gallagher, Nature (London) 192:881 (1961).
125. T. Barka and P. J. Anderson, Histochemistry, New York, Harper and Row, 1963, pp. 190-193.
126. R. D. Lillie, F. S. Daft, and W. H. Sebrell, Public Health Rept. 56:1255 (1941).
127. E. A. Porta and W. S. Hartroft, Lipid pigments in relation to aging and dietary factors. In Pigments in Pathology. Edited by M. Wolman, New York, Academic, 1969, pp. 191-235.
128. H. Pinkerton, Arch. Pathol. 5:380 (1928).
129. W. S. Hartroft, Science 113:673 (1951).
130. W. S. Hartroft, Fed. Proc. 22:250 (1963).
131. A. G. E. Pearse, Histochemistry Theoretical and Applied, 2nd ed., London, J. and A. Churchill, 1960, Chap. 34.
132. K. E. Mason and A. F. Emmel, Anat. Rec. 92:33 (1945).
133. A. M. Pappenheimer and J. Victor, Amer. J. Pathol. 22:395 (1946).
134. N. M. Sulkin, J. Gerontol. 12:430 (1957).
135. N. M. Sulkin and D. F. Sulkin, J. Gerontol. 22:485 (1967).
136. T. Miyagishi, N. Takahata, and R. Iizuka, Acta Neuropathol. 9:7 (1967).
137. N. Nishioka, N. Takahata, and R. Iizuka, Acta Neuropathol. 11:174 (1968).
138. J. Victor and A. M. Pappenheimer, J. Exp. Med. 82:375 (1945).
139. W. G. B. Casselman, J. Exp. Med. 94:549 (1951).
140. K. S. Chio, U. Reiss, B. Fletcher, and A. L. Tappel, Science 166:1535 (1969).
141. A. L. Tappel. In Pathobiology of Cell Membranes. Edited by B. F. Trump and A. U. Arstilla, New York, Academic, 1975, pp. 145-170.

142. W. Zeman, J. Neuropathol. Exp. Neurol. $\underline{33}$:1 (1974).
143. D. Armstrong, S. Dimmitt, D. E. Van Wormer, Arch. Neurol. $\underline{30}$:144 (1974).
144. I. Molenaar, C. E. Hulstaert, and J. Vos, Proc. Nutr. Soc. $\underline{32}$:249 (1973).

8   EFFECT OF VITAMIN E ON IMMUNE RESPONSES

ROBERT P. TENGERDY
Colorado State University
Fort Collins, Colorado

I.	Introduction	429
II.	Effect of Vitamin E on Immune Responses	430
	A. Humoral Immunity	430
	B. Cellular Immunity	434
III.	Disease Protection by Vitamin E	435
IV.	Interaction of Vitamin E, Vitamin A, and Selenium	439
V.	Implications for Cancer Immunotherapy and Alleviating of Aging Disorders	441
	A. Cancer	441
	B. Aging	442
VI.	Conclusions	442
	References	443

I. INTRODUCTION

Vitamin E has been plagued from the time of its discovery with exaggerated claims about its possible or wished role in human and animal health. This is undoubtedly due to a large degree to the elusive nature of the biological functions of this vitamin or rather to our ignorance about it. In light of this, it is particularly important to separate in this review the experimentally verifiable facts from conjectures and speculations. Even when the experimental facts clearly demonstrate a point, it must be remembered that all the available data collected so far were obtained in experiments with small animals, mice, rats, rabbits, guinea pigs, and chickens, and thus great caution must be exercised in extrapolating conclusions to humans.

Another important distinction should be made. Vitamins are usually present in diets at levels that prevent nutritional deficiency symptoms. If the vitamin is consumed at much higher dosages, at some level, it may be proper to talk about the pharmacological action of the vitamin. This distinction may be arbitrary, at least until the recommended daily allowance of a vitamin is defined for optimal metabolic functions rather than for lack of deficiency symptoms.

In this report we are concerned with the quantitative effect of so-called pharmacological doses of vitamin E on immune responses and disease resistance, accepting the premise that a minimal level of vitamin E is absolutely necessary for these processes, i.e., that vitamin E-deficient animals would have impaired immune responses and disease resistance.

Resistance to infectious diseases (these are the diseases considered mainly in this review) depends on many factors, some related to the host that is infected, some related to the parasite that infects. In the disease resistance of the host, the immune state of the animal is an important but not the only important factor. One should bear in mind that the innate resistance of the host, the so-called general health, may be equally important. Disease resistance also depends on environmental effects such as nutrition and environmental, behavioral, or mental stress. Finally, the pathogenicity and virulence of the invading parasitic microorganism greatly influence host resistance. These factors have to be taken into consideration in the final evaluation of the effect of vitamin E on disease resistance, because vitamin E may affect some of these factors.

When we mention vitamin E in this report, the compound [dl] tocopheryl-acetate is understood if not otherwise indicated. This compound was used in most of our investigations, and as far as it can be determined, in most other reported works.

II. EFFECT OF VITAMIN E ON IMMUNE RESPONSES

A. Humoral Immunity

According to the reasoning expressed in the introduction, a distinction will be made between the effect of vitamin E deficiency on humoral immunity and the pharmacological effect of large doses of vitamin E on immunity.

Vitamin E deficiency, like other vitamin deficiencies, may lead to a decreased immune response. In general, nutritional deficiencies lead to a complex array of metabolic dysfunctions; therefore, to single out the precise cause of immunological impairment would be next to impossible. The role of nutrition in acquired immunity has been reviewed extensively by Axelrod [1].

From a practical point of view the pharmacological effect of vitamin E is much more interesting, because, as it will be seen, it produces a positive effect and thus holds a promise for therapeutic applications.

Some early observations indicated that vitamin E might be an immunostimulant in pharmacological doses. Segagni noted in 1955 that vitamin E
supplemented rabbits produced antibodies earlier to typhoid vaccine,
O-streptolysin, and staphylococcus toxoid than rabbits on normal diets,
but the peak antibody levels were not higher than those of the controls [2].
Solarino reported in 1957 that vitamin E, pantothenic acid, riboflavin,
p-aminobenzoic acid, and nicotinic acid stimulated antibody production in
rabbits to vaccines of Vibrio cholerae, Salmonella typhi, and to heterologous erthrocytes [3]. No explanation was offered for the observed effect
in these early reports.

In 1970 we began investigating the immunostimulatory property of
vitamin E in some detail. We found that vitamin E significantly enhanced
humoral antibody formation in young and adult chickens and mice [4-6].
The effective dietary vitamin E supplement was 130-150 mg/kg diet, added
to diets which contained 35-60 milligrams of vitamin E per kilogram of
food. It was particularly interesting to note that the greatest antibody
enhancement was found in 1 week-old hypoxic chickens hatched either at
natural or simulated high altitudes [4]. This suggested the first clue
about the possible mode of action of vitamin E. Vitamin E as an antioxidant or redox agent may have acted synergistically with hypoxia in
creating favorable reducing conditions that stimulated immunopoietic
cellular development and proliferation.

Since synthetic antioxidants are known to replace vitamin E in reversing many E deficiency symptoms, their potential effect on antibody formation was tested in mice. We used two different antigens: sheep red blood
cell (SRBC), a particulate antigen, and tetanus toxoid, a soluble antigen,
because these antigens stimulate antibody production by different mechanisms [6].

An illustrative example of one of the many similar experiments is
shown in Table 1. Mice were maintained on a normal diet, Wayne Lab
Block chow (WLB), which contains about 35 milligrams of vitamin E per
kilogram of food, and on a vitamin E-deficient diet (Nutritional Biochemicals Co., now ICN Pharmaceuticals, Cleveland, Ohio). To these diets
vitamin E, N-N-diphenyl-p-phenylene diamine (DPPD), a synthetic antioxidant, or both were supplemented in graded amounts. In the table
only the doses are shown that gave maximum response.

The mice were immunized with SRBC. The number of antibody-
forming cells, plaque-forming cells (PFC) in the spleen was counted by
the local hemolytic effect of antibody-producing cells on surrounding SRBC
in an in vitro single cell suspension tissue culture test, the PFC test.
The relative level of antibody in the blood serum was determined by
hemagglutination titration (HA). After the serum is treated with
2-mercaptoethanol (ME) only the IgG antibody remains active; thus from
the HA titration with or without ME the relative amounts of IgM and IgG
antibodies in the serum can be estimated.

TABLE 1 Effect of Vitamin E and DPPD[a] on Humoral Immunity

Diet	Spleen weight	PFC[b] per 10^6 cells	HA[c] $\log_2$ titer	
			Without ME[d]	With ME
Vitamin E-deficient diet[e]	0.059 ± 0.007	419 ± 25	5.0 ± 1.2	<1
Vitamin E-deficient diet + 222 mg DPPD/kg	0.073 ± 0.010	562 ± 32	6.5 ± 1.2	<1
WLB[f] Chow	0.096 ± 0.021	1225 ± 85	7.0 ± 0.2	3.0 ± 0.2
WLB Chow + 222 mg DPPD/kg	0.123 ± 0.032	5461 ± 292	7.3 ± 0.4	3.5 ± 0.2
WLB Chow + 2035 mg vitamin E/kg	0.114 ± 0.024	7863 ± 295	7.9 ± 1.2	4.1 ± 0.9

[a] DPPD = N, N-diphenyl-p-phenylene-diamine; an antioxidant; $P < 0.01$ between controls and treatment groups.
[b] PFC = plaque-forming cells.
[c] HA = hemagglutination.
[d] ME = 2-mercaptoethanol.
[e] Nutritional Biochemicals Co., now ICN Pharmaceuticals, Cleveland, Ohio.
[f] WLB = Wayne Laboratory Blocks.

It can be seen from the table that mice on the vitamin E-deficient diet had a very low PFC response and no IgG response. DPPD supplemented at twice the level that was used by others for reversing some vitamin E deficiency symptoms [7] failed to restore the PFC or IgG responses. On the normal diet DPPD enhanced the PFC, IgM, and IgG responses, but this effect was always less than that found with vitamin E supplementation, especially for IgG production. The immunostimulatory effect of both DPPD and vitamin E was accompanied by an increase in spleen weight, indicating increased cell proliferation. These data suggest that the antioxidant action of vitamin E may contribute to immunostimulation, but this may not be the sole explanation of its activity.

The data in Table 1 were taken 4 days after immunization, the time of the maximal PFC response. Detailed kinetic studies [9] revealed that HA titers reached their peak on or around the seventh day; by that time the titer of the vitamin E-supplemented groups was usually 2-4 $\log_2$ units higher than the controls.

The effect of vitamin E and DPPD on antibody production was similar with the two antigens used for immunization, SRBC and tetanus toxoid [6]. Tetanus toxoid is a completely foreign antigen for the mouse in the sense that the mouse has never been exposed to this antigen previously, whereas SRBC is not completely foreign, because the mouse is exposed to SRBC-like antigens during its normal life. For this reason tetanus toxoid gives a true primary immune response, characterized by an initial IgM production, while SRBC gives a mixed IgM and IgG response. The main effect of vitamin E in both cases appeared to be the stimulation of both IgM and IgG antibody production, with an early shift from IgM to IgG production.

These results were corroborated later in in vitro antibody production experiments [8]. Mouse spleen cells were cultured with SRBC in single cell suspension cultures in the presence of emulsified [dl]-α-tocopheryl-acetate, and the PFC response was measured 5 days later. The PFC count was two to four times higher in the presence of vitamin E. Similar enhancement was found with 2-mercaptoethanol and somewhat less with DPPD and butylated hydroxy-toluene (BHT), another good antioxidant. Vitamin E had to be well emulsified (solubilized) for this effect.

The next experiment in vitro gave a hint for the possible mechanism of immunostimulation by vitamin E [8]. When the spleen cells were separated into an adherent (macrophage-like) cell population and a nonadherent (lymphocyte-like) cell population, the nonadherent cells could produce antibody under vitamin E or other antioxidant stimulation. Normally the cooperation of the adherent cell population is necessary for an immune response. This result may be interpreted either as an apparent macrophage bypass or as a true enhancement of the remaining few macrophage-type cells in the nonadherent population, enabling them to perform more efficiently. In any case vitamin E seems to be involved in cell cooperation in the immune response. A further analysis of the cell types involved in the two populations (T and B lymphocytes, macrophages) should decide the target cell(s) of the vitamin E stimulation.

An indirect hint for explaining the immunostimulatory role of vitamin E comes from the recent observation by Machlin and others that prostaglandin levels were higher in vitamin E deficient rats than in controls [44]. This supports the hypothesis that vitamin E inhibits prostaglandin synthesis from arachidonic acid.* Prostaglandins stimulate cyclic AMP production, which is a suppressor of many immunological cellular activities, such as IgE-mediated histamine release from mast cells, mitogenic transformation and cytotoxicity of lymphocytes, formation of erythrocyte rosettes of T lymphocytes, lysosomal enzyme release during phagocytosis, and chemotactic activities of neutrophils [45]. If excess dietary vitamin E would prove to suppress prostaglandin or cyclic AMP levels, it would give a strong clue for explaining its immunostimulatory effect, and perhaps other biological functions. It seems worthwhile to direct future research in this direction.

In summary, vitamin E increases the efficiency of antibody production in animals whose immune response functions normally. The mechanism of this immunostimulation is largely unknown, but an antioxidant effect on one or more cell types of the immunopoietic system seems to be involved.

B. Cellular Immunity

Vitamin E increased the delayed-type hypersensitivity (DTH) tuberculin reaction in guinea pigs by increasing the size of erythema on the abdomen skin from 62 mm^2 in the control to 237 mm^2 in the treated animals [9]. The effective dose of added vitamin E was 60 mg/kg diet. In a similar tuberculin test in mice the dietary supplementation of either 1 ppm selenium or 120 mg/kg vitamin E or the combination of the two gave significantly increased foot pad thickness compared to controls. The best results were obtained with the 120 mg/kg vitamin E supplement, which doubled the footpad thickness. The results of these skin tests have not been corroborated yet with other more accurate measurements of DTH, and there is some doubt that humoral, Arthus type, reactions may obscure skin test interpretations. Vitamin E-supplemented mice were not protected against challenge by virulent Mycobacterium tuberculosis, an infection in which

---

*Some more recent evidence further supports this hypothesis. Dogs fed diets high in PUFA but deficient in vitamin E and selenium rapidly developed a severely depressed lymphoproliferative response to mitogens. Vitamin E completely restored the response. (Sheffy, B. E. and Schultz, R. D. Fed. Proc. 38:2139, 1979.) Vitamin E actually decreased PG levels in chicken organs and enhanced antibody production. (Tengerdy, R. P. and Brown, J. C. Poultry Sci. 56:957, 1977; Likoff, R. O. et al. Fed. Proc. 37:829, 1978.)

cellular immunity plays a protective role. This casts doubt on the stimulation of an effective cellular immunity by vitamin E. The evaluation of a
cellular effect is further complicated by the possible enhancement of
blocking antibodies by vitamin E that may antagonize cellular immunity
[10]. The evaluation of the effect of vitamin E on cellular immunity must
await in vitro and in vivo proofs of action on T and B lymphocytes, macrophages, and associated cells.

III. DISEASE PROTECTION BY VITAMIN E

An important practical question emerges from the above investigations:
does the elevated antibody level afford increased protection against infectious diseases? The answer is not an automatic yes, because frequently
antibody titers are poorly or not at all correlated with disease protection.
If the increased antibody production promotes a more effective phagocytosis, this might lead to an increased disease protection.

Some experiments do support the disease protecting role of vitamin E.
Chicks raised on vitamin E-supplemented diets (150-300 mg/kg) had
increased protection against E. coli infection [11]. Chicks on a
normal diet had 25-30% mortality rate, while those on the vitamin E diet
had 0-10% mortality. The increased protection corresponded with elevated
HA titers (2-3 $\log_2$ units), suggesting that the higher antibody level contributed to the increased protection.

Similar protection was found by Julseth in young turkeys, cold and
light stressed at 5 days of age, and challenged with E. coli at 3 weeks of
age [12]. Vitamin E supplemented at 100 mg/kg diet decreased mortality
from 31 to 8% resulting from the cold-light stress and from 40 to 8%
resulting from the E. coli infection.

There are current experiments underway at Colorado State University
with Newcastle virus vaccination and Brucella infections that may throw
more light on the role of vitamin E in disease protection. In such experiments G. R. J. Law (personal communication) found that vitamin E may
give increased protection to newly hatched chicks against Brucella abortus
infection through passively transferred maternal antibody. The maternal
antibody from B. abortus sensitized hens passed through the egg yolk and
and absorbed by the chicks. Since the eggs also had an elevated vitamin E
level, which might have stimulated the active immunopoietic development
of the chick embryo, a double protective effect may have operated in this
experiment. Increasing disease protection of sensitive young chicks by
maternal vaccination is an attractive potential therapeutic use of vitamin E.
C. F. Nockels (personal communication) noted an increased antibody titer
in guinea pigs infected with Venezuelan equine encephalitis virus, if the
guinea pigs were injected intramuscularly with 33 mg/kg b.w. of [dl]-α-
tocopherol, prior to the virus infection. The acetate form, either injected
or supplemented in the diet, was without effect. Furthermore the injected

[dl]-α-tocopheryl acetate caused some local muscle damage. This shows that the chemical form and route of administration may be important in the therapeutic application of vitamin E and vary with host and disease agent.

The mechanism of disease protection was scrutinized in mice infected with Diplococcus pneumoniae type I (DpI) [13]. A dietary supplement of 120 or 180 milligrams of vitamin E per kilogram of diet increased survival of nonimmunized mice from 20 to 80% when challenged with 20 organisms and of mice immunized with 0.6 ng DpI polysaccharide (SI) from 15 to 70% when challenged with 20,000 organisms (Fig. 1). The phagocytic index, the ratio of DpI cells phagocytized in treatment groups versus the control, was four times higher on the vitamin E-supplemented diet than on normal diet. The fourfold increase in survival and phagocytosis was greater and more significantly than found previously in antibody titers and PFC count.

Phagocytosis was enhanced by vitamin E even in the absence of immune phenomena. Inert carbon particles were cleared faster from the blood of vitamin E-supplemented mice than normal mice (Fig. 2). These data strongly support the idea that increased phagocytosis by vitamin E plays a major role in disease protection.

There is a striking parallel between these results and those obtained by Bliznakov and others on the nontoxic stimulation of the reticuloendothelial system by various members of the ubiquinone group and related compounds. They observed a significant stimulation of the cellular phagocytic activity as well as humoral antibody formation [14-18]. The compounds were generally administered intravenously as emulsions; the mode of preparation of this emulsion, particularly the particle size, as well as the dose of ubiquinone were critical for the biological effect. In these studies, coenzyme Q_{10} (CoQ_{10}) proved to be the most effective stimulator of phagocytic activity. CoQ_{10} had a protective role in cancer; it increased the number of survivors in Friend leukemia virus-infected mice and in 3,4,9,10-dibenzpyrene-induced tumors [18].

CoQ_{10} administered to mice intravenously in a dose of 150 μg in emulsion doubled the primary hemolytic antibody titer (4 days) against sheep erythrocytes. Curiously, vitamins E and K were without effect in these experiments, but this may be attributed to the low dose used [15].

CoQ_{10} combined with low doses of chloroquine (an antimalarial drug) prolonged survival time and reduced parasitemia in blood-transferred Plasmodium berghei (the parasite causing malaria) infection in mice [16].

In our experiments with the DpI in mice, Heinzerling found that vitamin E (180 mg/kg) increased the CoQ_{10} level in the plasma, liver, kidney, and spleen by 30-40% over controls [9]. He also found an increased [14C]phenylalanine incorporation into the above organs in vitamin E-supplemented mice [9]. Since phenylalanine is a precursor of CoQ_{10}, a possible direct stimulation of CoQ_{10} biosynthesis might be suspected. The 14C incorporation, however, was not specific for CoQ_{10}.

More significant is perhaps the finding that in vitamin E-supplemented mice there is an increased accumulation of 3H-labeled [dl]-α-tocopheryl

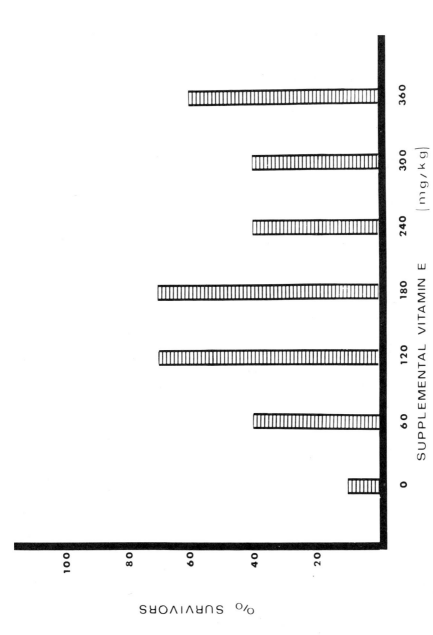

FIG. 1 Protection of mice from D. pneumoniae type I (DpI) infection by vitamin E. Mice were immunized with 0.5 ng DpI polysaccharide and challenged 1 week later with 20,000 DpI. Survivors in each group of 10 were counted 5 days later. (From Ref. 13.)

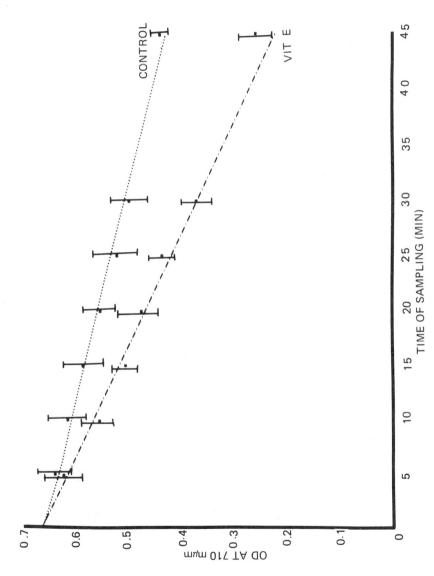

FIG. 2   Effect of vitamin E on the rate of carbon clearance from blood.   (From Ref. 13.)

acetate in the thymus and the spleen [9]. It is possible that this excess vitamin E may increase the efficiency of some cellular functions, e.g., by protecting ubiquinones from oxidation.

This idea would be in line with present concepts on ubiquinone/ vitamin E interactions, according to which vitamin E is likely to protect the isoprenoid side chain of ubiquinones from oxidation rather than being involved directly in ubiquinone biosynthesis [20, 21].

Other experiments also support the view that vitamin E may act through ubiquinone. Russian researchers reported that injections of vitamin E into rats significantly increased the ubiquinone content in the liver by 30% and in the kidney by 12.4% [19]. A combination of vitamins E and A caused even greater enhancement.

Another line of reasoning suggests that vitamin E itself cannot promote phagocytosis. A direct effect of vitamin E on phagocytic activity would seem contrary to recent views on phagocytic killing of bacteria. According to Shohet and coworkers during phagocytosis the killing of bacteria may be partially dependent on peroxides generated via bacterial lipid peroxidation [22]. Such peroxidation may be promoted by a ubiquinone, a prooxidant but certainly not by α-tocopherol, an antioxidant. The phagocytosis-promoting effect of vitamin E is thus compatible with the idea that vitamin E helps maintain high ubiquinone levels in phagocytic cells and the ubiquinones directly promote phagocytosis.

The disease protective effect of vitamin E in the cases studied so far is restricted to bacterial infections in which opsonizing antibody and increased phagocytosis play the protective role. The failure of vitamin E to increase protection against a virulent M. tuberculosis infection [9] seems to indicate that vitamin E may not have a protective role in diseases involving cellular immunity.

Since disease resistance involves many host and parasite factors besides the ones discussed above, it would be unwise to exclude the possibility that vitamin E may affect such factors perhaps by entirely different mechanisms.

In summary, vitamin E increases the protection of animals against certain bacterial infections in which humoral immunity and phagocytosis play a protective role. The mechanism of increased protection is not known, but in the case of increased phagocytosis ubiquinone may be the mediator of action.

IV. INTERACTION OF VITAMIN E, VITAMIN A,
    AND SELENIUM

There are interactions among the various biological functions of vitamins E, A, and selenium. These interactions have been discussed in detail in section IV of this book. Here we will consider the particular effect of these interactions on immune responses and disease protection. As before, we will consider interactions of these compounds only at pharmacological doses, disregarding the effects at the deficiency level.

Vitamin A, when administered at very high doses, is an immunostimulant having adjuvant effect in humoral immune responses [23, 24]. Cohen and Cohen reported that 1000 IU vitamin A injected daily into mice for 4 successive days significantly increased the number of antibody-forming cells in mice immunized with SRBC [25]. The immunosuppressive effect of hydrocortisone was also prevented by vitamin A. Since vitamin A decreases the stability of lysosomal membranes, whereas hydrocortison increases it, it is suggested that lysosomal alterations in immunocytes may be responsible for the observed effect.

In searching for the potential interaction between vitamins E and A in immune stimulation and disease protection, we tested the effect of the two vitamins in protecting chickens from E. coli infection [26]. The supplementation of either vitamin E (300 mg/kg diet) or vitamin A (60, 000 IU/kg diet) to a standard chick ration increased the protection of 6 week-old chickens against repeated exposure to E. coli by decreasing mortality from 40 to 5%. The combination of the two vitamins, however, did not give as much protection as either vitamin alone. Vitamin E or A did not protect the chickens from weight loss and severe morbidity due to infection, but slightly increased the rate of their recovery. Apparently there is no synergistic effect between vitamin A and E in promoting immune responses, rather, an antagonistic effect may exist.

Edwin and others observed earlier that an inverse relationship exists between dietary vitamin A and tissue α-tocopherol and ubiquinone levels in vitamin A and E deficient rat tissues [27]. Increased vitamin A addition decreased α-tocopherol and ubiquinone levels, but α-tocopherol addition increased tissue vitamin A and ubiquinone levels. It appears then that α-tocopherol influences both vitamin A and ubiquinone levels, and vitamin A may inversely affect tocopherol levels. This experiment was performed with vitamin A- and/or vitamin E-deficient animals and not at the pharmacological levels used in the immunological experiments; thus, a direct comparison cannot be made. Nevertheless the fact that the ubiquinone tissue levels are influenced by vitamin E and A interactions may explain the lack of synergism between vitamin E and A in disease protection, if ubiquinone has a role in the protection.

Another important biological interaction exists between vitamin E and selenium. According to Diplock, Baum, and Lucy, α-tocopherol, a membrane-bound redox substance, protects selenide from oxidation in membrane-bound nonheme iron proteins [28]. Selenium is also part of glutathione peroxidase that reduces hydroperoxides in tissues. Vitamin E acts as a chain breaker in peroxidation and thus acts synergistically with selenium [29].

In view of this interaction it is interesting to see what effect selenium has on immune responses. Spallholz and others reported that when

1.0-3.0 ppm sodium selenite was supplemented to normal Purina Chow or to a low selenium basal torula yeast diet that contained an adequate level of vitamin E (60-70 mg/kg diet), the hemagglutination titer of mice against sheep red blood cell increased by 5-7 $\log_2$ units [30,31]. The effect was greater on the natural Purina diet than on the semisynthetic diet. The immune response was expectedly poor on the semisynthetic diet which was deficient in both vitamin E and selenium. Selenium addition (0.1 ppm) alone did not restore normal immune response, but vitamin E addition (70 mg/kg) did. These levels of selenium or vitamin E are contained in normal mouse diets. Similar results were obtained by Burenshtein on antibody formation in rabbits [32]. Selenium and vitamin E synergistically stimulated antibody production.

These results indicate that selenium potentiates vitamin E but does not replace it in immunostimulation. In this respect the results are similar to the ones obtained with the synthetic antioxidant DPPD [6]. The antibody stimulated by selenium was mainly IgM, just as in stimulation by DPPD, although a delayed (after 14 days) shift to IgG production was observed [31].

In all of the immunological studies reviewed here it was evident that the immunostimulating effect of vitamin E was always better in natural diets than in synthetic diets. This suggests that other nutritional interactions may potentiate vitamin E or are needed independently for an optimally functioning immune response.

V. IMPLICATIONS FOR CANCER IMMUNOTHERAPY AND ALLEVIATING OF AGING DISORDERS

A. Cancer

Can vitamin E and related factors contribute to immunological protection against cancer? Since vitamin E enhances humoral immune responses and perhaps affects cellular immune responses too, the potential use of vitamin E in immunotherapeutic treatments, especially in viral cancer vaccines, is tempting to consider.

Vitamin E [33-35], other antioxidants [36], selenium [37,38], and ubiquinones [18] have been implicated in the prevention and/or cure of some forms of cancer. In view of the immunostimulatory effect of these agents, and the possible role of immunity in cancer surveillance and therapy [39], the anticancer properties of these agents should be looked upon from this point of view.

In preliminary experiments we have found that dietary supplementation of 180 milligrams of vitamin E per kilogram of diet slightly decreased the size of implanted mammary carcinoma tumors in C3H mice, and in some cases retarded or prevented the reappearance of tumors after a combined radiation treatment and BCG immunotherapy. These results are, however, very tentative as yet.

We must understand first the precise role of T and B lymphocytes, macrophage, and soluble lymphokine factors in cancer immunity, and the effect of vitamin E, selenium, and other interrelated nutritional factors on these cells and cell products before the role of vitamin E in cancer immunity can be understood.

B. Aging

A decreased functioning of the immune system is known to occur in old age, manifested by a decreased resistance to infectious diseases, a higher incidence of cancer and autoimmune diseases [39, 41]. The intriguing question is, can the deterioration of the immune system be slowed down by an immunostimulant such as vitamin E? There are no data yet on the effect of vitamin E on the immune system of aging animals but at this writing a long-term experiment is being conducted in Harman's laboratory (personal communication). Looking at the aging problem from an immunological point of view deserves a serious consideration, taking into account not only the effect of a single factor such as vitamin E but many interrelated effects that may contribute to slowing down the deterioration of the immune system.

VI. CONCLUSIONS

What does all this mean? There are established facts, conjectures, and speculations presented here. It is a fact that vitamin E, supplemented in pharmacological doses to normal well-balanced diets increases humoral antibody production, especially IgG production, against a variety of particulate or soluble antigens. This effect was repeatedly reproduced in chickens, mice, turkeys, guinea pigs, and rabbits, and the effect was also demonstrated in vitro in mouse spleen cultures. The effect is a quantitative one, the efficiency of an already well-functioning system is increased by promoting an increased proliferation of antibody-producing cells. Selenium and synthetic antioxidants also effect the immune system but do not completely replace vitamin E in its immunological effect.

It is also a fact that vitamin E increases disease protection in chickens against E. coli infection and in mice against D. pneumoniae infection. It remains to be seen, however, if such a protection prevails under field conditions and in economically important infectious diseases. Many promising laboratory results have been unsuccessful in the field.

The mode of action of disease protection in the limited cases studied so far is still a conjecture; macrophage activation through ubiquinone and increased antibody production seem to be involved.

The interpretation of the interaction of vitamin E, selenium, and vitamin A in promoting antibody biosynthesis and disease protection is speculative. Selenium potentiates vitamin E in its immunological action but does not replace it. The immunological effect, at least, correlates with other biological interactions of selenium and vitamin E. The apparent antagonism between vitamins E and A in immunological effects is puzzling and waits further elucidation; the answer may be sought in basic metabolic and nutritional studies.

The projections for the potential use of vitamin E and related compounds in cancer protection and protection from some aging disorders are speculative and need to be investigated.

REFERENCES

1. A. E. Axelrod. In Modern Nutrition in Health and Disease. Edited by R. S. Goodhart and M. E. Shils, Philadelphia, Lea and Febiger, 1973.
2. E. Segagni, Minerva Pediatr. 7:985, 1074, 1124 (1955).
3. G. Solarino, Int. Zeit. Vitamin Forsch. 27:373 (1957).
4. R. P. Tengerdy, R. H. Heinzerling, and C. F. Nockels, Infection Immun. 5:987 (1972).
5. R. P. Tengerdy and R. P. Happel, WHO Bulletin 48:279 (1973).
6. R. P. Tengerdy, R. H. Heinzerling, G. L. Brown, and M. M. Mathias, Intern. Arch. Allergy 44:111 (1973).
7. H. H. Draper and A. S. Csallany, Proc. Soc. Exp. Biol. Med. 99:739 (1958).
8. P. A. Campbell, H. R. Cooper, R. H. Heinzerling, and R. P. Tengerdy, Proc. Soc. Exp. Biol. Med. 146:465 (1974).
9. R. H. Heinzerling, The Effect of Vitamin E on Immunity, ph.D. Thesis, Colorado State University, Fort Collins, Colorado, 1974.
10. I. Hellstrom and K. E. Hellstrom. In Progress in Immunology II. Edited by L. Brent and J. Holborow, Amsterdam, North Holland, 1974, p. 147.
11. R. H. Heinzerling, C. F. Nockels, C. L. Quarles, and R. P. Tengerdy, Proc. Soc. Exp. Biol. Med. 146:279 (1974).
12. D. R. Julseth. Evaluation of Vitamin E and Disease Stress on Turkey Performance, M.S. Thesis, Colorado State University, Fort Collins, Colorado, 1974.
13. R. H. Heinzerling, R. P. Tengerdy, L. L. Wick, and D. C. Lueker, Infection and Immun. 10:1292 (1974).
14. E. Bliznakov, A. Casey, and E. Premuzic, Experientia 26:953 (1970).
15. A. C. Casey and E. G. Bliznakov, Chem. Biol. Interactions 5:1 (1972).
16. E. G. Bliznakov. In The Reticuloendothelial System and Immune Phenomena. Edited by N. R. Di Luzio, New York, Plenum, 1971, p. 315.

17. E. G. Bliznakov and A. D. Adler, Pathol. Microbiol. 38:393 (1972).

18. E. G. Bliznakov, Proc. Natl. Acad. Sci. USA 70:390 (1973).

19. H. A. Donchenko, A. Dyadychiv, and Ye. K. Vounyanko, Ukr. Biochem. Zh. 43:609 (1971).

20. K. Folkers, Amer. J. Clin. Nutr. 27:1026 (1974).

21. R. E. Olson, Fed. Proc. 24:85 (1965).

22. S. B. Shohet, J. Pitt, R. L. Baehner, and D. G. Poplack, Infection and Immun. 10:1321 (1974).

23. D. W. Dresser, Nature (London) 217:527 (1968).

24. M. M. Azar and R. A. Good, J. Immunol. 106:241 (1971).

25. B. E. Cohen and K. Cohen, J. Immunol. 111:1376 (1973).

26. R. P. Tengerdy and C. F. Nockels, Poultry Sci. 54:1292 (1975).

27. E. Edwin, J. Bunyan, J. Green, and A. Diplock, Br. J. Butr. 16:135 (1962).

28. A. T. Diplock, H. Baum, and T. A. Lucy, Biochem. J. 123:721 (1971).

29. A. L. Tappel, Amer. J. Clin. Nutr. 27:960 (1974).

30. J. E. Spallholz, J. L. Martin, M. L. Gerlach, and R. H. Heinzerling, Proc. Soc. Exp. Biol. Med. 143:685 (1972).

31. J. E. Spallholz, J. L. Martin, M. L. Gerlach, and R. H. Heinzerling, Infection Immun. 8:841 (1973).

32. T. F. Burnshtein, Zdravookhr. Beloruss. 18:34 (1972).

33. K. K. Carroll and H. T. Khor, Cancer Res. 30:2260 (1970).

34. D. Harman, J. Gerontol. 26:451 (1971).

35. D. Harman, Clin. Res. 17:125 (1968).

36. L. W. Wattenberg, J. Natl. Cancer Inst. 48:1425 (1972).

37. R. J. Shamberger, J. Natl. Cancer Inst. 48:1491 (1972).

38. J. R. Harr, J. H. Exon, P. D. Whanger, and P. H. Weswig, Clin. Toxicol. 5:187 (1971).

39. R. T. Smith and M. Landy, eds. Immunology of the Tumor-Host Relationship, New York, Academic, 1974.

40. D. Harman, J. Amer. Geriatrics Soc. 17:721 (1969).

41. R. L. Walford, The Immunologic Theory of Aging, Baltimore, Williams & Wilkins, 1969.

42. J. Miguel, First Rocky Mountain Symposium on Aging, Colorado State University, Fort Collins, Colorado, 1971.

43. D. B. Menzel, First Rocky Mountain Symposium on Aging, Colorado State University, Fort Collins, Colorado, 1971.

44. L. J. Machlin. In Tocopherol, Oxygen and Biomembrane. Edited by C. de Duve and O. Hayaishi, New York, Elsevier, 1978.

45. L. Brent and J. Holborow, eds. Progress in Immunology II, Vol. 2. Amsterdam, North-Holland, 1974, p. 59.

9 VITAMIN E AS AN IN VIVO LIPID STABILIZER AND ITS EFFECT ON FLAVOR AND STORAGE PROPERTIES OF MILK AND MEAT

WILBER L. MARUSICH

Hoffmann-La Roche Inc.
Nutley, New Jersey

I. Introduction 445
II. Milk Off-Flavor (Oxidized Flavor) 446
III. Poultry Meat—Whole and Further Processed 449
IV. Pork and Pork Products 462
V. Recent Developments 465
References 466

I. INTRODUCTION

Mammals and birds require exogenous antioxidants in general for the stabilization of tissue lipids, and in particular for the lipoprotein components of cellular and subcellular membranes. Tocopherols are the prime natural lipid-soluble antioxidants. The role of tocopherols at the molecular level appears to be nonspecific; however, from an overall physiological standpoint, the tocopherol molecule may be unique in its ability to satisfy all the specifications of a biologically active lipid antioxidant. Chemical antioxidant substitutes as ethoxyquin (1,2-dihydro-6-ethoxy-2,2,4-trimethyl quinoline), N,N' diphenyl-phenylenediamine (DPPD), butylated hydroxy toluene-2,6-di-tertiary butyl 4-methylphenol (BHT), and butylated hydroxy anisole, a mixture of 2- and 3-tert-butyl-4-methoxyphenol (BHA), all possess some physiological limitations. These may include inefficient absorption from the intestine, inadequate transfer across the placenta, insufficient deposition in the target tissue, or extremely rapid tissue clearance [1,2].

The requirement for α-tocopherol (vitamin E) is primarily related to the proportion of polyunsaturated fatty acids consumed in the dietary lipids and the effectiveness of vitamin E as an antioxidant associated with the in vivo prevention of lipid peroxidation [3,4]. The majority of evidence supports this concept; however, a few researchers have interpreted the low peroxide level of tissue lipids in animals receiving supplemental vitamin E as due to an inhibition of absorption of oxidized fatty acids from the intestinal tract [5-7].

In this chapter, the biochemical effect of vitamin E is associated with its capacity to protect easily oxidizable substances against oxidation, primarily in adipose tissue and in cell membranes. The peroxides that are found are not of exogenous origin but are formed by auto-oxidation in vivo.

Vitamin E as used here is synonymous for both d- and dl-α-tocopherol (free tocopherol) and the esters (d- and dl-α-tocopheryl acetate). The d- and dl-α-esters are much more stable to in vitro oxidation, thus they are the preferred form for feed supplementation. Tocopheryl acetate (d- or dl-) has no activity as an in vitro antioxidant; however, it is readily hydrolyzed in the animal to nonesterified or free tocopherol which is the potent in vivo antioxidant.

II. MILK OFF-FLAVOR (OXIDIZED FLAVOR)

Oxidized flavor is a very unpleasant off-flavor in milk and is one of the oldest problems related to milk quality. This flavor defect is variably described as "tallowy," "metallic," or "cardboard." Chemically, the oxidized flavor is a consequence of the oxidation of the milk fat, and the reaction is catalyzed most often by small quantities of copper that may get into the milk either by way of the feed or by contamination during milk handling and processing [8,9]. The results obtained by King and coworkers [10-12] further suggest that the amount of copper associated with the fat-globule membrane has more influence on oxidative stability than the total copper content of the fat globule. In turn, the oxidized flavor in the milk is attributed to oxidation of phospholipids [13] which are concentrated in the fat-globule membrane. The fatty acids of the phospholipids are more unsaturated, and hence, more susceptible to oxidation than are those of the triglycerides [14-16].

Control of oxidized flavor has emphasized elimination of potential copper contamination, with stainless steel replacing most other fabricating metals for dairy equipment. Creamline milk has also been practically eliminated as a product since homogenized milk is more resistant to oxidized flavor [8]. Prevention or reduction of the oxidized flavor by the direct addition of chemical antioxidants to milk has not been considered a practical solution due to existing philosophies concerning the "wholesomeness" of milk. In nearly all countries it is forbidden to add anything to milk [8]. Vitamin E has been shown, however, to be effective when added directly to milk [17-20]. King [17] reported that the addition of vitamin E directly to milk required less than 1% of the amount required as a dietary supplement to provide the same protective effect. The direct addition of vitamin E per se to milk, however, also is not presently permitted [8, 9, 17, 21].

The tocopherol content of milk varies with the season primarily because the ration of the cow is richer in tocopherols in the summer than in the winter [22-24]. As early as 1937, Anderson [25] observed that when cows were fed good quality alfalfa hay they gave a more stable milk than when fed poor quality alfalfa. Cows on green feeds or pasture give more stable milk than those on dry feeds [26-32]. High quality alfalfa and lush green pastures provide substantial quantities of mixed tocopherols. Krukovsky et al. [33] found a significant correlation between the tocopherol content of milk and its ability to resist oxidized flavor development. Tocopherol supplementation of the cows' ration increases the tocopherol content of the milk fat [34-37] and the oxidative stability of milk [8, 9, 24, 35-42]. Typical data are shown in Table 1 as gathered by Dunkley et al. [35]. They found that daily supplements of vitamin E increased the milk tocopherol concentration which produced a significant increase in stability of the milk to copper-induced oxidized flavor, as determined by the thio-barbituric acid (TBA) test and sensory scores.

Werner [9] reported that the direct addition of vitamin E was effective in preventing the development of oxidized flavor when added at only several-fold higher levels than the "normal" content of the milk. She was not able, however, to show any direct correlation between the tocopherol content of the milk and the oxidative stability of the milk expressed by the TBA values. She also showed that the antioxidant BHA was not transferred to

TABLE 1   Intake of Vitamin E and Oxidative Stability of Milk Fat

Parameter	Control [a]	Supplemented [a]
Vitamin E intake (IU/cow/day)	66	818
α-tocopherol (mg/100 g milk fat)	2.79	5.65 [b]
TBA increase after 2 days	83	25 [b, c]
Flavor score after 2 days	3.2	1.9 [b, d]

[a] Copper added at 0.1 mcg/g fluid milk.
[b] Significantly different (P < 0.05).
[c] The lower the number, the lesser development of rancidity.
[d] The lower the number, the lesser the degree of "off-flavor." 0 = no oxidized flavor; 4 = strong oxidized flavor.
Source: From Ref. 35.

the milk and had no effect on the tocopherol content or the oxidative stability of the milk.

Erickson et al. [39] found the tocopherol concentration to be at least 3 times higher in the lipid of the fat-globule membrane than inside the fat globule. During lipid oxidation, the tocopherol associated with the fat globule membrane was lost more rapidly. Thus, the membrane tocopherol content is more important than that inside the fat globule for determining the oxidative stability of milk. Studies with intravenously injected tocopherol by Erickson et al. [38] showed that as little as 1.5 g free tocopherol or acetate ester in emulsified form caused a marked increase in milk tocopherol and oxidative stability. When the milk lipids were fractionated by a churning procedure, changes in oxidative stability of the milk correlated with the tocopherol in the membrane lipids (from buttermilk) more closely than with those inside the fat globule (butter oil).

In these numerous trials cited, both d- and dl- α -tocopherol or the respective acetate esters were used with equal success and generally reflected the biological activity of the various forms of vitamin E [43-46].

Adams [47] concluded, from both research data and field experience, that high level supplementation of dairy rations with vitamin E (1000-2000 IU per head daily) has successfully controlled oxidized off-flavor in milk.

Tikriti [48] reported that supplementation of a tocopherol-poor ration with 1000 mg α-tocopheryl acetate/cow/day prevented the development of oxidized flavor. The minimum effective level of supplementation was related to the degree of copper contamination of the milk. Over supplementation was largely wasted and the minimal daily supplement (1000 mg) was more effective than intermittent larger doses, either orally or intramuscularly. The transfer of α-tocopherol to milk was poor (<4.0%) but directly related to the plasma concentration. Dunkley et al. [36] had also previously found that intermittent administration of relatively large doses (6000 mg α-tocopheryl acetate) was not a practical method for control of oxidized flavor in milk.

In summary, it can be concluded that the continuous supplementation of the cow's ration with tocopherol is feasible as a practical method of delaying the development of oxidized flavor in milk based on TBA values, flavor scores, and induction period tests. The responses to tocopherol are both rapid and marked; an increase in the tocopherol content of milk results in a decrease in the susceptibility to develop oxidized flavor. The effect is quite reproducible and predictable—the more tocopheryl acetate in the ration, the greater the tocopherol content of milk; the greater the tocopherol content in milk, the more resistant the milk is to oxidized flavor. The direct addition of α-tocopherol would be most efficient. However, as noted, this approach is not currently permitted.

III. POULTRY MEAT—WHOLE AND FURTHER PROCESSED

Flavor components of poultry are becoming increasingly important as
more and more poultry products are marketed frozen after extended
freezer storage [49-53]. In addition, the increased emphasis on further
processing and the development of new products utilizing all or part
poultry meat makes acceptable fresh flavor preservation and retardation
of off-flavor development of paramount importance.

This discussion is appropriate for both chicken and turkey. Currently,
frozen turkeys and turkey products represent a larger portion of total
turkey production as compared to chicken; however, as the broiler industry changes from the present fresh market to the frozen product, a major
concern will be maintaining quality to ensure continued acceptability.

Mountney et al. [54] reported that there was enough difference in the
flavor of frozen chicken stored 3 months from fresh chicken to indicate a
preference for the fresh. Hanson et al. [55] found flavor changes occurred
more rapidly in the meat than the coating in precooked frozen, coated
(breaded) chickens. Quick-frozen broilers lost flavor after only 51 days
storage at -23°C, according to Stewart et al. [56]. The breast and leg
meat of chickens stored at 0°C were significantly less intense in flavor
after only 5 weeks of storage than controls based on the findings of
van den Berg [57]; off-flavors were also noted. In addition, processed
products also reflect the adverse effects of storage [58-61].

A number of factors may affect poultry flavor in both fresh and stored
products, one of the more important being dietary components [62-80].
Fish oils are particularly rich in the long-chained linolenates which are
readily assimilated and deposited in the carcass of poultry [75-80]. It is
the increased tissue deposition of the long-chained linolenates, particularly
20:5, 22:5, and 22:6 which has been correlated with the development of
fishy flavor in poultry [75, 77, 79, 80, 82, 83, 85-92]. Klose et al. [65, 93]
and Kummerow et al. [94] found that the problem was not unique to the
inclusion of fish oils or fish meals in the diet since linseed oil could also
impart a fishy flavor in poultry.

As early as 1926, Carrick and Hauge [62] reported that the feeding of
cod-liver oil to broilers adversely affected flavor. Asmundson et al. [63]
observed a similar effect in turkeys when fed 2-5% fish oil; Marbel et al.
[64] reported off-flavors in turkeys due to feeding of cod-liver oil and
white fish meal. These effects have been confirmed by many investigators
over the years [65-92].

There have been numerous reports that vitamin E supplementation
(levels above those required to prevent nutritional diseases) significantly
reduces fishy flavor in poultry fed fish oils and fish meals; however, the
vitamin E did not affect the uptake and deposition of linolenates by the
bird [70, 79, 80, 85, 86, 91, 95, 96].

Laksesvela [70] reported that the taste and odor of fresh chicken meat were significantly improved when broilers were fed 50 IU vitamin E/kg feed with from 6 to 15% of regular herring meal compared to unsupplemented controls. High levels of vitamin E (170 IU/bird ingested during the last 5 days prior to slaughter) also improved the taste of the fresh meat. Dreosti et al. [96] also confirmed the beneficial effect of vitamin E on chicken flavor when fed rations containing large quantities of fish meal.

Opstvedt [95] demonstrated a relationship between the quality of the flavor of broiler meat and its stability towards oxygen (as measured by the TBA value) and shown in Fig. 1, and the flavor score in relation to the tissue concentration of vitamin E (Fig. 2).

The effect of feeding fish meal (0-10% of the diet) with and without supplemental vitamin E (22 IU E/kg of feed) on fishiness and rancidity in precooked, sliced, frozen turkey meat was investigated by Webb et al. [97] through the use of TBA numbers and taste panels. The authors concluded that the inclusion of vitamin E in high-level fish meal rations reduced the magnitude of TBA numbers and severity of off-flavors. Typical data are shown in Table 2.

Crawford et al. [80] had shown that 200 mg dl-α-tocopheryl acetate per kg diet afforded optimum protection against the development of fishy

TABLE 2   TBA Numbers and Taste Panel Scores for Cooked Turkey Thigh Meat Held in Frozen Storage for 8 Months

Supplement to basal ration	TBA number [a]	Fishy flavor score [b]	Rancid flavor score [b]
None (control)	3.21a [c]	7.58c [c]	6.38ab [c]
Control plus 22 IU E/kg	3.16a	7.90c	7.08c
5% Fish meal	3.76a	6.21b	6.27ab
5% Fish meal plus 22 IU E/kg	3.33a	7.40c	6.73bc
10% Fish meal	5.44b	4.83a	5.92a
10% Fish meal plus 22 IU E/kg	3.96a	5.29a	6.06ab

[a] The higher the number, the greater the chemically determined oxidative rancidity.
[b] The higher the score, the more desirable the taste.
[c] Means within a vertical column followed by different letters differ significantly at the 0.05 level of probability.
Source: From Ref. 97.

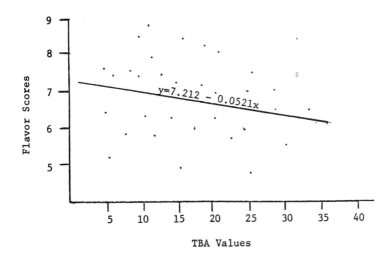

FIG. 1   Relationship between flavor scores and TBA values of broiler meat. The higher the flavor score, the more desirable the taste. (From Ref. 95.)

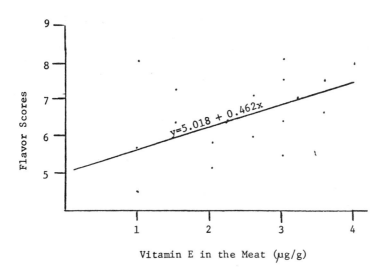

FIG. 2   Relationship between the flavor scores and the vitamin E content of broiler meat. The higher the flavor score, the more desirable the taste. (From Ref. 95.)

flavor in turkeys when as much as 2% tuna oil was fed. Crawford and Kretsch [91] reported on the flavor of breast meat from turkeys that had been fed 2% tuna oil with and without vitamin E supplements, and cooked in air or under nitrogen with a slight vacuum. Cooking under nitrogen prevented the development of fishy flavor nearly as well as the dietary dl-α-tocopheryl acetate supplements. Others have investigated the problem [98-100]. Lineweaver [101] found that when tocopherol is added to a diet containing fish oil, the level of fishiness is reduced even though the fatty acid composition of the turkey fat is not altered. When fishy birds are removed from fish-oil diets, the time required to eliminate fishiness is reduced from about 5 weeks to about 2.5 weeks if the nonfish diet is supplemented with tocopherol.

Prevention of peroxide accumulation in the fat of rats by feeding tocopherols had been shown in the early 1940s with the conclusion drawn that the normal source of tissue antioxidants was the tocopherols of the feed [102, 103]. Experiments with hog fat had indicated a similar relationship between the keeping quality of the fat and the presence of tocopherols [104]. Dam and Granados [105] showed that certain of the body lipids in vitamin E-deficient chicks underwent lipoperoxide formation in vivo, and that it could be prevented by supplementing the ration with vitamin E.

Criddle and Morgan [106, 107] were the first to study the effect of graded doses of tocopherol upon the production of peroxides and the development of rancidity in stored turkey carcasses. They determined the peroxide number for the fat under the skin and for the abdominal fat before and after frozen storage and found the values progressively greater with storage and decreasing amounts of tissue tocopherol. The acceptability of meat and fat and the detection of rancidity by a taste panel fell in the same order as the peroxide numbers. Kummerow et al. [108] also observed significantly lower peroxide values for the fat of turkeys fed a tocopherol concentrate. Hood et al. [109] reported the same protective effect in broiler chickens. Mecchi et al. [110-112] found that the stability of chicken fat was increased two to threefold and four to sixfold for turkey fat when 0.1% α-tocopheryl acetate was added to the ration. In spite of the increase in turkey-fat stability, the chicken fat still had a twofold greater stability than the turkey fat. They found the tocopherol content to be much higher in chicken tissue than in turkeys held under the same dietary conditions. When tocopherol was added to the turkey fat (in vitro) in order to raise the level to that of the chicken fat (in vivo), then the stability, indicated by induction period for rancidity development, was the same for fats from the two species. The stabilizing effect of tocopherol supplements was confirmed by chemical analysis (development of peroxides) in stored frozen carcasses using the iodometric method of Pool et al. [113]. Organoleptic scores on cooked birds by a panel of eight judges supported the chemical tests run initially and after storage.

Mecchi et al. [112] further evaluated the effect of vitamin E when fed for only 1-2 weeks to both chickens and turkeys at 0.1% as a d-α tocopherol acetate concentrate. They found the 1- and 2-week feeding of vitamin E resulted in increased tocopherol content and markedly improved stability in chickens, but only slightly in turkeys. Some of their values are shown in Table 3 and compared to more recent data obtained by Marusich et al. [114] 20 years later (Tables 4 and 5). Direct comparisons of tissue α-tocopherol concentrations should not be attempted as the levels and length of supplementation were markedly different. It can be seen, however, in comparing the tissue concentrations (Tables 3-5) that chickens are much more efficient in absorbing and depositing α-tocopherol compared to turkeys. Table 5 is presented to show that over the first 8 weeks, the ingestion of vitamin E in relation to body weight is comparable for the chicken and turkey. The substantially lower liver and breast muscle concentrations found for the turkey must be due to far less efficient absorption and deposition of vitamin E and/or a greater physiological utilization of vitamin E as compared to the chicken. Thus, the dietary level of vitamin E required to protect tissues from rancidity will be markedly higher for the turkey than for the chicken.

Additional studies were reported showing the positive effect of tissue concentrations of α-tocopherol on retarding the rate of rancidity development in the carcass lipids of both broilers [72, 95, 115-117] and turkeys [97, 118-124] under various storage conditions. Webb et al. [116] studied the effect of feeding dl-α-tocopheryl acetate, ethoxyquin, and BHT on rancidity development in prefried broiler parts using both a chemical test (TBA numbers) according to the procedure of Tarladgis et al. [125] and taste panel evaluations. A good correlation was obtained between increased TBA number and increased off-odor and/or off-flavor. Feeding of 220 IU vitamin E per kilogram of feed (220 mg/kg $\cong$ 0.022%) for 12 days preslaughter held TBA numbers significantly below those of the control group. Panel taste scores were also significantly better and confirmed the TBA number results on the prefried, frozen broiler parts (Table 6). Feeding BHT at 0.01, 0.02, or 0.04% of the ration did not significantly reduce rancidity development. Ethoxyquin at 0.04% did reduce TBA numbers and the effect was detected by the taste panel.

Marusich et al. [114] studied the effect of dietary concentrations of vitamin E on rancidity development during refrigerated storage at 1°C (34°F) on uncooked broiler carcasses, based on TBA numbers and related tissue concentrations of α-tocopherol to the retardation in development of rancidity. In Table 7 we see the results of feeding 0, 60, 140, 180 or 220 IU vitamin E per kilogram of feed for the last 5 days prior to slaughter. Supplementation with 140 IU E/kg (total 160 IU E/kg) or more for 5 days did induce adequate breast-muscle concentrations of α-tocopherol and also held the TBA number low for 17 days. This is about the

TABLE 3 Stability of Extracted Skin Fat in 24 Week-Old Birds

Mixed tocopherol concentrate supplement (%) [a]	Length of feeding (wk)	Chicken		Turkey	
		Tocopherol content (mg/100 g)	Induction period (hr)	Tocopherol content (mg/100 g)	Induction period (hr)
None	—	2.8	16	1.2	1.7
0.22	1	4.3	31	1.9	3.1
0.22	2	5.7	55	2.3	13.0

[a] Concentrate contained 45% by weight d-α-tocopheryl acetate, so 0.1% or 1360 IU E/kg feed were fed.
Source: From Ref. 112.

TABLE 4   Liver and Breast-Muscle Concentrations of α-Tocopherol in Chickens and Turkeys

Species	Vitamin E supplement (IU/kg)	Tissue α-tocopherol (mg/100 g)					
		Liver			Breast muscle		
		4 wk	6 wk	8 wk	4 wk	6 wk	8 wk
Chicken [a]	40	2.98	2.78	2.51	0.43	0.47	0.50
Turkey [b]	37	0.60	0.63	0.59	0.14	0.13	0.14

[a] Average data for three male chickens at both 4 and 6 weeks and for six male birds at 8 weeks.
[b] Average data for 10 turkeys (5 females, 5 males) at each time period.
Source: From Ref. 114.

maximum time that birds can be held at 1°C before developing pronounced bacterial spoilage. This dietary level (160 IU E/kg) is in basic agreement with that of Webb et al. [116] where they fed 220 IU E/kg for 12 days. Table 8 presents a summary of tissue α-tocopherol concentrations and TBA values for broilers after 6 or 8 weeks continuous feeding of lower concentrations of supplemental vitamin E. TBA measurements show that a total dietary concentration of 40 IU E/kg fed continuously is required to prevent development of rancidity and achieve a tissue (breast-muscle) α-tocopherol concentration of 0.5 mg/100 g in 8 week-old market-weight birds.

Based on liver and breast-muscle α-tocopherol concentrations and TBA numbers run on breast-muscle, it was shown that dl-α-tocopherol was as effective as dl-α-tocopheryl acetate [114]. In turn, d-α-tocopheryl acetate was equal to dl-α-tocopheryl acetate [126] when all were fed on an IU basis, thus confirming previous data on the relative biological efficacy of the d- and dl-α-isomers [127-134].

Off-flavor in turkeys is presently a far more serious problem than with chickens due to the more common practice of freezing most turkeys prior to retail sale. Also, turkey meat currently enters into further processing to a greater extent and in a greater variety of precooked items than chicken meat.

Webb et al. [122] studied the effect of tocopherol supplementation in turkeys on the stability of both precooked frozen turkey meat and of mechanically deboned turkey (MDT) meat. Vitamin E was fed at 22 and 220 IU/kg, or the ingested weekly total was injected subcutaneously once per week for 5 weeks. All supplements except the 22 IU/kg feed resulted

TABLE 5   Relationship of Vitamin E Ingested to Body Weight Over 0-8 Weeks in Chickens and Turkeys

	Vitamin E supplement (IU/kg)	Total E intake per period (IU)			Average E intake per day (IU)			Average E intake/day/kg b.w. (IU)		
		1-28 days	29-42 days	43-56 days	1-28 days	29-42 days	43-56 days	1-28 days	29-42 days	43-56 days
Chicken[a]	40	48.2	54.0	66.6	1.72	3.86	4.76	3.88	3.31	2.57
Turkey[b]	37	31.1	54.3	84.5	1.11	3.88	6.04	3.28	3.68	2.92

[a] Average data for 12 birds at 4 weeks, 9 birds at 6 weeks, and 6 birds at 8 weeks (all male chickens).
[b] Average data for 10 turkeys (5 females, 5 males) at each time period.
Source: From Ref. 114

TABLE 6   TBA Numbers and Rancidity Development of Precooked Frozen Broiler Parts

Dietary supplement	Mean TBA number [a]	Rancidity development [b]
None (control basal ration)	1.47a [c]	7.40A [c]
220 IU E/kg for last 12 days	0.34b	8.45B
10% animal fat for last 12 days	1.39a	7.86A
10% animal fat plus 220 IU E/kg for last 12 days	0.57b	8.46B

[a] The lower the number, the lesser the degree of rancidity.
[b] The lower the number, the least desirable (1) to most desirable (10).
[c] Means within a vertical column followed by different small or capital letters differ significantly ($P < 0.01$) or ($P < 0.05$), respectively.
Source: From Ref. 116.

in lower TBA numbers than the controls for the samples tested initially and after 4 months freezer storage of precooked frozen turkey. Flavor preference and off-flavor followed the TBA values, with only the 22 IU/kg vitamin E samples being detectably more rancid. Breast-tissue was more resistant to oxidative rancidity than thigh-muscle held under identical conditions. The MDT meat was far more susceptible to oxidative changes at refrigerated temperatures than the whole carcass, however, the MDT meat also definitively reflected the retarding effect of supplemental vitamin E on rancidity development.

Hayse et al. [123] reported that 4 weeks of prior supplementation with 220 IU/kg vitamin E was necessary to significantly delay the development of TBA-reactive compounds in MDT meat when held at refrigerator temperatures.

The effect of vitamin E on turkey carcasses stored under refrigeration (1°C) was studied by Marusich et al. [114]. All supplemental levels of vitamin E delayed the onset of rancidity with 200 IU/kg feed for 4 weeks or 400 IU/kg for 3 weeks, yielding the optimal effects based on TBA values being held below 0.75 for at least 7 days when stored at 1°C. These data are shown in Table 9. These studies [114] with turkeys show that concentrations of tocopherol in liver and breast-muscle are only 1:5 to 1:3, respectively, those of broiler chickens fed similar dietary concentrations (see Tables 4 and 5). As noted, Mecchi et al. [110-112] had previously reported similar effects (see Table 3). Thus, turkeys require markedly

TABLE 7 Liver and Breast-Muscle α-Tocopherol Content and Breast-Muscle TBA Number of Market-Weight Broilers Fed a Commercial-type Ration Continuously, Supplemented with Additional Vitamin E for the last 5 Days

Vitamin E (IU/kg)			E ingested per bird in 5 days (IU)	α-Tocopherol (mg/100 g tissue)[b]		TBA number (breast-muscle)[b,c]
Basal[a]	Added	Total		Liver	Breast-muscle	
20	0	20	10.6	1.58	0.38	0.85
20	60	80	43.4	4.34	0.40	0.50
20	140	160	84.1	7.78	0.59	0.47
20	180	200	107.4	11.25	0.62	0.40
20	220	240	139.6	12.74	0.69	0.30

[a] Contained 19.7 IU/kg vitamin E.
[b] Average data for two groups of 4 male birds per treatment.
[c] After 17 days storage of whole carcasses at 1°C.
Source: From Ref. 114.

TABLE 8 Liver and Breast-Muscle α-Tocopherol Content and Breast-Muscle TBA Number of Broilers Fed a Commercial-type Ration for up to 8 Weeks with Graded Concentrations of Vitamin E

Ration vitamin E content (IU/kg)			Liver α-tocopherol (mg/100 g)		Breast muscle α-tocopherol (mg/100 g)		TBA number of breast-muscle at day determined (d)	
Basal[a]	Added	Total	6 wk[b]	8 wk[c]	6 wk[b]	8 wk[c]	6 wk[b]	8 wk[c]
16	0	16	1.19	1.06	0.18	0.20	1.08, 6 d	0.86, 5 d
16	4	20	1.30	1.65	0.24	0.27	0.84, 11 d	0.85, 6 d
16	14	30	2.01	2.19	0.34	0.39	0.27, 14 d	0.70, 11 d
16	24	40	2.78	2.51	0.47	0.50	0.17, 14 d	0.50, 14 d
16	44	60	3.84	3.20	0.63	0.62	0.17, 14 d	0.36, 14 d

[a] Contained 15.9 IU/kg vitamin E.
[b] Average data for 9 male birds.
[c] Average data for 6 male birds.
Source: From Ref. 114.

TABLE 9   Dietary Intake and Tissue Levels of Vitamin E Related to Breast-Muscle TBA Values

Vitamin E supplement (IU/kg)			Average weight (kg)[b]	Feed intake (kg)	Vitamin E intake		
Basal[a]	Added	Total			Total (IU)	Average (IU)	Daily (IU/kg b.w.)
Hen Data							
Supplements fed for last 4 weeks (16-20 weeks of age)							
50	0	50	4.975	6.147	307	11.0	2.2
50	100	150	5.068	5.605	841	30.0	5.9
50	200	250	5.487	6.454	1614	57.6	10.9
50	400	450	4.913	5.529	2488	88.9	18.1
Supplements fed for last 3 weeks (17-20 weeks of age)							
50	100	150	5.244	4.430	665	31.7	6.0
50	200	250	5.463	4.929	1232	58.7	10.7
50	400	450	5.175	4.129	1858	88.5	17.1
Tom Data							
Supplements fed for last 4 weeks (20-24 weeks of age)							
50	0	50	9.805	10.727	536	19.1	1.9
50	100	150	9.519	10.400	1560	55.7	5.9
50	200	250	10.700	10.567	2642	94.4	8.8
50	400	450	10.306	9.923	4465	159.5	15.5
Supplements fed for last 3 weeks (21-24 weeks of age)							
50	100	150	11.969	7.250	1088	51.8	4.3
50	200	250	10.369	7.017	1754	83.5	8.0
50	400	450	10.000	6.723	3025	144.0	14.4

[a] Ration contained 50 IU vitamin E per kilogram feed.
[b] For supplementation period.
[c] 8-Day TBA value.
Source: From Ref. 114.

| α-Tocopherol content | | TBA values (days) | | | |
Breast-muscle (mg %)	Lipid (mg/g)	2	4	7	9
0.105	0.135	0.63	0.71	1.64	—
0.130	0.145	0.35	0.63	0.81	0.87
0.185	0.285	0.34	0.44	0.62	0.84
0.205	0.300	0.24	0.30	0.39	0.82
0.115	0.135	0.43	0.41	0.76	0.76[c]
0.125	0.210	0.31	0.66	0.72	0.65
0.155	0.290	0.29	0.28	0.40	0.86
0.075	0.090	0.55	0.98	—	—
0.150	0.200	0.44	0.56	0.92	1.32
0.195	0.320	0.16	0.34	0.36	0.35
0.225	0.245	0.09	0.15	0.20	0.40
0.110	0.170	0.33	0.70	0.77	—
0.150	0.150	0.09	0.59	0.87	1.20
0.220	0.235	0.08	0.25	0.55	0.39

higher levels of supplemental vitamin E than broiler chickens to delay the
onset of rancidity. dl-α-Tocopherol proved to be no more effective than
the acetate ester when both were fed to turkeys on a IU basis [126].

The weight of evidence indicates an overall excellent correlation
between TBA values and the α-tocopherol content of poultry meat. In turn,
the tissue content reflects the dietary vitamin E levels. Jacobson and
Koehler [135] reported a good correlation between taste panel scores and
TBA numbers for frozen, cooked turkeys. Dawson and Schierholz [136]
noted that the stability of turkey meat as measured by TBA numbers was
adversely influenced by cooking, grinding, and storage, and the combination resulted in maximum lipid oxidation. Dawson et al. [137] have
attempted to solve the problem by the direct addition of three approved
chemical antioxidants [138] for use in processing poultry products. TBA
values were effectively controlled by all three antioxidants; however, panel
flavor scores were not well correlated.

In a trial with ducks, Klinger and Stadelman [139] found that injection
of α-tocopherol or combinations of citric acid, polyphosphates, propyl
gallate, and BHA prior to cooking offered some protection against oxidation
during cooking, storage, and reheating based on TBA tests, but were not
completely confirmed by the taste panel evaluations.

In summary, both chicken and turkey meats, fresh, precooked, or
further processed and held refrigerated or frozen, benefit from the dietary
addition of vitamin E based on both objective (TBA number) and subjective
(taste panel) measurements. Continuous supplementation with lower concentrations or short-term feeding of substantially higher levels prior to
slaughter are both effective. Both free tocopherol and its acetate ester
are effective and equal on an IU basis. The tissue α-tocopherol content is
correlated with the dietary levels fed and these, in turn, are related to the
TBA number and off-odor and off-flavor formation. Turkeys require
higher dietary concentration of vitamin E and feeding for a longer time than
chickens to achieve effective protection against rancidity development.

IV. PORK AND PORK PRODUCTS

Pork is especially susceptible to fatty acid oxidation which markedly
decreases palatability. It has been observed over many years that when
feeds containing unsaturated and easily oxidized fats are fed, pigs are
able to deposit these fats in the muscle and adipose tissue, resulting in
increased oxidation of pork-tissue and fat. This increased oxidation is, in
turn, the most important cause for the development of off-flavor, discolor-
ation, and reduced keeping quality. This oxidation, like that in milk and
poultry, can be inhibited by vitamin E. Direct addition of one or more of
several tocopherols to the pigs' ration has been shown by numerous

workers [104,140-157] to counteract the unfavorable effects of the unsaturated fatty acids.

The earliest studies with swine and vitamin E were those of Chipault et al. [104] in 1945, Burr et al. [140] in 1946, and Carpenter and Lundberg [141] in 1949. Chipault et al. [104] showed that the prevention of peroxide accumulation in hog fat by feeding tocopherol indicated that the relationship holds between the keeping quality of the hog fat and the presence of vitamin E and unsaturated fatty acids. Burr et al. [140] emphasized the need to add vitamin E to swine rations to significantly stabilize the fatty tissues. Carpenter and Lundberg [141] found the induction period for oxygen absorption to be much shorter in fat from hogs which had not received supplementary tocopherol as compared to those which had received a total of 31 g in 12 weeks. Palmer et al. [142] in 1952 studied the deterioration of flavor in frozen pork as it relates to fat composition, storage temperature, length of storage, and packaging treatment. They found that pork containing unsaturated carcass fat as a result of feeding soybeans became rancid when stored at temperatures above -17.6°C, but not when stored below that temperature.

Dammers et al. [143] concluded from their studies that 40 mg vitamin E fed daily in the ration was the minimum quantity required to give pork a satisfactory keeping quality. Duncan et al. [145] and Leat [146] conducted similar feeding experiments and also showed that the stability of the pork was improved. Zaehringer et al. [147] found a highly significant (P < 0.01) positive correlation (r = 0.86) between the amount of tocopherol supplement fed and the concentration of tocopherol found in the fresh loin. Bratzler et al. [158] had observed a similar effect with weanling barrows. Zaehringer et al. [147] noted that the concentration of tissue tocopherol decreased significantly (P < 0.01) during frozen storage; in turn, the TBA values determined by the method of Turner et al. [159] increased significantly (P < 0.01) during frozen storage. Judges' scores for all palatability factors showed a highly significant decrease (P < 0.01) during frozen storage with the first serious loss of quality appearing after 9 months. No significant (P > 0.01) differences in palatability due to the amount of tocopherol supplemented were found, however. Their findings confirmed previous data from the same group [144].

A number of reports from Scandinavia [148-150,152,153,155-157) have confirmed the beneficial effect of vitamin E supplementation on pork-tissue stability and palatability. Hvidsten and Astrup [148] reported that daily supplementation with 50 IU vitamin E from 20 to 90 kg (total supplement per pig, 5000 IU) improved the keeping quality of the pork as measured by TBA number [160] and induction period [161] using both d- and dl-αtocopheryl acetate. They further observed that when the distinct off-flavor of the pork was produced by a ration high in marine fats, the off-flavor was diminished by adding vitamin E. However, this effect of added vitamin E was scarcely detectable if the ration only produced a faint off-flavor.

Typical data are shown in Table 10 [148] after feeding 50, 100, and 200 IU vitamin E per head per day for the last 32 days prior to marketing. TBA numbers and induction-period time reflected the positive effect of supplemental vitamin E. They also found that a given quantity of vitamin E may have a greater effect when supplemented for only the last month prior to slaughter, than when it is evenly distributed over the entire growing period.

From a series of feeding trials run at the Institute of Animal Nutrition, Agricultural University of Norway [148,153,162,163], Astrup [157] concluded that (1) vitamin E is effectively transferred from the ration to the fat of the pig; (2) the stability of the fat towards oxygen has been increased based on both TBA values and the induction period; and (3) the taste of the pork has been improved. The off-taste scores were found to be significantly related to the data on stability towards oxygen, and they confirmed the more direct evidence that vitamin E improves the quality of the taste of pork. Astrup [157] also states that there is no upper limit to be observed when vitamin E is used as a stabilizing agent; in fact, the higher the level used, the better are the results. No undesirable side effects have ever been reported following the administration of massive doses to swine.

In the area of further processing or further handling of pork, Keskinel et al. [151] reported increases in TBA values immediately following the grinding operation and a rapid increase in TBA number during storage at

TABLE 10   Effect of Feeding Graded Concentrations of Vitamin E to Swine

Parameter	IU vitamin E per head per day for last 32 days [a]			
	0	50	100	200
Vitamin E (mcg/g) back fat	5.2	6.9	9.4	9.4
Vitamin E (mcg/g) lard fat	4.6	5.9	8.4	9.9
TBA number-back fat	11.7	9.0 [b]	6.2	3.9
TBA number-lard fat	10.8	6.6	5.2	3.9
Induction period (days)-back fat	5.3	5.2 [b]	7.2	7.8
Induction period (days)-lard fat	4.8	6.5	6.8	8.8

[a] Average data for four animals.
[b] Only values not statistically significant at the 5% level when compared to control ration.
Source: From Ref. 148.

5°C. Grau and Fleischmann [154] claimed that a certain German "cold cut," cervelatwurst, is improved organoleptically if the pigs from which it is made have been supplied with supplemental vitamin E.

Thus, we note the same basic findings for pork and pork products as have been documented for milk, chicken, and turkey meat, and further processed products. Supplemental vitamin E improves shelf life, aids in resisting rancidity development and thus helps prevent off-odors and off-flavors. These data support the antioxidant theory for the function of vitamin E [164-167]. The tocopherols are nature's choice of antioxidants playing an important intracellular role, relating especially to the stabilization of ingested fats and to those products resulting from the metabolic synthesis and degradation of lipids. Vitamin E thus functions as a general protector of structural lipoproteins and of oxidizable lipid components of enzymes.

The weight of evidence supports the following general summarization: α-tocopherol is deposited into milk, liver, fat, and muscle tissue in proportion to the amount ingested. The concentration in tissue is directly related to the log-dose of the intake.

Development of rancid off-flavor in milk, poultry, and pork products after storage is reduced in proportion to the amount of tocopherol deposited in the tissues. This protective effect is related to the antioxidant effect of tocopherol as measured by a reduction in malonaldehyde (TBA test) in these products.

Estimated requirements to achieve the effect with vitamin E are as follows:

Dairy cows:	500-2000 IU vitamin E/head each day continuously
Chickens:	30-50 IU E/kg feed continuously or 150-250 IU E/kg for about 1 week prior to slaughter
Turkeys:	100-200 IU E/kg feed for 1 month prior to slaughter or 50-100 IU E/kg continuously
Swine:	50 IU E/kg feed continuously or 100-200 IU E/head each day for 1 month prior to slaughter

RECENT DEVELOPMENTS

Since this manuscript was prepared, Bartov and Bornstein [168-171] and Bartov [172] have published a series of papers assessing vitamin E and several other antioxidants for their effect on the stability of broiler meat and adipose tissue. Most recently, Uebersax et al. [173] reported on the stability of turkey breast and thigh meat as well as mechanically deboned turkey meat used in loaves after refrigerated storage at 4°C or frozen storage at -18°C. Vitamin E had been administered to the turkey in the feed or by subcutaneous injection.

REFERENCES

1. S. Krishnamurthy and J. G. Bieri, J. Nutr. 77:245 (1962).
2. H. H. Draper, J. Amer. Oil Chem. Soc. 45:244 (1968).
3. O. A. Roels, Present Knowledge in Nutrition, 3rd ed. Nutrition Foundation, New York, 1967, p. 84.
4. J. Glavind, Br. J. Nutr. 24:19 (1972).
5. J. Bunyan, E. A. Murrell, J. Green, and A. T. Diplock, Br. J. Nutr. 21:475 (1967).
6. J. Bunyan, J. Green, E. A. Murrell, A. T. Diplock, and M. A. Cawthorne, Br. J. Nutr. 22:97 (1968).
7. J. Green and J. Bunyan, Nutr. Abst. and Rev. 39:321 (1969).
8. R. L. King, Proc. Maryland Nutr. Conf. p. 13 (1967).
9. H. Werner, Acta Agric. Scand. (Suppl.) 19:29 (1973).
10. R. L. King and W. L. Dunkley, J. Dairy Sci. 42:420 (1959).
11. R. L. King, J. R. Luick, I. I. Litman, W. G. Jennings, and W. L. Dunkley, J. Dairy Sci. 42:780 (1959).
12. R. L. King and W. F. Williams, J. Dairy Sci. 46:11 (1963).
13. L. M. Smith and W. L. Dunkley, J. Dairy Sci. 42:896 (1959).
14. C. H. Lea, J. Sci. Food Agr. 8:1 (1957).
15. L. M. Smith and E. L. Jack, J. Dairy Sci. 42:767 (1959).
16. E. N. Frankel, L. M. Smith, and E. L. Jack, J. Dairy Sci. 41:483 (1958).
17. R. L. King, J. Dairy Sci. 51:1075 (1968).
18. C. Kanno, M. Hayashi, and K. Yamauchi, Agr. Biol. Chem. (Jap.) 34:878 (1970); Through CA 73, #97:460t (1970).
19. C. Kanno, K. Yamauchi, and T. Tsugo, Agr. Biol. Chem. (Jap.) 34:886 (1970); Through CA 73, #97:461u (1970).
20. C. Kanno, K. Yamauchi, and T. Tsugo, Agr. Biol. Chem. (Jap.) 34:1652 (1970); through BA 52, #48:578 (1971).
21. H. E. Gallo-Torres, Int. J. Vit. Nutr. Res. 42:312 (1972).
22. R. Abderhalden, Biochem. Z. 318:47 (1947).
23. P. L. Harris, M. L. Quaife, and W. L. Swanson, J. Nutr. 40:367 (1950).
24. W. F. Shipe, Proc. Cornell Nutr. Conf., p. 108 (1964).
25. J. A. Anderson, 25th Ann. Rept. Int. Assoc. Dairy and Milk Inspectors, p. 223 (1937).
26. V. N. Krukovsky, J. Agr. Food Chem. 9:439 (1961).
27. W. L. Dunkley, L. M. Smith, and M. Ronning, J. Dairy Sci. 43:1766 (1960).

28. K. M. Narayanan, C. P. Anantakrishman, and K. C. Sen, Ind. J. Dairy Sci. 9:87 (1956).
29. J. Nielsen, A. N. Fisker, A. H. Pedersen, I. Prange, E. Sundergaard, and H. Dam, J. Dairy Res. 20:333 (1953).
30. J. K. Loosli, V. N. Krukovsky, G. P. Lofgreen, and R. B. Musgrave, J. Dairy Sci. 33:228 (1950).
31. V. N. Krukovsky, F. Whiting, and J. K. Loosli, J. Dairy Sci. 33:791 (1950).
32. V. N. Krukovsky, G. W. Trimberger, K. L. Turk, J. K. Loosli, and C. R. Henderson, J. Dairy Sci. 37:1 (1954).
33. V. N. Krukovsky, J. K. Loosli, and F. Whiting, J. Dairy Sci. 32:196 (1949).
34. A. P. DeLuca, R. Teichman, J. E. Rousseau, M. E. Morgan, H. D. Eaton, P. MacLeod, M. W. Dicks, and R. E. Johnson, J. Dairy Sci. 40:877 (1957).
35. W. L. Dunkley, M. Ronning, and L. M. Smith, Proc. 17th Int. Dairy Congr. (Munich) A:223 (1966).
36. W. L. Dunkley, A. A. Franke, M. Ronning, and J. Robb, J. Dairy Sci. 50:100 (1967).
37. W. L. Dunkley, M. Ronning, A. A. Franke, and J. Robb, J. Dairy Sci. 50:492 (1967).
38. D. R. Erickson, W. L. Dunkley, and M. Ronning, J. Dairy Sci. 46:911 (1963).
39. D. R. Erickson, W. L. Dunkley, and L. M. Smith, J. Food Sci. 29:269 (1964).
40. W. L. Dunkley and W. G. Jennings, J. Dairy Sci. 34:1064 (1951).
41. A. A. Franke, W. L. Dunkley, J. R. Luick, and M. Ronning, J. Dairy Sci. 49:7 (1966).
42. G. J. Smith and W. L. Dunkley, J. Dairy Sci. 45:170 (1962).
43. W. L. Dunkley, A. A. Franke, and J. Robb, J. Dairy Sci. 51:531 (1968).
44. W. L. Marusich, G. Ackerman, and J. C. Bauernfeind, Poultry Sci. 46:541 (1967).
45. W. L. Marusich, G. Ackerman, W. C. Reese, and J. C. Bauernfeind, J. An. Sci. 27:58 (1968).
46. W. L. Marusich and J. C. Bauernfeind, Poultry Sci. 50:506 (1971).
47. R. S. Adams, Penn. State Dairy Nutr. Newsletter (Aug. 1966).
48. H. H. Tikriti, Dissert. Abstr. Int. 31:No. 4, 1717B (1970).
49. K. D. Naden and G. A. Jackson, Calif. Agric. Exp. Sta. Bull. No. 734 (1953).
50. B. D. Raskopf, Tenn. Univ. Agric. Exp. Sta. Bull. No. 331 (1961).
51. H. D. Smith, Maryland Univ. Agric. Exp. Sta. Bull. No. 417 (1961).
52. E. A. Sauter, M. V. Zaehringer, and C. A. Rickard, Poultry Sci. 41:103 (1962).
53. F. E. Cunningham, Worlds' Poultry Sci. J. 31:136 (1975).

54. G. J. Mountney, R. E. Branson, and W. C. Hurley, Poultry Sci. 39:287 (1960).
55. H. L. Hanson, L. R. Fletcher, and H. Lineweaver, Food Technol. 13:221 (1959).
56. G. F. Stewart, H. L. Hanson, B. Lowe, and J. J. Austin, Food Res. 10:16 (1945).
57. L. van den Berg, A. W. Kahn, and C. P. Lentz, Food Technol. 17:91 (1963).
58. E. O. Essary and P. J. Rogers, Poultry Sci. 47:1670 (1968).
59. C. S. Martinsen and A. F. Carlin, Food Technol. 22:223 (1968).
60. H. L. Hanson and L. R. Fletcher, Food Technol. 12:40 (1958).
61. L. E. Dawson and E. Bouwkamp, World's Poultry Sci. J. 25:331 (1969).
62. C. W. Carrick and S. M. Hauge, Poultry Sci. 5:213 (1926).
63. V. S. Asmundson, T. H. Jukes, H. M. Fyler, and M. L. Maxwell, Poultry Sci. 17:147 (1938).
64. D. R. Marble, J. E. Hunter, H. C. Enandel, and R. A. Dutcher, Poultry Sci. 17:49 (1938).
65. A. A. Klose, H. L. Hanson, E. P. Mecchi, J. H. Anderson, I. V. Streeter, and H. Lineweaver, Poultry Sci. 32:82 (1953).
66. S. J. Marsden, L. M. Alexander, G. E. Schopmeyer, and J. C. Lamb, Poultry Sci. 31:451 (1952).
67. S. J. Marsden, L. M. Alexander, J. C. Lamb, and G. S. Linton, Poultry Sci. 36:635 (1957).
68. M. T. Swickard, E. H. Montague, E. F. Dochterman, and S. J. Marsden, Poultry Sci. 31:126 (1952).
69. M. T. Swickard, A. M. Harkin, and S. J. Marsden, Poultry Sci. 32:726 (1953).
70. B. Laksesvela, J. Sci. Food Agric. 11:128 (1960).
71. J. O. Hardin, J. L. Milligan, and V. D. Sidewell, Poultry Sci. 43:858 (1964).
72. W. M. M. A. Janssen and A. C. Germs, Acta Agric. Scand. (Suppl.) 19:72 (1973).
73. W. M. M. A. Janssen, Plattelands Post 26:8 (1970).
74. M. G. Schrieber, G. E. Vail, R. M. Conrad, and L. F. Payne, Poultry Sci. 26:14 (1947).
75. D. Miller and P. Robisch, Poultry Sci. 48:2146 (1969).
76. D. Miller, E. H. Gruger, Jr., K. C. Leong, and G. M. Knobl, Jr., Poultry Sci. 46:438 (1967).
77. D. Miller, E. H. Gruger, Jr., K. C. Leong, and G. M. Knobl, Jr., J. Food Sci. 32:342 (1967).
78. H. M. Edwards, Jr., J. E. Marion, and J. C. Driggers, Prox. XII World's Poultry Congress, p. 182 (1962).
79. L. Crawford, D. W. Peterson, M. J. Kretsch, A. L. Lilyblade, and H. S. Olcott, Fish. Bull. 72:1032 (1974).

80. L. Crawford, M. J. Kretsch, D. W. Peterson, and A. L. Lilyblade, J. Food Sci. 40:751 (1975).
81. T. S. Neudoerffer and C. H. Lea, Br. J. Nutr. 20:581 (1966).
82. J. Opstvedt, E. Nygard, and S. Olsen, Acta Agric. Scand. 20:185 (1970).
83. D. Miller, K. C. Leong, and P. Smith, Jr., J. Food Sci. 34:136 (1969).
84. K. C. Leong, G. M. Knobl, D. G. Snyder, and E. H. Gruger, Jr., Poultry Sci. 43:1235 (1964).
85. G. M. Dreosti, Fishing Ind. Res. Inst. Mem. No. 197 (South Africa) (1970).
86. A. Atkinson, R. P. van der Merwe, and L. G. Swart, Agroanimalia 4:63 (1972).
87. A. Atkinson, L. G. Swart, R. P. van der Merwe, and J. P. H. Wessels, Agroanimalia 4:53 (1972).
88. G. C. Mostert, G. M. Dreosti, L. G. Swart, A. Atkinson, and E. S. van Zyl, Afr. J. Agric. Sci. 11:295 (1968).
89. G. C. Mostert, G. M. Dreosti, A. Atkinson, L. G. Swart, and E. S. van Zyl, Agroanimalia 1:123 (1969).
90. G. M. Dreosti, R. P. van der Merwe, A. Atkinson, and L. G. Swart, Fishing Ind. Res. Inst. Prog. Rep. No. 131 (South Africa) (1970).
91. L. Crawford and M. J. Kretsch, Fish. Bull. 74:89 (1976).
92. J. M. Kretsch, Nutritional Sciences (Ph.D. thesis), Studies of some compounds which contribute to fishy flavor in roasted turkeys fed a basal diet and tuna oil supplement. Univ. of California, Berkeley, July 1975.
93. A. A. Klose, E. P. Mecchi, H. L. Hanson, and H. Lineweaver, J. Amer. Oil Chem. Soc. 28:162 (1951).
94. F. A. Kummerow, J. Hite, and S. Kloxin, Poultry Sci. 27:689 (1948).
95. J. Opstevedt, Acta Agric. Scand. (Suppl.) 19:64 (1973).
96. G. M. Dreosti, R. P. van der Merwe, and A. Atkinson, Fishing Ind. Res. Inst. Ann. Rep. (South Africa) 23:69 (1969).
97. J. E. Webb, C. C. Brunson, and J. D. Yates, Poultry Sci. 52:1029 (1973).
98. A. M. Harkin, C. Kitzmiller, G. L. Gilpin, and S. J. Marsden, Poultry Sci. 37:1328 (1958).
99. J. L. Fry, P. Van Walleghem, P. W. Waldroup, and R. H. Harms, Poultry Sci. 44:1016 (1965).
100. A. Holdas and K. N. May, Poultry Sci. 45:1405 (1966).
101. H. Lineweaver, Minutes, Pacific Egg and Poultry Association's Scientific Advisory Committee Meeting, February 26, 1975, Anaheim, California.

102. R. H. Barnes, W. O. Lundberg, H. T. Hanson, and G. O. Burr, J. Biol. Chem. 149:313 (1943).

103. H. T. Hanson, R. H. Barnes, W. O. Lundberg, and G. O. Burr, J. Biol. Chem. 156:673 (1944).

104. J. R. Chipault, W. O. Lundberg, and G. O. Burr, Arch. Biochem. 8:321 (1945).

105. H. Dam and H. Granados, Acta Physiol. Scand. 10:162 (1945).

106. J. E. Criddle and A. F. Morgan, Fed. Proc. 6:27 (1947).

107. J. E. Criddle and A. F. Morgan, Proc. Soc. Exp. Biol. Med. 78:41 (1951).

108. F. A. Kummerow, G. E. Vail, R. M. Conrad, and T. B. Avery, Poultry Sci. 27:635 (1948).

109. M. P. Hood, R. S. Wheeler, and J. B. McGlamery, Poultry Sci. 29:824 (1950).

110. E. P. Mecchi, M. F. Pool, and A. A. Klose, Poultry Sci. 32:915 (1953).

111. E. P. Mecchi, M. F. Pool, G. A. Behman, M. Hamachi, and A. A. Klose, Poultry Sci. 35:1238 (1956).

112. E. P. Mecchi, M. F. Pool, M. Nonaka, A. A. Klose, S. J. Marsden, and R. J. Lillie, Poultry Sci. 35:1246 (1956).

113. M. F. Pool, H. L. Hanson, and A. A. Klose, Poultry Sci. 29:347 (1950).

114. W. L. Marusich, E. DeRitter, E. F. Ogrinz, J. Keating, M. Mitrovic, and R. H. Bunnell, Poultry Sci. 54:831 (1975).

115. J. Opstvedt, E. Nygard, and S. Olsen, Acta Agric. Scand. 21:125 (1971).

116. J. E. Webb, C. C. Brunson, and J. D. Yates, Poultry Sci. 51:1601 (1972).

117. J. E. Webb, C. C. Brunson, and J. D. Yates, J. Food Sci. 39:133 (1974).

118. W. C. Mickelberry, Poultryman 37(15):9 (1967).

119. L. D. Pickett, B. F. Miller, and R. E. Moreng, Poultry Sci. 47:1493 (1968).

120. W. W. Marion, Turkey World, 47(4):25 (1972).

121. R. W. Webb, W. W. Marion, and P. L. Hayse, J. Food Sci. 37:496 (1972).

122. R. W. Webb, W. W. Marion, and P. L. Hayse, J. Food Sci. 37:853 (1972).

123. P. L. Hayse, W. W. Marion, and R. J. Paulson, Poultry Sci. 53:1934 (1974).

124. J. V. Spencer and J. A. Verstrate, Poultry Sci. 54:1820 (1975).

125. B. G. Tarladgis, B. M. Watts, M. T. Younathan, and L. Dugan, Jr., J. Amer. Oil Chem. Soc. 37:44 (1960).

126. W. L. Marusich, E. F. Ogrinz, and M. Mitrovic, Hoffman-La Roche, Animal Health Res. Dept., unpublished data, 1975.

127. E. M. Hume, Nature 148:472 (1941).
128. M. Joffe and P. L. Harris, J. Amer. Chem. Soc. 65:925 (1943).
129. P. L. Harris and M. I. Ludwig, J. Biol. Chem. 179:111 (1949).
130. P. L. Harris and M. I. Ludwig, J. Biol. Chem. 180:611 (1949).
131. W. J. Pudelkiewicz, L. D. Matterson, L. M. Potter, L. Webster, and E. P. Singsen, J. Nutr. 71:115 (1960).
132. L. Friedman, W. Weiss, F. Wherry, and O. L. Kline, J. Nutr. 65:143 (1958).
133. L. D. Matterson, Feedstuffs 34:(1), Jan. 6 (1962).
134. L. D. Matterson and W. J. Pudelkiewicz, J. Nutr. 104:79 (1974).
135. M. Jacobson and H. H. Koehler, J. Agric. Food Chem. 18:1069 (1970).
136. L. E. Dawson and K. Schierholz, Poultry Sci. 54:1753 (1975).
137. L. E. Dawson, K. E. Stevenson, and E. Gertonson, Poultry Sci. 54:1134 (1975).
138. Code of Federal Regulations, Title 9, Part 381.147, Chapter III, Sub-Chap. C, Jan. 1 (1973).
139. S. D. Klinger and W. J. Stadelman, Poultry Sci. 54:1278 (1975).
140. Q. O. Burr, W. O. Lundberg, and J. R. Chipault, Oil and Soap 23:382 (1946).
141. L. E. Carpenter and W. O. Lundberg, Ann. N.Y. Acad. Sci. 52:269 (1949).
142. A. Z. Palmer, D. E. Brady, H. D. Naumann, and L. N. Tucker, Missouri Agric. Exp. Sta. Bull. No. 492 (1952).
143. J. Dammers, K. Stolk, and G. Van Wieringen, Vers Land kund Ond 64:5 (1958).
144. M. V. Zaehringer, S. V. Bring, C. A. Rickard, and W. P. Lehrer, Jr., Food Technol. 13:313 (1959).
145. W. R. H. Duncan, G. A. Garton, I. McDonald, and W. Smith, Br. J. Nutr. 14:371 (1959).
146. W. M. F. Leat, Proc. Nutr. Soc. 20:III (1961).
147. M. V. Zaehringer, C. A. Rickard, and W. P. Lehrer, Jr., J. An. Sci. 22:592 (1963).
148. H. Hvidsten and H. N. Astrup, Acta Agric. Scand. 13:259 (1963).
149. H. N. Astrup, Tidskr. Det Norske Landbruk 70:101 (1963).
150. H. N. Astrup, Tidskr. Det Norske Landbruk 71:3 (1964).
151. A. Keskinel, J. C. Ayres, and H. E. Snyder, Food Technol. 18:101 (1964).
152. S. Thomke, O. Dahl, and K. A. Persson, Acta Agric. Scand. 15:262 (1965).
153. H. Hvidsten, H. N. Astrup, and L. Aure, Fiskeridir. Skr. 4:No. 9 (1965).
154. R. Grau and O. Fleischmann, Z. Lebensmittelunters. Forsch. 130:270 (1965).

155. H. N. Astrup and A. Langebrekke, Z. Tierphysiol. Tierernähr. Futtermittelk. 21:15 (1966).

156. T. Homb and H. N. Astrup, Schweizer Landw. Mh. 9-10:439 (1968).

157. H. N. Astrup, Acta Agric. Scand. (Suppl.) 19:152 (1973).

158. J. W. Bratzler, J. K. Loosli, V. N. Krukovsky, and L. A. Maynard, J. Nutr. 42:59 (1950).

159. E. W. Turner, W. D. Paynter, E. J. Montie, M. W. Bessert, G. M. Struck, and F. C. Olson, Food Technol. 8:326 (1954).

160. E. Askoe and J. Madsen, Acta Agric. Scand. 4:266 (1954).

161. O. Dahl, Svenska Svinavelsforeningens Tidskrift No. 6:102 (1956).

162. K. Breirem, Bondevennen 66:27 (1963).

163. T. Homb, A. Lyso, and H. N. Astrup, Z. Tierphysiol. Tierernähr. Futtermittelk. 22:203 (1967).

164. J. Glavind, Acta Agric. Scand. (Suppl.) 19:105 (1973).

165. A. L. Tappel, Vit. Horm. 20:493 (1962).

166. A. L. Tappel, Fed. Proc. 24:73 (1965).

167. K. E. Mason and M. K. Horwitt, in The Vitamins: Chemistry, Physiology, Pathology, Methods. W. H. Sebrell, Jr. and R. S. Harris, eds., Vol. 5, 2nd ed. Academic, New York, 1972, p. 272.

168. I. Bartov and S. Bornstein, Br. Poultry Sci. 17:29 (1976).

169. I. Bartov and S. Bornstein, Br. Poultry Sci. 18:47 (1977).

170. I. Bartov and S. Bornstein, Br. Poultry Sci. 18:59 (1977).

171. I. Bartov and S. Bornstein, Br. Poultry Sci. 19:129 (1978).

172. I. Bartov, Br. Poultry Sci. 18:553 (1977).

173. M. A. Uebersax, L. E. Dawson, and K. L. Uebersax, Poultry Sci. 57:937 (1978).

10 COUNTERACTION OF ENVIRONMENTAL EFFECTS

Part 10A / Protection Against Environmental Toxicants   474

Part 10B / Free Radical Damage and Protection:
       Relationship to Cellular Aging and Cancer   495

Part 10A/   Protection Against Environmental Toxicants

DANIEL B. MENZEL
Duke University Medical Center
Durham, North Carolina

I.	Introduction	474
II.	Effects of Peroxidation on Cell Membranes	475
III.	Oxidizing Air Pollutants as Initiators of Lipid Peroxidation	480
IV.	Protection Against Air Pollutant Intoxication by Vitamin E	482
V.	Biological Properties of Ozone-Catalyzed PUFA Peroxides	483
VI.	Other Toxicants Producing Lipid Peroxidation	484
VII.	A Hypothetical Role for Vitamin E in Lipid Peroxidation Toxicities	487
VIII.	Summary	491
	References	492

I. INTRODUCTION

There are few more important opportunities to examine the antioxidant
theory of action of vitamin E than that afforded by the toxicity of oxidizing
air pollutants. Ozone and the various oxides of nitrogen occur in virtually
all of the cities of the world. Ozone levels in rural areas of the United
States are elevated by air pollution drifting from urban centers [1]. Photochemical reactions with terpenes expired by trees appear to be natural
sources of ozone and nitrogen dioxide [2] analogous to hydrocarbons
expelled by motor vehicles. Yet we know little about the geological history
of these oxidizing air pollutants and their interaction with biological systems through peroxidation.

It is interesting to note that "peroxides" are under speculation as
potential intermediates in recent experiments searching for life on Mars.
Peroxides, being a highly reactive chemical species, could serve as
prebiotic hydroxylases.

Peroxides and other highly reactive oxygen species, such as superoxide anion and singlet oxygen, might have served to shape the evolution of
all cells.

The evolution of the biological membrane may represent an attempt at "antioxidant" capacity by three-dimensional organization. The mammalian cell membrane is organized with the peroxidizable polyunsaturated fatty acids predominantly at the interior of the membrane. Oxygen, having a permanent dipole, is more soluble in aqueous than in hydrocarbon phases and therefore is excluded from the hydrophobic region of the membrane. Such an arrangement naturally limits the rate of oxidation of the polyunsaturated fatty acids of membranes and is in effect an antioxidant. In support of this concept, disaggregation of the isolated subcellular fractions rich in membranes by chaotrophic agents promotes a rapid peroxidation of the unsaturated fatty acids of the membrane.

Molenaar et al. [3] have emphasized the membrane-associated effects of vitamin E deficiency and lead us to suggest that in the membrane will be found those key reactions through which vitamin E exerts its vitamin effects [4]. Some predictions of peroxidation effects on membranes can be made on the basis of current theories of mammalian membrane structure.

II. EFFECTS OF PEROXIDATION ON CELL MEMBRANES

Nicholson [5] has presented a heroic and comprehensive review in support of the Singer and Nicholson [6] fluid mosaic model of cell membranes. This hypothesis suggests that membranes are composed of a lipid bilayer arranged as suggested above to orient the polar head groups of the phospholipids of membranes toward the aqueous medium of all cells and turn the hydrocarbon tails of the fatty acid residues inward. A model of a membrane adapted to the following discussion on peroxidation is shown in Fig. 1.

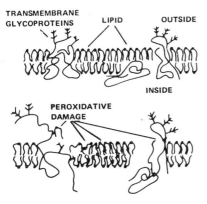

FIG. 1   Potential alterations of normal membrane structure by lipid peroxidation. Cross-linking reactions are shown as bars between membrane molecules.

An important aspect of the mosaic theory is the intercalation of proteins on top of, through, and on the bottom of the lipid bilayer. Most of the proteins in plasma membranes exposed to the exterior of the cell are glycosidated and many of the ionic characteristics of the cell are mediated by the glycosyl groups.

Communication between cells may be mediated by the recognition of specific glycosyl prosthetic groups of membrane-bound proteins [5]. Glycosyl prosthetic groups react with plant lectin proteins and the distribution of lectins such as wheat-germ agglutinin serves to map the distribution of the surface receptor protein(s). Hormones such as insulin affect the cell by interaction with an external receptor whose conformation is modified by the interaction with the hormone. Adenyl cyclase activation subsequently occurs generating cyclic adenosine 5'-monophosphate (cAMP) to carry out the final action of the hormone on the cell. Hormone receptors appear to be present in disaggregated and aggregated distributions on the cell surface as shown by lectin-mapping. Aggregation of receptors appears to be associated with hormone action. More than one membrane-bound protein may be necessary for formation of the hormone receptor. Aggregation and disaggregation in the plane of the plasma membrane are thought to be essential for normal activity of the cell according to the fluid mosaic hypothesis.

Complete fluidity does not appear to occur. A complex network of microtubules and microfilaments extends from the interior surface of the membrane deep within the cell. The normal commerce of the cell—the recognition of other cells, uptake of nutrients, and release of cell contents— appears regulated via the complex ultramicroanatomy of the membrane. A simplistic view of such an aggregating and disaggregating receptor system is shown in Fig. 2. Keeping in mind that the externally observable membrane proteins are literally the "tips of the iceberg" of the ultramicroanatomy of the cell, one can speculate that peroxidation could have profound effects upon the behavior of the cell.

Peroxidation of cell membranes is probably restricted to the hydrophobic region of the alkyl residues of the fatty acids attached to the phospholipids of the lipid bilayer of cell membranes. Peroxidation of hydrocarbons is supposed to proceed via the scheme below [Eqs. (1-4)] which predicts that alkyl-free radicals, $\underline{1}$, rapidly react with molecular oxygen to form hydroperoxyl-free radicals, $\underline{2}$ [Eq. (2)].

$$RH + X\cdot \rightarrow \underset{\underline{1}}{R\cdot} + XH \tag{1}$$

$$R\cdot + O_2 \rightarrow \underset{\underline{2}}{RO_2\cdot} \tag{2}$$

$$RH_2\cdot + RH \rightarrow RO_2H + R\cdot \tag{3}$$

$$RO_2\cdot + \underset{\underline{3}}{AH} \rightarrow AO_2H + A\cdot \tag{4}$$

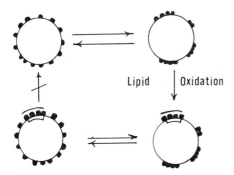

FIG. 2 Membrane receptors for hormones or other agents are shown here undergoing continuous association and disociation. Four membrane proteins are shown here aggregating to form a single receptor. Peroxidation of membrane lipids (indicated by the arc) in their immediate environment results in a change in membrane viscosity or covalent reactions, which restricts the proteins to a permanent association. Dissociation to a random random distribution or resting state of the cell is not possible.

where RH represents an unsaturated fatty acid and AH the phenolic antioxidants. Hydroperoxyl free radicals, 2, are the propagating species. Reactions eliminating peroxyl free radicals should then terminate the chain reaction and the peroxidation of alkenes [Eq. (4)]. Phenolic antioxidants, 3, or water, serve as excellent reactants with hydroperoxyl free radicals.

It is unlikely that such a short-chain length reaction could be sustained for any length of time with its major reactant scavenged by water. Water is present in biological systems at concentrations far in excess of that needed to scavenge a trace reactant. Consequently, peroxidation once initiated as in Eq. (1) should be propagated predominantly in the hydrophobic plane of the membrane.

Chain termination can occur by removal of the propagating peroxyl free radicals by organic compounds. In biological systems the tocopherols have been proposed as the principal, if not the exclusive, scavengers of peroxyl free radicals [Eq. (4)]. Returning to the model of the membrane, termination could be envisioned to result in a two-dimensional region of the membrane having distinctly different properties than those of the unperoxidized region.

Hypothetical reactions are depicted in Fig. 1, in which reactions between lipid molecules, between lipids and proteins, and between proteins are shown. Lipid-lipid interactions are likely to dominate due to the restriction of the chain reaction to the plane of the membrane and to the larger molar fraction of lipid than protein in membranes. Peroxidation of neat unsaturated fatty acids results in a remarkable increase in viscosity and ultimately the transformation of the liquid fats into a solid. If the

Singer-Nicholson hypothesis is correct, drastic changes in the mobility of membrane proteins would have profound alterations in properties of the membrane.

In early studies of model systems of peroxidation, polymerization of ribonuclease was observed [7]. Much of the polymerization could be accounted for on the basis of malonaldehyde cross-linkage between ribonuclease monomers. Malonaldehyde arises during the metabolism of arachiodonic acid, as well as from nonenzymatic peroxidation of polyunsaturated fatty acids. The pathways of arachidonic acid metabolism are shown in Fig. 3 [8] where malonaldehyde has been proposed to arise from prostaglandins G_2 and H_2 forming 12-L-hydroxy-5, 8, 10-hepta-decatrienoic acid (HHT) as a result. Other polymerization reactions between proteins could result by the combination of protein free radicals.

Peroxidation of a region of a cell membrane is likely to immobilize the proteins intercalated in the region or to cause major changes in their conformation. The cell cannot then return to its resting or disaggregated state short of membrane resynthesis. The formation of Heinz bodies in human and murine erythrocytes by fatty acid ozonides is indirect evidence for the formation of perturbations in cellular membranes by ozone-initiated peroxidation. Incubation of red blood cells (RBC) with ozonides prepared from oleic, linoleic, linolenic, or arachidonic acids resulted in the formation of Heinz bodies [9]. Heinz bodies are thought to be polymers of hemoglobin linked to the interior of the plasma membrane by disulfide bridges. Methemoglobin is formed on incubation of RBC with fatty acid ozonides and the soluble thiol content of the cells also falls to extremely low levels. As most of the thiol content of RBC is reduced glutathione (GSH), the observed decrease probably represents a rapid loss in GSH). Provision of glucose does not prevent Heinz body formation. Ozonides catalyze the disulfide linked polymerization of proteins in purified model systems and may promote Heinz body formation specifically by this mechanism. Injection of ozonides and peroxides into rats produces lung edema much like that produced by ozone (O_3) inhalation [10, 11]. Heinz bodies are present transiently in RBC of mice exposed to O_3, but are removed from RBC by the spleen. Heinz body formation can be prevented in human RBC by prior ingestion of vitamin E [10]. Ingestion of up to 200 IU vitamin E per day as d, 1-α-tocopheryl acetate provided a marked protection to RBC which were subsequently treated in vitro with fatty acid ozonides.

Using wheat-germ agglutinin (WGA), alveolar macrophages (AM) isolated from the lungs of rabbits which were exposed to O_3 and nitrogen dioxide (NO_2) agglutinated and formed rosettes with rabbit and sheep RBC more readily than did AM^2 isolated from control animals [12]. In this assay WGA served as a bridge between the two types of cells. Wheat-germ agglutiuin possesses two binding sites for the N-acetylglucosamine residues of the glycosyl prosthetic groups of plasma membrane proteins. WGA binding is thus a means for mapping the distribution and availability of surface proteins having N-acetylglucosamine residues accessible to the

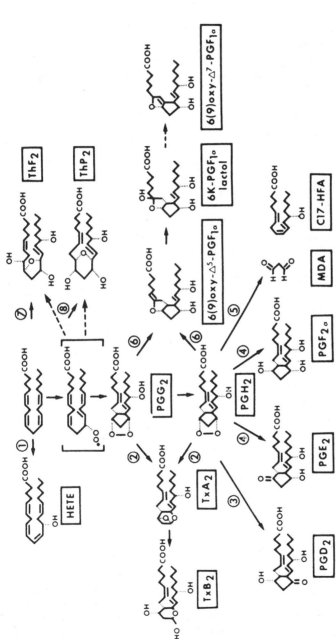

FIG. 3   Pathways of oxidative metabolism of arachidonic acid. Arachidonic acid (AA) is converted by cycloxy-genase to PGG$_2$ through the cyclization of AA hydroperoxyl free radical. PGG$_2$ is reduced to PGH$_2$. Other pathways shown are: (1) lipoxygenase; (2) thromboxane synthetase; (3) PGH-PGD isomerase; (4) prostaglandin isomerase (PGE$_2$ formation) and reductase (PGF$_2$ formation); (5) malonaldehyde (MDA)–C$_{17}$ hydroxy fatty acid formation (probably nonenzymatic); (6) 6(9) oxy cyclase (prostacyclin or PGX synthetase); (7) tetrahydrofuran (ThF$_2$) formation; and (8) tetrahydropyran (ThP$_2$) formation. (From C. R. Pace-Asciak, Prostaglandins 13:811, 1977, with permission.

solvent. The greater agglutination of AM from O_3- and NO_2-exposed
rabbits probably represented a redistribution of receptors to "clusters."
The O_3 and NO_2 effects are lost slowly, at the same rate as membrane
resynthesis. This supports the idea of immobilizing or "freezing" membranes through peroxidation. Lead ingestion produces perturbation of the
membrane leading to peroxidation and increased rigidity (see Sec. VI).

III. OXIDIZING AIR POLLUTANTS AS INITIATORS
OF LIPID PEROXIDATION

The inventory of the pollutants found in urban air is not complete, but two
components that are well identified and studied are ozone and nitrogen
dioxide. Ozone is at least 10-14 times more toxic. Both NO_2 and O_3 occur
in the atmosphere at concentrations of 0.05-1.00 ppm. Generally, equal
amounts of each are present at any one time. Since both are the results of
a complex series of photochemical reactions in the atmosphere, it is not
possible to predict the exact concentration of each likely to occur at any
one time.

When unsaturated fatty acids are exposed to either O_3 or NO_2, rapid
peroxidation results. Nitrogen dioxide reacts readily with olefins by
addition to the ethylene group [Eq. (5)]. A free-radical species, 4, has
been reported on the basis of electron-spin resonance spectroscopy [13].

$$\text{RCH} = \text{CHR'} + \text{NO}_2 \rightarrow \overset{\text{NO}_2}{\underset{\underline{4}}{\text{RCH} - \text{CHR'}}} \tag{5}$$

$$\underline{4} + \text{RH} \rightarrow \overset{\text{NO}_2}{\text{R·} + \text{RCH}_2\text{CHR'}} \tag{6}$$

$$\text{R·} + \text{O}_2 \rightarrow \text{RO}_2\text{·} \tag{7}$$

$$\text{RO}_2\text{·} + \text{RH} \rightarrow \text{RO}_2\text{H} + \text{R·} \tag{8}$$

$$\text{RO}_2\text{·} + \text{AH} \rightarrow \text{RO}_2\text{H} + \text{A·} \tag{9}$$

The NO_2-catalyzed autoxidation of linoleic acid is inhibited by the phenolic
antioxidants, d,1-α-tocopherol, BHT, and BHA [14,15]. Once the antioxidant is consumed in the reaction with hydroperoxyl free radicals [Eq.
(9)], the rate of autoxidation is the same regardless of the initiating concentration of NO_2. The induction period is proportional to both the concentration of NO_2 to which the thin films of linoleic acid are exposed and to

the amount of antioxidant present. Emulsions of linolenic acid behave in a
very similar manner to anhydrous thin films.

The autoxidation of unsaturated fatty acids by O_3 is, however, much
more complex. O_3 also adds directly across ethylene groups [Eq. (10)],
but the reaction is ionic in nature due to the dipole of O_3.

$$>C=C< \; + \; \overset{+}{O}\text{-}O\text{-}\overset{-}{O} \longleftrightarrow \overset{+}{O}=\overset{-}{O}\text{-}\overset{-}{O} \; \longrightarrow \; \underset{\underset{5}{>C\text{—}C<}}{\text{⬠}} \tag{10}$$

Once addition has occurred, the initial adduct, $\underline{5}$, can decompose to the
Criege zwitterion, $\underline{6}$, and an aldehyde, $\underline{7}$. These reactants recombine in
aprotonic solvents to form the conventional ozonide, $\underline{8}$.

$$\underset{5}{\text{⬠}} \; \longrightarrow \; \underset{6}{-\overset{O\text{-}\overset{-}{O}}{\underset{|}{C}}+} \; + \; \underset{7}{H\overset{O}{\overset{||}{C}}^{-}} \; \longrightarrow \; \underset{8}{\text{⬠}} \tag{11}$$

Ozonides are powerful oxidizing agents, but are sufficiently stable to be
isolated by thin-layer chromatography and are characterized by a strong
infrared absorbance at 9 μ.

A competing reaction is possible with alcohols, carboxylic acids, and
water. Peroxides result from such reactions.

$$-\underset{|}{\overset{OO^{-}}{\underset{|}{C}}}+ \; \underset{\underset{HOH}{RCO_2H}}{\xrightarrow{ROH}} \; -\underset{|}{\overset{OOH}{\underset{|}{C}}}\text{-OR} \; \text{or} \; -\underset{|}{\overset{OOH}{\underset{|}{C}}}\text{-OCOR} \; \text{or} \; -\underset{|}{\overset{OOH}{\underset{|}{C}}}\text{-OH} \tag{12}$$

Ozone-catalyzed autoxidation of polyunsaturated fatty acids is only
partially inhibited by phenolic antioxidants [14]. The products of the
reaction also differ depending upon the amount of water present and the
type of reaction vessel used to carry out the reaction. For instance,
Pryor et al. [16] used a microimpinger or sparger to bubble air containing
trace amounts of O_3 through neat methyl linolenate and found predominately
peroxidic products, while Roehm, Hadley, and Menzel [14] using thin films
of methyl linoleate found mostly ozonides and few peroxides. When neat
arachidonic acid was exposed to a stream of air containing 3 ppm O_3 in a
fashion similar to that of Pryor et al. peroxides were formed within sec-
onds of exposure to O_3 [17]. Addition of $\underline{d},\underline{1}$-$\alpha$-tocopherol to the mixture
in molar ratios of from $\underline{1}$:100 to 1:1000 retarded the reaction equally well.

Ozone catalyzes a complex series of reactions in aqueous emulsions
of methyl linoleate, which are also only partially inhibited by phenolic
antioxidants [14]. The products of autoxidation were mostly peroxidic and
too complex for characterization by conventional thin-layer chromatography.

IV. PROTECTION AGAINST AIR POLLUTANT
INTOXICATION BY VITAMIN E

Most of the evidence for the formation of peroxides in vivo during O_3 or NO_2 exposure is indirect [14,15,18,19]. Using ultraviolet absorption spectra, diene conjugation resulting from oxidation of polyunsaturated fatty acids (PUFA) has been reported. Unfortunately, some products of the reaction of PUFA with NO_2 have absorption maxima near those of diene conjugates of PUFA and may interfere with diene conjugation as an estimate of peroxidation. Increased amounts of TBA-reactive substances in the lung have been reported [20]. In these assays prostaglandin-like endoperoxides were likely to be isolated and detected as TBA-positive reactants. The detection of TBA reactants in the lung represents the best direct evidence that O_3 exposure results in the formation of PUFA peroxides.

Vitamin E profoundly affects the morbidity of rats and mice exposed to O_3 and NO_2 [15,20-22]. Rats depleted of vitamin E are much more susceptible to both NO_2 and O_3 than when given 100 mg/kg diet of d,l-α-tocopheryl acetate. The PUFA content of the lungs of these rats was altered by O_3 and NO_2 exposure [22]. Following exposure to NO_2 the total lung unsaturated fatty acid content declined. O_3 exposure had more complex effects on the lung lipids and mimicked the changes in PUFA composition found on vitamin E depletion alone [22]. PUFA derived metabolically from linolenic acid or oleic acid declined sharply while the arachidonic acid content rose despite depletion of vitamin E and simultaneous O_3 exposure. Depletion of vitamin E and O_3 exposure should have decreased the arachidonic acid content through oxidation. Since the lung does not carry out elongation and desaturation of fatty acids, but does synthesize saturated fatty acids up to and including stearic acid, some of the changes in the lung PUFA content may be due to inhibition of serum acyl transferases by O_3 [23]. Other researchers have reported increases in tissue arachidonic acid, however, in tissues other than the lung during vitamin E deficiency.

When mice are fed a low or high PUFA diet major alterations in their lung fatty acids can be achieved [24,25]. The alterations in lung fatty acid composition take place independent of the level of dietary vitamin E supplied. The lung fatty acids attain a constant composition after about 3 weeks of feeding. Arachidonic acid does not increase with vitamin E depletion as it does in rats. In these experiments, most of the alterations in lung PUFA reflect the difference in linoleic acid content of the diets. Continuous exposure of these groups of animals, having been fed either a high PUFA diet (5% corn oil) or a low PUFA diet (5% lard) and either 0, 10.5, or 105.0 mg/kg d,l-α-tocopheryl acetate for 6 weeks, to 1 ppm O_3 resulted in a major delay in mortality (LT_{50}) only in those groups receiving 105 mg vitamin E acetate/kg diet (equivalent to 100 milligrams free tocopherol per kilogram of diet). Despite the higher peroxidizability index (PI) of the PUFA-fed groups there was no increased mortality in those animals having a higher lung PI. Levels of less than 105 mg vitamin E acetate/kg diet had no effect on mortality. An exponential relationship appears to govern the protection effect of vitamin E in RBC hemolysis [26] and in the formation of peroxides in the lungs of ozone-exposed rats [20]. In mice, prevention of the morbidity of O_3 is achieved by vitamin E at 10.5 mg/kg and 105 mg/kg.

Arachidonic acid is the primary precursor of prostaglandins, thromboxanes, and similar vasoactive compounds in the lung. The lung rapidly metabolizes these compounds. Ozone inhibits the lung prostaglandin synthetase, presumably the cycloxygenase, noncompetitively [27]. The uptake and elimination of preformed prostaglandin E_2 is not affected by O_3, but the metabolism to its 15-keto analog is inhibited by O_3 [28]. Ozone exposure may result in a redirection of the flow of arachidonic acid to other products.

Vitamin E appeared to be depleted more rapidly in rats exposed to 1 ppm O_3 than in those exposed to clean air [22]. When two groups of rats had been equilibrated for the same length of time to a diet containing 100 mg/kg d,l-α-tocopheryl acetate, red cells taken from one group receiving no further supplementation with vitamin E and exposed to O_3 were more susceptible to the dialuric acid hemolysis test than another group of littermates also deprived of vitamin E but breathing clean air. Direct measurements of vitamin E depletion by O_3 exposure have been difficult to demonstrate.

There is increased synthesis of arachidonic acid during vitamin E deficiency in rats but not in mice. Mice are more like humans in the symptoms evidenced during vitamin E deficiency and may be a better model. Few debilitating syndromes occur and the requirement for vitamin E appears very low. A true threshold level for vitamin E may exist under conditions of exposure to oxidant stresses. The levels of O_3 and NO_2 used in studies of vitamin E protection are well within the range of oxidants occurring throughout the industrialized world and, therefore, are directly applicable to large segments of the industrialized world's population.

V. BIOLOGICAL PROPERTIES OF OZONE-CATALYZED PUFA PEROXIDES

The biological activity of peroxides formed by ozone initiated oxidation of arachidonic acid has been examined using smooth muscle strips and human platelets [17]. Human platelets are particularly sensitive to the action of endoperoxides formed from arachidonic acid, PGG_2, and PGH_2 (see Fig. 3). These endoperoxides are rapidly converted to thromboxane A_2 (TXA2) which is thought to initiate platelet aggregation. Only a few nanograms of TXA2 are needed to aggregate human platelets. It seems likely that the compounds detected by the TBA reaction in autoxidizing PUFA are in reality cyclic peroxides. Assuming one mole equivalent of malonaldehyde per mole of endoperoxide, peroxides formed by 2 ppm O_3 had biological activity

equivalent to authentic prostaglandin endoperoxides formed by the prostaglandin cycloxygenase. About $1.5-3.0$ nmol ozone peroxides (EC_{50}, an
effective concentration for 50%, 1.65 nmol in 0.4 ml) were required to
aggregate human platelets compared to $0.03-0.82$ nmol PGG_2. Half-
maximal contraction of rabbit aortic spiral strips was obtained with
1.95 nmol ozone peroxides. Prostaglandin-like activity was found with rat
fundus strips also. Smooth muscle bioassays were performed in the
presence of a mixture of inhibitors which prevent the contraction of these
smooth muscles by any known, nonprostaglandin biological agents. Rabbit
aortic spirals in particular are exquisitely sensitive to prostaglandins and
TXA_2. When incubated with human platelet microsomes, a potent source
of thomboxane synthetase, ozone-formed peroxides were not found to be
substrates for human platelet thromboxane synthetase as are PGG_2 and PGH_2.

When vitamin E was included in the reaction mixture, peroxide formation was decreased, but more importantly, the peroxides formed had little
biological activity. In the presence of vitamin E, the activity of ozone-
formed peroxides on both smooth-muscle bioassays and platelet aggregation was essentially abolished. Prior incubation with vitamin E or addition
of vitamin E after peroxides had been formed by ozone-initiated autoxidation, had no effect on the biological activity of peroxides. Vitamin E thus
appears to function by converting the peroxides formed by O_3 into those
having less biological activity in these assays.

Pryor et al. [16] have provided evidence for the formation of the dinor-
PGG_2-like compound from the O_3-catalyzed peroxidation of methyl linolenate. Presumably, the peroxides formed in our experiments from
arachidonic acid are isomers of PGG_2 or PGH_2. Because of the large
number of potential stereoisomers and the isomerization through free
radicals, the endoperoxides are not likely to be the same stereoisomers as
naturally formed PGG_2 or PGH_2. Nonetheless, the arachidonic acid
endoperoxides have potent biological activity.

VI. OTHER TOXICANTS PRODUCING LIPID PEROXIDATION

The oxidizing air pollutants are not the only toxicants which can produce
lipid peroxidation. Considerable debate rages about whether or not lipid
peroxidation is the major toxic lesion in carbon tetrachloride, halocarbon,
and ethanol hepatotoxicity (see Ref. 29 for review). There seems little
doubt that halogenated compounds react within hepatocytes to produce
covalently linked compounds with cellular constituents and lipid peroxidation. Apparently an enzymatic dehalogenation is responsible for the
production of a halogen free radical and a carbon free radical. This free
radical reaction is catalyzed by microsomes, but the identity of the enzyme
has not been conclusively demonstrated. Both halogen and carbon residues
from carbon tetrachloride, for example, are incorporated into covalently
bound constituents within the cell of intoxicated animals. Confusion exists

as to whether lipid peroxidation occurs simulataneously with or secondary to the dehalogenation reaction. Vitamin E and several antioxidants provide protection against the hepatotoxicity of carbon tetrachloride. Some of the confusion derives from the variety of methods that have been used to measure lipid peroxidation under these circumstances. The TBA reaction, diene conjugation, and alterations in the total content of unsaturated fatty acids have been used in studies of carbon tetrachloride intoxication. DiLuzio [30] proposed that ethanol initiates lipid peroxidation and has provided evidence that vitamin E protects against ethanol-induced fatty livers. As evidence for lipid peroxidation, he performed iodimetric titrations to measure lipid peroxides extracted from the liver [31] Some of the apparent divergent results are clarified by assuming that the TBA reaction represents the formation of endoperoxides by the Dahle et al. mechanism which is discussed in Sect. VII. Oxidation of fatty acids having less than three ethylene groups will not produce TBA-positive endoperoxides, whereas diene conjugation can be detected in the absence of cyclization to an endoperoxide. There is little similarity in the dietary fat-fed animals prior to exposure to toxicants and thus the PUFA composition is different in different experiments. Comporti et al. found that N,N'-diphenyl-p-phenylene (DPPD) prevented hepatic necrosis from carbon tetrachloride intoxication but did not prevent diene conjugation [32]. If peroxidation were to proceed to cyclic compounds as suggested by our studies of ozone-initiated peroxidation and by those of Pryor et al. then tissues of animals having a low content of PUFA could undergo sufficient peroxidation to be detected by diene conjugation but not produce enough peroxides to cause major changes in cell function. Only minor changes in fatty acid composition have ever been detected evan at doses of carbon tetrachloride that produce massive hepatic necrosis, making interpretation of changes in hepatic PUFA difficult.

An important function of prostaglandins is in the regulation of the cyclic nucleotide content within the cell. Cyclic AMP affects membrane stability and cyclic guanosine 5'-monophosphate (cGMP) affects exocytosis. Cyclic peroxides induced by ethanol or CCl_4 could mimic the action of prostaglandin on cyclic nucleotides to produce changes in cell permeability and triglyceride accumulation. The role of DPPD, vitamin E, and other antioxidants in the prevention of such toxic effects could be twofold: first, the redirection of the end products of peroxidation away from cyclic peroxides towards hydroperoxides capable of being detoxified by glutathione peroxidase or other cellular mechanisms; and second, the conventional concept of inhibition of peroxidation per se.

Levander and his co-workers reported a protection effect of vitamin E on lead intoxication in rats [33-36]. This work is provocative as it relates several aspects of lipid peroxidation. Vitamin E deficiency exacerbates the anemia caused by lead intoxication by what appears to be an oxidative mechanism. Red cells from lead-intoxicated animals are more susceptible to peroxidative hemolysis than are those from control animals. Similarly,

RBCs from vitamin E-deficient animals are more susceptible to peroxidative attack than those from vitamin E-supplemented animals. The combined onslaught of both vitamin E deficiency and lead intoxication renders cells very susceptible to oxidative attack.

When lead acetate is given in the drinking water, lead appears to be incorporated in the interior of red blood cells making them more rigid and less deformable as measured by their ability to pass through 3 μm diameter pores in polycarbonate filters [34]. This lack of ability to deform is also seen in RBCs with Heinz bodies. Alterations in the fluidity and deformability of RBC obtained from lead-intoxicated animals is particularly apparent at lower pHs similar to that of the interior of the spleen. Defective RBCs are normally removed by the spleen. The removal of Heinz bodies is often referred to as the "pitting" of red cells by the spleen in an attempt to remove the defective parts from the RBC. The lack of deformability by red cells from vitamin E-deficient, lead-intoxicated animals leads to their sequestering in the spleen, and subsequent splenomegaly and anemia.

Levander and co-workers [34] showed that incubation of red cells from animals which were lead intoxicated and deficient in vitamin E produced TBA reactants concommitant with a decrease in red cell filterability. Fatty acid composition of the red cell membrane was manipulated by feeding the animals dietary fats of differing unsaturation. Little difference in filterability was noted, however, regardless of the dietary fat. Unfortunately the fatty acid composition of the red cell membrane was not measured in these experiments, and we do not know the extent to which changes in dietary fat were reflected in the red-cell lipid composition. It is known, however, that the red cell exhibits asymmetry in the distribution of phosphatides between the exterior and interior surfaces of the membrane. Unsaturated fatty acid containing phospholipids tend to be situated at the interior surface of the plasma membrane, and thus, the total unsaturation of the phospholipid of the red cell membrane at the interior surface may not have been significantly altered. Lead may perturb the interior surface and the total PUFA subject to peroxidation may, coincidentally, be the same in red cells from animals fed high and low PUFA-containing diets. Such an explanation is particularly attractive since the effects of lead in vivo are greater than those in vitro and may represent the binding of lead to specific receptors on the interior of the red cell membrane [34].

In contrast to ozone intoxication, glutathione peroxidase does not appear to play a singificant role in the protection of the red cell against the oxidative attack of lead since selenium deficiency did not affect susceptibility [36]. Protection by selenium could be found only at toxic levels of selenium.

The studies of Levander and his co-workers point to the concept that perturbation of cell membrane can result not only in functional alterations of the cell but also in changes of the ability of the cell membrane to withstand peroxidative attack. Lead and other divalent cations are known to "tan" cell membranes, making them more rigid. Simultaneously, the more rigid membranes appear to be more susceptible to peroxidative attacks. Removal of vitamin E from the membrane by feeding E-deficient diets reveals more receptors on the RBC membrane for binding of lead, presumably on the interior of the plasma membrane.

VII. A HYPOTHETICAL ROLE FOR VITAMIN E IN LIPID PEROXIDATION TOXICITIES

Pryor et al. [16] have extended the mechanism for the autoxidation of PUFA PUFA proposed by Dahle et al. [37] to the peroxidation of PUFA by trace amounts of O_3. This mechanism centers around the observation that malonaldehyde is formed by peroxidation of PUFA having three or more double bonds, but not by peroxidation of fatty acids having one or two double bonds. Hydrogen abstraction of 9 (Fig. 4) can result in any one of the isomeric free radicals. Oxygen reacts rapidly with alkyl free radicals so that the hydroperoxides 11 and 12 are likely to result at high oxygen tension. The allylic free radical 10 having a double bond β, γ to the peroxyl free radical is of special interest. The radical 10 can undergo further reactions. Cyclization will lead to an alkyl free radical γ to the original peroxyl free radical. The free radical at γ is likely to react with molecular oxygen and then to abstract a hydrogen from another molecule of fatty acid to lead to 13. A less likely reaction is with a molecule of fatty acid leading to 14 and another alkyl free radical.

The radical 10 may cyclize to form a prostanoic acid nucleus, 15, which can again react first with molecular oxygen and then with another molecule of fatty acid to yield the stable bicyclic endoperoxide hydroperoxides 16 and 17. By analogy with the enzymatically produced endoperoxide hydroperoxide, PGG_2, the hydroperoxides of 16 and 17 might be reduced rapidly in the cell to give the corresponding PGH-like compounds.

The cyclization of the free radical 10 to a prostanoic acid derivative is analogous to the Nugteren–Samuelsson mechanism for the formation of prostaglandins by the enzyme cycloxygenase. Porter et al. [38] have recently confirmed this mechanism by the preparation of the corresponding fatty acid hydroperoxide and cyclization of the peroxide to dinor PGE_2 following chemical generation of the peroxyl radical 10. The formation of the free radical 10 is then essential for cyclization and further conversion to either the enzymatically or chemically derived endoperoxide.

Under the acid conditions of the TBA assay, the cyclic peroxides 13, 16, and 17 would give a positive TBA test [39]. Through this mechanism, which is substantiated by mass spectra of the critical endoperoxide 15 (see Pryor et al.), the TBA test is more likely to give different results depending upon the fatty acid composition of the peroxidizing lipid. Animal tissues are likely to have higher concentrations of the tri- and tetraenoic acids necessary for formation of the β, γ-allylic peroxydylic radical, 10. These fats then should provide a better correlation between oxygen uptake and TBA value, for example. Plant fats on the other hand contain mostly

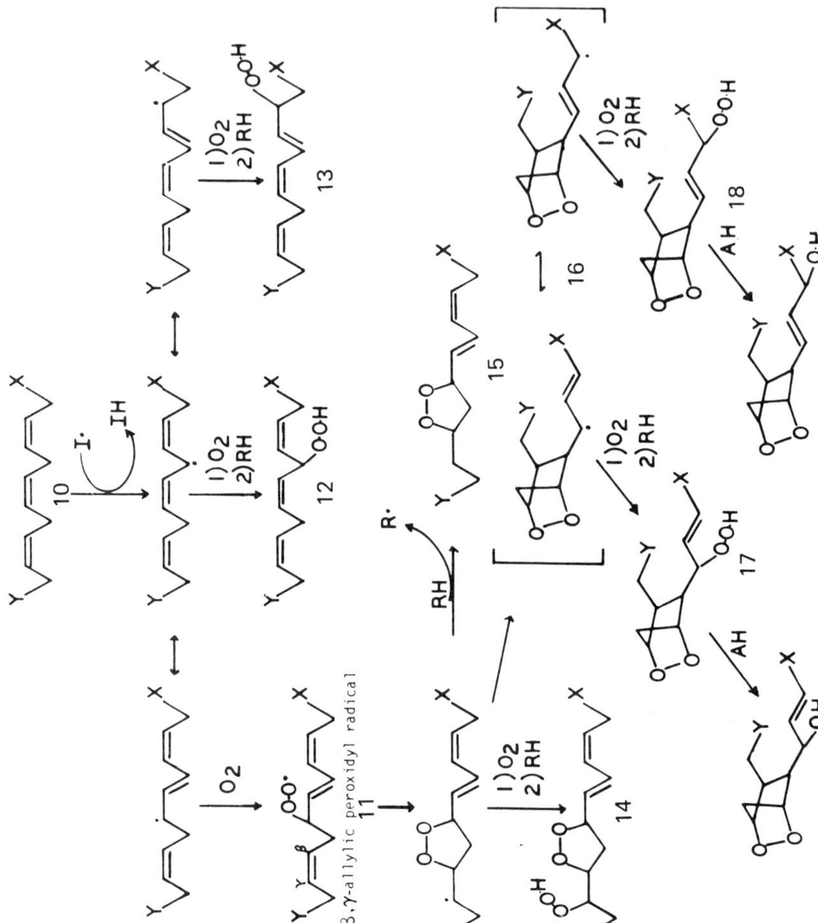

FIG. 4.

mono- and dienoic acids and would not provide on peroxidation such a correlation between TBA value and oxygen uptake. It is important to emphasize the fact that the formation of peroxide end-products such as illustrated in this scheme are likely to occur only at low levels of product formation. Generally conversions greater than 5% of the total substrate result in complex raction mixtures and reactions between products as well as the autoxidation of the original substrate.

Interpretation of the biological significance of TBA values has been further complicated by the failure of some investigators to control adequately the reaction conditions of the TBA test. Transition metals are known to decompose peroxides into hydroxyl and alkoxyl free radicals, thereby supporting further autoxidation of unreacted fatty acids that may be present in the reaction mixture. When the reaction is carried out in the prescence of a chelating agent such as citric acid buffer and a phenolic antioxidant such as BHT, reproducible TBA values can be obtained from autoxidizing reaction mixtures including neat arachidonic acid. Hydroperoxides formed through the mechanism such as 11 and 12 will yield $\omega 3$ and $\omega 6$ hydroperoxides from the nonessential and essential fatty acid series in animal tissues, respectively. These hydroperoxides are decomposed to ethane and petane respectively by transition metals especially iron [40]. Ethane and pentane evolution have been used as indirect measures of tissue autoxidation in carbon tetrachloride intoxication and vitamin E deficiency [41-43]. Phenols are known to react only poorly with alkyl free radicals and are not likely to compete with the rapid reaction of molecular oxygen with alkyl free radicals to form peroxyl free radicals. That vitamin E inhibits both ethane and pentane evolution argues for an intimate relationship between vitamin E and the cyclic peroxidation of PUFA. Diplock and Lucy [44] have proposed close conformational association between vitamin E and arachidonic acid.

A scheme combining some of these concepts in peroxidation toxicity is shown in Fig. 5. Free radical initiation is likely to occur by abstraction of one of the hydrogens of the methylene group. Initiation could be from a variety of natural or unnatural means. Examples discussed here center mainly around ozone and nitrogen dioxide; organic solvents and anesthetic agents containing halogen are also well known as agents for initiating lipid peroxidation in the liver.

The initial radical is unlikely to survive due to the rapid rate of reaction with molecular oxygen. The peroxyl free radical resulting from reaction with molecular oxygen becomes a key intermediate determining the lesion ultimately observed, although it may be transient itself. We have long supposed that such peroxyl free radicals abstract hydrogen from other relatively stable compounds and have little prostaglandin-like activity (Anderson, Roycroft, and Menzel, unpublished results). Either the hydroperoxide or the peroxyl free radical may be reduced by glutathione

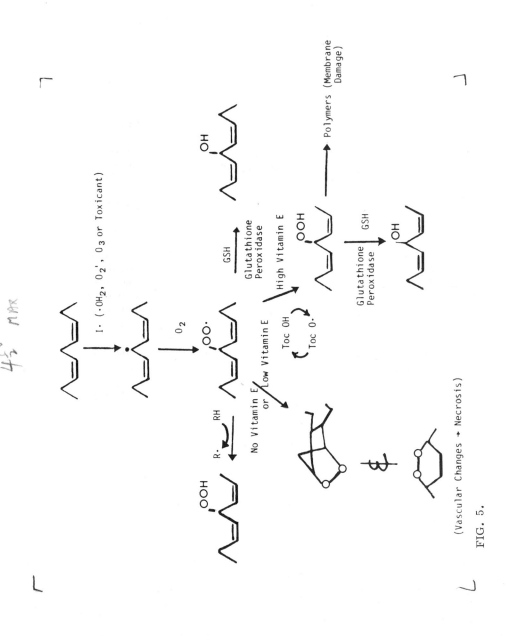

FIG. 5.

peroxidase to the corresponding alcohol as a detoxification mechanism. Indeed, glutathione peroxidase activity increases after exposure of rats to ozone, suggesting the induction of a protection mechanism [20]. Glutathione peroxidase, a soluble enzyme, may, however, be restricted in its activity on membrane-bound peroxides.

In the presence of little or no vitamin E in the tissue, β,γ -allylic peroxyl free radicals may spontaneously cyclize to form either bicyclic or monocyclic peroxides. The cyclization reaction need not be enzymatically catalyzed and the stereochemistry need not be identical to the enzymatic product. Spontaneously formed endoperoxides have significant potency as noted above for at least two classes of receptors, smooth muscles and platelets. Tocopherol can react with the peroxyl free radical to form a hydroperoxide in preference to cyclization to an endoperoxide. In this view, vitamin E provides its essential function by direction of peroxidation to hydroperoxides. While still reactive, hydroperoxides are more stable than endoperoxides and are over 10^3 times less potent than are endoperoxides on prostaglandin receptors. The biological function of hydroperoxides is not fully known, but they may serve as chemotactic agents for phagocytes (Menzel, Hatch, Gardner, and Graham, unpublished observations). Hydroperoxide decomposition could lead to polymerization of lipids, thereby drastically altering membrane viscosity. Hydroperoxides would also be substrates for glutathione peroxidase. Molenaar et al. [3] have pointed to the important role for vitamin E in the maintenance of the vascular integrity of animals. Evidence is now accumulating that vitamin E has a function in platelet integrity [45-47]. The interaction of platelet aggregates with blood vessel walls may become the locus for the formation of atherosclerotic plaques.

VIII. SUMMARY

Lipid peroxidation resulting from inhalation of ozone and nitrogen dioxide may prove to be a valuable tool for an understanding of the basic mechanism of action of vitamin E at the molecular level. The TBA reaction, once shunned as being highly unreliable, may, in fact, present a valuable indicator of the total amount of potent products formed during peroxidation. Very little is known of the biological activity of nonenzymatically formed endoperoxides. Because of the great biological potency of the naturally formed fatty acid endoperoxides, PGG_2 and PGH_2, and the multiplicity of their metabolic products, this line of investigation may indeed prove fruitful. The uniqueness of vitamin E (d-α-tocopherol) may be associated with the cyclization reaction. The ability to react with unsaturated fatty acid peroxyl free radicals in some manner to prevent their further conversion to endoperoxides may be the key to the biological function of vitamin E.

The end products of peroxidation that have been lumped together in the generic term "peroxides" may be highly important to the ultimate effect of the toxicants. This is particularly underscored in halocarbons and ethanol hapatotoxicity and in ozone and nitrogen dioxide pulmonary toxicity. These considerations have led us to suggest that vitamin E functions by determining the nature of the end products formed and that properties of the end products, e.g., hydroperoxide, monocyclic peroxide, or bicyclic endoperoxide, are the critical determinants in the effect of lipid peroxidation on these specific cell types. We have not touched at all on other drugs that are known to induce peroxidation, but the phenomenon might well be a general one extending to a wide variety of toxic reactions that occur through environmental, industrial, and drug intoxication, in which vitamin E may have a critical role in the fate of the intoxicated animals. The level levels of dietary vitamin E in humans may have greater clinical significance than previously supposed.

ACKNOWLEDGMENTS

This work was supported by USPHS Grants ES00798 and HL16264 and by a contract from the U.S. Environmental Protection Agency. I wish to thank Ms. Elaine Smolko for her editorial assistance.

REFERENCES

1. S. M. Bruntz, W. S. Cleveland, T. E. Graedel, D. K. Kleiner, and J. L. Warner, Science 186:257 (1974).
2. D. Lillian, in Photochemical Smog and Ozone Reactions. Edited by B. Weinstock. Washington, D.C., Amer. Chem. Soc., 1972, p. 211.
3. I. Molenaar, C. E. Hulstaert, J. Vos, and F. A. Hommes, in Therapeutic Aspects of Nutrition. Edited by J. H. P. Jonxis, H. K. A. Visser, and J. A. Troelstra. Leiden, Stenfert Kroese, 1973, p. 40.
4. D. B. Menzel, in Free Radicals in Biology, Vol. II. Edited by W. A. Pryor. New York, Academic, 1976, p. 181
5. G. L. Nicolson, Biochim. Biophys. Acta 457:57 (1976).
6. S. J. Singer and G. L. Nicolson, Science 175:720 (1972).
7. D. B. Menzel, Lipids 2:83 (1967).
8. C. R. Pace-Asciak, Prostaglandins 13:811 (1977).
9. D. B. Menzel, R. J. Slaughter, A. M. Bryant, and H. O. Jauregui, Arch. Environ. Health 30:296 (1975).
10. D. B. Menzel, R. J. Slaughter, A. M. Bryant, and H. O. Jauregui, Arch. Environ. Health 30:234 (1975).

11. R. Cortesi and O. S. Privett, Lipids 7:715 (1972).
12. J. G. Hadley, D. E. Gardner, D. L. Coffin, and D. B. Menzel, International Conference on Photochemical Oxidant Pollution and Its Control: Proceedings, Vol. I, 505 (1977).
13. J. R. Rowlands and E. M. Gause, Arch. Intern. Med. 128:88 (1971).
14. J. N. Roehm, J. G. Hadley, and D. B. Menzel, Arch. Environ. Health 23:142 (1971).
15. J. N. Roehm, J. G. Hadley, and D. B. Menzel, Arch. Intern. Med. 128:89 (1971).
16. W. A. Pryor, J. P. Stanley, and E. Blair, Lipids 11:370 (1975).
17. J. H. Roycroft, W. B. Gunter, and D. B. Menzel, Toxicol Lett., in press.
18. H. V. Thomas, P. K. Mueller, and R. L. Lyman, Science 159:532 (1968).
19. B. D. Goldstein, C. Lodi, and C. Collinson, Arch. Environ. Health 18:631 (1969).
20. C. K. Chow and A. L. Tappel, Lipids 7:518 (1972).
21. J. N. Roehm, J. G. Hadley, and D. B. Menzel, Arch. Environ. Health 24:237 (1972).
22. D. B. Menzel, J. N. Roehm, and S. D. Lee, J. Arric. Food Chem. 20:481 (1972).
23. K. Kyei-Aboagye, M. Hazucha, I. Wyszogrodski, D. Rubinstein, and M. E. Avery, Biochem. Biophys. Res. Commun. 54:907 (1973).
24. D. H. Donovan, S. J. Williams, J. M. Charles, and D. B. Menzel, Fed. Proc. 36:1158 (1977).
25. D. H. Donovan, S. J. Williams, J. M. Charles, and D. B. Menzel, Toxicol. Lett., in press.
26. J. G. Bieri and R. P. Evarts, J. Amer. Dietet. Assoc. 66:134 (1975).
27. D. B. Menzel, W. G. Anderson, and M. B. Abou-Donia, Res. Commun. Chem. Pathol. Pharmicol. 15:135 (1976).
28. W. B. Gunter, M. B. Abou-Donia, and D. B. Menzel, Pharmacologist 18:244 (1976).
29. G. L. Plaa and H. Witschi, Ann. Rev. Pharmacol. Toxicol. 16:125 (1976).
30. N. R. DiLuzio, Life Sci. 3:113 (1964).
31. G. H. Kalish and N. R. DiLuzio, Science 152:1390 (1966).
32. M. Comporti, A. Benedetti, and A. Casini, Biochem. Pharmacol. 23:421 (1974).
33. O. A. Levander, V. C. Morris, D. J. Higgs, and R. J. Ferretti, J. Nutr. 105:1481 (1975).
34. O. A. Levander, V. C. Morris, and R. J. Ferretti, J. Nutr. 107:363 (1977).
35. O. A. Levander, R. J. Ferretti, and V. C. Morris, J. Nutr. 107:373 (1977).

36. O. A. Levander, V. C. Morris, and R. J. Ferretti, J. Nutr. 107:378 (1977).

37. L. K. Dahle, E. G. Hill, and R. T. Holman, Arch. Biochem. Biophys. 98:253 (1962).

38. N. A. Porter, R. Isaac, M. Funk, J. H. Roycroft, and D. B. Menzel, Proceedings, 1976 Intra-Science Symposium, in press.

39. N. A. Porter, J. Nixon, and R. Isaac, Biochim. Biophys. Acta 441:506 (1976).

40. D. H. Donovan and D. B. Menzel, in preparation.

41. C. J. Dillard, E. E. Dumelin, and A. L. Tappel, Lipids 12:109 (1976).

42. D. G. Hafeman and W. G. Hoekstra, J. Nutr. 107:656 (1977).

43. D. G. Hafemen and W. G. Hoekstra, J. Nutr. 107:666 (1977).

44. A. T. Diplock and J. A. Lucy, FEBS Lett. 29:205 (1972).

45. L. J. Machlin, R. Filipski, A. L. Willis, D. C. Kuhn, and M. Brin, Proc. Soc. Exp. Biol. Med. 149:275 (1975).

46. W. C. Hope, C. Dalton, L. J. Machlin, R. J. Filipski, and S. M. Vane, Prostaglandins 10:557 (1975).

47. M. Steiner and J. Anastasi, J. Clin. Invest. 57:732 (1976).

Part 10B/ Free Radical Damage and Protection:
Relationship to Cellular Aging and Cancer

JUDIE R. WALTON* AND LESTER PACKER
University of California
Berkeley, California

I.	Introduction	495
II.	Sources of Free Radicals	498
III.	Free Radicals and Cellular Aging	500
	A. Cross-Linking	501
	B. Repair	501
	C. Copper	501
	D. Lipopigments	502
	E. Vitamin E Deficiency	504
IV.	Free Radicals and Cancer	505
V.	Antioxidants and Cellular Aging	506
	A. Cultured Cells as Model Systems	506
	B. Lower Animal Models	508
	C. Mammalian Models	508
VI.	Antioxidants and Cancer	510
	A. Some Possible Modes of Protection	510
	B. Tumor Levels of Endogenous Protectors	511
VII.	Conclusion	511
	References	512

I. INTRODUCTION

At a recent Gordon Research Conference on the chemistry of aging, the opening session was devoted to defining this subject area. After a lengthy discussion the following definition was produced:

> The beginning of aging is due to the accumulation of biological effects and events, the sum of which causes the function of a given organ system, either in whole or in part, to pass the point of optimum potential function, in a given environment.

---

*Present affiliation: Lawrence Livermore Laboratory, Livermore, California.

495

Having satisfied ourselves with such a comprehensive definition, laughter was evoked when someone erased the word "aging," and replaced it with "disease." We can paraphrase this definition of aging or disease. as follows:

> In a given environment, cells suffer a certain amount of damage: if the rate at which damage accumulates exceeds the cells' genetic potential to correct it by division, biosynthesis, or repair, the damage will be cumulative.

Thus we are led to question, Where and how does the damage occur and how can we protect against it in a given environment?

Many hypotheses have been advanced to account for cellular aging. Although no single explanation is sufficient, for several years a free radical hypothesis has appeared to be most attractive. This has stemmed from our long-standing interest in the mechanism of the free radical system of biological oxidation catalysts involved in mitochondrial electron transport and from an appreciation of the sophisticated membrane organization developed to prevent the spread of molecular damage by these catalysts (cf. Ref. 1).

Recently, Smith [2] pointed out that the free radical, mutation, error, cross-linking, and immunological hypotheses for aging could all be considered under a single umbrella as related aspects of what he termed a genetic alteration theory. Free radical damage can be considered to play a central role by causing molecular damage to information macromolecules, resulting in amplification and spread of damage (Fig. 1). Damage to the biosynthetic and repair functions could result from free radicals from such different sources as ionizing radiation, visible or ultraviolet radiation, environmental pollutants, metabolically generated radicals, genetic defects in peroxide-scavenging enzymes like glutathione peroxidase, or from depletion of radical-scavenging molecules of the hydrophobic or aqueous phase. If, in a given environment, free radical damage cannot be repaired or corrected at a rate faster than it is generated, the damage will be amplified through errors and, eventually, visible accumulation of the damage will arise.

The World Health Organization has estimated that 75% of the incidence of human cancer is caused by environmental factors [3], and Boyland has suggested that 90% of human cancer may result from endogenous and environmental chemical carcinogens [4]. The widespread production of free radicals by environmental agents and their involvement in experimental carcinogenesis lend importance to the further understanding of how free radical species interact with tissue components to cause cellular and organismic degeneration.

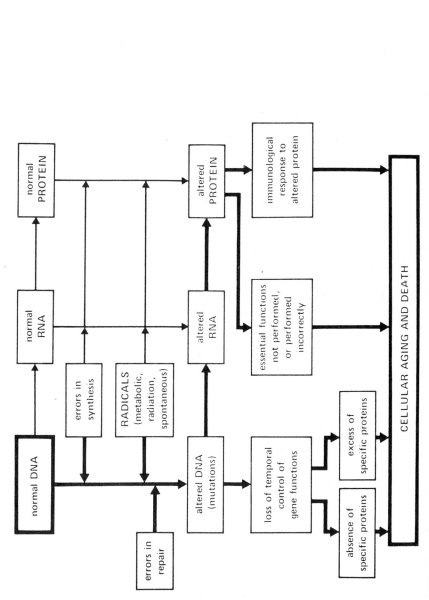

FIG. 1   Scheme showing the central role that free radicals may play in molecular damage to informational macromolecules related to cell aging and death.   (Frcm Ref. 2.)

In this chapter we shall consider some of the evidence for environmental free radical damage, and its prevention, as it related to cellular aging and cancer.

II. SOURCES OF FREE RADICALS

Certain environmental agents are themselves free radicals or serve to generate low, but continual, levels of free radicals in vivo. The physical relationship of free radical-generating agents to specific biological tissues, e.g., restriction of visible and ultraviolet light to surface structures, determines which cells will be exposed. It is, perhaps, significant that wrinkles and change of skin texture, features that we commonly use as an index to estimate chronological age [5], occur primarily on parts of the body ordinarily exposed to light.

Free radicals and peroxides are also generated within our internal environment. The stomach and small intestine are most likely to be exposed to lipid hydroperoxides originating from the oxidative rancidity of foods [6]. The lungs, blood, and heart are exposed to high concentrations of O_2 which generates free radicals in vivo [6]. These tissues are likewise exposed to nitrogen dioxide and ozone, atmospheric pollutants that also cause damage through free radical mechanisms (see Chap. 5/E.1). Ionizing radiation produces many of its biological effects through the induced disociation of water and H_2O_2 formation [7]:

$$H_2O \rightarrow H\cdot \ + \ HO\cdot$$

$$2\ HO\cdot \rightarrow H_2O_2$$

$HO\cdot$ is also a product of lipid oxidation and it is among the most reactive of free radicals exposed to human beings. In the reduction of O_2 to water by the respiratory chain, biological oxidation involves catalysts of hydrogen and electron transfer (flavins, quinones, nonheme iron–sulfur, and cytochromes) that exist as free radicals themselves during electron transport [8]. Damage to membrane phospholipids may be initiated by hydrogen abstraction via electron-transport catalysts so as to form free radicals of unsaturated fatty acid side chains of phospholipids. Another source of such damage is the formation of superoxide ions during biological oxidations [10]. An illustration of how damage may be propagated within the lateral plane of a membrane is depicted in Fig. 2. Here hydrogen abstraction is shown to lead to a free radical of a fatty acid chain of a membrane phospholipid; this may form a peroxy compound by oxygen addition. These radical species are highly reactive compounds which may damage adjacent proteins and lipids. Reduction of radicals by dl-α-tocopherol will break the chain

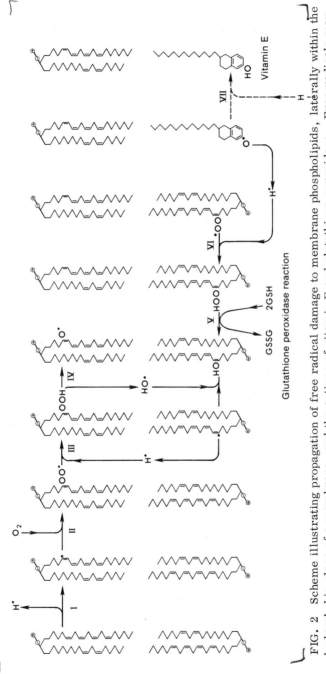

FIG. 2 Scheme illustrating propagation of free radical damage to membrane phospholipids, laterally within the hydrophobic plane of a membrane, and the actions of vitamin E and glutathione peroxidase. Free radicals may arise from endogenous sources as from hydrogen abstraction by electron transport, or exogenously from substances in the environment or photochemical mechanisms.

of events preventing lipid decomposition. One of the major decomposition products of the polyunsaturated fatty acids is a bifunctional aldehyde, malondialdehyde, which cross-links and polymerizes lipids and proteins [6].

The chain-breaking action of tocopherol on this system relates to its ability to partition into the membrane's lipid phase, and to reduce lipid radicals. In stopping radical propagation, vitamin E itself becomes a free radical. Because the unpaired electrons are delocalized over its chromanol ring, it thereby halts the spread of free radical reactions. Its ability to quench lipid radicals may be related to the rate of lateral diffusion of membrane phospholipids which is on the order of 10^{-8} cm/sec [10]. Lateral diffusion for dl-α-tocopherol is unknown, but is likely to be of the same order of magnitude as phospholipids. It is also possible that some of the tocopherol radicals formed may be regenerated if they are reduced by electron transport prior to degradation.

The cell has several endogenous mechanisms for protection against oxidative or free radical damage. Free radicals and free radical-generating systems are scavenged in both the lipid and aqueous phases, e.g., by vitamins E and C, respectively. Peroxide byproducts of oxidative reactions are decomposed by catalases and peroxidases. Superoxide radicals are quenched by superoxide dismutase. A clear example of the damage that can result in the absence of protection against free radicals is afforded by glutathione peroxidase. In an inherited disorder, severe or moderate deficiency of this enzyme results in failure to decompose the peroxides that accumulate during metabolism, leading to erythrocyte damage and hemolytic anemia [11]. As this enzyme requires selenium for activity, selenium deficiency is also harmful [12].

III. FREE RADICALS AND CELLULAR AGING

In 1968, Harman [13], a proponent of a free radical hypothesis of aging, enumerated some of the changes that would be expected to occur with age. These included accumulative oxidative alterations in the long-lived molecules of collagen, elastin, and chromosomal material; breakdown of mucopolysaccharides through oxidative degradation; changes in membrane characteristics due to lipid peroxidation; accumulation of metabolically inert material such as ceroid and age pigment through oxidative polymerization reactions involving lipids, particularly polyunsaturated lipids and proteins; and arteriolocapillary fibrosis [13]. Considerable evidence has accrued to substantiate some of these changes, but insufficient information is available to determine whether they are of primary or secondary importance to organismic aging. Also, there is insufficient knowledge at the molecular level to evaluate involvement of free radicals on a quantitative basis.

A. Cross-Linking

Cross-linking is considered to be an important factor in mammalian aging. Random cross-linking between macromolecules would be expected to immobilize them, causing loss of function. Bjorksten has suggested that, of the cross-linking mechanisms, lipid peroxidation by itself could suffice to cause the changes observed with age in the body proteins and nucleic acids [14]. Although most cross-linking studies have been concerned with collagen, elastin and other cytoplasmic or extracellular proteins, evidence now exists for an age-related increased binding of chromosomal proteins to each other and to DNA [15]. DNA-protein adducts [2] may partly account for reported decreases in the percentage of DNA transcribed with increasing age in mice and rats [16]. Following up on insights gained from radiation biology, it seems safe to predict that a new field is now emerging, focused upon determining mechanisms of cross-linking of DNA by agents other than radiation. Some consequences of free radical-induced cross-linking of proteins and other molecules to DNA are illustrated in Fig. 1.

B. Repair

The cell may compensate for defective proteins by turnover and biosynthesis. Defective DNA is repaired by several mechanisms, namely, excision or prereplication repair [17], strand-break repair [18], and postreplication repair [19]. A correlation exists between excision repair capacity of fibroblast tissues with ultraviolet-induced DNA damage and their lifespan within placental mammals [20]. Also, though repair of DNA damage does not appear to change significantly as cells age in culture [21], it has been reported that cultures derived from patients afflicted with progeria (a disease characterized by premature symptoms of old age before the end of the individual's second decade), were reported to be normal in excision repair, but defective in strand-break repair [22]. However, this finding has not been substantiated [23].

While defective single strands of DNA might be subject to these kinds of repair, it has been pointed out that DNA damage by cross-linking agents may involve corresponding sites on both strands of the helix so that after excision, no template remains for DNA replication [24]. Painter et al. have also described some other conditions for nonrepairable strand breaks in mammalian DNA [25].

C. Copper

This cation is a potent catalyst of lipid peroxidation. Total serum copper concentrations increase almost linearly as a function of human age from 123.7 mg/100 ml at 20 years to 144.6 mg/100 ml at 60 years of age [26].

Persons with a history of myocardial infarction have a significantly higher serum copper level. Copper-catalyzed increases in serum lipid peroxidation may accelerate other age-associated processes, including atherosclerosis and arteriolocapillary fibrosis [26]. It is interesting that vitamin E has been successfully used clinically to improve microcirculation in the treatment of intermittent claudication [27], and other antioxidants can prevent experimentally induced atherosclerosis [28].

D. Lipopigments

Lipopigments or "age pigments" have been identified in many animal cells; they often increase linearly with age, and they have been reported to occasionally occupy as much as 50% of the cytoplasmic volume of some postmitotic cells [29]. They accumulate at the rate of 0.6-1.0% of the total myocardial volume per decade in human cardiac tissue [30]. The related pigments lipofuscin and ceroid have been implicated in many studies of cell senescence. It is generally accepted that they originate from subcellular organelles undergoing peroxidation reactions [31]. Ceroid can accumulate in visible amounts within a few days to several months but lipofuscin formation generally occurs over a period of months to years. Their composition is similar except that ceroid contains higher concentrations of acidic lipid polymers while lipofuscin is richer in neutral lipid polymers [32]. Also, lipofuscin has a high concentration of zinc and is resistant to chelating agents or cation-exchange resins, while ceroid contains more iron and calcium and can be dissolved by metal chelation [32]. Tappel and his colleagues have shown that lipofuscin and ceroid have qualitatively similar maximum fluorescence emission spectra at 440-460 nm with a maximum excitation at 265 and 375 nm [33].

Lipopigment accumulation is characteristic not only of aged cells (e.g., Fig. 3), but also of several conditions that involve peroxidative damage: (1) Wilson's disease (a disorder of copper metabolism, see Ref. 34), (2) thalassemia major [35] and hemochromatosis [36] (both associated with high levels of circulating or stored iron), (3) hypoxia [37], and (4) vitamin E deficiency. Drosophila flies exposed to 100% oxygen at 1/3 atmospheric pressure for 4 days suffer a loss of viability and shortening of lifespan by 25%. Accumulation of dense bodies resembling age pigment are observed to form in their tissues. Thus, oxygen toxicity in Drosophila shares some of the characteristics of accelerating aging [38].

It is difficult to imagine an efficiently functioning cell in which lipopigment occupies much of its cytoplasmic volume. Lipofuscin accumulation in cells could impede the diffusion and transport of essential metabolites and macromolecules [39]. Indeed, the lipofuscin accumulation is reminiscent of glycogen-storage diseases [40], in which a genetic defect of a hydrolytic enzyme causes accumulation of intracellular glycogen particles that bring about cell death and, in infants, the disease itself. Nevertheless,

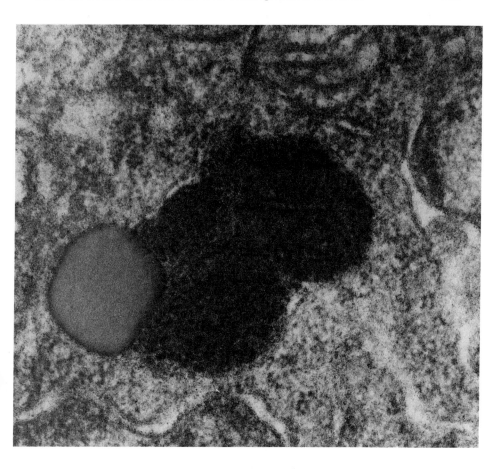

FIG. 3   Lipofuscin deposit in aged rat cardiac muscle (X 121,000).

it remains to be established whether lipofuscin deposits in long-lived cells actually contribute to their senescence and death. Deamer and Gonzalez [41] correlated accumulation of autofluorescent material in cultured human fibroblasts with the inability to synthesize DNA. Also, chickens fed a vitamin E-deficient diet high in polyunsaturated fatty acids developed acute necrotizing encephalopathy [42]. In these animals, dense ceroid-like bodies began to accumulate in some epithelial cells of brain capillaries within 1 week, and after 2 weeks dense bodies occupied large segments of the endothelial cytoplasm. This was followed by swelling and fragmentation of the cells, denudation with focal degeneration of the capillary wall, edema, and plugged vascular channels—conditions rapidly followed by death. These findings, while not definitive, provide circumstantial evidence that progressive accumulation of the fluorescent material contributes to the degeneration of cells.

E. Vitamin E Deficiency

Vitamin E deficiency has been related to aging in mammals because such animals have a shortened lifespan [43], increased susceptibility to disease and accumulations of age pigment in long-lived postmitotic cells [44]. To what extent these changes are due to the loss of the antioxidative action of vitamin E is unknown.

In vitamin E deficiency, the polyunsaturated fatty acid content of membranes is decreased. This has been attributed to selective peroxidative destruction of polyunsaturated fatty acids, particularly arachidonic acid [45]. When the vitamin E-deficient diet is high in linoleic acid or other polyunsaturated fatty acids that are susceptible to lipid peroxidative reactions, symptoms of vitamin E deficiency, including lipopigment accumulation, are enhanced. Thus, a hemolytic anemia characteristic of vitamin E deficiency in premature infants is most effectively corrected by administering vitamin E and lower dietary levels of linoleic and arachidonic acids [46].

Mitochondria of vitamin E-deprived animals [47, 48] show changes in normal ultrastructure. Protrusions of their membranes into adjacent mitochondria and mitochondrial coalescence can be seen by electron microscopy. After 150 days of vitamin E deprivation, the average mito-chondrial volume is 60-80% greater than the controls. Such abnormal mitochondria may contribute to intracellular lipopigment deposits since mitochondrial membranes are often detected within forming lipopigment (e.g., Ref. 49). In vitamin E-deficient cells, some investigators have observed proliferation of peroxisomes (microbodies) [48]. Because hydrogen peroxide decomposition is an important function of these organelles it was suggested that increase in their numbers might be a mechanism whereby the cell compensates for the loss of vitamin E's antioxidative action [48].

Vitamin E has been implicated in the metabolism of mitochodria (see Chap. 5, Sec. E.3). Although vitamin E can function as an activator in the enzymatic reduction of cytochrome c by reduced nicotinamide adenine dinucleotide (NADH) [50], it has not yet been established that it can be oxidized and reduced by the mitochondrial respiratory chain. However, in photosynthetic electron transport there is evidence of oxidation-reduction of vitamin E by photosystem II activity [51]. Vitamin E has also been reported to decrease membrane fluidity and alter phosphate permeability [52]. It may affect prostaglandins biosynthesis (and hence cyclic AMP metabolism) by preventing the peroxidation of arachidonic acid to pro-staglandins [53].

IV. FREE RADICALS AND CANCER

Many chemical carcinogens and/or their intermediates may either be free radicals themselves or else may be activated by free radicals. In evidence of this, harmful environmental agents often can be detected by their ESR signals [54]; these include exhaust fumes, tobacco tars, cigarette smoke, charred foods, chimney smoke, etc.

Polycyclic hydrocarbons have a strong tendency to abstract an electron from an alkali metal, thereby forming relatively stable free radicals. Carcinogenesis seems particularly associated with a high π-electron density in the 9, 10 position (K-region) of the phenanthrene nucleus and a low π-electron density in the neighboring L-region [55]. Certain polycyclic hydrocarbons, which are initially inactive, become altered to reactive carcinogens during oxidation by the liver microsomal electron transport system [56]. Nagata et al. [57-59] have used ESR to detect free radicals of these carcinogens in tissue homogenates. Benzo[α]pyrene is metabolized via a free radical mechanism to 6-OH-benzopyrene with concomitant formation of H_2O_2 [60]. 6-OH-Benzopyrene reacts covalently with nucleic acids of in vitro cell-free systems and induces strand breakage [61]. This carcinogen causes morphological transformation of Syrian hamster cells [62] and rat fibroblasts [63]. Interestingly, transformation efficiency has a positive correlation with increasing age of the cell culture [63].

By painting a wide range of substances on animal skin and then exposing them to light, Epstein and co-workers [64] found that those compounds that have carcinogenic activity also behave as photosensitizers giving rise to reactive intermediates similar to those produced internally in liver by the action of mixed-function oxidases on polycyclic hydrocarbons. Boyland and Sims [65] first suggested that ring hydroxylation of polycyclic hydrocarbons proceeds via the formation of highly reactive epoxides. Jerina and his colleagues [66] have demonstrated the epoxide intermediate in hydroxylation of naphthalene, and Grover, Hewer, and Sims [67, 68] found epoxides during oxidation of benzopyrene, phenanthrene, and benzo[α]anthracene. These intermediates can rapidly react covalently with DNA. Ames et al. have shown that the active forms of a large number of carcinogens are potent frameshift mutagens in bacteria [69].

Although there have been some unsuccessful attempts to produce tumors directly with stable free radicals or with peroxides or organic hydroperoxides, it has been suggested that the free radicals tested were too stable and consequently relatively inert [70].

Vithayathil et al. [71] administered p-dimethylaminoazobenzene, thioacetamide, and 2-acetylaminofluorene to rats and detected transitory

signals at g = 2.035 ± 0.002 before recognizable tumors developed, suggesting that ESR spectroscopy may become clinically useful for early
detection of tumors. Triplet signals have been found in some tumors, but
not in corresponding normal tissues at g = 2.07 [72] and at g = 2.003 [73].
The triplet signals were ascribed to an unshared electron on a nitrogen
atom and Emanuel et al. [72] concluded that "some new rather stable
paramagnetic complex absent from normal tissues seems to be involved in
the metabolism of tumor cells." Quantitative changes in ESR signals of
tumor tissue [74-76] have also been observed. For example, a decreased
intensity of the signal occurs in hepatoma tissue in the region g = 2.25 of
the microsomal fraction associated with cytochrome P_{450}; this finding is
consistent with its decreased drug metabolism [76].

V. ANTIOXIDANTS AND CELLULAR AGING

Efforts directed at extending the lifespan of animals often utilize cells in
culture and lower animals as model systems, where stochastic events are
reduced and death is more likely to result from cell senescence. Although
the causes of aging in short-lived animals may not be identical to those that
occur in humans and other mammals, fundamental mechanisms of cellular
aging are probably common among animal species. For example, lipopigment accumulation, probably the most conspicuous age-associated subcellular change, has been found in cells ranging from primitive coelenter-
ates [77] and mollusks [78] to humans and other mammals [79].

If free radical injury also constitutes a major environmental source of
aging, increased dietary concentrations of suitable forms of antioxidants
and free radical scavengers should afford some protection against this kind
of damage and contribute to an organism's ability to express its genetic
potential in terms of a maximum lifespan. Several studies have already
shown that dietary supplementation of vitamin E or other antioxidants can
significantly increase lifespan and retard changes that are known to occur
at predictable times in cultured cells, lower animals, and mammals
[80-96].

A. Cultured Cells as Model Systems

Diploid mammalian and human cells can undergo only a limited number of
population doublings in vitro. Cultured human lung diploid cells (WI-38)
have a documented lifespan of 52 ± 10 population doublings (the Hayflick
limit, see Ref. 80). Macieira-Coelho [81] and Cristofalo et al. [82] have
reported that addition of 5 μg/ml hydrocortisone to the medium extends
WI-38 cell lifespan by 5-40%. Packer and Smith [83] reported a series of
experiments where the number of population doublings was increased to

about 112-117 (in the absence or presence of hydrocortisone) by supplementation of the culture medium with vitamin E. Todaro and Green [84] reported that rat fibroblasts supplemented with 20 mg/ml albumin above the amount present in serum permitted the cells to grow to 100 population doublings. These findings, particularly the two latter observations, are difficult to reproduce, apparently due to nutritional fluctuations. A further complication is that control cultures are occasionally very long-lived. Nevertheless, such experiments show that the mitotic potential of diploid fibroblasts in culture may not be rigidly limited and can be altered by dietary manipulation.

More reproducible results are obtained with antioxidant protection of cultured cells exposed to environmental stress. Deamer (personal communication) has found that confluent WI-38 cells, which have been maintained in a low serum medium (0.1%), show appreciable accumulation of fluorescent material after 7 weeks and morphologically resemble senescent cells. However, cells held under these conditions in the presence of 100 μg/ml vitamin E do not show these changes. It is noteworthy that the 10% fetal calf serum normally used in cell culture media has a concentration of vitamin E that is on an order of magnitude lower than that present in human plasma (10 μg/ml). Malondialdehyde formation is inhibited in WI-38 cell lipid if cells are grown in the presence of either dl-α-tocopherol or solubilized preparations of Hoffman-La Roche vitamin E acetate [85].

Addition of vitamin E to the culture medium also affords these cells partial protection against oxygen toxicity induced by 50% oxygen exposure. Indeed, human WI-38 cells grow more rapidly and undergo more population doublings if grown at 10% O_2 [86]. Thus, in the tissue culture environment, it appears that oxygen toxicity may affect fibroblast cell lifespan. Other recent studies from our laboratory (Packer and Fuehr) indicate that seleno-dl-methionine supplementation also allays cell death brought about by exposure of cells to 50% oxygen.

Riboflavin-induced photosensitization to visible light causes damage to WI-38 cells; this photokilling can be prevented by supplementing cells with 100 μg/ml vitamin E during growth prior to visible light exposure [87]. Further studies using rat liver mitochondria have implicated flavin photosensitized reactions [88]. Inhibition of flavin-linked enzymes was accelerated in liver mitochondria from vitamin E-deficient rats.

Bland et al. [89] have also shown that α-tocopherol significantly protects red blood cells against oxygen and light exposure by prohibiting the formation of cholesterol hydroperoxide in the membranes which apparently labilizes them, resulting in cell deformation and abnormal budding.

B. Lower Animal Models

As a model for aging studies, Epstein et al. [90,91] used the free-living
nematode Caenorhabditis briggsae, an organism composed mainly of
postmitotic cells. During its lifespan, they noted that a progressive age-
dependent accumulation of pigment granules with acid phosphatase activity
occurred particularly in the intestinal epithelium. Pigment granules
eventually occupied most of the cytoplasmic volume and appeared to cause
the breakdown of the entire tissue. Near the end of the life cycle, extensive damage to muscle cells and nerve complexes impaired the round-
worms' motility. Addition of dl-α-tocopherol quinone to the medium
increased the 50% survival of treated animals by 11 days over the
35 ± 2 days typical of control populations, prolonging the lifespan of the
cells by approximately 30%. The vitamin E-treated nematodes also showed
a delay in the onset of detectable lipofuscin and a reduction in the quantity
of pigment detected [91]. Experiments of this type are usually conducted
under static and crowded culture conditions. It would be interesting to
learn whether the effect of vitamin E on lifespan would be improved or
reduced by repeating such experiments in perfused and sparsely populated
conditions where the lifespan of controls are about fourfold longer.

Bolla and Brot [92] confirmed the α-tocopherol quinone-induced life
extension under static culture conditions in another species of nematode,
Turbatrix aceti. In studies correlating enzyme changes with age they found
a constant decline in specific activities of DNA polymerase and aldolase
and a sharp increase in those of elongation factor 1 and RNA polymerase at
5 and 15 days, respectively, before the activities ultimately declined.
These researchers also observed a progressive accumulation of totally or
partially inactive enzyme molecules detected as antigenically cross-
reacting material. Evidence of the occurrence of inactive enzymes, i.e.,
errors in protein synthesis, accompanying aging has been reported elsewhere [93-95], but their causal relevance to aging is still in dispute.
Inclusion of α-tocopherol quinone in the medium prolonged nematode lifespan by 17% and also altered the time at which the activity of those enzymes
peaked. For example, specific activities of RNA and DNA polymerase
declined in the vitamin E-treated animals at a later age than in the controls
[92].

It has recently also been reported that Drosophila melanogaster
responded to vitamin E treatment by showing a 15% increase in its lifespan
and a marked reduction in the accumulation of lipofuscin [96].

C. Mammalian Models

Tappel et al. [33] showed that high concentrations of vitamin E, administered to mice in conjunction with other antioxidants [selenium, butylated
hydroxytoluene (BHT), methionine, and ascorbic acid] decreased the

age-pigment accumulation in heart and testis. This mixture of antioxidants was used in an effort to obtain maximum protection against free radical damage since, in certain tissues where exposure to oxidants is high, vitamin E cannot by itself completely inhibit peroxidation by means of its chain-breaking reactions. Vitamin E was chosen as the key antioxidant for inhibiting damage by lipid peroxidation [97], butylated hydroxytoluene for its chain-breaking synergism with vitamin E [98], ascorbate and methionine for their ability to scavenge free radicals in the aqueous phase of the cell [99], and selenium, a cofactor for glutathione peroxidase, to stimulate maximum activity of that enzyme system [12]. Reduction of lipid peroxides to nontoxic, hydroxy fatty acids by selenium-glutathione peroxidase produces a sparing effect on vitamin E and prevents decomposition of peroxides into free radicals capable of reinitiating peroxidation [6]. Although it was established [33] that the progressive accumulation of fluorescent lipopigment could be slowed by increasing dietary antioxidants, there was no increase in lifespan. Attempts to optimize protection with antioxygenic nutrients and antioxidants could be hampered by several factors: nutritional imbalances as caused by the levels of methionine, vitamin E, and selenium used; by difficulties in detoxifying the high doses of the synthetic antioxidant butylated hydroxytoluene; and by the increased susceptibility of old animals to infectious diseases in both control and treated animals.

Harman [100] reported a prolongation of the half-survival time (but not mean lifespan) of AKR mice fed antioxidants other than vitamin E. One percent weight cysteine-HCL extended the time by 14.5%, 1% wt hydroxylamine-HCL by 8.3%, and 2% wt hydroxylamine-HCL by 17.0%. Also, a 45.0% increase in the 50% survival time of LAF mice occurred with 0.5% butylated hydroxytoluene and a 29.2% increase with 2-mercaptoethylamine-HCL [13]. Kohn [101], in a similar study, showed that antioxidants increased the 50% survival time of mice only when the control lifespan values were suboptimal. This was interpreted to indicate that antioxidants do not directly inhibit aging, but inhibit some harmful environmental or nutritional factors such as the oxidation of essential dietary nutrients.

Two other antioxidants, nordihydroguaiaretic acid [102] and ethoxyquin have also been reported to increase the half-time survival of mice. Comfort et al. [103] suggested that antioxidant prolongevity may be related to the increased ability of these compounds to induce activity of hepatic enzymes responsible for detoxification of nutrients. Walker et al. [104] showed that a marked decrease in the activity and inducibility of the drug-metabolizing enzymes occurs with age. Mice fed a diet containing 0.5% nordihydroguaiaretic acid, ethoxyquin, or butylated hydroxytoluene, however, had increased liver weights, microsomal protein, and cytochromes P_{450} and b_5. From days 81 to 440, the microsomal protein of these animals remained at about double the control level. N-Propyl gallate, an antioxidant which does not extend the lifespan, did not induce these hepatic changes [104].

VI. ANTIOXIDANTS AND CANCER

Persons residing in geographical areas naturally rich in selenium exhibit a significantly lower death rate from cancer [105]. Such observations have encouraged attempts to slow tumor growth in experimental animals by including vitamin E, selenium, or other antioxidants in the diet. Several interesting developments have emerged. For example, chemical transformation of hamster cells can be inhibited by antioxidants [106]. Also, after feeding mice a diet including a mixture of antioxidants, it is possible to prevent the formation in irradiated skin of cholesterol-α-oxide, a carcinogenic photoproduct of ultraviolet light. This finding may eventually provide a basis for preventive measures against ultraviolet light-induced skin cancer [107].

Harman [108] has shown that, of two experimental groups of rats to which 7,12-dimethyl-benz[α]anthracene (DMBA) was administered by stomach tube, those which received a dietary supplementation of 20 mg vitamin E had a 40.0% incidence of tumors compared with a 73.6% incidence of tumors in animals receiving only 5 mg vitamin E. Similar protection was afforded by vitamin E and selenium following topical application of DMBA to mice [109]. Dietary vitamin E also decreases the number of malignant growths resulting from feeding with the carcinogens 3-methyl-4'dimethylaminobenzene [110] and methylcholanthrene [111].

Besides vitamin E and selenium, other dietary antioxidants show some protection against cancer. Harman noted that inclusion of hydroxylamine-HCL in the diet markedly decreased the incidence of spontaneous tumors [100]. This antioxidant also gave a 20% extension of survival time to mice innoculated with Ehrlich ascites tumor [112]. Butylated hydroxyanisole and ethoxyquin were effective in inhibiting carcinogenic effects of diethylnitrosamine and 4-nitroquinoline-N-oxide in mouse lung [113] and benzo[α]pyrene on the forestomach of the mouse [114].

In a novel finding, Snipes et al. [115] have reported that infection of lipid-containing viruses is inhibited following their incubation with 0.1 mM butylated hydroxytoluene. This has been interpreted as a structural effect of butylated hydroxytoluene on the membrane, causing decreased viral attachment. The effects were not evaluated in terms of butylated hydroxytoluene's known radical-scavenging properties.

A. Some Possible Modes of Protection

The molecular mechanisms of antioxidant protection against cancer are not well understood. Antioxidants may prevent the activation of various carcinogens to epoxides which are more effective than the parent compound in producing malignant transformation [116]. Antioxidant agents would be expected to inhibit peroxidation reactions which affect DNA molecules in many deleterious ways. These include covalent reaction of carcinogens with DNA [117] and destruction of pyrimidine moieties [118]. Shamberger [119] has shown that cells cultured with DMBA had 63.2% more chromosome breakage than those cultures which contained both DMBA and vitamin E in the incubation medium.

The results of Snipes et al. [115] suggest that membrane structural modifications with hydrophobic molecules may have anticancer activity, particularly with regard to viral cancer. A promising direction for future research should be to load cellular membranes with appropriate types of hydrophobic molecules, which would reduce viral infection and sequester potentially damaging environmental free radicals.

B. Tumor Levels of Endogenous Protectors

The concentrations of endogenous molecules which normally afford protection against free radicals have been studied in neoplasms. In general, tumor tissue possesses high antioxidant activity and low peroxidant activity [120]. Thus, it has been observed that tumor tissues peroxidize less readily than their normal counterparts. Although increased peroxidation occurs in the liver, adipose tissue, and brain of tumor-bearing animals, lipid peroxides are not detected in the tumors themselves [121]. This has been ascribed to the high antioxidant concentrations in tumors [122].

Tumors generally have decreased catalase activity [123-126]. Rats bearing ascites hepatoma cells were shown to have a lower incorporation of [^{14}C]leucine into liver catalase both in vivo and in vitro, suggesting that the decrease of catalase in tumor-bearing rats is caused by a depression of its synthesis [126].

In chronic leukemia and carcinoma, glutathione peroxidase is significantly less than normal [127]. Correlation of low peroxidase levels with high putrescine levels in leukemia, Morris hepatoma, and Ehrlich ascites tumors has led to the interpretation that putrescine binding and inhibition of tissue peroxidase may be an important step in the transformation process. Decreased peroxidase would result in elevated tissue peroxides and these in turn would lead to increased free radical formation ultimately damaging nucleic acids, enzymes, and other cellular constituents to result in carcinogenesis and/or mutagenesis [128].

VII. CONCLUSION

Analysis of the current evidence leads us to infer:

1. That optimization of the cellular environment should delay the degenerative changes of senescence and may result in a modest

extension of lifespan by enabling an organism to approach its full genetic potential in a given environment. Further research is needed on (a) identifying the toxic effects of pollutants and other ambient factors in our environment such as light and oxygen, on the components of our diet that contain damaging free radical substances, and on (b) identifying where and at what levels damage is generated in a particular environment.

2. That future experiments on antioxidant protection against cancer and cellular aging are highly promising and warrant further investigation. Such studies will provide information on what combination of antioxidants in a particular environment afford maximum protection.

REFERENCES

1. L. Packer, D. W. Deamer, and R. L. Heath, in Advances in Gerontological Research. Edited by B. L. Strehler. New York, Academic, 1967, pp. 77-120.
2. K. C. Smith, in Cellular Aspects of Ageing: Concepts and Mechanisms. Edited by R. G. Cutler. Basel, Krager, 1976.
3. World Health Organization, Prevention of Cancer (Ser. 276). Geneva, Technical Report Service, 1964.
4. E. Boyland, Prog. Exp. Tumor Res. 11:222 (1969).
5. B. L. Strehler, Environ. Res. 1:46 (1967).
6. A. Tappel, Amer. J. Clin. Nutr. 27:960 (1974).
7. G. Stein and J. Weiss, Nature 161:650 (1948)
8. B. Commoner, J. J. Heise, B. B. Lippincott, R. E. Norberg, J. V. Passoneau, and J. Townsend, Science 126:57 (1957).
9. I. Fridowich, Adv. Enzymol. 41:35 (1974).
10. P. Devaux and H. M. McConnell, J. Amer. Chem. Soc. 94:4475 (1972).
11. T. F. Necheles, M. H. Steinberg, and D. Cameron, Br. J. Haematol. 19:605 (1970).
12. J. T. Rotruck, A. L. Pope, H. E. Ganther, A. B. Swanson, D. G. Hafeman, and W. G. Hockstra, Science 179:588 (1973).
13. D. Harman, J. Gerontol. 23:476 (1968).
14. J. Bjorksten, J. Amer. Geriatr. Soc. 16:408 (1968).
15. G. B. Price and T. Makinodan, Gerontologia 19:58 (1973).
16. R. G. Cutler, Exp. Gerontol. 10:37 (1975).
17. B. S. Strauss, Life Sci. 15:1685 (1974).
18. C. D. Town, K. C. Smith, and H. S. Kaplan, Curr. Top. Rad. Res. Quart. 8:351 (1973).

19. A. R. Lehmann, J. Mol. Biol. $\underline{66}$:319 (1972).
20. R. W. Hart and R. B. Setlow, Proc. Natl. Acad. Sci. USA $\underline{71}$:2169 (1974).
21. J. M. Clarkson and R. B. Painter, Mut. Res. $\underline{23}$:107 (1974).
22. J. Epstein, J. R. Williams, and J. B. Little, Proc. Natl. Acad. Sci. USA $\underline{70}$:977 (1973).
23. J. D. Regan and R. B. Setlow, Biochem. Biophys. Res. Commun. $\underline{59}$:858 (1974).
24. J. Bjorksten, in Theoretical Aspects of Aging. Edited by M. Rockstein, M. L. Sussman, and J. Chesky. New York, Academic, 1974, pp. 43-59.
25. R. B. Painter, B. R. Young, and H. J. Burki, Proc. Natl. Acad. Sci. USA $\underline{71}$:4836 (1974).
26. D. Harman, J. Gerontol. $\underline{20}$:151 (1965).
27. H. T. G. Williams, D. Fenna, and R. A. Macbeth, Surg. Gynecol. Obstetr. $\underline{132}$:662 (1971).
28. R. B. Wilson, P. M. Newberne, and N. S. Kula, Exp. Mol. Pathol. $\underline{21}$:118 (1974).
29. J. Miquel, A. L. Tappel, C. J. Dillard, M. M. Herman, and K. G. Bensch, J. Gerontol. $\underline{29}$:622 (1974).
30. B. L. Strehler, in The General Physiology of Cell Specialization. Edited by D. Mazia and A. Tyler. New York, McGraw-Hill, 1963, pp. 116-148.
31. K. S. Chio, U. Reiss, B. Fletcher, and A. L. Tappel, Science $\underline{166}$:1535 (1969).
32. A. N. Siakotos and N. Koppang, Mech. Age. Dev. $\underline{2}$:177 (1973).
33. A. Tappel, B. Fletcher, and D. W. Deamer, J. Gerontol. $\underline{28}$:415 (1973).
34. S. Goldfischer, Amer. J. Pathol. $\underline{46}$:977 (1965).
35. L. Goldberg and J. P. Smith, J. Pathol. Bacteriol. $\underline{80}$:173 (1960).
36. C. B. Hyman, B. Landing, R. Alfin-Slater, L. Kozak, J. Weitzman, and J. A. Ortega, Ann. NY Acad. Sci. $\underline{232}$:211 (1974).
37. N. M. Sulkin and P. Srivanij, J. Gerontol. $\underline{15}$:2 (1960).
38. D. E. Philpott, K. G. Bensch, and J. Miquel, Aerospace Med. $\underline{45}$:283 (1974).
39. P. Gordon, in Theoretical Aspects of Aging. Edited by M. Rockstein, M. L. Sussman, and J. Chesky. New York, Academic, 1974, pp. 61-81.
40. H. G. Hers and F. V. Hoof, in Lysosomes in Biology and Pathology, Vol. 2. Edited by J. T. Dingle and H. B. Fell. New York, Elsevier, 1973, pp. 19-40.
41. D. W. Deamer and J. Gonzalez, Arch. Biochem. Biophys. $\underline{165}$:421 (1974).
42. W. A. Yu, M. C. Yu, and P. A. Young, Exp. Mol. Pathol. $\underline{21}$:789 (1974).

43. K. E. Mason and I. R. Telford, Arch. Pathol. 43:363 (1947).
44. L. Einarson and A. Ringsted, in Effect of Chronic Vitamin E
     Deficiency on the Nervous System and Skeletal Musculature in Adult
     Rats. Copenhagen, Levin and Munksgaard, 1938, p. 163.
45. L. A. Witting, Lipids 2:109 (1967).
46. F. A. Oski and L. A. Barness, J. Pediatrics 70:211 (1967).
47. N. M. Sulkin and D. Sulkin, in Fifth International Conference on
     Electron Microscopy, Proceedings. Philadelphia, 1962, p. VV-8,
     Abstr.
48. U. N. Riede, C. Stitny, S. Althaus, and H. P. Rohr, Beitr. Pathol.
     145:24 (1972).
49. G. Gopinath, Acta Anat. (Basel) 89:14 (1974).
50. A. Nason and I. R. Lehman, Science 122:19 (1955).
51. R. Sicher and N. I. Bishop, Plant Physiol. 56:abstract 48 (1975).
52. F. A. Hommes, D. J. Mastebroek-Helder, and I. Molenaar, Nutr.
     Metab. 19:263 (1976).
53. W. C. Hope, C. Dalton, L. J. Machlin, R. J. Filipski, and F. M.
     Vane, Prostaglandins 10:557 (1975).
54. W. Gordy, in Information Theory in Biology. Edited by H. P. Hockey,
     R. L. Platzman, and H. Quastler. Oxford, Pergamon, 1958, p. 353.
55. A. Pullman and B. Pullman, Adv. Cancer Res. 3:117 (1955).
56. R. S. Umans, S. A. Lesko, and P. O. P. Ts'o, Nature 221:763 (1969).
57. C. Nagata, Y. Tagashira, M. Kodama, and A. Imamura, Gann 57:437
     (1966).
58. C. Nagata, M. Kodama, and Y. Tagashira, Gann 58:493 (1967).
59. C. Nagata, M. Inomata, M. Kodama, and Y. Tagshira, Gann 59:289
     (1968).
60. P. O. P. Ts'o, J. C. Barrett, W. J. Caspary, S. A. Lesko, and
     R. S. Lorentzen, in Aging, Carcinogenesis and Radiation Biology:
     The Role of Nucleic Acid Additive Reactions. Edited by K. C. Smith.
     New York, Plenum, 1976, pp. 373-398.
61. P. O. P. Ts'o, W. J. Caspary, B. I. Cohen, J. C. Leavitt, S. A.
     Lesko, R. J. Lorentzen, and L. M. Schechtman, in Chemical
     Carcinogenesis, Part A. Edited by P. O. P. Ts'o and J. A. DiPaolo.
     New York, Dekker, 1974, p. 113.
62. L. Schechtman, S. Lesko, R. Lorentzen, and P. Ts'o, Proc. Amer.
     Assoc. Cancer Res. 15:66 (1974).
63. C. Lasne, A. Gentil, and I. Chouroulinkov, Nature 247:490 (1974).
64. S. S. Epstein, M. Small, H. L. Falk, and N. Mantel, Cancer Res.
     24:855 (1964).
65. E. Boyland and P. Sims, Biochem. J. 97:7 (1965).
66. D. M. Jerina and J. W. Daly, B. Witkip, P. Zaltzman-Nirenberg,
     and S. Udenfriend, Biochem. J. 97:7 (1965).

67. P. L. Grover, A. Hewer, and P. Sims, Biochem. Pharmacol. 21:2713 (1972).
68. P. L. Grover, A. Hewer, and P. Sims, FEBS Lett. 18:76 (1971).
69. B. N. Ames, W. E. Durston, E. Yamasaki, and F. D. Lee, Proc. Natl. Acad. Sci. USA 70:2281 (1973).
70. T. F. Slayter, in Free Radical Mechanisms in Tissue Damage. London, Pion Pty., Ltd., 1972.
71. A. J. Vithayathil, J. L. Ternberg, and B. Commoner, Nature 207:1246 (1965).
72. N. M. Emanuel, A. N. Saprin, V. A. Shabalkin, L. E. Kozlova, and K. E. Krugljakova, Nature 222:165 (1969).
73. M. J. Brennan, T. Cole, and J. A. Singley, Proc. Soc. Exp. Biol. 123:715 (1966).
74. D. W. Nebert and H. S. Mason, Cancer Res. 23:833 (1963).
75. T. F. Slayter and J. W. R. Cook, in Cytology Automation. Edited by D. M. D. Evans. Edinburgh, Livingstone, 1969, p. 108.
76. J. D. Wallace, D. H. Driscoll, C. G. Kalomiris, and A. Neaves, Cancer 25:1087 (1970).
77. M. A. Brock, J. Ultrastruc. Res. 32:118 (1970).
78. I. Szabo and M. Szabo, Arch. Molluskenk. 65:11 (1933).
79. B. L. Strehler, D. D. Mark, A. S. Mildvan and M. V. Gee, J. J. Gerontol. 14:430 (1959).
80. L. Hayflick, Exp. Cell Res. 37:614 (1965).
81. A. Macieira-Coelho, Experientia 22:390 (1966).
82. V. J. Cristofalo, J. Kabakjan, D. Kobler, and B. Baker, Ninth Intl. Cong. Gerontol. 3:17 (1972).
83. L. Packer and J. R. Smith, Proc. Natl. Acad. Sci. USA 71:4763 (1974).
84. G. J. Todaro and H. Green, Proc. Soc. Exp. Biol. Med. 116:688 (1964).
85. L. Packer, Protein and Other Adducts to DNA: Their Significance to Aging, Carcinogenesis, and Radiation Biology, Intl. Symp. Proceedings, Williamsburg, Va., May 1975, pp. 519-536.
86. L. Packer and K. Fuehr, Nature 267:423 (1977).
87. O. M. Pereira, in Riboflavin Sensitized Visible Light Effects on Human Diploid Fibroblasts in Culture (Thesis). Berkeley, University of California, 1975.
87a. L. Packer and K. Fuehr, Nature 267, 423 (1977).
88. B. B. Aggarwal, Y. Avi-Dor, H. M. Tinberg, and L. Packer, Biochem. Biophys. Res. Commun. 69:362 (1976).
89. J. Bland, P. Madden, and E. J. Herbert, Physiol. Chem. Phys. 7:69 (1975).
90. J. Epstein, S. Himmelhoch, and D. Gershon, Mech. Age. Dev. 1:245 (1972).

91. J. Epstein and D. Gershon, Mech. Age. Dev. 1:257 (1972).

92. R. Bolla and N. Brot, Arch. Biochem. Biophys. 169:227 (1975).

93. H. Gershon and D. Gershon, Proc. Natl. Acad. Sci. USA 70:909 (1973).

94. R. Holliday and G. M. Tarrant, Nature 238:26 (1972).

95. C. M. Lewis and R. Holliday, Nature 228:877 (1970).

96. J. Miquel, Gerontol. Soc. Abstr. (1975).

97. W. A. Pryor, Chem. Eng. News 49:35 (1971).

98. J. R. Chipault, in Autoxidation and Antioxidants, Vol. 2. Edited by W. O. Lundberg. New York, Interscience, 1962.

99. A. L. Tappel, Amer. J. Clin. Nutr. 23:1137 (1970).

100. D. Harman, J. Gerontology. 16:247 (1961).

101. R. R. Kohn, J. Gerontology. 26:378 (1971).

102. N. P. Buu-Hoc and A. R. Ratsimamanga, Comp. Rend. Biol. 153:1180 (1959).

103. A. Comfort, I. Youhotsky-Gore, and K. Pathmanathan, Nature 229:254 (1971).

104. R. Walker, A. Rahim, and D. V. Parke, Proc. Roy. Soc. Med. 66:780 (1973).

105. R. J. Shamberger and C. E. Willis, Crit. Rev. Clin. Chem. 2:211 (1971).

106. L. Piekarski and M. Koniewicz, Neoplasma (Bratisl.) 22:251 (1975).

107. W.-B. Lo and H. S. Black, Nature 246:489 (1973).

108. D. Harman, Clin. Res. 17:125 (1969).

109. R. J. Shamberger and G. Rudolph, Experientia 22:116 (1966).

110. R. W. Swick and C. A. Baumann, Cancer Res. 11:774 (1962).

111. S. L. Haber and R. W. Wissler, Proc. Soc. Exp. Biol. Med. 111:774 (1962).

112. D. Harman, Clin. Res. 4:54 (1956).

113. L. W. Wattenberg, Fed. Proc. 31:2363 (1972).

114. L. M. Wattenberg, J. Natl. Cancer Inst. 48:1425 (1972).

115. W. Snipes, S. Person, A. Keith, and J. Cupp, Science 188:4183 (1975).

116. R. J. Shamburger, J. Natl. Cancer Inst. 48:1491 (1972).

117. C. E. Morreal, T. L. Dao, K. Eskins, C. L. King, and J. Dienstag, Biochim. Biophys. Acta 169:224 (1968).

118. M. S. Melzer and R. V. Tomlinson, Arch. Biochem. Biophys. 115:226 (1966).

119. R. J. Shamberger, F. F. Baughman, S. L. Kalchert, C. E. Willis, and G. C. Hoffman, Proc. Natl. Acad. Sci. USA 70:1461 (1973).

120. E. A. Neyfakh and V. E. Kagan, Biokhimiia 34:692 (1969).

121. C. W. Shuster, Proc. Soc. Exp. Biol. Med. 90:423 (1955).

122. E. D. Lash, Arch. Biochem. Biophys. 115:332 (1966).

123. V. E. Price and R. E. Greenfield, J. Biol. Chem. 209:363 (1954).

124. T. Higashi, K. Kashiwagi, and K. Warabioka, Gann 59:461 (1968).
125. E. T. Nishimura, T. Y. Kobara, J. P. Kaltenbach, and W. B. Wartman, Arch. Biochem. Biophys. 97:589 (1962).
126. K. Kashiwagi, T. Tobe, T. Higashi, and K. Warabioka, Gann 63:57 (1972).
127. J. Hopkins and G. R. Tudhope, Br. J. Haematol. 25:563 (1973).
128. D. Armstrong, S. Dimmitt, and D. VanWormer, in Protein and Other Adducts to DNA: Their Significance to Aging, Carcinogenesis and Radiation Biology, Int. Symp., Williamsburg, Va. May 1975, p. 80 (Abstr.).

11 HUMAN HEALTH AND DISEASE

Part 11A / Deficiency States, Pharmacological Effects,
    and Nutrient Requirements   520

Part 11B / Interpretation of Human Requirements for
    Vitamin E   621

Part 11A/ Deficiency States, Pharmacological Effects,
and Nutrient Requirements

PHILIP M. FARRELL

University of Wisconsin
Madison, Wisconsin

I.	Introduction	520
II.	Deficiency States	523
	A. Definition of Vitamin E Deficiency	523
	B. Premature Infants	526
	C. Malabsorption	540
III.	Possible Pharmacological Effects	579
	A. General	579
	B. Safety of High Doses	584
	C. Cardiovascular Disease	586
	D. Other Proposed Pharmacologic Uses	594
IV.	Nutritional Requirements	598
	A. Survey Status	598
	B. Recommended Dietary Allowances	604

I. INTRODUCTION

Despite over 50 years of intensive study and wide acceptance as an essential nutrient for lower animals, the status of vitamin E in human nutrition remains unsettled, if not enigmatic. This, of course, is very much in contrast to the other fat-soluble vitamins where the path from discovery to application in clinical medicine was generally traversed in the span of a decade [1]. As discussed under Biochemical Function in Chapter 5, the tocopherol family has also proven uniquely elusive in regard to delineation of specific biochemical functions at the cellular level. In fact, a comprehensive review of the literature on vitamin E in human health and disease conveys the strong impression that virtually all aspects of this nutrient's role in human beings are controversial.

It is ironic that the lack of a readily apparent role for tocopherol in human nutrition and the generation of doubts regarding its value in clinical practice have occurred despite a great abundance of supporting data for nutritional essentiality in animals (see Chapter 6). And yet it is the bizarre array of diverse syndromes encountered with vitamin E in animals that contributes to the complex and sometimes confusing picture of tocopherol requirements in humans. Further complicating our understanding of vitamin E in human nutrition are the many sound observations that implicate other, structurally unrelated components which can, at the very least, exert a sparing influence on tocopherol requirements [2,3].

Vitamin E deficiency in humans secondary to nutritional deprivation is a rare occurrence. It is difficult, in fact, to produce experimentally a vitamin E deficiency state in adult human beings because of the considerable tissue storage of the vitamin leading to an extended period of diminished intake before depletion occurs. On the other hand, deficiency of vitamin E, as disclosed by low plasma tocopherol levels and erythrocyte hemolysis in the presence of hydrogen peroxide, does occur in association with intestinal malabsorption syndromes of various etiologies. In addition, prematurely delivered newborns, who begin life with marginal stores at best, and who also exhibit transient malabsorption, are commonly subject to vitamin E deficiency. Although vitamin E depletion in humans is encountered infrequently, there are several disorders in children and adults which bear superficial resemblance to tocopherol deficiency syndromes of animals. Such resemblances have repeatedly raised the suggestion that a clinical counterpart has been discovered in humans. Nonetheless, when disorders such as genetic (Duchenne) muscular dystrophy have been subjected to more careful and objective scientific scrutiny, and when such patients have been treated with vitamin E, the results have been uniformly disappointing.

The elusive search for a clinical correlate of tocopherol deficiency in humans has been based to a large extent on our understanding of nutritional deprivation experiments in animals. Therefore, it is useful to recount briefly the salient features of vitamin E deficiency in lower animals. Perhaps the most notable aspects are the marked degree of species specificity and the great diversity of tissue and organ functions affected by diminished tocopherol levels [4]. In many instances, particularly in rapidly growing animals, disorders such as muscular degeneration and encephalomalacia occur in an acute fashion over a matter of several days to a few weeks [5,6]. In human beings, however, rapid development of vitamin E deficiency does not apparently occur due to the resistance of tissue stores to depletion as well as the abundant presence of the vitamin in foodstuffs. Additionally, young growing animals, the usual subjects for tocopherol depletion studies, are generally placed on diets that are virtually devoid of all antioxidants and which contain a limited variety of nutrient sources as compared with most human diets. It is conceivable that this laboratory practice may promote an isolated, severe vitamin E deficiency state in circumstances where possible compensatory mechanisms (e.g., increased tissue glutathione) cannot become operative.

Because of the pronounced differences in nutritional status between animals under study and humans available for clinical investigations of vitamin E deficiency, it has become necessary to search for somewhat insidious pathological processes in humans, possibly leading to subclinical manifestations. However, the efforts of investigators to uncover specific clinical signs of human tocopherol deficiency have met with frustration in many instances. This further distinguishes vitamin E from the other fat-soluble vitamins where dramatic manifestations of the deficiency state may develop (e.g., severe hemorrhage in vitamin K deficiency and rickets in vitamin D deficiency).

In view of this unsettled picture, it is not at all surprising that a diversity of opinion exists with respect to the efficacy of treatment with vitamin E. This situation has prevailed not only for circumstances where supplementation of nutritionally adequate patients is at issue, but also in some clinical settings where this has been extended to subjects who are clearly deficient based on analysis of blood samples. Although the latter approach is disconcerting to nutritional scientists, physicians are generally reluctant to prescribe a medication without an established efficacy. In the case of vitamin E, the failure of investigators to establish a direct correlation between vitamin E deficiency and a clinical syndrome in humans, as well as the lack of effect of vitamin E in the treatment of those human diseases which bear some resemblance to vitamin E-deficient animals, have led a number of pharmacologists to conclude that there is no compelling evidence that vitamin E has any therapeutic use [7, 8]. The disappointing results of most therapeutic trials and the failure to confirm observations in isolated case reports partially justify such a conclusion. Thus, the search for a tocopherol associated disorder in humans and an established value for the vitamin in clinical practice continues and could remain elusive until an essential biochemical mechanism in cellular metabolism can likewise be delineated.

In order to discuss the role of vitamin E in human health and disease, it becomes necessary to divide the relevant nutritional data into two broad categories: (1) findings in patients with chemically proven vitamin E deficiency and (2) observations on subjects who possess normal circulating tocopherol levels but who have been placed on therapeutic trials ("megavitamin E" supplementation) because of diseases with a possible relationship to antioxidant deficiency. It is the purpose of this review to discuss vitamin E deficiency in humans in a comprehensive fashion with attention to all aspects from prenatal nutrition to possible effects on adult longevity. Previous reviews [9-13] have dealt with various aspects of vitamin E deficiency in humans and have generally drawn the analogy between tocopherol depletion in animals and expected manifestations in humans. For various reasons discussed previously, comparisons with deprived animals may not be appropriate. An attempt has therefore been made in this chapter to consider human vitamin E deficiency as a separate subject. Especially emphasized in other reviews is the so-called "Elgin

Project," in which a limited number of adult male volunteers nutritionally depleted for 3 years were found to show low plasma tocopherol levels but little in the way of symptoms [14-16]. In addition, previous review articles tend to stress data obtained from the study of small populations of E-deficient subjects. Accordingly, deliberate efforts have been made herein to highlight results obtained from large series of deficient patients and in large clinical trials. Some degree of selection is necessary, however, in order to condense the several hundred publications which have appeared on this subject. Therefore, those studies with carefully controlled variables will be selectively emphasized, particularly in Sec. III on proposed pharmacological uses.

Finally, it should be noted at the outset that although a more coherent picture is emerging, the role of vitamin E in human nutrition remains complex and at times confusing—leading the author to apologize in advance for inclusion of material which may prove difficult to interpret and place in clinical perspective. Nonetheless, it is hoped that the descriptions and critical interpretations made in the discussion of human vitamin E deficiency states will, despite their shortcomings, serve not only to emphasize the many gaps that exist in our knowledge of the role of vitamin E deficiency in human beings, but also to support our fundamental need for the antioxidant.

II. DEFICIENCY STATES

A. Definition of Vitamin E Deficiency

Vitamin E deficiency is defined herein as a low blood tocopherol level or evidence of in vitro hemolysis of erythrocytes exposed to hydrogen peroxide or other oxidants.

The terms "subclinical deficiency" or simply "deficiency" (unqualified) are used in this context to indicate that laboratory evidence of low tocopherol levels in humans is not necessarily equivalent to biological tocopherol deficiency. Discussion of conditions in human beings leading to such a state can be conveniently divided into five categories: (1) premature infants, (2) malabsorption states, (3) abetalipoproteinemia, (4) protein-calorie malnutrition, and (5) experimental deprivation (the Elgin Project). Some may view the distinction between the first three as somewhat arbitrary, in view of the long appreciated disturbances in intestinal digestion and/or absorption affecting both prematures [17] and patients with abetalipoproteinemia [18]. Nonetheless, other factors contribute to tocopherol deficiency in the latter two groups and thus, the usefulness of separate categorization.

Prior to considering deficiency states, however, it is worthwhile to comment briefly on expected normal blood vitamin E levels and the distribution of plasma or serum tocopherol concentrations in the United States population. This will permit a quantitative definition, albeit an arbitrary one, of what constitutes deficiency. Evaluation of nutritional status with respect to vitamin E has depended upon measurement of either the blood level of total tocopherols or α-tocopherol or on the identification of erythrocyte hemolysis following in vitro exposure to hydrogen peroxide. The peroxide hemolysis test is a convenient procedure but lacks specificity [19, 20] and has not led to a uniformity in results between various studies. In general, total plasma tocopherol concentrations in excess of 0.5 mg/dl have been regarded through the years as "sufficient" [9-13]. It has recently become appreciated, however, that interpretation of blood tocopherol levels may be fraught with difficulty in the absence of simultaneously determined triglyceride or total lipid concentrations. In fact, because of the relationship now known to exist between vitamin E and plasma lipids, the significance of an isolated blood tocopherol concentration in humans has become uncertain.

The relationship of lipid levels to tocopherol levels becomes most important of course when one evaluates the nutritional status of subjects who are likely to show widely varying blood lipids, e.g., young children and patients with hyperlipidemia. Horwitt et al. [21] have especially stressed the importance of simultaneous determination of blood lipids and expression of circulating vitamin E levels as the ratio of tocopherol to total lipid. Using a simple turbidimetric method for lipids [22] and the micromethod of Quaife et al. [23] for total tocopherols, it was possible for Horwitt and associates to determine this ratio on less than 0.5 ml serum or plasma. Their results indicate that in fasting subjects, a ratio of 0.8 mg tocopherol per gram of total lipid may be considered the lower limit of normal. Using this ratio as the guideline, it becomes apparent that subjects exhibiting low blood lipids are not necessarily deficient in vitamin E. Similarly, it is now evident that levels of tocopherol above 0.5 mg/dl, which in former years were considered adequate, may occasionally prove low if related to a high blood lipid content.

A further issue in measurement of plasma vitamin E relates to the question of contribution by isomers other than α-tocopherol [8, 24, 25]. The α-vitamer in plasma accounts for greater than 95% of the total vitamin E activity upon correction for the concentration and activity of β-, γ-, and δ-tocopherols [25]. However, the presence of the latter isomers, particularly γ-tocopherol, has become increasingly important in recent years. This is attributable to the fact that the American diet has undergone various changes and now includes foods relatively higher in γ-tocopherol (e.g., soy bean oil) than the products consumed in the 1950s and early 1960s [24]. Since the γ-isomer contributes 10-20% of total

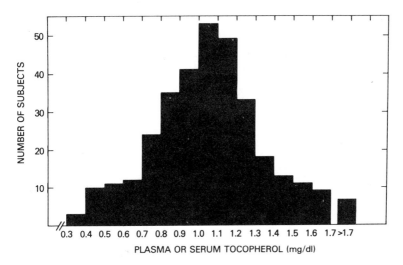

FIG. 1 The distribution of total tocopherol values in adult serum. (Data from Refs. 27 and 28 on 329 adult subjects were combined to produce this histogram.)

tocopherols in plasma [25] but is only about 10% as active as the α-form in vivo (based on nutritional bioassays) [26], blood vitamin E status is best assessed by performing chromatographic separation of the isomers and determining both α- and γ-tocopherol levels.

Unfortunately, data available from population surveys (discussed in more detail in Sec. IV) deal almost exclusively with total plasma or serum tocopherol values without information on blood lipids. The results of two such surveys in adults by Harris et al. [27] and Bieri et al. [28] are shown in Fig. 1. From these results, it may be concluded that the normal level of total tocopherols in plasma averages 1.05 mg/dl but that the range is wide. The values essentially follow a normal distribution with the two standard deviation ranges being 0.50-1.6 mg/dl serum. Since the normal lipid concentration in adult serum averages 0.6 g/dl, it may be calculated that the mean ratio of total tocopherols to lipids in adult serum is 1.8 mg/g. This is approximately twice the level which Horwitt et al. [21] consider minimal based on estimates of blood tocopherol levels and lipids in the Elgin Project. On the other hand, limited surveys on infants and young children have disclosed lower plasma total tocopherols. In McWhirter's [29] series of children from 4 months to 6 years of age, for instance, total tocopherols averaged 0.64 and ranged from 0.2 to 1.3 mg/dl plasma. Similarly, Levine et al. [30] have noted an average of

0.53 and a range of 0.30-0.93 mg/dl plasma in 2-10 year-old children.
These relatively lower levels are in agreement with, but not entirely
attributable to, the lower blood lipid content in children [30,31].

With regard to assessing the vitamin E status of potentially deficient
subjects, most of the studies, even those published recently, have been
based on measurement of plasma tocopherol alone rather than the ratio
between tocopherol and lipids. It therefore becomes necessary in this
review to consider clinical observations in such patients solely on the
basis of blood tocopherol concentrations reported in the literature. For
practical purposes, the author has regarded a level of total tocopherols
less than 0.5 mg/dl serum or plasma as being consistent with vitamin E
deficiency. This arbitrary definition is supported by the finding that
plasma tocopherol concentrations below this level correlate with development of erythrocyte hemolysis in vitro. It must be kept in mind, however,
that many of the studies of vitamin E deficiency states may contain subjects who, because of lower blood lipids, are in reality not deficient in
vitamin E. Thus, levels less than 0.5 mg/dl in infants and young children
should probably be regarded as only suggestive of deficiency. Conversely,
patients with high blood lipids may be deficient in spite of a total tocopherol level above 0.5 mg/dl.

B. Premature Infants

1. General

Neonates delivered prematurely because of various circumstances [32]
have been the subjects of a number of human vitamin E deficiency studies.
These infants have, of course, been denied a full period of gestation and
thus have not developed adequate tissue stores of several nutrients. Nor
have they attained maturity with respect to the functioning of many important organs such as the gastrointestinal tract and the bronchopulmonary
system [33,34]. Observations on the vitamin E status of premature
infants and the effects of tocopherol deficiency deserve considerable attention in this review since these findings have perhaps lent the strongest
support for an essential role of tocopherol in humans. Indeed, proponents
of human vitamin E supplementation must largely resort to data from
prematures in support of their claims.

That the premature infant is a useful model of human vitamin E deficiency and in a somewhat analogous state to animals utilized for experimental studies of tocopherol depletion is indicated by the following:
(1) tissue stores of vitamin E in premature neonates are limited as
inferred from Filer's tocopherol measurements in human fetuses of
various gestational ages [35]; (2) fat adsorption is faulty owing to
"immaturity" of the gastrointestinal tract and associated organs of importance in the digestion process [17,31]; (3) artificial feedings, low in

tocopherol content as compared with breast milk (until recently), must be utilized and in some cases are poorly tolerated [36]; (4) a rapid period of growth occurs during infancy; and (5) the practice of medicinal iron supplementation enhances the susceptibility of prematures to antioxidant deficiency [37].

Prior to discussing vitamin E levels during infancy, prenatal nutrition deserves brief consideration. There is strong evidence that plasma vitamin E levels in pregnant women rise during advancing gestation [38-40]. As shown in Table 1, several groups of investigators have reported increased plasma vitamin E levels in pregnancy, particularly during the third trimester. From the list, it is apparent that on the average circulating tocopherol concentrations in pregnant women are approximately 50% higher than values found in nonpregnant females. This increase is probably attributable to concommitant elevations in blood lipids. Comprehensive study, however, is required to evaluate other contributing factors.

The relationship between maternal and fetal blood tocopherol levels has also been studied by several investigators [21,38,40-42] who obtained fetal blood samples from the umbilical cord at delivery. As early as 1946, Straumfjord and Quaife [38] noted that maternal levels were considerably higher than those of the fetus. They reported that the mean ratio of plasma vitamin E in the mother to that in the fetus was 5.0. Subsequently, a number of other investigators, as listed in Table 1, verified this finding with most of the observed ratios approximating 4. The study of Leonard et al. [43] disclosed a nearly constant ratio of 4:1, independent of the mother's absolute plasma vitamin E concentration. These data have been interpreted by some as suggesting poor placental transport of tocopherol; however, this question has not been studied directly and requires further examination.

2. Discovery of Tocopherol Deficiency in Prematures

The crisis in newborn care associated with an alarming increase in retrolental fibroplasia in the late 1940s provided the occasion for the first demonstration that neonates are deficient in vitamin E. Owens and Owens [44] first called attention to this state of malnutrition in 1949 when they reported that the serum total tocopherol concentration averaged 0.25 mg/dl in a group of 46 premature infants 2-8 weeks old. Shortly thereafter, Moyer [45] confirmed this observation and conclusively established that blood vitamin E levels of newborns are low in comparison to adults. In a series of 53 term infants and 32 premature infants, all of whom had uncomplicated hospital courses, it was noted on the day of delivery that no significant differences were present in the serum tocopherol concentrations of the two groups; term infants averaged 0.24 and prematures 0.22 mg/dl serum. Of further interest, Moyer observed that whereas full term neonates showed a significant increase in blood tocopherol levels during the

TABLE 1   Maternal Vitamin E Levels During Pregnancy and Maternal-
Fetal Tocopherol Relationships as Determined at Delivery

A. Maternal tocopherol [a]	N [b]	Gestation (weeks)	Reference number
1.17 ± 0.19	11	8-24	38
1.62 ± 0.31	12	26-36	38
0.89 ± 0.02	74	8-13	39
1.04 ± 0.02	240	14-18	39
1.09 ± 0.01	258	19-22	39
1.16 ± 0.02	273	23-26	39
1.21 ± 0.02	273	27-30	39
1.26 ± 0.02	276	31-34	39
1.32 ± 0.02	149	35-38	39
1.40 ± 0.05	32	39-24	39
0.62 ± 0.26[c]	108	8-13	40
0.77 ± 0.27[c]	250	14-27	40
0.96 ± 0.29[c]	503	28-42	40

B. Maternal tocopherol	Fetal tocopherol	Maternal/fetal ratio	Reference number
1.60 ± 0.51	0.61 ± 0.31	2.6	41
1.70 ± 0.34	0.34 ± 0.12	5.0	38
1.21 ± 0.24	0.29 ± 0.02	4.2	21
1.71 ± 1.20	0.41 ± 0.22	4.2	42
1.05 ± 0.26[c]	0.26 ± 0.10[c]	4.0	40

[a] Mean ± standard deviation in milligrams per deciliter serum or plasma;
values represent total tocopherols unless otherwise noted.
[b] Number of subjects evaluated.
[c] Serum α-tocopherol determined after chromatographic separation.

first week of life, concentrations in the low birthweight infants did not rise
until after 3 months of age. Moyer's study was soon followed by that of
Wright et al. [46] who confirmed the deficiency state of prematures. Subsequently, a number of investigators have reported low blood tocopherol
concentrations in premature infants as listed in Table 2. Noteworthy is
the consistency of results and the relatively narrow range found in
reported series of prematures.

Demonstration of low blood tocopherol levels was soon followed by the
discovery of György et al. [47] that erythrocytes of neonates showed

abnormal susceptibility to hydrogen peroxide. This was found to be the case for full-term infants and prematures, both of whom developed a resistance to peroxide-induced red blood cell (RBC) hemolysis upon dietary supplementation with large doses of vitamin E. Gordon and de Metry [48] subsequently confirmed and extended the observation that RBCs of premature infants tended to hemolyze in the presence of oxidants. Thus, it became possible to utilize either the level of serum tocopherol or the degree of erythrocyte hemolysis in dilute hydrogen peroxide as an index of neonatal vitamin E nutrition in newborns.

In monitoring serum tocopherol values during the first several months of life, Wright et al. [46] and Mackenzie [49] noted that the levels not only remained low in prematures for approximately 3 months but also that the concentrations actually decreased in many infants during this period. Comparison of dietary vitamin E intake and the persistance of abnormal hemolysis tests suggested that an inverse relationship existed between the two. More revealing was the direct comparison between serum tocopherol levels and peroxide-induced hemolysis in samples of blood from individual

TABLE 2 Blood Tocopherol Levels Reported in Premature Infants

Mean plasma or serum tocopherol (mg/dl)	Range	Reference number
0.25	—[a]	44
0.22[b]	0.40–0.46	45
0.26[c]	0.02–0.56	45
0.28	—[a]	46
0.20	0.06–0.39	49
0.26[b]	—[a]	50
0.20[c]	—[a]	50
0.32	0.12–0.50	51
0.25	0–0.41	52
0.22	0.09–0.32	53
0.25[d]	—[a]	54
0.38[e]	—[a]	54

[a] Data not reported.
[b] Blood samples obtained at birth.
[c] Blood samples obtained 2 days to 2 months postnatally.
[d] Blood obtained 3 weeks postnatally from premature infants of 28-32 weeks gestational age.
[e] Blood obtained 3 weeks postnatally from premature infants of 32-36 weeks gestational age.

prematures. Such an approach, as reported by Mackenzie [49], led to the demonstration that circulating tocopherol concentrations correlated significantly with the tendency of red cells to hemolyze in vitro. The relationship, however, was found to be an imperfect one, possibly because of the rather large number of variables which can affect the erythrocyte hemolysis test [14, 55, 56]. Nonetheless, results in the early 1950s strongly suggested that a serum tocopherol level of 0.5 mg/dl was essential for complete protection of the RBC membrane against oxidant stress [57].

The vitamin E deficiency state of prematures over the first few months of life can, as mentioned previously, be attributed to several factors. These include: (1) limited tissue storage at birth, (2) relative dietary deficiency, (3) intestinal malabsorption, and (4) rapid growth. After development of mature digestive and absorptive capability, tocopherol absorption improves and blood vitamin E levels rise [54]. It is noteworthy, however, that prematures of early gestational age weighing 1000-1500 g at birth show tocopherol malabsorption until 2-3 months of age. The severity of vitamin E loss by this group is such that even oral supplementation with large doses of water-miscible α-tocopherol may fail to increase the blood levels significantly [54].

3. Possible Effects of Tocopherol Deficiency in
   Prematures: Retrolental Fibroplasia

The discovery that prematures were chemically deficient in vitamin E led to a search for a corresponding vitamin E deficiency syndrome which might bridge the gap between experimental studies in laboratory animals and practical application of vitamin E therapy in medicine. A number of clinical problems and pathological findings in newborns superficially resemble some of the manifestations of vitamin E deficiency found in lower animals. These include a hemorrhagic tendency, resembling exudative diathesis, and encephalomalacia, which may occur as a terminal event particularly in low birthweight infants. Early attempts to uncover a counterpart in prematures of the experimental vitamin E deficiency syndromes focused on three disturbances: (1) encephalomalacia, (2) increased vascular fragility, and (3) retrolental fibroplasia. More recently, investigations have pursued hematologic aspects of vitamin E deficiency.

Encephalomalacia akin to the disorder found in antioxidant-deficient chicks [6] can be dismissed as a likely possibility in view of the single case report claiming such a relationship [58]. The second of these, increased capillary fragility, was studied as early as 1951 by Minkowski [59] and others [60]. Their results, however, are difficult to interpret and are unconvincing as far as a specific role for vitamin E is concerned. To the author's knowledge, neither of these possibilities are under active study currently.

On the other hand, a relationship between hypovitaminosis E and
retrolental fibroplasia (RLF) continues to be pursued to the present day.
RLF is a condition affecting retinal blood vessel growth and is characterized in severe stages by cicatricial changes or scar tissue formation in
the retinal vasculature. Retinal scarring and consequent blindness are
preceded by more minor disturbances such as arterial vasoconstriction
[61]. After the vasoconstructive phase, the disease becomes primarily a
proliferative vaculopathy [61]. The presence of relatively large amounts
of α-tocopherol in the retinal outer segment of vertebrate eyes has been
documented by Dilley and McConnell [62]. Because full development of the
retinal vessels in the fetus is not generally complete until term gestation,
prematurely delivered newborns possess an enhanced susceptibility to
stresses, such as high oxygen tension, which are now known to damage
the retinal vasculature.

As mentioned previously, the possibility that vitamin E deficiency in
prematures leads to or aggravates retrolental fibroplasia was explored
concommitant with the discovery that these neonates are low in circulating
tocopherol. Prior to the time that Kinsey [63] indisputably associated the
excessive use of oxygen as the incriminating factor in RLF, Owens and
Owens [44] conducted a clinical trial in prematures with oral supplements
of α-tocopheryl acetate. Their results, although seemingly promising on
superficial analysis, are difficult to interpret in retrospect because of the
inadequately controlled nature of the study, particularly the lack of oxygen
monitoring. The report of Owens and Owens [44] was followed up by
Kinsey and Chisholm [64] who, after 3 years of evaluation, concluded that
treatment with vitamin E had little or no effect on the incidence of
retrolental fibroplasia. The latter investigators also noted in their report
that because of the considerable year-to-year variability in the incidence
of RLF, attempts to associate vitamin E deficiency and retinal scarring by
retrospective assessment of case histories (a common approach to the
problem) was unlikely to produce convincing data.

In contrast to the relatively disappointing results with tocopherol supplementation, a dramatic decrease in RLF incidence occurred in the few
years after the first vitamin E trial, once it became widely appreciated
that the disease was a manifestation of oxygen toxicity. During the decade
following the resolution of the etiology of retrolental fibroplasia, concern
for the possible role of vitamin E deficiency declined and further clinical
trials were not conducted.

Interest in the possible relationship of vitamin E to retinal oxygen
toxicity, however, was rekindled by the advent of neonatal intensive care
centers. These facilities began to appear in the 1960s and were largely
designed to provide maximum environmental and metabolic support and
intensive respiratory care for premature newborns suffering from pulmonary immaturity or hyaline membrane disease [34, 65, 66]. Such infants

are commonly managed with assisted ventilation which is provided by elaborate mechanical respirators. In this form of treatment, patients frequently receive high oxygen concentrations in association with greater than normal inspiratory pressures [67].

Not surprisingly, the great need to provide adequate tissue oxygenation in infants with hyaline membrane disease led to excessive use in some instances and development of retrolental fibroplasia. Thus, an apparent resurgence in RLF occurred in the late 1960s [68,69]. Reawakening of interest in this disease and the possible role of vitamin E is evidenced by the somewhat recent commencement of controlled clinical studies for the purpose of further characterizing RLF, determining the safe limits of oxygen, and evaluating potential therapeutic agents such as tocopherol. Because the early vascular changes associated with hyperoxia are extremely subtle, more sophisticated instrumentation is being employed in present ophthalmoscopic examinations. This has led in turn to more frequent detection of acute stages which in former years were "preclinical" and commonly went undetected. Fortunately, the early stages of the disease are nearly always reversible [70]. Because such changes represent a developmental phase of the disease rather than the classical membranous or cicatricial RLF, some ophthalmologists prefer other terms for the early vasculopathy such as "pre-retrolental fibroplasia" or "retinopathy of prematurity" [68,71,72].

The possible therapeutic use of vitamin E in preventing or ameliorating retrolental fibroplasia is currently under investigation by Johnson and co-workers [73]. They are utilizing a parenteral form of α-tocopheryl acetate in a water-miscible base [74] and are employing the indirect ophthalmoscope with frequent and careful evaluation of optic fundi. The initial dose of vitamin E given is 30 IU/kg and is administered intramuscularly as soon as possible following delivery. This is followed by injections of 15 IU/kg every 6-12 hr "until a serum E level in the range of 2 mg/100 ml is achieved." Such a schedule amounts to a rather large total dose, i.e., nearly 200 IU/kg in the first week of life. However, the approach of Johnson et al. [73] clearly eliminates the problems of poor intestinal absorption and delay in achievement of sufficient levels. Further, it insures vitamin E sufficiency in the first few days of life when exposure to oxygen for treatment of hyaline membrane disease is greatest.

In their first report, Johnson et al. [73] concluded that vitamin E reduces the incidence, severity, and duration of the early stages of RLF. This preliminary conclusion, however, was based entirely on differences in infants with hyaline membrane disease less than 1.5 kg birthweight and the group only included 16 vitamin E-treated neonates and 17 given placebo; the reported RLF incidence figures were 38 and 71%, respectively (p < .06). Curiously, there were no differences in infants of 1.5-2.0 kg birthweight and there was an apparent increase in RLF incidence in

25 vitamin E-treated infants greater than 2 kg as compared with 20 in a corresponding placebo group. Because of the small number of patients less than 1.5 kg and because of the unusually high RLF incidence (71%) in the control group, further information will be required to assess the significance of the findings initially reported by Johnson et al.

Preliminary results from another study have recently been recorded by Curran et al. [72]. These investigators are utilizing even more sophisticated monitoring devices including photographic methods of indirect ophthalmoscopy and fundus florescein angiography of retinal vessels. This equipment used in a serial fashion permitted them to evaluate very early vascular responses to oxygen in 75 premature infants under 2 kg birthweight. From their observations, Curran and associates reported that no correlation could be established between vitamin E levels and retinal vascular changes and that "retinopathy of prematurity" is a common developmental and nonspecific response of the immature retina which is nearly always reversible.

Therefore, it must be concluded that at present the evidence is mixed with respect to the possible beneficial effects of vitamin E therapy in relationship to prevention or amelioration of retrolental fibroplasia. Available evidence, however, strongly indicates that there are no major advantages or dramatic effects of vitamin E on the cicatricial form of RLF, the disorder of such great clinical importance during the period from 1943 to 1954. Nonetheless, there remains the possibility that the effects of tocopherol treatment might be manifest in the early stages of retinal vasculopathy, the significance of which, aside from alerting one as to the potential for development of RLF, remains to be determined.

4. Possible Effects of Tocopherol Deficiency in
   Prematures: Anemia of Prematurity

Hemolytic anemia represents another reported manifestation of hypovitaminosis E in premature infants. Investigations dealing with this possibility must be viewed against the background of the rapidly changing hematologic system of the newborn. Indeed, as Oski and Naiman [75] have stated, "during the first few weeks of life, there are more diagnostic problems with hematologic aspects than at any time thereafter." Profound alterations and hematologic adjustments take place from birth until several months of age as the erythrocyte population undergoes a "switchover" from cells containing fetal hemoglobin to those predominantly composed of adult hemoglobin. Since the possible role of vitamin E in the infant's hematologic system can only be interpreted in relationship to the marked erythrocyte changes regularly taking place, considerable background information is included in this discussion.

Normal full term infants show a fall in hematologic indices, especially during the second and third months of life, at which time the hemoglobin

value may fall to 11.4 ± 0.9 g/dl [75]. Infants delivered prematurely
experience a decline in hemoglobin concentration which significantly
exceeds that of term neonates. Levels as low as 6-8 g/dl blood are commonly observed and a mean ± S.D. of 9.6 ± 14 g/dl has been reported for
2 month-old prematures [76]. This more pronounced "anemia of prematurity" also begins relatively earlier in life (at approximately 6 weeks
of age) and tends to vary in proportion to the degree of immaturity, i.e.,
those of younger gestation age are likely to develop a more severe anemia.
The marked fall in hemoglobin level is usually found in prematures who
except for their anemia are otherwise normal. Because of this, the
regularity of its appearance, and other considerations [76], it is often
referred to as the state of "physiologic anemia." Many etiologies have
been proposed to account for this phenomenon but it remains poorly
understood to this day [75, 76]. Further complicating the interpretation of
hematologic status in infants are 1) sex differences (females display
lower cord hemoglobin levels in cord blood than males), and 2) the
spontaneous correction of anemia recognized to occur in premature infants
after 3 months of age [75].

The possible relationship between vitamin E deficiency and the
hematologic disturbances of prematurity was first noted by Hassan et al.
[51] who exaggerated the antioxidant deficiency state of a group of prematures by feeding formulas high in polyunsaturated fatty acid (PUFA).
The studies of Oski and Barness [52, 53], however, have had the most significant impact on our assessment of the role vitamin E deficiency might
play in prematures, if not generally in humans. Oski and Barness
initially recognized the association of anemia and vitamin E deficiency in
eleven low birthweight infants, all of whom were subsequently treated at
44-77 days of age with vitamin E. Following oral administration of
200-800 mg α-tocopherol over 1-4 days, serum tocopherol levels rose to
normal, erythrocyte hemolysis in vitro decreased, and mean hemoglobin
level rose from 7.6 to 9.8 g/dl with the mean reticulocyte count falling
from 8.2 to 3.9%. These changes were statistically significant and were
manifest 10 days from the start of therapy on the average. In a subsequent
prospective trial, Oski and Barness [52, 53] found that 13 infants supplemented orally from 3 days of age with either 9 mg/day α-tocopherol in
Tween 80 or 15.7 mg/day of water-miscible α-tocopheryl acetate showed
less of a fall in hemoglobin and less prominent reticulocytosis in comparison to 12 vitamin E-deficient prematures. It should be noted, however, that there was considerable overlap in all hematologic indices in the
two groups studied. Further, the vitamin E treated group did in fact
develop anemia with a minimal mean hemoglobin of 9.2 g/dl, as compared
to a corresponding figure of 7.7 g/dl in the tocopherol-deficient group.
Autologous [51Cr]RBC survivals were measured in two infants with low
serum tocopherol levels and found to be "shortened" to half-lives of 11 and

15 days. Unfortunately, the survival of erythrocytes from vitamin E-treated patients was not reported. It was also observed by Oski and Barness [53] that red cell glutathione concentrations were markedly increased in vitamin E-deficient infants and were lower following therapy.

The above observations and accompanying red cell morphological disturbances led Oski and Barness to draw the following conclusions: (1) vitamin E deficiency in the premature infant is associated with an anemia; (2) the anemia in these infants is hemolytic in nature; (3) the abnormality responds to tocopherol treatment as characterized by a rise in hemoglobin and a fall in the reticulocyte count; and (4) provision of supplementary vitamin E from birth reduces the severity of anemia and prevents the marked reticulocytosis observed in infants of low birthweight. A further finding of Barness and associates [77], arising in studies designed to define the minimum amount of vitamin E required to "prevent anemia," relates to the poor absorption of the orally administered tocopherol in prematures. This will be addressed in more detail in Sec. II.C.g.

Subsequent to the findings of Oski and Barness, several groups have investigated the relationship of vitamin E deficiency to erythrocyte function in prematures. Ritchie et al. [78] reported a group of seven such infants studied during the second month of life who showed widespread edema, anemia, reticulocytosis, thrombocytosis, and tocopherol levels averaging 0.18 mg/dl serum. Erythrocyte survival was determined in one infant with both [^{51}Cr] and [^{32}P]diisopropylfluorophosphate (DF[^{32}P]) monitoring techniques. These results, as compared to normal values for adults, revealed marked shortening of the survival time (^{51}Cr-$t_{1/2}$ = 16.8 days; DF[^{32}P]-$t_{1/2}$ = 27.3 days). Following administration of 100 mg/day α-tocopherol for 6 weeks DF[^{32}P] survival determination was again carried out and found to be considerably improved to a $t_{1/2}$ value of 42 days. Unfortunately, however, erythrocyte survivals in control neonates were not measured by Richie et al.

In another prospective trial, Chadd and Fraser [79] followed hematologic indices for several weeks and found that hemoglobin levels were significantly higher 8-10 weeks after birth in infants provided vitamin E supplements. Additionally, Lo and associates [80] reported a statistically significant rise in hemoglobin levels and fall in reticulocyte counts in 6-8 week-old prematures after 2 or 3 weeks of oral treatment with 10 mg/day of α-tocopherol.

Perhaps the most extensive studies of the hematologic effects of vitamin E deficiency in premature infants have been conducted by Gross and Melhorn [37, 54, 81-84]. These investigators evaluated 235 prematures in an intensive care nursery between 1968 and 1971 and controlled the study for gestational age and medications other than tocopherol. As illustrated graphically in Fig. 2, their work confirmed and extended the observations of Oski and Barness [52, 53] with respect to (1) the pattern of fall in

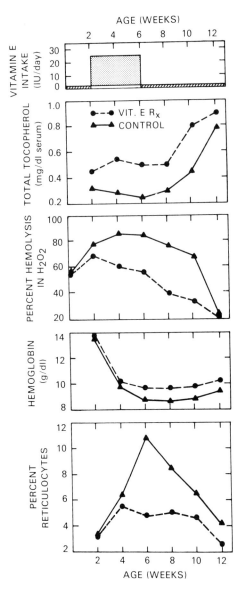

FIG. 2 Serum tocopherol levels and hematologic indices in premature infants of 1000–1500 g birthweight (28–32 weeks' gestation). Both the control group (triangles–solid line) and the tocopherol treated group (circles–broken line) were fed a commercial formula providing approximately 2 IU/day vitamin E. As shown, the treated group received an additional 25 IU/day as water-miscible α-tocopheryl acetate from the second through the sixth week of life. (Data from Ref. 54.)

erythrocyte indices, (2) the poor intestinal absorption of vitamin E in immature infants, and (3) the hematologic effects of tocopherol supplementation. In particular, Gross and Melhorn reported that while infants on standard formula exhibit a 51% decline in mean hemoglobin concentration at 8 weeks of age, if of either 28-32 weeks gestation or of 32-36 weeks gestation, corresponding prematures supplemented with 25 IU/day of water-miscible α-tocopheryl acetate show less pronounced decreases of 45 and 46%, respectively. These differences were reflected in values observed with the in vitro erythrocyte hemolysis test. Although the magnitude of improvement in terms of absolute hemoglobin concentration only amounted to 1 g/dl blood, the differences were highly significant (p < .001) in both groups of prematures. Additionally, lower reticulocyte counts were noted in the vitamin E-supplemented group (mean ± SD = 4.9 ± 1.9%) as compared with the untreated controls (8.7 ± 2.2%). From studies on the interplay of tocopherol and iron, it was demonstrated that the administration of large amounts of medicinal iron exaggerates the "hemolytic process" [37]. This has subsequently been confirmed by Williams et al. [85]. Thus, although Gross and Melhorn did not conduct RBC survival studies, their hematologic data clearly substantiated the original findings of Oski and Barness.

On the other hand, Panos et al. [86] were unable to confirm the improvement in hemoglobin concentration in vitamin E-supplemented prematures, despite the demonstration that such therapy led to increased blood tocopherol levels. Their study, which focused on 47 infants at approximately 10 weeks of age, included measurement of [51Cr]RBC survival in 27 infants, as well as survival studies before and after vitamin E supplementation in 14 infants. In addition to their inability to document improvement in hemoglobin concentration, Panos and co-workers were also unable to confirm the reduced reticulocytosis noted by others. Rater, the opposite, viz., increased reticulocytosis, was reported to occur after vitamin E supplementation. Perhaps the most significant finding by these investigators was that no improvement in [51Cr]RBC survival was evident after vitamin E administration. Specifically, "shortened" RBC half-lives were noted in tocopherol-deficient infants and no significant differences were detected upon vitamin E treatment in 12 of the 14 infants so studied.

Similarly negative hematologic results were reported by Goldbloom and Cameron [87] who studied 44 premature infants for 6 months after birth on either low tocopherol diets or those fortified with vitamin E. The latter group of subjects failed to show an increased mean hemoglobin concentration and did in fact develop the typical "anemia of prematurity." In another negative trial, Sartain et al. [88] found no improvement in hematologic indices of prematures fed tocopherol-supplemented formula. In addition, Hashim and Asfour [89], from a study of term infants receiving either a formula inadequate in vitamin E as compared to PUFA or alternatively tocopherol-fortified evaporated milk, reported that vitamin E-deficient infants do not develop an exaggerated anemia; rather, they show spontaneous improvement in hemoglobin levels at rates comparable to controls.

Because all hemolytic anemias may result in hyperbilirubinemia, especially in newborns, another approach to assessing the role of vitamin E has been to monitor serum bilirubin levels in neonates treated with tocopherol. Interestingly, neither Richards et al. [90] nor Abrams et al. [91] were able to show a significant effect of the vitamin on the degree of hyperbilirubinemia developed in infants given daily supplements of α-tocopheryl acetate. The doses utilized by these investigators were sufficiently large to raise serum tocopherol levels and reduce the hemolytic tendency in vitro. Although Abrams and co-workers [91] pointed out that the course of neonatal hemolysis and hyperbilirubinemia could perhaps be more favorably influenced if large doses of vitamin E were given to the mother in late gestation, a clinical trial by Tateno [41] using this approach yielded negative results.

Therefore, from this consideration of all the studies which could be found in the pre-1976 literature bearing on the status of the erythrocyte in vitamin E-deficient prematures, it is clear that significant discrepancies are present and that several questions need to be addressed more extensively. Those investigators who claim hematologic improvement after supplementation with vitamin E can demonstrate statistically significant increases in blood hemoglobin concentration at approximately 8-10 weeks of age. The tocopherol effect is accompanied by reduced reticulocytosis according to both Oski and Barness [52, 53] and Gross and Melhorn [54]. This suggests that an enhanced hemolytic tendency occurs in association with vitamin E deficiency. Nonetheless, it should be noted that even with tocopherol supplementation reticulocytosis along with anemia both become manifest, and thus tocopherol does not <u>correct</u> the hematologic disturbances of prematurity. Furthermore, the hemoglobin differences between vitamin E-treated and control infants are small in every series (approximately 1 g/dl blood) and considerable overlap characterizes all the hematologic data obtained in treated versus nontreated infants.

The question then remains as to whether or not the typical anemia of prematurity is truly a reflection of vitamin E deficiency, and if so, how significant a role might tocopherol play in alleviating this disturbance. A hemolytic disease is best defined as a disorder in which the red cell lifespan is shortened. Shortening of red cell survival does not always result in overt anemia if increased erythrocyte destruction is compensated for by increased production. However, in the case of the premature infant, inadequately developed erythropoietic mechanisms are available when he is forced to respond to a shortened red cell survival. Thus, prematures are likely to develop anemia in the face of prolonged hemolysis. The most reliable procedures for establishing in vivo hemolysis unequivocally are the various isotopic methods where "tagged" red cells are injected and their destruction monitored. Thus, it is pertinent to review briefly some of the basic studies on red cell survival in neonates, irrespective of whether vitamin E status was assessed.

A variety of methods have been utilized in attempts to define the life-span of neonatal red cells [75]. The standard technique of determining erythrocyte survival, as recommended by the Panel on the Diagnostic Applications of Radioisotopes in Hematology of the International Committee for Standardization in Hematology [92], involves measuring the loss of [^{51}Cr] or DF[^{32}P]-labeled red cells from the patient's own circulation (autologous technique). Because of the ethical considerations, particularly the desirability of avoiding radiation exposure, most RBC survival studies in neonates have been carried out in the heterologous fashion whereby erythrocytes are transfused into adults. Monitoring the disappearance of labeled neonatal red cells accordingly, Hollingsworth [93] calculated a mean half-life of 20 days for term newborns as compared to a figure of 27 days for normal adult cells. Foconi and Sjolin [94], also using the heterologous technique, arrived at a $t_{1/2}$ of 22.8 days for term infants as compared with 27.5 days for adult cells treated similarly. Kaplan and Hsu [95] subsequently employed both autologous and heterologous transfusions and compared the [^{51}C]half-life for term infants with data obtained in prematurely delivered newborns. They reported a range of 21-35 days for the former group with 9 of 11 subjects showing $t_{1/2}$ figures in the normal adult range of 25-35 days. In contrast, six prematures of the same age showed half-lives less than 20 days. Gilardi and Miescher [96] also demonstrated that while the survival of erythrocytes in term infants was near normal at birth (mean $t_{1/2}$ = 24 days, adult mean = 30 days) premature infants showed a shortened half-life with a mean survival of 16 days. The dissimilarity between term and premature infants, however, was not noted by Kaplan and Hsu [95] in subjects of 3-8 weeks of age.

Some concern has been raised as to whether or not [^{51}Cr] is an appropriate labeling agent for neonatal red cells. It has been suggested that this isotope elutes more rapidly from newborn erythrocytes as compared to adult red cells [75, 97]. It has been further shown by Pearson and Vertrees [98] that the difference in elution rates may be attributable to the high fetal hemoglobin content of newborn erythrocytes. This is consistent with the fact that the fetal hemoglobin molecule contains α- and γ-polypeptide chains rather than the β-subunits to which chromium preferentially binds.

The conclusions warranted from the foregoing studies, none of which documented the vitamin E status of the infants, are as follows: (1) the use of [^{51}Cr] tagging and monitoring of erythrocytes in infancy does not produce results that can be directly compared to adult RBC survival figures; (2) taking the former into account, normal term infants appear to have a similar or slightly shortened RBC lifespan as compared with figures for adults; and (3) prematures, in comparison to term infants, show considerably reduced erythrocyte survival, especially in the first week of life.

In view of the fact that hemolytic disease is defined as a disorder in which the red cell lifespan is shortened, and hemolytic anemia as shortened RBC survival in association with an incompletely compensated acceleration of red cell production, the three studies in premature infants where both vitamin E status and RBC survival have been documented deserve further discussion. To restate the pertinent observations: (1) Oski and Barness [52] found shortened [^{51}Cr]RBC half-lives (11 and 15 days) in two tocopherol deficient infants; (2) Richie et al. [78] found a reduced [^{51}Cr]RBC survival (16.8 days) in one infant and confirmed this with DF[^{32}P] labeling; and (3) Panos et al. [86] reported shortened [^{51}Cr]t$_{1/2}$ figures (mean = 11 days) in 27 vitamin E-deficient infants. Repeat determination of erythrocyte survival after vitamin E treatment revealed improvement in the infant studied by Richie et al. but no change in 12 of 14 patients so evaluated by Panos and co-workers. The latter observation of course casts considerable doubt on the proposed "antihemolytic effect" of tocopherol in vivo. Further, it should be indicated once again that complete correction of a presumed antioxidant defect and prevention of anemia cannot be validly claimed since prematures do develop low hemoglobin values on continuous tocopherol therapy. Other factors such as hemodilution [76] and diminished erythropoietin response [99] must be at least partially responsible for the "anemia of prematurity."

Establishing the efficacy of α-tocopherol in the anemia of prematures will depend upon sound demonstration that erythrocyte survival is improved following treatment of deficient infants with vitamin E. In view of the lack of such data at present and the various discrepancies in the literature cited previously, the author is forced to conclude that differences in hemoglobin concentration reported by some investigators, although statistically significant, are not firmly convincing. The failure of other workers to verify these findings, the fact that anemia develops even on tocopherol therapy, and the failure thus far to provide the necessary RBC survival data, all indicate that further study will be required to establish a clinically significant role for tocopherol in the anemia of prematurity [76,100].

C. Malabsorption

1. General

A second category of human subjects who manifest vitamin E deficiency include patients with various forms of intestinal malabsorption or as more properly termed, "malassimilation." This is a heterogeneous group in which the intestinal loss of nutrients can be ascribed to a number of different disturbances in digestive or absorptive capability. In fact, vitamin E deficiency has been associated with disturbances affecting nearly every component of the gastrointestinal tract including stomach (post-gastrectomy), liver (cirrhosis), pancreas (cystic fibrosis, chronic pancreatitis, and pancreatic carcinoma), and intestinal mucosa per se (gluten enteropathy, tropical sprue, regional enteritis, and ulcerative colitis). A common feature of these enteropathies is the persistent inability to absorb dietary fat to the extent (greater than 95%) found in normal individuals. As discussed in Chapter 5A and 5B under absorption and transport, the uptake and transfer of vitamin E across the epithelial cell membrane of the small intestine is considered to be dependent on the coincidental absorption of lipids. Thus, whatever the cause of the steatorrhea, if it is of sufficient duration and magnitude, vitamin E deficiency would likely ensue as a consequence of tocopherol malabsorption.

2. Cystic Fibrosis

a. Nature of the disease: Of those patients with enteropathies leading to chronic steatorrhea, subjects with pancreatic exocrine insufficiency, especially cystic fibrosis (CF), have been of particular interest to investigators concerned with tocopherol deficiency in humans. There are a number of reasons why CF patients are appropriate for extensive study and have been the focus of many investigators: (1) they represent the largest available group of human subjects in caucasian populations with severe steatorrhea [101]; (2) they manifest a prolonged, permanent digestive defect which cannot be corrected, but only ameliorated, by pancreatic replacement therapy (powdered preparations of hog pancreas given in tablet or capsule form) [102-104]; and (3) cystic fibrosis patients are largely found in the pediatric age group which, by analogy to animal experimentation, appears to represent the ideal population for studies of tocopherol depletion in humans. Since many patients with cystic fibrosis manifest pancreatic insufficiency from birth, tocopherol deficiency appears to develop early in life after the tissue stores are exhausted and when the nutritional demands for growth are greatest. Furthermore, in the absence of supplementation using 2-10 times the recommended dietary allowance of tocopherol in a water-miscible form, chemical evidence of vitamin E deficiency is invariably present in CF patients with pancreatic achylia [105]. Thus, these patients may provide the closest analogy to nutritional experiments on vitamin E deficiency in animals and probably represent the best available models of profound, chronic vitamin E deficiency in humans.

It should be recognized that "cystic fibrosis of the pancreas," as the disease was originally misnamed [106], is a complex, generalized disease of metabolism affecting numerous organs, if not every tissue in the body [102]. Its salient features deserve brief review in this treatise prior to discussion of observations relating to vitamin E deficiency. The cardinal characteristics of the disease are pancreatic achylia, chronic obstructive pulmonary disease, and an elevated content of electrolytes in eccrine sweat gland secretions. This triad, plus a family history of cystic fibrosis, forms the basis for diagnosis. Not all patients, however, manifest pancreatic insufficiency. Approximately 15% of those with three of the above four criteria sufficient for diagnosis have been found to show unimpaired pancreatic function [102, 106]. As noted subsequently, such patients do not have steatorrhea and are not deficient in vitamin E.

Another feature of cystic fibrosis deserving comment is the potential pathological involvement of multiple organs of importance in the assimilation of foodstuffs. For example, a wide variety of intestinal complications occur in this disease [107, 108] and as many as one-third of C F patients manifest hepatic dysfunction on careful examination [109]. It is conceivable, therefore, that a number of factors in addition to the lack of the lipase-rich, alkaline pancreatic juice contribute to tocopherol malabsorption. Two of these possible factors are impaired bile acid secretion in patients with extensive biliary cirrhosis and disturbed transport of nutrients across the intestinal mucosa per se. Not surprisingly, considerable variation exists from patient to patient in the extent of malabsorption [103]. Additionally, it has been observed that individual patients, for reasons not entirely clear, will show significant day-to-day variability in terms of the magnitude of fecal fat excretion.

Relative to the subsequent discussion on vitamin E therapy in cystic fibrosis, it should be mentioned that investigators commonly encounter a number of difficulties in attempting to evaluate new therapeutic modalities in CF patients. Of special concern in this regard are: (1) the great variability of the basic disease process and associated course, both depending for the most part on the extent of bronchopulmonary obstruction and infection [102]; (2) the large number of medications required daily by these patients for optimal management; and (3) the profound psychological trauma of this lethal disease which promotes a sense of desperation and unusual cooperativity in some patients and parents. Because of the latter, virtually any new treatment if offered optimistically by the physician can result in subjectively apparent beneficial effects that are not demonstrable objectively.

In any event, cystic fibrosis patients have been carefully studied with respect to plasma and tissue tocopherol levels as well as in regard to the effects of vitamin E deficiency. Findings in these patients therefore, together with those in premature infants, deserve major emphasis in this article.

b. Occurrence and Degree of Tocopherol Deficiency: To the author's knowledge, the first report describing vitamin E deficiency in cystic fibrosis patients, as well as in other subjects with malabsorption, appeared in 1949 and resulted from a survey of 200 hospitalized patients by Darby et al. [110]. Although these investigators did not publish blood tocopherol values for individual subjects, they mentioned that CF patients were found to show circulating levels of less than 0.5 mg/dl serum. Two years subsequently, Filer et al. [111] reported serum total tocopherol values of 0.04, 0.11, 0.24, 0.36, and 0.58 mg/dl in five subjects with cystic fibrosis. Neither of these studies provided information on the possible effects of vitamin E deficiency in such children.

It was largely through the efforts of Nitowsky, Gordon, and associates [50, 60, 112, 113] that patients with cystic fibrosis were firmly identified as vitamin E deficient and then characterized in terms of the possible consequences of this malnourished state. Their studies, which commenced in the mid-1950s, included both measurement of plasma tocopherol and evaluation of erythrocyte hemolysis in the presence of hydrogen peroxide. In 13 CF patients, aged 2 months to 10 years, Nitowsky et al. [50] found that virtually all determinations of blood tocopherol revealed levels less than 0.5 mg/dl. The mean concentration of 0.15 mg/dl found in these subjects was significantly less than the mean values of 0.84 in normal adults, 0.58 in children of 6-24 months of age, and 0.73 in children of 2-12 years of age. A number of CF patients, in fact, showed undetectable circulating vitamin E.

Assessment of RBC hemolysis in these 13 patients with cystic fibrosis disclosed abnormal peroxide susceptibility in all but one determination. In comparing the relationship between plasma tocopherol level and erythrocyte hemolysis in individual subjects, Nitowsky and co-workers [50] noted a great variation in the two parameters with wide scatter of the data and imperfect correlation in untreated patients. Nonetheless, after supplementing these malnourished subjects with α-tocopheryl succinate and repeating the blood analyses, Nitowsky et al. were able to establish a statistically significant, inverse correlation (r = -0.67) between plasma tocopherol levels of less than 0.5 mg/dl and positive erythrocyte hemolysis tests. This was in accord with their data comparing the two indices in both full-term infants and prematures and established a serum total tocopherol concentration of 0.5 mg/dl as the statistical "cross-over point" for peroxide hemolysis test results.

Following the pioneer series of studies by Nitowsky, Gordon, and associates [50, 60, 112, 113], a number of investigators have measured tocopherol concentrations in blood from patients with cystic fibrosis. A list of published values is shown in Table 3. From these results, it is evident that all surveys have disclosed vitamin E deficiency and that reasonably good agreement exists with respect to the average concentration of circulating tocopherol in this form of pancreatogenous steatorrhea. It is equally apparent, however, that such patients display a relatively wide range of blood vitamin E concentrations, particularly in comparison to premature infants. This is in agreement with the marked variation in extent of fat malabsorption manifested by CF patients [103]. In order to compare the severity of impaired digestion to the degree of vitamin E deficiency, Farrell et al. [121] have measured plasma α-tocopherol levels and various indices of malabsorption in individual CF patients. Their findings, shown in Fig. 3, indicate that reductions in plasma α-tocopherol are closely related to results obtained in assessing two of the best indices of malabsorption, viz., fecal fat excretion during balance studies and the serum carotene level. Such a correlation has also been detected in comparing plasma tocopherol values with serum cholesterol concentrations [117], another measure of malabsorption, though less useful clinically than fecal fat and serum carotene determinations. Therefore, it may be concluded that vitamin E deficiency in CF patients with steatorrhea occurs to an extent determined by the degree of malabsorption. It should be emphasized, however, that cystic fibrosis in the absence of significant pancreatic involvement (as indicated by normal duodenal fluid, fecal fat content, and serum carotene concentration), is not accompanied by vitamin E deficiency.

In addition to vitamin E levels in plasma, Underwood and Denning [117] measured tissue α-tocopherol concentrations in liver and skeletal muscle from CF patients with pancreatic achylia. Comparing these figures to values in control subjects, as shown in Table 4, reveals that CF patients manifest substantial reductions in both tissues. It has been

TABLE 3   Blood Tocopherol Levels Reported in Cystic Fibrosis Patients

Mean plasma or serum tocopherol (mg/dl)	Range	Number of patients	Reference number
0.27	0.04-0.58	5	111
0.11	0.01-0.97	31	114
0.15	0-0.47	14	113
0.44	0.05-0.90	4	115
0.22	—[a]	10	116
0.24[b]	—[a]	11	117
0.22	0.01-0.74	19	118
0.30	0.10-0.60	10	119
0.25	—[a]	47	120
0.13[b]	0.02-0.41	50	105
0.24	0-0.74	9	29

[a] Data not reported.
[b] Represents plasma α-tocopherol determined after thin-layer chromatography.

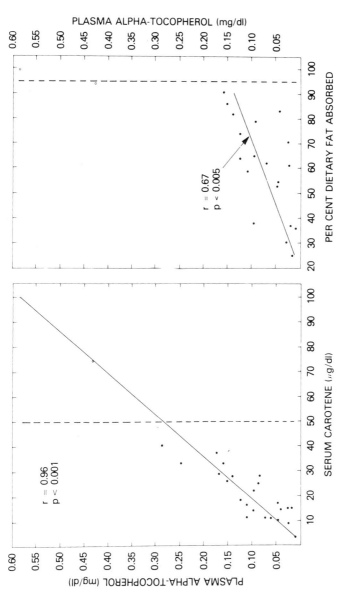

FIG. 3   The correlation between plasma α-tocopherol levels in cystic fibrosis patients and their degree of mal-absorption. The latter was evaluated by measurement of serum carotene concentration and fecal fat excretion during balance studies. The lower limits of normal for serum carotene (50 mg/dl) and fat absorption (95%) are indicated by the broken lines. Open circles represent two CF patients with intact or nearly intact pancreatic function as demonstrated by assay of duodenal contents. Data from P. M. Farrell and P. A. Sant'Agnese. [121]

TABLE 4   Cellular and Tissue Tocopherol Levels Reported in Cystic Fibrosis

Sample analyzed [a]	Number	α-Tocopherol content [b, c]	Reference number
Liver (μg/100 g)			
Control	18	1280 ± 340	117
Cystic fibrosis	10	350 ± 140	117
Skeletal muscle (μg/100 g)			
Control	6	1940 ± 370	117
Cystic fibrosis	7	262 ± 58	123
Erythrocytes (μg/dl)			
Control	5	251 ± 14	122
Cystic fibrosis	11	57 ± 8	122
Control	14	230 ± 13	122
Cystic fibrosis	5	42 ± 17	105

[a] Determinations were all performed using the method of Bieri [126].
[b] Mean ± SE figures are shown.
[c] All differences between values for control subjects and CF patients are statistically significant.

further observed that erythrocytes [105,122] and various other tissues from CF patients including lung, cardiac muscle, and adipose tissue [121] are similarly deficient in vitamin E.

c. Possible Effects of Tocopherol Deficiency: The possible consequences of vitamin E deficiency in cystic fibrosis patients were originally studied by Nitowsky, Gordon, and associates [50,61,112,113] and have more recently been pursued by Farrell et al. [105] as well as others [118,125].   In general, clinical studies have focused on the neuromuscular system, erythrocyte stability, and the morphology of the intestinal tract.

The neuromuscular system attracted the earliest attention due in part to the recognition that the myopathy of vitamin E deficiency in animals ("nutritional muscular dystrophy") can be readily produced under appropriate conditions in virtually every species which has come under study. Taking as their clue the prevailing clinical impression of the time that CF patients were characteristically weak with flabby and atrophic muscles," Nitowsky et al. [113] investigated 27 such subjects with vitamin E deficiency over a course of several years.   Creatinuria, a striking manifestation of muscle necrosis in genetic dystrophies and a common feature of acute nutritional myopathies in lower animals [127], was employed as the principal marker of muscle dysfunction. It was observed that 69% of the CF patients excreted excessive creatine as defined by a urinary output in 24 hr equal to at least 20% of the daily creatinine excretion. Excessive urinary creatine could be demonstrated when patients were placed on a creatine-poor diet and was shown to correlate well with increased plasma creatine levels, suggesting a prerenal etiology for the creatinuria. Consistent with the presumed muscle origin of pathological creatine excretion, Nitowsky and co-workers [113] found that biopsy samples of gastrocnemius muscle from tocopherol-deficient CF patients showed a tendency towards a lowered creatine concentration. Of particular interest was the finding that supplementation with α-tocopherol to normal plasma levels resulted in elimination of creatinuria in 12 of the 14 patients so studied. This change was accompanied by a lowering of plasma creatine and an apparent rise in the muscle creatine content in six patients biopsied subsequent to treatment. The frequent but variable occurrence of pathological creatinuria in tocopherol-deficient CF patients was confirmed by Farrell et al. [105] in a series of 25 subjects on low creatine diets. Such patients as a group were found to excrete 170 ± 29 mg/day (mean $\pm$ SE) as compared to a control level of 14 ± 2 mg creatine/day.

Excessive urinary creatine excretion, however, is not a specific index of muscle disease but may develop secondary to a number of conditions [128]. These include starvation, severe infection, hyperthyroidism, leukemia, and several maladies associated with generalized wasting and atrophying of skeletal muscles. Thus, the association of creatinuria and vitamin E deficiency in CF patients cannot be regarded as definitive evidence of myopathy, particularly since these subjects characteristically suffer from chronic infection which at times is accompanied by secondary muscle wasting [102, 106].

A more sensitive and specific index of skeletal muscle damage in humans is release of sarcoplasmic enzymes into the blood stream. Creatine phosphokinase (CPK) and aldolase are especially useful in this regard since their activities are markedly and invariably elevated in progressive muscular dystrophy of genetic origin [129]. The persistent rise in CPK has in fact become recognized as one of the most useful diagnostic criteria of Duchenne dystrophy [129] and can be utilized for detection of the carrier state [130]. Further, it has been found by Farrell et al. [131] that vitamin E-deficient chicks, as well as those with genetic dystrophy, show a striking elevation in plasma CPK. This alteration has also been noted by Bird and Carbello [132] in antioxidant-deficient guinea pigs and by Olson and Carpenter [127] in rabbits on tocopherol-deficient diets. The magnitude of increase in blood CPK is such that animals with nutritional or genetic dystrophy can be identified by this measurement in preclinical stages of the disorders where muscle involvement is minimal [127, 131, 133].

Because of the sensitivity and reliability of these enzyme determinations, Farrell et al. [105] measured serum CPK and aldolase activities in a series of 50 vitamin E-deficient cystic fibrosis patients. The survey disclosed only two subjects with significant enzyme elevations. Both of the patients were adolescents in a stage of active growth and both showed severe steatorrhea and extremely low levels of vitamin E in plasma and skeletal muscle. In addition, one 8 year-old boy with hepatic disease on cholestyramine therapy was found to show a markedly elevated CPK activity in association with virtually undetectable plasma α-tocopherol [134].

Unequivocal diagnosis of muscular degeneration depends, of course, upon morphological examination of biopsied tissue. Unfortunately, the lesions in vitamin E-deficient skeletal muscle, as described in over 20 different species of animals, tend to be focal and of varying severity such that their demonstration in small muscle samples is fraught with difficulty [135,136]. In some sections of muscle from animals with acute myopathy, fibers manifesting no damage are found, while in other sections, healthy fibers are evident and tend to be intermingled with those showing mild damage. Thus, many regions of skeletal muscle may require examination for accurate identification of pathological changes. Another difficulty in interpreting muscle lesions in animals has been the multitude of factors which influence the character and intensity of the lesions [135,136]. The age of the animal, developmental maturity of muscle fibers, acuteness or chronicity of the deficiency state, and apparent species differences in the degree of response to vitamin E deficiency, all contribute to a confusing picture when one attempts to compare alterations in lower animals to possible myopathological disturbances in humans.

In any event, limited investigations of muscle structure have been carried out in cystic fibrosis. In a retrospective review of necropsy tissue from 48 children with the disease, Oppenheimer [125] was able to study adequate portions of muscle from 10 patients and found abnormalities in only one of these. This patient had died at 24 months of age and showed pathological evidence of fat-soluble vitamin deficiencies, e.g., rickets and metaplasia of bronchial epithelium. The child also exhibited focal areas of muscle necrosis, hyalinization, and leukocyte infiltration—lesions similar to those of nutritional muscular dystrophy in animals. Unfortunately, tocopherol levels had not been measured in this patient, although there is no reason to doubt that he was vitamin E deficient.

More recently, muscle biopsies from the quadriceps femoris of four CF patients have been examined histologically and histochemically at the National Institutes of Health [137]. All of the patients were vitamin E-deficient as disclosed by markedly decreased plasma α-tocopherol levels and virtually undetectable concentrations in muscle specimens. Two patients also had elevated plasma CPK and aldolase activities, as mentioned previously. Histologically, the architecture of muscle fibers was intact but mild abnormalities were noted on histochemical evaluation. These consisted primarily of darkly staining type II fibers with the esterase procedure. Neither necrosis nor fragmentation of muscle fibers was evident.

Although further assessment of muscle morphology is clearly needed, it must be concluded that at the most, only minor abnormalities of a subtle nature are present in vitamin E-deficient human muscle. This is in keeping with the results of serum CPK and aldolase measurements indicating that muscle enzyme "leakage" associated with necrosis is an uncommon occurrence in CF patients. It must be stressed, however, that extensive examination of serial sections from multiple skeletal muscles will probably be required to clarify the morphological state of vitamin E-deficient human muscle.

The question arises as to the muscular strength of vitamin E-deficient CF patients and the effect of tocopherol supplementation on muscle function in these subjects. This issue has been carefully investigated by Levin et al. [138] and by Darby et al. [118]. Both groups were unable to document by objective techniques a significant degree of muscular weakness in these patients. The results of muscle testing following treatment with tocopherol to normal plasma levels were likewise unrevealing. Specifically, Levin and associates in a well-controlled evaluation of the strength of eight different muscle groups found that subjects supplemented with tocopherol showed no differences as compared to those given placebo. Darby et al. further observed that the physical endurance of CF patients was not improved upon treatment with vitamin E.

In view of the observation that vitamin E deficiency in animals also leads to cardiomyopathy in appropriate circumstances, a brief comment is in order on the histopathology of heart musculature in CF patients. The alteration observed in vitamin E-deficient animals of myocardial necrosis and fibrosis have also been sought in CF patients and reported to be present in nine isolated cases. These have been reviewed by McGiven [139]. The pertinent reports describe degeneration of cardiac muscle fibers and emphasize the focal nature of the abnormality as is also found in antioxidant deficient animals. The patchy foci of fibrosis are accompanied by adjacent areas of actively degenerating muscle fibers according to McGiven [139]. Kintzen [140] also found vacuolation of the degenerating fibers and considerable interstitial edema. In addition, Oppenheimer and Esterly [141] noted changes of myocarditis in two of five abnormal cardiac specimens. Although an accurate estimate of the incidence of these lesions cannot be provided, Nazelof and Lancret's review [142] of 44 cases of cystic fibrosis suggests that as many as 10% might display evidence of cardiomyopathy:

Since children and young adults with cystic fibrosis have low blood lipids and are therefore unlikely to develop coronary arterial occlusion, the finding of cardiomyopathy in such patients is even more significant. That is, one would not expect to find pathologic changes in heart muscle from these patients. Thus, the abnormalities likely represent a primary muscle disturbance, rather than secondary lesions occurring as a result of vascular occlusion.

Nonetheless, the lack of data on plasma and cardiac muscle tocopherol concentrations in the reported CF patients, the absence of a controlled study with supplemented subjects, and the lack of supporting data in other vitamin E-deficient conditions leaves one unable to conclude definitively on the possible involvement of tocopherol deficiency in these myocardial lesions.

Erythrocyte stability represents a second area of research interest relative to the role of vitamin E deficiency in cystic fibrosis. Investigators have pursued the possible protective effect of tocopherol on oxidant-exposed red cells both in vitro and in vivo. As mentioned previously, it has been demonstrated that red blood cells from CF patients show a reduced content of the vitamin (see Table 4).

Abnormal hemolysis in vitro of CF erythrocytes incubated in dilute solutions of hydrogen peroxide was first reported by Gordon et al. [143]. Virtually all preparations of red cells from tocopherol-deficient CF patients in their series showed greater than 10% hemolysis during a 3-hr incubation. The degree of hemolysis, although showing some variability at a given level of plasma tocopherol, was related linearly to blood vitamin E levels less than 0.5 mg/dl. Gordon, Nitowsky, and associates [50, 60, 112, 113, 143], however, did not provide evidence suggesting that hemolysis occurred in vivo in these patients. Binder et al. [115] subsequently reported the results of erythrocyte hemolysis tests on blood from six CF patients, as well as from a number of other subjects with steatorrhea. Curiously, four of the subjects with cystic fibrosis showed "negative hemolysis tests" as defined by Binder and associates to be less than 20% hemoglobin release in 2% hydrogen peroxide over 3 hr. Although their patients were not described in detail, the presence of normal serum tocopherol levels in two suggests that they were being supplemented with vitamin E.

In order to define further the degree of hemolysis and its relationship to plasma α-tocopherol levels in blood from CF patients, Farrell et al. [105, 121, 144] measured the two parameters in the same sample of blood from a number of subjects. With several modifications in the peroxide hemolysis procedure of Gordon et al. [143] and Horwitt et al. [14], it was possible to improve the reproducibility of the test and demonstrate that almost no hemolysis (mean $\pm$ SE = 0.5 $\pm$ 0.2%, range = 0-2%) occurred in

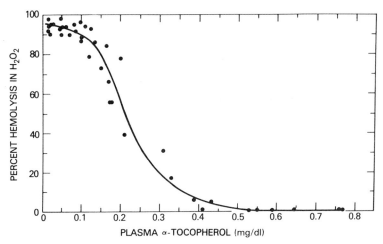

FIG. 4   The relationship between the degree of peroxide-induced hemolysis and plasma α-tocopherol level in cystic fibrosis patients. The sigmoid
curve was drawn to approximate the apparent trend of the data. (Unpublished date of P. M. Farrell and P. A. di-Sant'Agnese. [121]

blood samples showing a plasma α-tocopherol content of greater than
0.45 mg/dl. On the other hand, red cell suspensions from vitamin E-
deficient CF patients were invariably found to show abnormal hemolysis
in vitro. Figure 4 illustrates the relationship between the degree of
hemolysis and the plasma α-tocopherol concentration. The sigmoidal
pattern evident in the data was previously observed by Bieri and Poukka
[145] in a study of vitamin E-deficient rat blood cells incubated with
dialuric acid. The resistance to oxidant damage in the region of the curve
corresponding to plasma α-tocopherol levels of 0.35-0.50 mg/dl suggests
there is generally an excess of circulating tocopherol in comparison to the
amount required for prevention of severe hemolysis.

Although the results of in vitro studies with blood from CF patients
have thus established the increased susceptibility of erythrocytes to
oxidant damage, the most significant clinical issue is whether or not red
cells function adequately in vivo. Does abnormal hemolysis occur in the
blood stream and do hematologic abnormalities develop as a consequence?
As discussed previously for premature infants, the monitoring of the disappearance of [51Cr]-labeled red cells represents the recommended
approach to identifying hemolytic disease [92]. Such a procedure is sufficiently senstive to permit the detection of subtle degrees of hemolysis.
Farrell et al. [121] have recently employed the [51Cr]RBC procedure
carried out in the autologous fashion to assess erythrocyte stability in 19

TABLE 5   Erythrocyte Survival in Vitamin E-Deficient Cystic Fibrosis
Patients[a]

Group	Number	[51Cr]RBC half-life (days) Mean ± SE	Range
Control	28	28.0 ± 0.5	25-35
Vitamin E deficiency	19	22.4 ± 0.9[b]	16-29
After vitamin E treatment	6	27.6 ± 0.9[c]	25-31

[a] Farrell et al. [105] and [121].
[b] P < 0.001 as compared to the control subjects.
[c] Mean ± SE survival of this group prior to treatment was 19 ± 1 days;
p < 0.001 as compared to the pretreatment value.

patients with low blood tocopherol levels. As provided in Table 5, data
from these measurements indicated that the vitamin E-deficient red cells
were abnormal in terms of survival with a mean $t_{1/2}$ of 22 days. Three
subjects were particularly low with figures of less than 18 days, but
several showed normal survivals. In what apparently represents the only
other assessment of [51Cr]RBC survival in cystic fibrosis, Goldbloom
[114] reported that one patient with markedly diminished serum tocopherol
showed a red cell half-life of 25 days. Six CF patients studied by Farrell
and associates were available for repeat [51Cr]RBC survival measurements after supplementation with oral tocopherol. This group exhibited a
significant increase in $t_{1/2}$ from 19 to 27 days after treatment (see
Table 5). The findings before and after vitamin E therapy in one such
patient are shown in Fig. 5 to illustrate the impressive difference observed
when his plasma α-tocopherol level was increased to normal.

It should be noted, however, that the average degree of shortening of
RBC survival in the 19 deficient patients studied by Farrell et al. [105] is
not sufficient to produce frank hemolytic anemia ([51Cr]RBC $t_{1/2}$ values in
hemolytic diseases approximate 5-15 days). Further, Farrell and associates found that their group of vitamin E-deficient patients showed no
clinical evidence of hemolysis and no change in hematologic indices upon
supplementation with vitamin E. This indicates that reduced red cell
survival was adequately compensated for by accelerated erythropoietic
mechanisms in these subjects. Nonetheless, the demonstration of a
shortened [51Cr]RBC survival in unsupplemented CF patients, and especially the finding that erythrocyte stability in vivo could be corrected upon

adequate tocopherol therapy, provides strong evidence that these subjects, and hence humans in general, require vitamin E for maintenance of normal red cell function. Even though vitamin E deficiency in humans is not accompanied by frank hemolytic anemia, it is reasonable to speculate that diminished antioxidant levels and a shortened red cell lifespan place a burden on the erythropoietic system. Because of this and other considerations, it has been recommended that cystic fibrosis patients be supplemented with vitamin E [105].

Since CF patients have a generalized defect in fat absorption and an associated alteration in the tissue content and distribution of polyunsaturated fatty acids (PUFA), the question may be raised as to the precise need of such patients for vitamin E. The results of several investigators [122, 146-149] indicate that circulating monoenoic fatty acids (palmitoleate and oleate) are elevated in cystic fibrosis and that linoleic acid levels are significantly decreased causing a reduction in total plasma PUFA. The studies of Underwood et al. [122] are especially relevant to a consideration of red cell requirements and function, since they measured both tocopherol and fatty acids in erythrocytes. As in the case of serum or plasma, the major changes in red cells were an increase in monoenoic acids and a decrease in linoleic acid. The decrease in RBC linoleate was

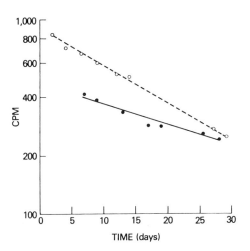

FIG. 5   The survival of ^{51}Cr-labeled red cells before (open circles) and after (filled circles) oral supplementation with vitamin E in a cystic fibrosis patient. [^{51}Cr]RBC survivals were determined 10 months apart during which time the patient received 100-200 IU water-miscible α-tocopherol acetate. Before supplementation, plasma α-tocopherol was 0.11 mg/dl peroxide hemolysis 88%, and [^{51}Cr]RBC half-life 16 days; corresponding after Vitamin E treatment were 0.65 mg/dl, 0.8%, and 28.5 days.

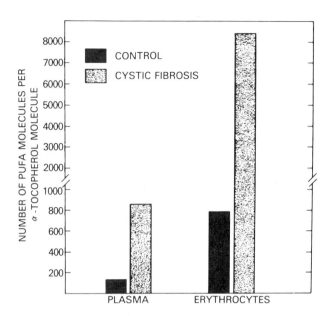

FIG. 6   Vitamin E/PUFA ratios in plasma and erythrocytes from control subjects and cystic fibrosis patients.   Mean figures shown were calculated from data reported by Underwood et al. [122].

compensated for by slight increases in more highly unsaturated fatty acids such that the peroxidizable index [150] was maintained at a level similar to that of control red cells.

From their data, Underwood et al. [122] were able to calculate the ratio of α-tocopherol to PUFA in red cells from unsupplemented patients. The results of such calculations are shown in Fig. 6.   In comparison to the E:PUFA ratio needed to prevent hemolysis in rats, which approximates 1 mol tocopherol/1000 mol PUFA [151], it is apparent that CF erythrocytes are markedly deficient by almost a full order of magnitude on the average.   It is equally evident from the individual figure reported by Underwood and associates that considerable variability exists with respect to the E:PUFA ratios in CF red cells.   This wide range of vitamin E concentrations in comparison to PUFA levels might account for the variability noted in measuring [^{51}Cr]RBC survival in vivo.   In any event, the data of Fig. 6 support the concept that erythrocytes in cystic fibrosis patients are highly susceptible to oxidants and that there is indeed a requirement for supplementary tocopherol.

Although Underwood and associates were only able to examine red cell preparations from three CF patients who had been supplemented to normal plasma and RBC tocopherol concentrations, a brief comment is in order on fatty acid levels in this group. When compared to erythrocytes of 20 unsupplemented patients, those of treated subjects contained significantly greater total PUFA. This change was due to a general increase in long chain, highly unsaturated fatty acids and should be studied further.

In view of the lack of a clinically evident hemolytic anemia in cystic fibrosis, one might inquire as to the level of other compounds which are known to exert a protective effect on the erythrocyte membrane. Although limited information is available in this regard, it is noteworthy that Shapiro and associates [152] have observed that red cells from CF patients exhibit significantly increased glutathione as well as an elevated glutathione reductase activity. In addition to glutathione, selenium levels have also been determined in cystic fibrosis. Underwood and co-workers [122] found that selenium concentrations ranged from 10 to 20 μg/dl (mean = 13.1) in CF plasma; these figures are comparable to those reported for normal human blood.

The morphology of the intestinal tract and other smooth muscle-containing tissues has been of interest to investigators concerned with aspects of vitamin E deficiency in cystic fibrosis. As discussed in Chapter 6, an acid-fast pigment referred to as ceroid or lipofuscin accumulates in the smooth muscle and may become disseminated throughout the reticuloendothelial system in association with prolonged vitamin E deficiency in animals. Examination of necropsy tissue from CF patients greater than 2 years old has invariably revealed the presence of ceroid pigment. This was first noted by Blanc and associates [153] when they reviewed microscopic sections of small intestine. They reported in 1958 that the pigment was present to a greater extent in specimens from CF patients as compared with sections of intestine from autopsied children without malabsorption. Careful histological study permitted these investigators to quantitate the extent of lipofuscin formation and correlation this with the presumed degree of antioxidant deficiency.

Subsequently, Kerner and Goldbloom [154] conducted an extensive retrospective survey of postmortem material collected from 57 CF patients who died between 3 days and 16 years of age. Tissues examined included esophagus, stomach, duodenum, jejunum, ileum, appendix, colon, urinary bladder, trachea, lungs, and liver. The overall amount of ceroid pigment accumulation was found to relate to the age at death. No sections from subjects living less than 2 years showed the pigment, whereas the largest quantities were found in the older patients. In terms of lipofuscin distribution, smooth muscle of the gastrointestinal tract contained the heaviest deposits, but areas of abnormal accumulation in all the above tissues were found upon careful examination of the sections. Since the major clinical problem in cystic fibrosis is chronic obstructive pulmonary disease, it is of interest to note that smooth muscle of the trachea was involved in several patients. More recently, Borel and Reddy [155] have also detected excessive lipofuscin pigment in thyroid tissue from seven CF patients over 12 years of age.

In another approach to intestinal morphology, Farrell and associates [105] examined the ultrastructure of jejunal mucosa obtained by biopsy from vitamin E-deficient CF patients and compared its appearance to that of jejunum from normal individuals adequate in vitamin E. Electron microscopic examination of these samples revealed that the appearance of subcellular membranous structures, particularly mitochondria and endoplasmic reticulum, was unaltered in the tocopherol-deficient patients. Thus, despite the apparent susceptibility of membranes to oxidant damage, the integrity of these structures in jejunum is maintained in cystic fibrosis patients.

3. Other Malabsorption Syndromes

a. Disorders Associated with Tocopherol Deficiency: In comparison to the amount of attention directed toward vitamin E in cystic fibrosis, a relative paucity of information is available on tocopherol status in other malabsorptive states. This "other" group is comprised of a wide variety of enteropathies. A selective list of such disorders along with reported blood tocopherol values is provided in Table 6; however, a detailed discussion of these diseases is beyond the scope of this chapter. For such information, the reader is referred to the excellent reviews by Volwiler [156] on adult steatorrhea and by Morin and Davidson [157] on pediatric gastroenterology.

From the list presented in Table 6, it is evident that disturbances affecting a variety of components in the digestive or absorptive processes may precipitate tocopherol deficiency, given a sufficient period of time with increased fecal loss. Thus, as mentioned previously, it would appear that any pathological condition leading to prolonged steatorrhea will eventually cause vitamin E deficiency as a consequence of tocopherol malabsorption. Clinical investigations have not as yet defined the length of time necessary for development of tocopherol depletion but this would ostensibly depend upon the amount of tissue storage in comparison to the degree of steatorrhea. Bieri's work in animals [158] and limited clinically studies [115] suggest that several months are required to exhaust tissue stores in cases where intestinal transport is severely compromised.

In addition to being a heterogenous group with regard to etiology, the disorders presented in Table 6 vary widely in terms of the type and age of the population affected. This may account in part for the great variability in degree and apparent effects of tocopherol deficiency in these patients, as will be discussed subsequently. The majority of the enteropathies usually afflict adults who, by analogy to studies in animals, are theoretically not as vulnerable as growing children to the effects of antioxidant

TABLE 6   Enteropathies Associated with Vitamin E Deficiency

Condition	Mean plasma or serum tocopherol (mg/dl)	Range	Reference number
Biliary atresia	0.11	—a	50
Biliary cirrhosis	0	—b	159
Biliary obstruction (cause unspecified)		0-0.14	160
Celiac disease	0.64	—b	161
Celiac disease	0.06	—b	111
Celiac disease	0.20	0-0.35	29
Celiac disease	0.39	—a	120
Chronic pancreatitis	0.40	0.17-0.79	115
Gastrectomy	0.34	0.10-0.80	162
Gastrectomy	0.37	0.10-0.77	162
Gastrectomy	0.58	0.41-0.74	115
Intestinal lymphangiectasia	0.28	—a	120
Intestinal resection	0.31	—b	115
Nontropical sprue	0.25	0.12-0.32	163
Regional enteritis plus intestinal resection	0.27	0.15-0.39	115
Tropical sprue	0.28	—a	164
Ulcerative colitis	0.24	0.17-0.36	115
Whipple's disease	0.30	0.14-0.45	115

a Data not reported.
b Only one patient studied.

deficiency. Nonetheless, some of the earliest studies on blood tocopherol levels in these malabsorption syndromes were conducted in the pediatric population. Thus, the first recorded observation of a low blood vitamin E concentration was in a 5 year-old girl with celiac disease. Minot [161] described this patient in 1944 and reported a serum total tocopherol level of 0.64 mg/dl as compared to a mean figure of 1.0 mg/dl in the control group. Shortly thereafter, Darby et al. [163] surveyed a number of hospitalized children and adults, including several with steatorrhea of various etiologies, and found markedly reduced plasma tocopherol concentrations in 20 patients with sprue (nontropical variety). Levels as low as 0.12 mg/dl were observed in patients with active disease and a "flat" vitamin E absorption curve was noted upon administering 600 mg mixed tocopherols orally and monitoring blood levels for 12 hr. This was contrasted to healthy adults who showed a mean plasma total tocopherol level of 1.06 mg/dl and a mean maximal rise of 0.37 mg/dl after a similar dose of oral tocopherol. By studying a limited number of sprue patients serially, Darby et al. [163] were also able to demonstrate that plasma tocopherol concentrations parallel the clinical stage of the disease, i.e., the degree of steatorrhea. Further evidence for this close relationship between plasma tocopherol levels and the state of intestinal absorption in patients with mucosal abnormalities has been obtained by evaluating adults with sprue in long-term remission and children with celiac disease after introduction of a gluten-free diet [115,120,165]. These patients develop normal blood tocopherol levels several weeks after their intestinal status improves. Tropical sprue may also lead to vitamin E deficiency, as reported by Ramirez et al. [164].

Although Darby and co-workers [163] commented in 1946 that "some patients having liver disease, either hepatitis or cirrhosis "show low levels of circulating tocopherol, 10 years elapsed before hepatic disturbances were explored further in terms of vitamin E deficiency. Nitowsky et al. [50] studied two children with biliary atresia from 3 to 15 months of of age and reported an average total tocopherol concentration of 0.11 mg/dl plasma. Of equal interest was their observation that blood vitamin E levels in these subjects were refractory to orally administered preparations. More recently, Muller and Harries [160] measured serum tocopherol levels in 12 children with obstructive jaundice and confirmed the pronounced deficiency state of patients with hepato-biliary disease as shown in Table 6. Additionally, these investigators encountered great difficulty in attempting repletion by the oral route. Administration of large doses of water-miscible tocopherol, in fact, had no effect on serum concentrations.

Both Nitowsky et al. [50] and Muller and Harries [160] demonstrated that red blood cells from children with intrahepatic or extrahepatic biliary obstruction are abnormally susceptible to hydrogen peroxide in vitro. RBC suspensions showed 55 and 76% hemolysis, respectively, over a 3-hr period in the two patients followed by Nitowsky and associates, while those studied by Muller and Harries exhibited a mean hemolysis of 58% and a range of 12-93%. The latter workers were unable to correct the in vitro erythrocyte hemolysis while Nitowsky et al. succeeded by treating their patients with a parenteral preparation of vitamin E.

Another patient with fat malabsorption of hepatic etiology and associated vitamin E deficiency was described in detail by Woodruff [159] in 1956. This was an adult with biliary cirrhosis and evidence of steatorrhea for at least 5 years who showed undetectable tocopherol in serum, abnormal erythrocyte hemolysis, and no response to an oral test dose of 600 mg α-tocopherol. Long-term tocopherol supplementation by the oral route was again ineffective and intramuscular doses were required to produce a satisfactory rise in the blood tocopherol level. Several patients with liver disease were also studied by Binder et al. [115]. One subject, diagnosed as having "intra-hepatic cholestasis," was found to show tocopherol deficiency with a serum level of 0.066 mg/dl and an in vitro hemolysis test result of 44%.

The foregoing findings in patients with hepatic disorders led credence to the proposal of Muller et al. [120] regarding the paramount importance of bile acids in the absorption of tocopherol. One might therefore suspect that the use of cholestyramine resin, which produces steatorrhea by sequestering bile acids, might lead to vitamin E deficiency. Although data from one patient support this concept when cholestyramine was given over a period of years [134], it has been reported that short-term (6 months) therapy with the resin in several patients with familial type II hyperlipoproteinemia did not lead to vitamin E deficiency [166]. Nonetheless, since a 6-month evaluation of tocopherol levels may be insufficient and cholestyramine is being used with increasing frequency, further study is warranted to determine its effect on plasma tocopherol levels in humans.

Several other intestinal disorders characterized by long-term fat malabsorption were studied by Binder et al. [115] and found to be associated with vitamin E deficiency. As listed in Table 6, these include diseases involving either the small or large intestine. With regard to small bowel disease, regional enteritis was identified as a cause of tocopherol depletion in two of five patients studied, but both of these had previously undergone partial intestinal resection also. Disturbances of the jejunum in two patients and Whipple's disease in one subject have also been found to produce tocopherol deficiency (see Table 6). In addition, intestinal lymphangiectasia has been documented by Muller et al. [120] as a cause of low blood vitamin E levels.

Disturbances affecting the large intestine and leading to significant fecal fat loss are relatively uncommon. Severe ulcerative colitis, however, may cause steatorrhea and has come under limited study in terms of associated vitamin E status. Binder et al. [115] evaluated five ulcerative colitis patients with respect to either erythrocyte hemolysis tests or serum vitamin E levels. Three of these exhibited low serum tocopherols but all five subjects showed normal or borderline RBC hemolysis tests.

Adult patients with chronic pancreatitis were reported by Binder et al. [115] to exhibit varying serum tocopherol levels. Two were clearly deficient at 0.17 and 0.20 mg/dl with corresponding erythrocyte hemolysis figures of 35 and 41%. Curiously, an additional patient with chronic pancreatitis showed a low serum tocopherol level at 0.25 mg/dl but a normal erythrocyte hemolysis test and serum carotene level. Out of two patients evaluated with carcinoma of the pancreas, one was shown to be vitamin E-deficient on the basis of both a low serum tocopherol concentration and an abnormal degree of peroxide-induced RBC hemolysis. Surgical causes of vitamin E deficiency in human beings include gastrectomy [162], if the

portion of the stomach removed is extensive enough to produce significant
steatorrhea, and various intestinal resection procedures (see Table 6).

From the foregoing discussion, it is evident that patients with these
"other" forms of malabsorption present a variable picture in terms of their
vitamin E status. Thus, the question of why subjects with nonpancreatog-
enous steatorrhea show such great variability deserves consideration. A
comparison of blood tocopherol levels with the extent of steatorrhea would
be helpful in this regard. Unfortunately, most investigators have not systematically quantitated fecal fat excretion but have relied upon either the
serum carotene concentration or other, less useful indices of malabsorption. It is noteworthy that in contrast to results obtained in cystic fibrosis
patients, serum carotene levels according to Binder et al. [115] could not
be closely correlated with circulating tocopherol levels in patients comprising this other group of malabsorption syndromes. Rather, it appears
that in adults with steatorrhea, the important variables in determining
tocopherol status at any given time are (1) the nature of the disorder,
(2) its severity, and (3) the total duration of illness [115]. The latter
seems to be especially significant in view of the finding by Binder and
associates that no patient with malabsorption for less than 9 months manifested vitamin E deficiency.

To elucidate the relationship between fecal fat excretion and tocopherol
malabsorption in patients with disorders other than cystic fibrosis,
MacMahon and Neale [167] recently conducted a study with radioactively
labeled vitamin E. These investigators administered physiological doses
of tritiated α-tocopherol to 7 normal volunteer adults and 23 patients with
steatorrhea of various etiologies. In contrast to the control subjects who
absorbed between 55 and 77% (mean = 69%) of the oral dose, adults with
malabsorption due to biliary obstruction, celiac disease, chronic pancreatitis, and lymphangiectasia uniformly displayed excessive fecal loss of
tocopherol. Absorption of α-tocopherol was most severely impaired in
patients with biliary obstruction and somewhat less severely impaired in
patients with pancreatic exocrine insufficiency. As low as 6% of the
[^{3}H]tocopherol test dose was absorbed in one patient with obstructive
jaundice, and two such patients failed to show any radioactivity in the
plasma. In patients with diseases attributable to abnormal small intestinal
mucosa, the extent of tocopherol malabsorption varied with the severity of
the condition. As one might expect, the scatter was particularly prominent
in patients with nontropical sprue. Most noteworthy, however, was the
finding that the degree of tocopherol malabsorption could be statistically
correlated with the degree of steatorrhea, as illustrated in Fig. 7. Therefore, it may be concluded that adults with malabsorption of various
etiologies are susceptible to tocopherol depletion according to (1) their
degree of general fat malabsorption and (2) their duration of disease.

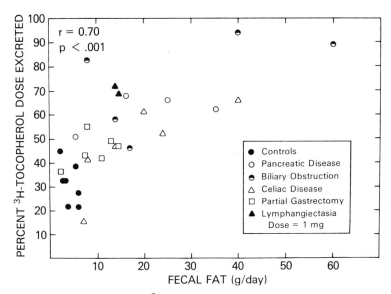

FIG. 7   The degree of [³H]tocopherol malabsorption in patients with various gastrointestinal disorders. Each subject was given a 1-mg dose of α-tocopherol containing 12-25 μCi of labeled vitamin. Feces were then collected for 6 days to determine the ³H-excretion pattern. (Data from Ref. 167.)

    b. Possible Effects of Tocopherol Deficiency: Limited investigations have been conducted on the effects of vitamin E deficiency in malabsorptive conditions other than cystic fibrosis. Because the diseases listed in Table 6 are not necessarily associated with persistent steatorrhea of long duration (hence prolonged tocopherol malabsorption), subjects with these disorders are presumably less appropriate than premature infants and cystic fibrosis patients for studying the effects of vitamin E deficiency in humans. The fact that they are primarily adults who are not actively growing also renders them less useful as investigational models of human antioxidant deficiency. Nonetheless, evidence has been sought attempting to demonstrate abnormalities similar to those reported in premature infants and CF patients, i.e., muscle dysfunction, erythrocyte hemolysis, and morphological disturbances in tissues containing smooth muscle.

    Regarding development of myopathy, retrospective surveys of the literature call attention to a case of sprue described in 1908 by Bramwell and Muir [168]. This patient showed muscle lesions and was probably deficient in vitamin E. Woodruff's patient with biliary cirrhosis and

pronounced tocopherol depletion was reported to have creatinuria, presumably as a result of muscle damage. Treatment with parenteral
vitamin E lowered the creatine excretion but not to the point of correcting
the abnormality [159]. Skeletal muscle removed from this subject at
autopsy showed extreme atrophy but no degeneration or other signs of
myopathy. Striated muscle from children with biliary atresia has also
been examined histologically. One such patient studied by Weinberg et al.
[169] showed foci of degeneration and necrosis plus hyalinization and
leukocytic infiltration—all consistent with findings in "nutritional dystrophy" of animals [135, 136]. On the other hand, muscle sections examined
extensively from another child with biliary atresia showed no lesions
[169]. Creatinuria was also found in the two patients with biliary atresia
studied by Nitowsky et al. [197]; however, the disturbance could not be
corrected with tocopherol injections given until normal plasma levels were
achieved. In the only other relevant report found by this author, Binder
and Spiro [171] commented that one of their malabsorption patients (cause
unspecified) had skeletal muscle lesions characterized by vacuolization
and proliferation of nuclei and marked variations in the size of the muscle
fibers. Otherwise, claims of muscular dysfunction are conspicuously
absent from the literature dealing with enteropathies and hepatobiliary
disorders associated with vitamin E deficiency. In view of the variable
findings on morphological examination of muscle and because creatinuria
may be a nonspecific sign of muscle atrophy [128], the data available at
present do not permit one to conclude that muscle disease commonly
occurs in patients with these other forms of malabsorption.

Almost equally scant are documented observations on erythrocyte
stability in malabsorption syndromes other than cystic fibrosis. As mentioned previously, abnormal RBC hemolysis in vitro was demonstrated in
the patients with either biliary atresia or biliary cirrhosis studied by
Nitowsky et al. [50] and Woodruff [159]. In addition, several of the
patients with low serum tocopherol levels followed by Binder et al. [115]
showed elevated erythrocyte hemolysis in the presence of hydrogen peroxide. Attempts to demonstrate correction of hemolysis by in vitro treating patients parenterally with vitamin E were successful in the two children
having biliary atresia, but not in the adult with biliary cirrhosis.

Limited data have been collected in regard to the possibility of significant hemolysis in vivo. On the basis of general observations and
clinical hematologic findings in patients with these other forms of malabsorption, one would not suspect hemolytic anemia. Binder et al. [115],
however, reported markedly shortened $[^{51}Cr]$RBC half-lives in three
vitamin E-deficient patients, two of which had chronic pancreatitis and one
of which had "idiopathic steatorrhea." The $t_{1/2}$ values of 8, 12, and
15 days were inconsistent with the observations that these subjects were
not anemic and that they showed normal reticulocyte counts, hepatoglobin

levels, bilirubin concentrations, and bone marrow morphology (most of which should be abnormal when RBC survival is shortened to the degree observed). This prompted Binder et al. [115] to conclude that the lowered [^{51}Cr]RBC survival figures were "a labeling artifact" possibly attributable to excessively rapid chromate elution from the tagged red cells. An unspecified number ("several") of other vitamin E-deficient patients evaluated by Binder and associates showed normal [^{51}Cr]RBC $t_{1/2}$ values.

In a careful study, Leonard and Losowsky [172] observed shortening of the mean red cell survival in a group of eight adults with malnutrition due to either steatorrhea (six subjects) or chronic alcoholism with poor diet. Seven of these patients showed abnormal [^{51}Cr]RBC half-lives (less than 25 days) and the mean ± SE of the group was 19.3 ± 5.4 days. None exhibited either anemia or reticulocytosis in keeping with the mild-to-moderate change in red cell survival data. Following oral plus intramuscular treatment with α-tocopherol and relabeling of red cells, it was observed that the $t_{1/2}$ values increased to the normal range in five subjects. Furthermore, the group as a whole showed a significantly greater (p < 0.025) posttreatment value of 24.9 ± 4.7 days (mean ± SE). The latter observation strongly implicates tocopherol deficiency as the cause of reduced erythrocyte lifespan in these patients.

Although the histopathologist may encounter difficulty in distinguishing the normal degree of ceroid pigment accumulation occurring with advanced age from that deposited excessively in adults with malabsorption, a variety of reports indicate that patients with disorders such as those listed in Table 6 commonly show abnormal ceroid deposition. As early as 1945, Pappenheimer and Victor [173] reported an abundance of this material in various tissues taken at autopsy from patients with sprue and other enteropathies leading to steatorrhea. Its distribution was essentially that reviewed previously for patients with cystic fibrosis. Blanc and associates [153] further demonstrated ceroid pigmentation in the small intestine of children with biliary atresia, and Braunstein [174] identified the material in 26 of 216 patients with chronic pancreatitis. None of the above investigations included measurements of plasma or tissue tocopherol but all authors concluded that antioxidant deficiency was the likely cause of lipofuscin accumulation. Binder et al. [115] did document chronic tocopherol deficiency in two patients who were found on examination of intestinal biopsy tissue to exhibit excessive ceroid pigment deposition in smooth muscle.

4. Abetalipoproteinemia

Although this hereditary disorder which leads to severe vitamin E deficiency could be categorized under other malabsorption syndromes, its unique features, particularly the striking absence of plasma betalipoproteins, justify a separate discussion. First described in 1950 by Bassen and Kornzweig [176], abetalipoproteinemia (ABL) has proven to be a fascinating disease producing what is apparently the most profound degree of tocopherol deficiency in humans. Because of its rarity (only 25 patients have been described to date), only limited data are available on the effects of tocopherol deficiency in ABL.

Clinical aspects of ABL have been reviewed in detail by Kayden [18] but deserve brief comment herein. ABL is transmitted as an autosomal recessive trait and generally becomes manifest during the infancy period with steatorrhea as an early symptom. Following several years of generalized growth retardation, neurological symptoms become evident including ataxia, apparent muscular weakness, and oculomotor disturbances. Underlying lesions in the central nervous system have been reported, particularly changes in the posterior columns and spinocerebellar long tracts of the spinal cord. Retinitis pigmentosa then develops in the later stages of the disease. The peculiar, "spiny" shape of the red blood cells in patients with ABL gave this disease its early name of acanthocytosis. Interestingly, despite their peculiar shape and mechanical fragility, acanthocytes seem to have a normal or near normal lifespan [18]. Both very low-density lipoproteins (VLDLS) and low-density lipoproteins (LDLS) are absent from the plasma of these patients, as indicated by various analytical techniques including ultra-centrifugation, electrophoresis, and immunoreactivity [176]. Extremely low concentrations of circulating lipids, particularly cholesterol and phosophlipids, reflect the absence of β-lipoproteins.

Gastrointestinal aspects of ABL are especially pertinent to our consideration of vitamin E deficiency and deserve further discussion. The amount of fecal fat excreted is variable and may in fact be normal at times when diets moderately restricted in fat content are utilized. Even when the degree of steatorrhea is mild, however, fat absorption remains fundamentally abnormal since the usual mechanism of chylomicron formation and uptake of resynthesized triglyceride into lymphatic channels is inoperative in ABL. From studies of pancreatic and biliary function, as well as from measurements of intestinal enzyme activities, there is no reason to suspect an accompanying digestive defect. This disorder thus affects fat absorption per se.

The steatorrhea and lipid transport abnormalities manifested by ABL patients have stimulated research on fat-soluble vitamin status. Shortly after Simon and Ways [177] reported that acanthocytes hemolyzed spontaneously in vitro, Kayden and Silber [178], using techniques sensitive enough to detect 0.05 mg/dl, reported that four children with absent β-lipoproteins had no measurable tocopherol in plasma. The apparent absence of circulating tocopherol in unsupplemented patients was confirmed by Bieri and Poukka [124] and also by Muller and Harries [160]. In all, a total of seven patients have been documented as showing a lack of detectable vitamin E in plasma or serum. Curiously, evaluation by Molenaar et al. [179] of two other patients with ABL has revealed the presence of tocopherol in plasma. Levels of 0.50 and 0.30 mg/dl were reported in these children before high-dose tocopherol supplementation, and 1.35 and 0.85 mg/dl after 4 months of treatment.

As one might suspect, erythrocytes from ABL patients are highly susceptible to peroxide-induced hemolysis [180]. This may be corrected with either massive oral doses of water-miscible tocopherol or with parenteral preparations of vitamin E. Although the absence of detectable tocopherol in these patients might lead one to speculate that the β-lipoprotein fraction serves as a transport system for plasma vitamin E, the fact that such patients can develop measurable tocopherol levels with supplementation as well as several other observations [181] render this unlikely.

Erythrocyte tocopherol levels were also measured by Bieri and Poukka [124] on blood samples of ABL patients receiving α-tocopheryl succinate in a daily oral dose of 750 mg. They observed that although α-tocopherol concentrations remained low in plasma, red cells were able to develop and maintain normal levels (mean = 0.21 mg/dl packed cells). It was further noted that treatment with vitamin E abolished erythrocyte hemolysis in vitro. The ratio of RBC tocopherol to its concentration in plasma was approximately fourfold greater in treated ABL patients as compared to normal subjects. Thus, plasma α-tocopherol levels cannot be considered a satisfactory index of the tissue concentration in patients with ABL receiving tocopherol supplements.

In addition, Bieri and Poukka [124] determined the fatty acid composition of acanthocytes. They found extremely low concentrations of linoleic acid but total PUFA approximating the levels present in normal red cells. The peroxidizable index was therefore unaltered. In keeping with observations on hemolysis testing, the ratio of tocopherol molecules to PUFA molecules in red cells from vitamin E-supplemented ABL patients was calculated to be greater than the minimum (1:1100) needed to protect the red cell membrane from oxidative damage [151].

Studies exploring the possible effects of vitamin E deficiency in patients with ABL are hampered by the small number of subjects available, as well as the severity and complexity of the disorder. The lack of evidence for hemolytic anemia has already been cited and there have been no reports of myopathy [18]. At least one patient, this a 9 year-old child, has been found to exhibit ceroid pigment deposition in the intestinal tract. The question arises as to the role of tocopherol deficiency in the neurological symptoms, but there is little information available regarding this possibility. Nonetheless, Kayden [18] does comment that two patients followed for 7 years on high-dose tocopherol therapy have shown no progression in neurological symptoms and nearly normal neuromuscular development during adolescence. In addition, Wallis et al. [182] reported that one 11 year-old child with ABL showed "a significant clinical improvement of muscular and neurological disturbances" when treated on a weekly to twice-weekly basis with 100 mg intramuscular injections of tocopherol. Certainly, further study is warranted on this important question.

Although the patients studied by Molenaar et al. [179] must be regarded as atypical in terms of plasma vitamin E level, ultrastructural study of jejunal biopsies has formed the basis for a proposed subcellular morphological disturbance in humans with vitamin E deficiency. Molenaar and co-workers reported that the membranes of mitochondria and endoplasmic reticulum could not be visualized, i.e., were totally absent, when routine preparations of mucosal cells were examined electron microscopically. Four months after tocopherol treatment, "a dramatic change" was evident with "a completely normal cellular ultrastructure." This cytological abnormality is clearly striking, and the response claimed after tocopherol therapy raises exciting possibilities. Confirmation is required, however, particularly in view of the normal ultrastructural findings on examination of jejunal biopsy tissue from CF patients with severe vitamin E deficiency [105].

5. Protein-Calorie Malnutrition

Infants and children with the severe form of protein-calorie malnutrition (PCM), viz., kwashiorkor, and a limited number with less severe malnutrition have been shown by a number of investigators to develop vitamin E deficiency. Tocopherol depletion in these patients can be attributed to both poor vitamin intake and impaired intestinal absorption. Their malabsorption in turn may be due to a combination of pancreatic insufficiency, decreased bile production, and diarrhea [183].

Little needs to be said in this review about the general features and clinical consequences of protein-calorie malnutrition, for these have been described in detail by others. In particular, an excellent monograph edited by Olson [184] has recently appeared defining the multiple metabolic disturbances as well as approaches to therapy in this condition. Nonetheless, a word about the anemia of protein-calorie malnutrition is in order since studies on the effects of vitamin E deficiency have largely focused on the erythropoietic system. In the absence of concomitant, severe deficiencies in iron or the B vitamins, acute PCM leads to a normochromic, normocytic anemia with a generally normal reticulocyte count [185]. There have been many reports of hypochromia and macrocytosis, however, and demonstrations of megaloblastic changes in the bone marrow.

Evaluation of the deficiency of a single nutrient, such as vitamin E in children with kwashiorkor, presents obvious difficulties to the clinical investigator. In addition to the problem of multiple deficiencies

accompanying protein-calorie starvation at the onset of studies, the control
of diet and environment may be extremely difficult in the hospital setting
where medical personnel make every attempt to improve the child's well-
being. Furthermore, the natural variation in severity of PCM and its
sometimes unpredictable clinical course require the investigator to employ
relatively large study populations—preferably randomly selected children
assessed in a double-blind fashion.

In any event, children of 5 months to 4 years of age with protein-
calorie malnutrition have come under intensive study with respect to
vitamin E status. Ever since 1957 when Schrimshaw and associates [186]
reported low blood tocopherol levels in patients with kwashiorkor, there
has been little dispute regarding the occurrence of vitamin E deficiency in
these subjects. At least seven other studies have verified this observation, as presented in Table 7. From the list of blood tocopherol values, it
is evident that the degree of deficiency varies, ostensibly in proportion to
the severity of generalized malnutrition. Indeed, McLaren et al. [187]
observed during a study of patients having protein-calorie malnutrition of
varying degrees of severity that the blood vitamin E levels are significantly lower in those who expire as compared to survivors (0.49 vs. 0.83 mg/
dl plasma, respectively).

Investigations exploring the possible effects of vitamin E deficiency in
protein-calorie malnutrition have, as mentioned previously, been directed
primarily toward hematologic aspects of the syndrome. Majaj et al. [188]
first claimed that the anemia of PCM responds favorably to vitamin E.
With observations on anemic, tocopherol-deficient monkeys [194] as their
clue, they studied hospitalized children of 6 months to 2 years of age in
Jerusalem. Data were gathered suggesting that tocopherol therapy is
associated with reticulocytosis and correction of low hemoglobin and
hematocrit values. These findings led Majaj et al. to propose that the
anemia in children with kwashiorkor was "vitamin E responsive." Review
of their experimental protocol, however, indicates that the investigation
was not sufficiently controlled, particularly with regard to administration
of other nutrients. For this reason, among others, Whitaker and associates [195] repeated the trial with 60 children hospitalized at the Chiang
Mai Medical School Hospital in Thailand. The patients were divided into
41 control subjects and 19 treated with vitamin E, but were not randomized
or studied in a blind fashion. Further, they were all given a high protein
diet during the hospitalization period along with various other therapeutic
measures. From the standpoint of validity assessing responses to tocopherol therapy, perhaps the most disconcerting aspect of their study is that
the vitamin E-treated group entered the protocol with an apparently greater
severity of malnutrition. This was suggested by their lower mean initial
hemoglobin value of 7.8 ± 1.9 g/dl (mean $\pm$ SD) as compared to $9.5 \pm$
1.9 g/dl in the control group. Whitaker et al. [195] reported that the

TABLE 7   Blood Tocopherol Levels Reported in Infants and Children with Protein-Calorie Malnutrition

Mean plasma or serum tocopherol (mg/dl)	Range	Reference number
0.43	0.33-0.65	188
0.28	0-0.91	189
_a	0.09-0.55	190
0.37	0.10-0.69	191
0.42	0.15-0.74	192
0.83	_a	187
0.49	_a	187
0.30	_a	193

a Data not reported.

control subjects showed a progressive fall in hemoglobin concentration over 40 days to a mean level of 8.3 g/dl. In contrast, patients receiving 250 mg/day vitamin E demonstrated a statistically significant increase in hemoglobin to 9.6 g/dl, as well as a rise in reticulocyte count.

The reports by Majaj et al. [188] and Whitaker et al. [195] aroused considerable interest in relationship to a possible bone marrow-stimulating effect of vitamin E. More carefully controlled studies were thus conducted by a number of investigators; however, none of these attempts to confirm the earlier two reports have produced data indicating that hemoglobin synthesis responds to vitamin E. On the contrary, investigations by Baker et al. [191], Halstead et al. [192], and Kulapongs [193] have served to strengthen the hypothesis that protein deficiency, and at times iron or folate deficiency, are the main factors relating to defective hematopoiesis in children with protein-calorie malnutrition. The study by Kulapongs is particularly noteworthy in that (1) the same population of Thai children were evaluated as in the trial of Whitaker et al. [195] and (2) the experimental design was excellent with proper use of controls. In contrast to the lack of uniform success with tocopherol therapy, reproducible responses can be elicited in the macrocytic anemia of PCM when folic acid is provided in pharmacologic amounts. Accordingly, it is appropriate to conclude that vitamin E can neither be incriminated as an important etiologic factor in the anemia of PCM, nor can it be reasonably promoted as a bone marrow stimulant.

In considering the anemia of protein-calorie malnutrition further, one might postulate a hemolytic etiology. The lack of significant reticulocytosis in most patients is against this hypothesis, as is the failure of

investigators to establish shortening of red cell survival. The studies of
Asfour and Firzli [196] can be cited as negative in regard to the latter.
Although these workers did not study severely malnourished subjects, but
rather infants and children in an orphanage with moderate malnutrition and
tocopherol deficiency, they clearly showed that the [^{51}Cr]RBC $t_{1/2}$ values
were in the normal range. Treatment of these patients with vitamin E to
normal blood levels did not lead to correction of the anemia, whereas iron
therapy was effective. In addition, Stekel and Smith [197], who did not
assess vitamin E status, reported that 12 Chilean infants with protein-
calorie malnutrition had normal [^{51}Cr]RBC half-lives (range = 25-40 days).

Attempts to define the precise cause of anemia in protein-calorie
malnutrition have lately centered on the hematopoietic hormone, erythropoietin. As stressed by Vilter [185], it appears that a reduced level of
this hormone is a major factor in the low hemoglobin state of children
with kwashiorkor. Since the anemia accompanying PCM is typically
normochromic and normocytic, proposals relating to erythropoietin deficiency are entirely consistent with its function. In support of this possibility, it has been observed that when kwashiorkor patients are given
protein, increased amounts of erythropoietin appear in the blood followed
by an increase in red cell production [198].

6. Experimental Deprivation

Aside from human vitamin E deficiency in developed countries occasioned
by malabsorption and instances associated with severely reduced food
intake in underdeveloped countries of the Middle and Far East, tocopherol
depletion in humans has only been comprehensibly investigated in a limited
number of adult males at the Elgin State Hospital in Illinois. Conducted
over a 6-year period by Horwitt and associates [5, 14-16, 199], the Elgin
Project provided important data which have proven useful for estimating
dietary tocopherol requirements in relationship to polyunsaturated fat
intake.

A word should be said about the purpose of this project to put the
experimental design and results in proper perspective. In order to establish people's need for exogenous tocopherol, it was clearly necessary to
demonstrate that the vitamin could not be synthesized in the body in
adequate quantities. The aim of the study, however, was not simply to
confirm that tocopherol is required as a nutrient and hence, fulfills the
definition of a vitamin. If this were the case, diets completely absent in
vitamin E could have been employed. Rather, a primary objective was to
determine the minimum level at which "signs of deficiency" could be prevented. Signs of deficiency at the time the project commenced could not
be defined on any basis other than a reduced circulating tocopherol level.
Indeed, a key question in the project was "What, if any, are the manifestations of vitamin E inadequacies in man?" [14]. The lack of sound, prior

knowledge regarding tocopherol deficiency states in humans led Horwitt and associates to be abundantly and properly cautious in dealing with these depleted subjects. Accordingly, as soon as suggestive evidence of pathology was present and before irreversible damage could likely develop, the investigators began supplementation with tocopherol.

Although Horwitt's group was unable to uncover firm evidence of a clinical syndrome attributable to tocopherol depletion, and thereby unequivocally establish a biological requirement for the vitamin, their data clearly defined human beings' chemical need. The literature contains several detailed descriptions of the Elgin Project design as well as the findings on tocopherol-deprived volunteers. For this reason, only a cursory review is included in this treatise and the reader is referred to other articles for more extensive information [14-16]. Briefly, 38 male subjects were carefully selected and divided into three groups as follows: (1) 19 receiving a basal diet providing 2-3 mg/day tocopherol and varying levels of polyunsaturated fat (see the caption to Fig. 8); (2) 9 subjects on the basal diet plus 15 mg α-tocopheryl acetate per day (control group); and (3) a second control group of 10 males on the regular hospital diet. Over the course of the study the number of volunteers in each group decreased continuously. During the initial 2-3 years, the period required for stabilization of laboratory parameters, 16 subjects could be followed in the first group and six in the second group.

The course of tocopherol depletion in response to dietary deprivation is illustrated in Fig. 8. On the basis of total tocopherol levels in plasma, it is evident that a period of approximately 2 years was required before vitamin E deficiency could be claimed, i.e., circulating concentrations less than 0.5 mg/dl plasma. This correlated well with the observed pattern of increased erythrocyte hemolysis since maximum susceptibility of red cells to peroxide was noted after 2 years of depletion. Thus, Horwitt et al. [14,15] succeeded in confirming earlier observations [47-49] indicating that the usual plasma:erythrocyte relationship of tocopherol was such that plasma concentrations less than 0.5 mg/dl are associated with a potential for oxidant damage to red cells under appropriate conditions in vitro.

Volunteers included in the group received 15 mg/day α-tocopheryl acetate showed an initial increase in plasma total tocopherol values, suggesting that they had been accustomed to consuming less than that dietary level prior to the study. Presumably due to an increase in tissue PUFA, plasma tocopherol concentrations began to decline after 4 months and stabilized after approximately 2 years on the basal plus E diet. Increasing PUFA intake further during the subsequent 20 months by feeding "tocopherol-stripped" corn oil instead of lard led to an additional decline in plasma vitamin E. When the vitamin was withdrawn 60 months into the study, however, plasma tocopherol concentrations declined more

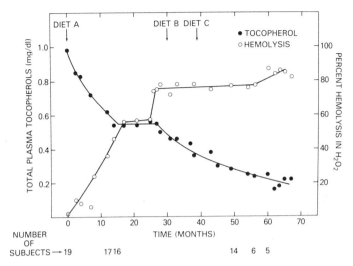

FIG. 8   The course of tocopherol depletion in adult subjects on diets providing approximately 2 mg total tocopherols per day. Diets A and B
included 60 g fat, 30 g of which was either "tocopherol-stripped" lard (A)
or corn oil (B). Diet C provided 90 g fat, 60 g of which was tocopherol-
stripped corn oil. Corresponding daily intakes of linoleic acid from lard
or corn oil approximated 3.3 g (diet A), 17 g (diet B), and 34 g (diet C).
(Adapted from Ref. 15.)

precipitously and an increased susceptibility of erythrocytes was noted
with the peroxide hemolysis test.

From these observations and others, Horwitt et al. [5,16] concluded
as follows: (1) tissue stores of tocopherol in adult males are sufficient to
prevent deficiency for 1-2 years when diets low but not absent in vitamin E
are fed; (2) the fatty acid composition of tissues can be altered by modi-
fying dietary fatty acids; (3) the precise requirement for vitamin E varies
as a function of the amount of polyunsaturated fat in the diet; and
(4) tocopherol requirements in humans, expressed on the basis of the
α-vitamer, range from a minimum of less than 5 mg/day to a maximum of
approximately 30 mg/day. The lower figure is a sufficient amount for
those consuming foods relatively low in unsaturated lipids, e.g., diets with
a large animal tissue component, and the 30 mg/day value is sufficient to
prevent deficiency with diets relatively high in unsaturates. These conclusions are clearly in accordance with findings from animal studies while
the relationship between increased vitamin E requirements and greater
consumption of PUFA was first defined [5,181]. It must be stressed,
however, that changes in tissue PUFA occur rather slowly with time, just

as plasma tocopherol concentrations tend to be maintained over several months. The resistance of tissue stores to depletion emphasizes the importance of average daily consumption over an extended time interval rather than the amount of vitamin E ingested on any given day.

As shown in Fig. 8, the results of the Eglin Project provided strong confirmation of the in vitro susceptibility of vitamin E-deficient erythrocytes to hydrogen peroxide. Despite the fact that Horwitt et al. [14] encountered some difficulty in quantitatively reproducing data with the peroxide hemolysis test, their findings on the relationship between plasma tocopherol concentrations and the degree of erythrocyte hemolysis unequivocally established the protective role of vitamin E in this regard. On the other hand, attempts to demonstrate that erythrocyte survival was compromised in vivo were less convincing [199]. Measurements of [^{51}Cr]RBC survival and reticulocyte counts were relied upon for this purpose; however, only a limited number of subjects were studied and those on the basal diet were apparently not reevaluated following tocopherol supplementation. Data obtained after ^{51}Cr "tagging" of red cells were used to calculate the $t_{1/2}$ value (the most widely used and accepted estimate of survival), and also the [^{51}Cr]RBC 95% life and the total erythrocyte lifespan. It must be stated that the latter two methods of calculating red cell survival offer both advantages and disadvantages. As Horwitt et al. [199] maintained, when differences expected are small, greater sensitivity is attained by the longer measurements; however, this is achieved at the expense of reduced accuracy and reproducibility.

Results from erythrocyte survival measurements by Horwitt and associates [199] in vitamin E-depleted subjects were variable. Three volunteers on the basal diet studied during the 31st month of the project showed [^{51}Cr]RBC $t_{1/2}$ figures of 27, 30, and 37 days, despite abnormal erythrocyte hemolysis in vitro. These half-lives are in the range of normal literature values and in fact are similar to the values of 29, 31, 36, and 32 days found in tocopherol-supplemented subjects. Such findings were obviously not significant, as the authors comment, but because the shortest half-life of 27 days was found in the subject with the highest peroxide susceptibility in vitro, the red cell survival determinations were repeated during the sixth year of the project. The second series included four depleted volunteers, one remaining on basal diet plus 15 mg/day α-tocopheryl acetate, and five subjects ingesting the hospital diet. Again, as shown in Table 8, [^{51}Cr]RBC $t_{1/2}$ values in the first group were not clearly abnormal and were certainly not in a range to influence the hematologic status of the subjects. Nor was the mean [^{51}Cr]RBC half-life in vitamin E-depleted subjects (25 days) found to be statistically different than the mean figure for controls (29 days). Nonetheless, calculation of the [^{51}Cr]RBC 95% life and the total red cell lifespan yielded data suggesting that vitamin E-deficient erythrocytes were compromised in vivo (see Table 8). Perhaps the strongest evidence gathered by Horwitt et al. [199] in support

TABLE 8 Erythrocyte Survival Data Measured with [^{51}Cr]RBC Monitoring Techniques in Adults Consuming Diets Adequate or Deficient in Vitamin E [a, b]

Group	Subject[c]	Plasma tocopherol (mg/dl)	[^{51}Cr]RBC survival (days)		
			$t_{1/2}$	95% life	Total life
Control					
	BE6	0.54	31	113	124
	HD4	0.50	34	114	128
	HD6	0.93	25	111	123
	HD7	0.62	25	103	121
	HD9	0.85	32	102	117
	HD10	0.75	30	104	121
Mean ± SE		0.70 ±	30 ± 1.5	108 ± 2.2	122 ± 1.8
Vitamin E deficient					
	B1[d]	0.18, 0.11	25, 26	91, 93	110, 113
	B3[d]	0.21, 0.07	24, 25	90, 91	106, 110
	B4	0.14	24	92	115
	B5	0.16	26	94	114
Mean ± SE		0.15 ± 0.005[e]	25 ± 0.48	92 ± 0.63[e]	112 ± 1.5[f]

[a] Values were determined during the sixth year of the Elgin Project as reported by Horwitt et al. [199].
[b] Diets are described in the text.
[c] Abbreviations: BE, basal diet supplemented with vitamin E; HD, hospital diet; B, basal diet.
[d] The first values shown for this subject were determined the 72nd month of the project and the second values during the 76th month; the average of the two determinations was used in calculating the group means.
[e] $p < 0.001$ as compared to the control group.
[f] $p < 0.005$ as compared to the control group.

of their proposal that RBC survival is reduced in human tocopherol deficiency was the observation that no overlap occurred in either the 95% life or the total lifespan values of erythrocytes in depleted volunteers, as compared to control subjects.

With regard to other hematologic indices, it was reported that anemia did not develop in the tocopherol-depleted subjects [199]. Reticulocyte counts were likewise normal in these subjects. Nonetheless, during the fifth year of the study when the basal group was evaluated before and after supplementation with 300 mg/day α-tocopheryl acetate, an apparent rise in circulating reticulocytes was observed. The change was statistically significant, although the levels before and after treatment were all within the normal range (reticulocyte counts of 0-1%). It must be stated in assessing these reticulocyte counts critically that they can neither be construed as supporting an erythropoietic role for tocopherol, nor can they be cited as evidence that the volunteers were subject to a greater hemolytic tendency when tocopherol deficient. If the latter were so, administration of vitamin E should have resulted in lower reticulocyte counts.

In addition to hematologic evaluation of tocopherol-deprived humans, Horwitt's group also attempted to uncover signs of myopathy using creatine excretion as the marker. Unfortunately, the failure to control dietary creatine intake, as well as the observation that control subjects showed creatinuria at times, precluded a valid assessment of this possibility [5].

In the long-term investigation of Horwitt and associates, volunteers kept on low tocopherol diets were not representative of the average male adult in the United States since they lived sedentary lives during the study. The relative inactivity of these hospitalized subjects could conceivably have influenced the need for tocopherol as well as the tissue levels of fatty acids. A more recent but shorter (13-month) trial of tocopherol deprivation was thus conducted by Bunnell et al. [200] in 35 male subjects engaged in strenuous labor. They were provided diets low in vitamin E by elimination of foods considered good sources of the vitamin. With an average daily intake of 9.4 mg total tocopherols (estimated to represent 4.5 IU/day), a progressive decline from 1.42 to 0.82 mg/dl plasma was observed in a subgroup of five subjects. The other 30 were given the low tocopherol diet plus 88 g/day polyunsaturated fat in the form of tocopherol-stripped safflower oil. This group showed a more rapid fall in mean plasma tocopherol concentration from an initial value of 1.01 mg/dl to a figure of 0.51 mg/dl at 5 months. Thereafter, the concentration remained relatively stable. Although Bunnell and associates did not assess peroxide-induced hemolysis, they did observe plasma tocopherol levels as low as 0.14 mg/dl. Interestingly, vitamin E-deficient subjects engaged in strenuous labor showed no muscular weakness or other physical symptoms. Although the observations of Bunnell et al. [201] raise the possibility that the stress of strenuous activity may lead to an increased requirement for vitamin E, it must be stated that the five volunteers receiving 9.4 mg tocopherol/day and a reasonable PUFA intake continued to maintain adequate plasma levels during the 13-month course of the study.

7. Overview and Approaches to Therapy

From this lengthy consideration of human vitamin E deficiency states, several generalizations and conclusions emerge as follows:

1. Tissue tocopherol stores are limited at birth such that satisfactory intake and absorption are especially important in the neonate if deficiency is to be avoided.

2. Tocopherol stores, once established in older individuals, are abundant and resistant to depletion. Thus, tissue vitamin E is not readily exhausted until deprivation has continued for a period of several months.

3. The large stores of tocopherol in adults makes them less than ideal subjects for exploring the effects of vitamin E deficiency in humans.

4. Contrariwise, growing children with vitamin E deficiency are more analogous to tocopherol-deprived animals in the usual laboratory setting.

5. Intestinal malabsorption states, if persistent and prolonged, will regularly lead to vitamin E deficiency in humans unless relatively large tocopherol supplements are administered.

6. Tocopherol deficiency in humans with prolonged steatorrhea develops to a degree commensurate with the extent of malabsorption.

7. A relatively large number of cystic fibrosis patients have been studied relative to the degree and effects of vitamin E deficiency, whereas only a limited number of subjects with other forms of malabsorption have been comprehensibly investigated.

8. Patients with abetalipoproteinemia, although fascinating for investigative purposes, are few in number and present a course sufficiently complicated that studies of vitamin E deficiency are pursued with great difficulty.

9. Infants and children with protein-calorie malnutrition show vitamin E deficiency in proportion to their severity of general dietary deprivation but do not respond dramatically to tocopherol supplementation.

10. Biliary atresia and other hepatobiliary disturbances cause profound tocopherol deficiency and have proven extremely difficult to treat with oral vitamin E supplements.

11. Therefore, from observations on patients with pancreatic achylia, hepatobiliary dysfunction, and impaired intestinal mucosal transport, it appears that bile acids are particularly important in the absorption of vitamin E. Ultimately, however, solubilization and uptake of tocopherol seems to depend on the combination of lipase-rich pancreatic juice, which liberates monoglycerides and fatty acids from dietary triglycerides, and the bile salts which transform these lipids into micelles containing "transportable" vitamin E for delivery to mucosal surfaces.

12. Possible hematologic effects of vitamin E deficiency in humans have come under closest scrutiny and offer the best supportive evidence

that tocopherol deprivation comprises the ability of the species to function in a normal manner.

13. Enhanced peroxide susceptibility of tocopherol-deficient red cells in vitro and a slightly shortened erythrocyte survival in vivo provide an indication that vitamin E exerts a protective effect in the bloodstream. Results of RBC survival studies, however, are variable. This suggests that compensatory factors (e.g., the glutathione system) or reduced needs (possibly due to lowered cellular PUFA) are operative in some subjects. Regardless of findings in vitro and in vivo with tocopherol-deficient red cells, diminished vitamin E does not alter the hematologic system to such an extent that frank hemolysis and anemia occur. Rather, the effect is a subclinical one with only insidious manifestations.

14. Observations on the neuromuscular system indicate that even in rapidly growing children, vitamin E deficiency does not produce the acute myopathy found in many animal species. Subtle pathological changes, however, are present in a small percentage of patients with malabsorption and associated vitamin E deficiency. Not only are the histological lesions mild, but one must also conclude that muscular performance and strength are unaffected in vitamin E-deficient children. Nonetheless, on the basis of isolated observations which require further study for confirmation, it is reasonable to speculate that tocopherol in humans may play a role in protecting stressed skeletal and cardiac muscle from oxidative damage.

15. Ceroid pigment accumulation has been detected in a number of vitamin E-deficient human organs, particularly those containing smooth muscle. Deposition of this material provides an indication that tocopherol protects such tissues from metabolic abnormalities which remain to be defined precisely.

Approaches to therapy will be discussed below only in relationship to deficient or potentially deficient patients (see Sec. III for a discussion of vitamin E supplements in nondeficient individuals). It is hoped that findings in vitamin E-deficient humans as reviewed herein will serve to emphasize that treatment of such patients should be encouraged. In view of the less than dramatic responses to vitamin E supplementation, it is not altogether surprising that completely satisfactory approaches to therapy in newborns and patients with malabsorption remain to be established.

With regard to prematurely delivered infants, particularly those of early gestational ages, Barness et al. [77] and subsequently Gross and Melhorn [54, 81] have shown that vitamin E is poorly absorbed for the first several weeks of life. This abnormality is illustrated in Fig. 9. Oral supplementation with relatively large doses of α-tocopheryl acetate, i.e., 5-25 IU/kg, has thus proven insufficient in newborns delivered 8-12 weeks prematurely [54]. It is not until they attain full maturity ex utero that these infants respond adequately to oral supplementation. In fact, the formulas provided for such patients nor the oral preparations of water-miscible

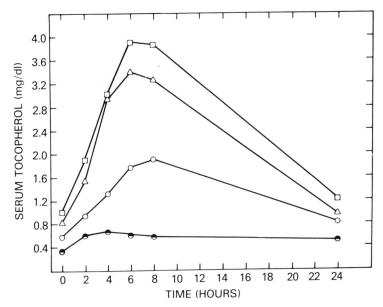

FIG. 9 Absorption of supplementary vitamin E in developing premature
infants of varying gestational age and children five to 16 years old. Each
infant received an oral dose of 25 IU/kg α-tocopherol acetate in a water-
miscible form at time zero. Gestational ages are indicated as follows:
28-37 weeks (half-filled circle), 32-36 weeks (open circle), 36-40 weeks
(triangles). Absorption patterns for children 5-16 years old (squares).

tocopherol presently on the market assure rapid repletion and correction
of the vitamin E deficiency state of the low birthweight infant. This indicates a need for an approved, parenteral preparation for physicians who
wish to treat successfully the vitamin E inadequacy of prematures.

A second category of patients who are resistant, if not refractory, to
the oral supplementation approach are those with biliary atresia and other
severe hepatobiliary disturbances leading to reduced bile acid secretion.
This group of patients provides a particularly difficult therapeutic challenge since in many instances they also receive cholestyramine resin in an
attempt to lower bilirubin levels. The efforts of Nitowsky et al. [50] and
Muller and Harries [160] to replete children with biliary obstruction, as
well as those of Woodruff [159] in an adult patient with biliary cirrhosis,
suggest that there is an absolute requirement for parenterally administered tocopherol in such subjects. Oral treatment has in fact failed to
raise blood vitamin E levels significantly in every patient described in the
literature to date fitting this category of disease.

Patients with abetalipoproteinemia are likewise difficult to supplement
orally. Nonetheless, once it became recognized that plasma levels in

these patients were not necessarily reflective of tissue concentrations, it was evident that massive doses of water-miscible tocopherol (e.g., 0.75-1.5 g/day of "emulsified" α-tocopheryl succinate) [124] suffice to increase erythrocyte vitamin E to normal levels and prevent hemolysis in vitro. It should be remembered by physicians treating patients with abetalipoproteinemia, however, that plasma tocopherol will likely remain low on the above regimen. Thus, the erythrocyte hemolysis test using hydrogen peroxide is a better index of the effectiveness of oral supplementation in ABL patients. Intramuscular injections of tocopherol (100-200 mg/week) have also been utilized in abetalipoproteinemia. Wallis et al. [182] reported that such treatment raised the plasma level of one patient to 0.74 mg/dl.

Cystic fibrosis patients with pancreatic insufficiency present less of a therapeutic challenge in regard to tocopherol supplementation. Nonetheless, in our experience [121], even CF patients require the routine use of water-miscible vitamin E preparations rather than the unmodified, fat-soluble forms. This is in accordance with the findings of Harries and Muller [116] who studied the absorption of both preparations in subjects with CF and demonstrated more efficient uptake of the water-miscible form. They found that in the absence of liver disease, daily doses of 1 mg/kg body wt were effective in correcting vitamin E deficiency within 2 months of treatment. Our results concur and indicate that for routine purposes, 25-50 IU/day is a satisfactory dose for children whereas 100-200 IU/day should be used in adolescents and young adults with CF.

As discussed previously, absorption of nutrients in CF may theoretically be affected by many factors. In keeping with findings in patients with biliary atresia and cirrhosis, it has been observed in our clinic [121] and also by Harries and Muller [116] that CF patients with hepatic involvement, which occurs in up to one-third of the cases [109], may be more difficult to replete with oral vitamin E. Such patients presumably suffer from a deficiency of bile salts in addition to their primary disturbance in the pancreatic component of digestion. Our experience indicates that CF patients with severe biliary cirrhosis poorly absorb tocopherol to such an extent that their plasma vitamin E concentrations cannot be raised to normal even with 1 g/day of the water-miscible preparations. Thus, a parenteral form of tocopherol is also required for these individuals.

Recently, an injectable vitamin E preparation has been described in the literature by Bauernfeind et al. [201] and Newmark et al. [74]. They report that the free alcohol form, rather than the acetate form, of α-tocopherol is more efficiently absorbed from tissues used for intramuscular injections. Although further investigation of this parenteral vitamin E preparation is required, results of limited trials by Johnson et al. [73] in premature infants have been encouraging and suggest that this agent may meet the requirements alluded to above. Such a preparation should prove useful in low birthweight infants and in patients having malabsorption with associated hepatobiliary disturbances. In addition, those with protein-calorie malnutrition accompanied by diarrhea and patients requiring total parenteral nutrition would likely benefit from injectable vitamin E. In any event, the parenteral approach to therapy should be studied further in the coming years and will probably become the method of choice in selected deficiency states.

III.   POSSIBLE PHARMACOLOGICAL EFFECTS

A. General

No aspect of vitamin E nutrition in human beings is currently more controversial, nor more popular among the lay public, than the possible pharmacologic role of tocopherol when taken in large dietary supplements ("megavitamin E therapy"). Impressed by the dramatic effects of vitamin E in correcting disorders of animals and encouraged by their resemblance to certain diseases in humans that defy therapeutic attempts, a number of physicians have conducted large dose trials of tocopherol for a variety of diseases. Although these clinical trials have advanced our knowledge of vitamin E in humans to some extent, they have caused considerable difficulty in interpreting the literature and have contributed to the development of a public fad for supplementary ingestion of the vitamin. Thus, despite the fact that human vitamin E deficiency is uncommon in the United States, there is good reason to believe that a large segment of the population is consuming large doses of tocopherol. Individuals taking these large amounts have generally initiated the "therapy" on their own accord without the recommendation of a physician. Just as in the case of megavitamin C ingestion, the popular fad for vitamin E has developed without scientific documentation of efficacy. Indeed, it is quite clear to those who have interviewed megavitamin E consumers [202, 203] that much of the recent popular interest has been generated by the appearance of articles in newspapers and magazines suggesting numerous medical conditions which may be alleviated by tocopherol.
    In general, the pharmacologic use of vitamins is a relatively recent development. The precise role of various essential nutrients in quantities far exceeding their daily requirements has not been established, nor have mechanisms been elucidated which explain the special physiological effects achieved. Nonetheless, widespread experience in the past several years indicates that beneficial effects may accrue from the administration of selected nutrients in doses equivalent to 10-100 times their usual intake. Examples of diseases which respond favorably to megavitamin therapy include vitamin D-resistant rickets, vitamin B_{12}-dependent methylmalonic aciduria, and the pyridoxine dependency states (a specific infantile

convulsive disorder and familial anemia) [204]. In addition, Pauling [205] has advocated the daily intake of vitamin E in gram quantities for prophy- laxis against the common cold. Finally, the analogy to the pharmacologic use of steroid hormones should be mentioned in view of the major role played by these agents in modern medical therapy. Glucocorticoids, nor- mally synthesized by the adrenal gland in small amounts and circulating in very low concentrations, are remarkably effective for the treatment of a wide spectrum of diseases [206] when administered in doses equivalent to 10-50 times their daily secretion rate. Molecular mechanisms explaining the effectiveness of megavitamin supplements remain to be elucidated. In the case of the B group vitamins which normally function as coenzymes such as pyridoxine and B_{12}, it is suspected that in the associated disease or dependency state, the affinity of the apoenzyme for its cofactor is altered due to a genetic mutation. Other possible mechanisms under study are discussed by Schriver [207].

The literature bearing on the pharmacologic use of vitamin E is volu- minous and replete with contradictory statements. Many case reports purporting to show evidence for therapeutic value do not represent con- trolled, scientific studies but rather are anecdotal descriptions at best. For this and other reasons, the author finds it necessary to select a limited number of such articles for discussion, especially those which present controlled studies involving relatively large groups of patients. It should be emphasized, however, that the attempt to select and summarize pertinent observations has been objective and that the conclusions cited are based on a critical survey of all reports which could be obtained dealing with megavitamin E supplementation.

For a detailed description of the early literature on the pharmacologic use of α-tocopherol in large doses, the reader is referred to the compre- hensive review by Marks [208]. In this article, the approach will be to focus on the most timely and seemingly most important aspect of mega- vitamin E research, viz., tocopherol "therapy" for cardiovascular disease. Relatively less attention will be given to the other disorders listed in Table 9 which, according to at least one claim per disease, are improved by the ingestion of tocopherol in large amounts. Finally, it should be mentioned that the author's tendency to discount the majority of claims for therapeutic usefulness of tocopherol is entirely attributable to the lack of documentary evidence from the proponents of megavitamin E supplementation.

From the list of diseases in Table 9, it is evident that vitamin E has been used primarily in disorders which are debilitating in terms of either physical or psychological impact. Typically, these conditions are not readily responsibe to present methods of management and thus present a frustrating challenge to physicians and patients. This aspect, probably more than any other, may account for the tendency to treat such patients

TABLE 9   Diseases Reported as "Responsive" to Pharmacologic Doses of Vitamin E

Collagen vascular diseases (e.g., lupus erythematosus)
Congestive heart failure
Cystic mastitis
Diabetic vasculitis
Fibrositis
Glomerulonephritis
Gravitational ulcers
Hypertension
Infertility
Inflammatory skin lesions
Intermittent claudication
Ischemic heart disease (arterioslcerotic heart disease)
Muscular dystrophy
Periodontal disease
Phlebitis
Purpura
Schizophrenia
Scleroderma
Spontaneous habitual abortion
Thalassemia

---

with unestablished agents such as vitamin E in large doses. It should be further stressed that the diseases listed in Table 9 are clearly distinguished from the vitamin E deficiency states described previously. Although plasma tocopherol levels have not generally been measured before or after treatment in megavitamin E studies, there is no reason to suspect from population surveys or evaluations of such patients that a reduction in blood or tissue tocopherol regularly accompanies any of these disorders.

The general pharmacology of vitamin E has been alluded to in previous subsections of this chapter and in other portions of the monograph. In particular, absorption from the gastrointestinal tract has been described in detail along with the metabolic fate of administered vitamin E. A number of tocopherol preparations for oral use are commercially available. These include capsules containing fat-soluble vitamin E [209] and those providing water-miscible forms of α-tocopheryl acetate in the presence of a variety of emulsifying agents [210]. Such capsules commonly contain 30, 50, 100, or 200 mg tocopherol, although larger doses are available from some manufacturers. Some preparations provide only the α-isomer, whereas mixed tocopherols are found in others. In addition to capsules, liquid preparations containing 50 IU/ml vitamin E may also be obtained, particularly from hospital pharmacies [210]. As mentioned previously, injectable forms of tocopherol are less available and in fact are approved for use in the United States only as investigational drugs. Injectable preparations can be utilized in other countries, however, and have occasionally been employed in clinical trials reported in the literature.

Previous discussion of the postulated functions of vitamin E has provided information relevant to potential pharmacologic actions. Although most attention has centered on either an antioxidant role or direct involvement with various enzyme systems, there are other possible biological effects which may be of importance in considering claims for efficacious use of vitamin E in the diseases in Table 9. In this context, however, it must be emphasized that tocopherols have no unequivocally established, intrinsic pharmacologic activities beyond those defined from correction of deficiency states in animals. The large body of evidence suggesting that vitamin E functions as a biological antioxidant, as reviewed elsewhere in this monograph, forms the basis for many of the present claims of therapeutic value. If oxidation of essential lipids and other substances occurs in tissues to the extent proposed by some investigators [213], vitamin E could indeed play a role in protecting cellular and subcellular membranes against free radical damage. Nonetheless, it remains to be proven that tocopherols afford such protection in the clinical setting.

Doses of vitamin E either self-prescribed or recommended by physicians vary widely. Those who report beneficial effects usually emphasize the necessity for sustained, daily dosage and feel that 200-600 mg/day α-tocopherol is effective [214, 215]. Some individuals, however, recommend an intake of 1000 IU or even 2000 IU vitamin E per day [216, 217]. A recent survey of megavitamin E consumers by Farrell and Bieri [202], in which 47 adults on self-prescribed tocopherol were interviewed, revealed an average intake of 400 IU/day.

Curiously, little information is available on the blood or tissue levels of tocopherol achieved by subjects with normal gastrointestinal function upon supplementary ingestion of vitamin E. In view of the limited capacity for tocopherol absorption from the alimentary canal, one might suspect considerable loss through fecal excretion. Indeed, it may be inferred from studies by Larsson and Haeger [215] and by Farrell and Bieri [202] that this appears to be the case. The former investigators measured plasma total tocopherol concentrations in patients with atherosclerosis receiving 300-600 mg α-tocopheryl acetate daily. These subjects, who had been taking the vitamin for 0.5-6 years, showed a mean of plasma tocopherol concentration of 3.07 mg/dl, as compared to a control group mean of 1.13 mg/dl. Larsson and Haeger also determined the tocopherol content of soleus muscle in a limited number of patients. A mean concentration of 32 μg tocopherol/g muscle was found in supplemented atherosclerotics and this value was approximately threefold greater than the levels noted in untreated patients or control subjects. For unknown reasons, however, a number of supplemented patients receiving "adequate doses of tocopherol" failed to show an increase in muscle vitamin E. The range of plasma tocopherol levels were also quite wide (0.6-5.8 mg/dl) and could not be correlated with the length of treatment.

The group of subjects consuming supplementary vitamin E who were studied by Farrell and Bieri [202] consisted mainly of federal employees at the National Institutes of Health. The 28 individuals selected for blood sampling ranged in age from 24 to 67 years and consumed the vitamin for 2.9 years on the average (range = 0.3-21 years). As mentioned previously, dosages averaged 400 IU/day with a range of 100-800 IU/day. Plasma α-tocopherol was found to be significantly (p < 0.001) elevated in the group of megavitamin E consumers with a mean ± SD of 1.34 ± 0.10 mg/dl, as compared to a control group of normal volunteers showing a level of 0.65 ± 0.14. Concentrations in the supplemented group varied widely, however, with one-fourth of the values falling within two standard deviations of the control mean. Plasma α-tocopherol levels did not correlate with either total daily dose or duration of treatment but did correlate with serum triglyceride values as shown in Fig. 10. In contrast to findings in patients with malabsorption, plasma tocopherol concentrations in megavitamin E consumers could not be related statistically to circulating carotenoid levels.

Prior to discussing the results of clinical trials where tocopherol was used in pharmacologic doses, it is perhaps worthwhile to comment on the statements of others who have previously reviewed the literature dealing with this topic. The nearly universal conclusion of individual authors and authoritarian groups is that claims for the therapeutic usefulness of large dietary supplements of vitamin E are unsubstantiated and unconvincing. Marks [208] for instance, in a thorough and critical appraisal of tocopherol treatment, noted very little in the way of sound, data-supporting efficacy, except for use in patients with intermittent claudication. Goodman and Gilman [7] likewise concluded that "there is no unequivocal evidence that vitamin E has any therapeutic use." In addition, a review of this issue by the Food and Nutrition Board [12, 218] has led to a statement that claims for the usefulness of megavitamin E ingestion are not adequately documented. Finally, from a comprehensive and impartial review of the literature, the Medical Letter on Drugs and Therapeutics [8] has recently concluded, that "there is no convincing evidence that large doses of vitamin E are effective for the prevention or treatment of heart disease or any other human disorder, except in premature infants and possibly in patients with diseases that impair fat absorption."

B. Safety of High Doses

Discussion of the pharmacology of vitamin E would be incomplete without some mention of the possible toxicity associated with ingestion of large doses. The toxicity of other fat-soluble vitamins, particularly vitamins A and D in children [219-221], has raised concern for the health of those who self-dose themselves with tocopherol. Although studies on the possible toxicity of vitamin E are extremely limited, assessment of data available in the literature leads to the impression that the likelihood of serious adverse effects from consuming 100-1000 IU/day appears to be very low [12, 214]. In the absence of careful studies on large populations of mega-vitamin E consumers, it is necessary to resort to isolated case reports. Some of these suggest the following as side effects: fatigue, dermatitis (either localized or generalized), various gastrointestinal symptoms, pruritis ani, acne, vasodilation, and impaired coagulation. These claims, however, are altogether unconvincing.

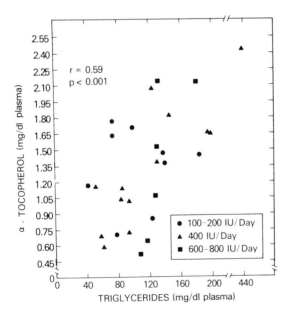

FIG. 10   α-Tocopherol levels and their relationship to serum triglycerides in subjects on megavitamin E supplementation. Note the lack of correlation between the daily dose of vitamin E and the level achieved in plasma. (Modified from Ref. 202.)

TABLE 10 Results of Selected Clinical Screening Tests in Vitamin E-
Supplemented Subjects [a]

Test	Megavitamin E group [b]	Control group [c]
Cholesterol (mg/100 ml serum)	216 (145-285)	200 (150-250)
Triglycerides (mg/100 ml serum)	126 (50-275)	100 (10-190)
Glucose (mg/100 ml plasma)	91 (52-128)	95 (70-120)
Albumin (g/100 ml serum)	4.1 (3.4-4.8)	4.1 (3.1-5.0)
Bilirubin (mg/100 ml serum)	0.5 (0.1-0.9)	0.6 (0.1-1.2)
Creatinine (mg/100 ml serum)	0.93 (0.61-1.2)	1.1 (0.7-1.5)
Thyroxin (μg/100 ml serum)	7.8 (3.4-12.2)	7.7 (4.6-10.7)
Hemoglobin (g/100 ml blood)	13.8 (12.2-15.4)	14.3 (12.5-16)
Reticulocyte count (% of RBC)	0.96 (0-2.2)	— (0-1.5)
White blood cell (WBC) count (cells/μl x 10^{-3})	5.9 (5.4-6.4)	7.7 (4.5-11)
Platelet count (platelets/μl x 10^{-3})	223 (107-339)	243 (150-334)
Prothrombin time (sec)	11.1 (9.7-12.4)	11.2 (10-12.5)
Partial thromboplastin time (sec)	32 (26-38)	31 (27-32)

[a] Figures shown represent the means followed by the 95% confidence
intervals in parentheses.
[b] This group consisted of 28 adults ranging in age from 24 to 62 years
(mean = 28) who were consuming 100-800 IU/day vitamin E for 4 months to
21 years (mean = 2.9 years).
[c] The control group consisted of 100-200 healthy adults.

In addition, it has been reported that various blood tests used for
clinical diagnostic purposes are altered in patients on high doses of
tocopherol. Careful assessment of this possibility by Farrell and Bieri
[202] failed to disclose alterations in 200 biochemical or hematologic
indices of health. In particular, the blood tests shown in Table 10 did not
reveal evidence of abnormalities in hepatic function, renal clearance,
thyroid gland function, the neuromuscular system, or bone marrow
activity. Additionally, review of the past medical histories of subjects
taking 100-800 IU/day vitamin E did not uncover any signs of toxicity [202].

Nevertheless, it is far from certain that chronic ingestion of tocopherol in large doses is entirely safe. There are several potential hazards suggested from laboratory studies with animals. In the chick for instance, depressed growth, interference with thyroid function, and increased requirements for vitamins D and K were found on high vitamin E dosage [222]. Further clinical investigations are therefore indicated on subjects ingesting supplementary tocopherol.

C. Cardiovascular Disease

1. Ischemic Heart Disease

Ischemic heart disease due to coronary arterial occlusion and manifested symptomatically as recurrent angina pectoris has emerged as the major health problem of middle-aged adult males in the United States. The physical and psychological impact of anginal chest pain is such that affected patients frequently become debilitated and economically unproductive. Although the advent in recent years of cardiac surgery techniques using vascular grafts offers a possible alternative, therapy for ischemic heart disease has traditionally depended upon the use of vasodilators such as nitroglycerin. In view of the serious nature of arteriosclerotic heart disease, it is not surprising that a number of agents such as vitamin E have come under study as "innovative" approaches to therapy.

Historically, the first claim that vitamin E could be useful in ischemic heart disease appeared in 1946 when in a brief report, Vogelsang and Shute [223] claimed that tocopherol in doses of 200-600 mg/day diminished, or in some instances completely abolished, anginal pain. One year subsequently, Shute et al. [224] reported 84 case histories of patients, 90% of whom showed reduced symptomatic manifestations of coronary occlusion after 12 weeks on vitamin E therapy. Since that time, Drs. Evan and Wilfrid Shute and their associates at the Shute Institute in London, Ontario have continued to be vociferous advocates of vitamin E treatment for cardiovascular disease [225]. Although it has now been 20 years since the Shutes first recommended α-tocopherol for angina, they have offered virtually nothing in the way of convincing new information in support of their claim. Thus, as reviewed below, the Shute Clinic appears to remain alone in advocating megavitamin E therapy for ischemic heart disease.

The dramatic claims of the Shute brothers led to early investigations attempting to confirm the purported efficacy of vitamin E. Negative reports were published within 1 year of the original article by Vogelsang and Shute [223] and continue to appear at the time of this writing. At least 17 reports contrary to their claim may be found in reviewing the literature [c.f., 226-230]. Some of these clinical trials were uncontrolled, as was the study of Shute and associates [224], whereas a number represent carefully controlled, double-blind investigations where placebo capsules were given randomly along with vitamin E. The common denominator of such investigations has been an unequivocal rejection of the claim that vitamin E is effective in the treatment of ischemic heart disease.

Relative to tocopherol therapy for anginal symptoms, the recent reports of Anderson [228] and Anderson and Reid [231] are particularly noteworthy since they describe a randomized, double-blind trial in a group of subjects in Toronto, Ontario; this population presumably corresponds closely to the patients of the Shute Clinic in terms of epidemiologic factors of importance in ischemic heart disease. In addition to assessing objectively the course of angina and carefully controlling the use of vitamin E versus placebo, Anderson [228] employed the extremely high doses (3200 IU/day) which have been advocated by the Shutes in recent years. The study criteria included evaluation of the following: (1) nitroglycerin consumption, (2) anginal status (by exercise testing and by severity of symptoms), (3) electrocardiograms, and (4) blood pressure. None of these parameters showed significant improvement in the group receiving vitamin E and no convincing evidence could be gathered in support of tocopherol ingestion for ischemic heart disease.

The study of Anderson can be criticized, however, because of the failure to determine circulating tocopherol levels, the small population of patients (20 in each group), and the greater mean nitroglycerin consumption in the vitamin E-treated subjects, suggesting the possibility of greater disease severity in this group. Further, as admitted by Anderson, the 9-week duration of the trial may not represent a sufficient time interval to establish favorable results. In this connection, the recent work of Haeger [232, 233] suggesting that several months of treatment are required for improved vascular flow in peripheral arterial disease may be pertinent. A previous double-blind trial of vitamin E supplementation for angina by Rinzler et al. [227], which also yielded negative results, may likewise be criticized for its short duration since the patients were only studied for 10-20 weeks.

In fairness to the Shutes and their associates, it must also be emphasized that because anginal pain is notoriously difficult to assess and since anxiety plays a prominent role in provoking symptoms of coronary insufficiency, major problems may be encountered in attempts either to establish or discount any antianginal medication. If the drug or its corresponding placebo is prescribed with enthusiasm by a physician, even the control group will tend to show signs of improvement. Thus, establishing a positive effect is at least as difficult as, and probably more so than, demonstrating nonefficacy. In addition, the natural course of ischemic heart disease and the symptoms thereof are sufficiently variable that large populations of subjects are required for satisfactory clinical trials. In this connection, the Shute Clinic is the only facility which has studied a large population of patients, purportedly 30,000 subjects. It is altogether regrettable that the physicians of this clinic have chosen the uncontrolled approach to medical research.

Another point which deserves comment in relationship to the difficulties encountered when attempting to establish a beneficial effect pertains to the lack of patient compliance. Widespread experience in clinical trials has demonstrated that no matter what degree of precaution is taken, participants in such studies cannot be relied upon to consume the drug according to the recommended schedule. Thus, there can be an inherent bias towards nonefficacy in any trial. Investigators studying megavitamin E supplementation should therefore always include assessment of blood tocopherol levels. It is only by this mechanism that clinical trials can exclude patients failing to comply with the study protocol.

Nonetheless, the abundance of evidence against the claim that vitamin E is effective for ischemic heart disease currently places the burden of proof on those who advocate its use for angina pectoris. Scientific caution therefore requires this author to conclude that vitamin E is of no proven value in the treatment of coronary occlusive disease. However, the persistent controversy over three decades indicates a need for further clinical research, particularly studies which are carefully controlled and include large populations of appropriate patients. The final rejection or acceptance of claims from the Shute Clinic will depend upon information derived from such investigations.

2. Peripheral Vascular Disease with Intermittent Claudication

Closely allied to the claim that megavitamin E supplementation is beneficial in ischemic heart disease are the recommendations of several physicians that tocopherol be prescribed for intermittent claudication. This symptomatic manifestation of arteriosclerotic, peripheral vascular disease may be as debilitating as recurrent angina pectoris. It afflicts the middle-aged and elderly population, particularly males, shows a variable course, and is typically treated in much the same fashion as arteriosclerotic heart disease (vasodilators, anticoagulants, and vascular surgery).

Vitamin E has been used for intermittent claudication by selective groups of physicians and clinical investigators ever since 1949 when Boyd et al. [234] presented supporting evidence in a limited group of patients. Subsequently, a large number of studies have been conducted addressing this issue and leading to a nearly continuous stream of reports. For a detailed discussion of the pertinent literature, the reader is referred to the comprehensive review by Marks [208] on the role of vitamin E in intermittent claudication. The following synthesis is based to a large extent on Marks' critical appraisal but also includes a number of more recent reports, particularly those describing objective trials where relatively large patient populations have been employed.

In general, a review of the literature on the possible pharmacological role of vitamin E in intermittent claudication leaves one with a considerably more favorable impression than is gained from reviewing studies on tocopherol treatment for ischemic heart disease. Similar difficulties are encountered, however, when investigators attempt to study vitamin E therapy for peripheral vascular disease. The predominant symptoms for instance are subjective in nature and the course shows considerable natural variability; at times, spontaneous improvement will occur without any treatment. Another difficulty encountered in assessing responses to treatment is that seasonal factors apparently modify the pain of intermittent claudication [209]. To reduce the effect of this latter variable, clinical trials should be of 1 or 2 years duration, or even longer is possible. The longer therapeutic trial period also tends to eliminate the variables introduced by the natural fluctuation in symptoms occurring during the course of the disease.

Studies showing a positive effect of supplementary tocopherol include the following: Boyd et al. [234] initially reported that 78% of 76 patients with moderately severe or severe claudication were improved with vitamin E therapy over a 6-month trial period. Subsequently, a controlled trial was conducted by Ratcliffe [235] which included objective assessment with a walking test. The results indicated that after 3 months of study, patients with moderate claudication receiving 400 mg/day tocopherol were improved in 34 of 41 cases, whereas only 5 of 25 untreated subjects showed improvement. This was followed by a trial lasting 40 weeks in which Livingstone and Jones [236] were able to document positive results in a double-blind study of 34 patients. In that group, 70% of the subjects receiving vitamin E (600 mg/day) showed signs of improvement, whereas only 10% receiving placebo showed a difference in disease manifestations. In addition, Williams et al. [237] reported improvement in 19 of 30 patients with femoral-popliteal occlusion after vitamin E therapy, whereas only 2 of 15 subjects on a placebo preparation showed improvement. More recently, Haeger [232, 233] has observed a significant increase in walking distance and arterial flow in patients with intermittent claudication receiving 300 mg α-tocopheryl acetate per day for 2-5 years.

On the other hand, negative studies have also been published along with negative anecdotal comments by physicians who conducted small trials [238]. Baer and Heine [239] and Hamilton et al. [240] both failed to observe improvement in double-blind trials conducted over a 3-month period. Unfortunately, the short duration of treatment precludes valid assessment of their results since the nature of the disease is such that a lag period of several months often occurs before improvement is noted with any modification in therapy. Indeed, even the proponents of tocopherol treatment for intermittent claudication emphasize the delay before significant responses are evident. For example, Haeger [232, 233] did not observe improvement

in walking distance until 3-4 months after vitamin E supplementation
began; likewise, a statistically significant increase in arterial flow was
not documented until after 12-18 months. Accordingly, the negative
reports of Baer and Heine [239] and Hamilton et al. [240] can be given
relatively less weight in comparison to other trials.

The investigations of Haeger [232,233] and Larsson and Haeger [215]
deserve further consideration herein since they provide objective assessment of tocopherol levels and functional responses to treatment. With
regard to ambulatory function, Haeger used a simple walking test where
distance traveled before the onset of calf pain is measured. He reported
a significantly increased walking distance in 33 patients treated with
vitamin E, whereas only 3 of 14 subjects managed by conventional approaches showed improvement. Arterial flow in the calf muscles of
patients with intermittent claudication was also measured by Haeger using
venous occlusion plethysmography. In these studies, the "first flow" after
release of obstruction [24] was chosen as the index of circulatory function.
The results in milliliters of blood flow per 100 grams of muscle per
minute, are reproduced graphically in Fig. 11. From such measurements
the following conclusions emerged: (1) initial flow was reduced in the
treated and control groups to a similar degree; (2) after 20-25 months, the
patients not receiving tocopherol showed a mild, further reduction in flow;
and (3) after the same period, subjects receiving 300 mg of α-tocopheryl
acetate per day demonstrated a significant increase in first flow. The
effect in the vitamin E-treated group is particularly impressive since 91%
(29 of 32 subjects) showed evidence of improved circulation after treatment.

The results of plasma and muscle tocopherol determinations by
Larsson and Haeger [215] have been described previously. Although not
all of the subjects receiving vitamin E demonstrated elevated plasma
tocopherol levels, 80% of the treated patients displayed values greater
than the 95% confidence interval of the control group, i.e., greater than
2 mg/dl plasma. Similarly, it was determined that some patients showed
no increase in soleus muscle tocopherol content, despite the fact that the
treated group as a whole manifested a statistically significant, threefold
increase in muscle tocopherol concentration. Larsson and Haeger were
further able to compare in 15 patients the clinical results from walking
tests with the levels of muscle tocopherol achieved. Interestingly, a
statistical relationship ($r = 0.55$) was noted between improvement in
ambulatory capability and the amounts of vitamin E per gram of muscle.
This correlation offers additional evidence in favor of tocopherol treatment
but requires confirmation.

In summary, it must be stated that although further clinical trials are
indicated, the majority of investigations support the use of vitamin E in
intermittent claudication of moderate severity, i.e., at least grade II of
the Boyd classification [234]. To recount the evidence in favor of this
recommendation:

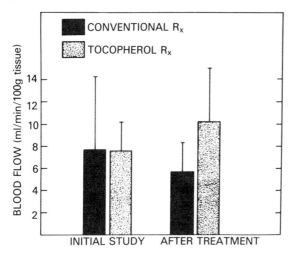

FIG. 11   The effect of vitamin E administration on arterial blood flow in the lower leg of patients with intermittent claudication. Venous occlusion plethysmography was utilized by Haeger [232] to measure "first flow" [241] and obtain these data; normal values in milliliters per minute per gram of tissue range from 14 to 40 (mean = 27). Vitamin E-treated subjects received 300 mg α-tocopheryl acetate per day for 20-25 months before reevaluation, while the control patients were given only vasodilator and anticoagulant medications.

1. Tocopherol has given satisfactory results in open clinical series where long periods of observation have been utilized.

2. Double-blind trials support the significant differences between treated and placebo groups.

3. Functional improvement, as evidenced by an increased walking distance, has been observed with treatment.

4. Arterial blood flow is improved after a sufficient period of treatment.

5. Correlation has been observed between dose and response.

6. As reviewed in Sec. III. B, toxicity has not been apparent in the dose ranges recommended.

7. There is limited evidence that lower morbidity and mortality result from the use of tocopherol in such patients [208].

3. Other Cardiovascular Disorders

Tocopherol therapy has also been evaluated in patients with congestive heart failure. However, Donegan et al. [242] and Levy and Boas [243] found that the course of a heterogenous group of patients with decompensated heart disease could not be favorably influenced by providing supplementary tocopherol. There has been insufficient follow-up of isolated reports that vitamin E is useful in the treatment of diabetic vasculitis, glomerulonephritis, congenital heart disease, and hypertension. Some physicians suggest that tocopherol sensitizes the myocardium to digitalis and thus might promote digitalis intoxication [244]; others discount this possibility [245].

Vitamin E has also been utilized in an attempt to lessen or prevent intravascular thrombus formation, particularly prior to and after extensive surgical procedures. Some investigators, notably Osner et al. [246,247], report favorable results, whereas others have failed to observe such a relationship. Since thrombus formation leading to pulmonary embolism is a major problem in bedridden, postoperative patients, tocopherol would have obvious importance if it were truly efficacious in this regard.

4. Possible Mechanisms of Action in Cardiovascular Disease

Those who discount the use of tocopherol in cardiovascular disease sometimes resort to the argument that vitamin E displays no mechanism of action which might account for beneficial effects. This position is only superficially sound in view of the fact that the whole issue of tocopherol's biological function remains to be resolved (see Chapters 5E.1 to 5E.3). Nonetheless, proponents of vitamin E therapy recognize the need to offer some potential mechanism of action which might facilitate blood flow and improve the circulation to relevant tissues such as cardiac muscle. In addition to a possible vasodilator effect, for which there is no evidence, other actions of tocopherol have been postulated in the literature which might influence the vascular system, albeit indirectly. For practical purposes, these may be divided into two categories: (1) a cholesterol-lowering effect and (2) an anticoagulation influence.

With regard to altering blood lipid concentrations, it is pertinent to mention that patients with intermittent claudication, as well as those with ischemic heart disease, tend to show elevations in various lipid constituents of serum such as cholesterol. Few clinical investigators, however, have addressed the issue of whether or not vitamin E administration in large doses might lower circulating cholesterol levels. Some have reported decreased levels [248], whereas other workers claim the opposite [249], and still others [250] have found no change. In their recent study of a group of volunteers ingesting large doses of tocopherol, Farrell and Bieri [202] found normal mean levels of serum cholesterol and triglycerides.

On the other hand, a number of studies bearing on coagulation factors during high-dose tocopherol supplementation have appeared in the literature. Evidence suggesting that vitamin E might interfere with the coagulation process surfaced as early as 1945 when Wolley and associates [251] reported that tocopherol shows "anti-vitamin K activity." Subsequently, Zierler et al. [252] reported that α-tocopheryl phosphate in physiological concentrations inhibits the action of thrombin in vitro. In this connection, it is pertinent to note that a coagulopathy associated with an apparent reduction in vitamin K-dependent clotting factors was observed by Corrigan and Marcus [253] in a patient voluntarily consuming 1200 IU vitamin E daily for 2 months. Discontinuation of tocopherol resulted in the development of a normal coagulation profile.

Perhaps the most provocative studies attempting to link tocopherol with reduced blood coagulability have come from investigators concerned with platelet function. Machlin and associates [254, 255] have reported that vitamin E-deficient rats show increased platelet aggregation. In addition, when the animals were maintained on deficient diets for at least 15 weeks, an elevated mean platelet count was noted. This observation is in agreement with that of Melhorn and Gross [81] who reported that tocopherol-deficient infants tend to show high platelet counts which can be reduced to normal levels following administration of vitamin E. Farrell and Bieri [202] examining a series of 28 adults on megavitamin E supplementation did not assess platelet aggregation but found only two subjects with reduced platelet counts. In another clinical study, Korsan-Bengtsen et al. [256] observed a highly significant prolongation of the plasma clotting time, but unaltered platelet numbers and adhesiveness, in nine males who ingested 300 mg/day α-tocopherol for 6 weeks. From the measurement of several clotting factors, they concluded that reduced platelet factor 3 activity was probably responsible for the alteration in clotting time.

Further in vitro studies addressing the possible role of vitamin E in platelet function have recently been reported by Steiner and Anastasi [257]. They found that addition of α-tocopherol to platelet suspensions resulted in a dose-dependent reduction in platelet aggregation. The "secondary wave" of aggregation was found to be completely inhibited by vitamin E. High levels of vitamin in vivo reduced platelet aggregation [257a]. When 1800 IU of vitamin E was consumed daily collagen-induced aggregation was reduced 50%.

The proposal that tocopherol is involved in platelet function is an attractive one since decreased platelet aggregation could conceivably explain several of the clinical observations relative to amelioration of cardiovascular disease by vitamin E. Further, there is evidence that lipid peroxides can accumulate in aged platelets, a phenomenon prevented by the presence of α-tocopherol [258]. In addition, recent data from Nordoy and Strom [259] indicate that platelets have a high content of vitamin E in comparison to plasma and red cells; this is in keeping with the large amounts of unsaturated fatty acids present in the lipid fraction of platelets.

Of further interest relative to the above is the proposal that peroxides are involved in the synthesis of prostaglandin E_2 from arachidonate and that this process may stimulate platelet aggregation [254]. Since antioxidants such as tocopherol are capable of interrupting peroxidation reactions, vitamin E could conceivably interfere with platelet aggregation through this mechanism.

Thus, data are being accumulated implicating vitamin E as a anticoagulation substance acting through blood platelets. Additional studies will be required, however, to confirm the initial findings and assess their clinical implications. Nonetheless, if this role of tocopherol as a potential anticoagulant becomes established, it could be utilized as a strong argument for the administration of vitamin E in selected vascular occlusive diseases.

D. Other Proposed Pharmacological Uses

1. Spontaneous Abortion

The long-appreciated disturbances in fetal development noted in animal pregnancies led to an early exploration of a possible use of vitamin E in pregnant women with a history of habitual, spontaneous abortion. Although this proposed prophylactic use of tocopherol was apparently accepted by many obstetricians in the 1940s and 1950s, sound evidence supporting such treatment is lacking. Because of the many interrelated variables and the necessity at times to intervene with established modes of management, considerable difficulty has been encountered in attempting to conduct controlled studies of vitamin E in pregnancy.

In 1940 Bacharach [260] analyzed the earliest data on the use of vitamin E therapy for habitual abortion and reported that the purported improvement in fetal outcome could be verified statistically in patients treated with tocopherol. Subsequently, Marks [208] from a review of other studies also concluded that the evidence favored tocopherol supplementation for pregnant women with habitual abortions. None of the clinical investigations cited by Bacharach or Marks, however, fulfill even the minimal criteria for a controlled trial.

Another approach to assessing the possible role of tocopherol in spontaneous abortion has been the determination of circulating vitamin E levels in groups of pregnant women with normal or pathological outcomes. As discussed previously, it has been established that blood tocopherol levels normally increase in a steady fashion from the first few weeks of pregnancy until delivery. An extensive survey by Ferguson et al. [39], in which 1611 pregnant women were evaluated, revealed that patients with previous spontaneous abortions and other pathological conditions did not show significant abnormalities in blood tocopherol. Other surveys have likewise disclosed a general lack of tocopherol deficiency in pregnant women [261].

On the other hand, a recent study by Vobecky et al. [40] suggests that pregnancies leading to abortions and stillbirths may be associated with unexpected decreases in serum tocopherol levels during late gestation. With serum tocopherol serving as the main index of nutrition, these workers undertook a longitudinal study to investigate the pattern of biochemical changes in pregnancies having pathological outcomes. Although the number of women evaluated was limited, it was observed that (1) their circulating tocopherol levels tended to fall in the third trimester, and (2) the group delivering stillbirths showed a significantly reduced mean serum tocopherol concentration (0.72 mg/dl) in late pregnancy.

In conclusion, it must be stated that further evidence is needed before one can recommend megavitamin E supplementation for pregnant women with a past history of spontaneous abortions.

2. Cystic Mastitis

Chronic cystic mastitis is a relatively common, benign lesion of the female breast which gives rise to symptoms of pain and tenderness. These manifestations vary in severity and may spontaneously regress in many instances. At times, the pain and tenderness appear and disappear in a cyclical fashion. Although cystic mastitis is a benign condition, its symptoms raise considerable concern on the part of those afflicted as does the evidence (albeit, highly contentious) suggesting an association with later development of mammary carcinoma [262].

The intense discomfort of some women with this disease has led to a number of therapeutic adventures of questionable basis, such as clinical trials with vitamin E. Although positive results with tocopherol therapy have been claimed [262, 263], the evidence is anecdotal at best and remains to be substantiated in a controlled trial. It should be further stressed that fibrocystic mammary disease is almost universally accepted as resulting from an exaggeration and distortion of the cyclic breast changes that normally occur in the menstral cycle. In fact, the term chronic cystic mastitis is a misnomer since the disease is not invariably chronic, not always cystic, and certainly not an inflammatory condition.

3. Thalassemia

Recent investigations in several countries have focused attention on the vitamin E status of patients with β-thalassemia major. In two series reported to date [264, 265], statistically significant reductions in circulating tocopherol have been documented in children with this disease. Zannos-Mariolea and associates [264] in Greece reported that 56 children with thalassemia major showed a mean ± SD tocopherol concentration in

serum of 0.53 ± 0.24 mg/dl in comparison to a group of normal children
who had a corresponding level of 0.83 ± 0.25 (p   0.001). Approximately
half of the thalassemia group showed tocopherol values less than 0.5 mg/dl.
Erythrocyte hemolysis in the presence of hydrogen peroxide was abnormal
in each thalassemia patient tested. The degree of hemolysis, however,
did not correlate with blood tocopherol levels and a large number of subjects with normal vitamin E status also demonstrated enhanced hemolysis
in vitro. Hyman et al. [265] subsequently evaluated 13 patients with
β-thalassemia major and reported a mean serum tocopherol content of
0.48 mg/dl in comparison to a control mean of 1.26 mg/dl (p < 0.01).
The association of thalassemia major and susceptibility of erythrocytes to
oxidative damage in vitro was also noted by Stocks et al. [266]. This is
apparently not the case for thalassemia intermedia and thalasemia minor
according to results obtained by Melhorn et al. [55] in a limited series of
patients. Serial biopsies of skin, liver, thyroid, and testes by Hyman
et al. [265] in thalassemic patients revealed many tissues with pigment
accumulation resembling ceroid deposition.

Assessment of the absorption of orally administered tocopherol has
been carried out in eight patients with thalassemia [265]. The results suggested that there was no defect in intestinal transport. This finding is
consistent with the notion that chronic disease per se and poor dietary
habits, rather than malabsorption, cause low vitamin E levels in these
patients. It is pertinent to mention in this regard that patients with
thalassemia major tend to have poor appetites and reduced food intake.
Another possible explanation for diminished blood tocopherol levels in
thalassemia is decreased circulating lipids, as has also been noted by
some investigators [266].

An important issue relative to vitamin E and β-thalassemia major
concerns the question of whether or not such patients should be treated
with supplementary tocopherol. The argument can be raised that excess
serum and tissue iron which occurs in thalassemia as a consequence of
multiple blood transfusions might increase the need for vitamin E.
Although controlled, long-term trials of vitamin E administration in pharmacologic doses remain to be carried out, Hyman et al. [265] comment
that "vitamin E therapy did not effect transfusion requirements" in a short-
term study. In addition, Modell et al. [268], after treating affected
children for periods up to 1 year with large doses of vitamin E, reported
that such a regimen had little effect on either the hemoglobin pattern or the
blood transfusion requirements. Modell and associates also comment that
the serum level of vitamin E showed no relationship to the severity of
hemolysis nor to the degree of iron overloading. Thus, there is no sound
basis at present for recommending tocopherol supplementation in thalassemia, but rather a need for further clinical research.

4. Wound Healing, Gravitational Ulcers, and Peridontal Disease

The above conditions are included under a single heading since they all can be discussed in relation to a proposed antiinflammatory property of vitamin E. As in the case of other diseases where pharmacologic doses of tocopherol have been studied, the information available on antiinflammatory activity is scant and comes largely from uncontrolled trials. Studies in animals by Ehrlich et al. [269] indicate that vitamin E given in large doses resembles corticosteroids in retarding wound healing as measured by tensile strength and accumulation of collagen. In addition, studies with infectious agents in rats support the concept that tocopherol interferes with the development of inflammatory lesions [270]. Corresponding effects in humans remain to be documented in a scientific fashion.

Stasis ulcers have been reported to benefit from supplementary tocopherol treatment as reviewed previously by Marks [208]. The positive reports have been unconvincing and include only a limited number of patients. Further, there have been negative trials of vitamin E for peripheral ulcers [271], leaving this possible role to be studied further.

The influence of vitamin E supplementation on human periodontal disease has been reviewed by Goodson [272]. The evidence for a beneficial effect of tocopherol includes reduced tooth mobility and a lowered sulcus fluid volume. These effects could presumably be attributable to an antiinflammatory action, if vitamin E possessed such activity. Further information on this possible role is also required before recommendations for treatment can be issued.

5. Exercise

Several reports have appeared relating supplementary tocopherol to improved athletic performance in humans as well as animals [273, 274]. The subjective nature of the evaluations in early studied, as well as the small doses utilized and the failure to allow for an athletic training effect, make it impossible to attach credence to this claim. More recently, Sharman et al. [275] conducted a double-blind trial using more objective techniques of evaluation and allowing for the effects of training on athletic ability. It was observed that a group of subjects receiving 400 mg α-tocopheryl acetate daily showed no improvement in muscular performance, whereas training had a significant effect. Because the study of Sharman and associates represents the most carefully designed and conducted trial addressing this issue, it must be concluded that the best available evidence does not support the hypothesis that megavitamin E supplementation leads to increased exercise tolerance.

6. Porphyria

Nair and associates [277] have reported that administration of supplementary vitamin E to a limited number of patients with porphyria resulted in
reduced excretion of porphyrin and its precursors. This occurred following a 6-week period in which water-miscible tocopherol was given in
dose of 100 mg/day. Subsequently, Watson et al. [277] have repeated the
evaluation but were unable to confirm their earlier findings. Further,
they point out that the effect observed in the patients of Nair and associates
was slight and probably not of clinical significance. In addition, Mustajoki
[278] failed to demonstrate any influence of vitamin E on porphyrin metabolism in five patients with porphyria. Therefore, the majority of the
evidence supports the position that tocopherol administration is ineffective
in this disease.

7. Pulmonary Oxidant Toxicity

It has been suggested that vitamin E may protect the bronchopulmonary
system from the toxicity associated with exposure to (1) oxygen in high
concentrations, (2) ozone, or (3) organic pollutants in the atmosphere
[279]. This possibility, to the author's knowledge, has not been studied
directly in humans.

8. Aging

The possibility that vitamin E supplements might retard the aging process
has come under consideration in relationship to the free radical theory of
aging [280]. Data addressing this proposal have been gathered in rodents
where the lifespan of the species is relatively short. Studies in humans,
however, have not been forthcoming and will be extremely difficult to
conduct.

IV. NUTRITIONAL REQUIREMENTS

A. Survey Status

The lack of a dramatic expression or consistent clinical syndrome in
vitamin E-deficient humans has been raised as an argument that there is
no biological requirement for tocopherol in human beings. This position
can no longer be considered tenable in view of the results of the Elgin
Project and the collective observations on premature infants and patients
with intestinal malabsorption. Thus, the relevant question for discussion
at this time is not whether humans require tocopherol, but rather how
much is needed to prevent "deficiency." In the absence of precise,
sensitive mechanisms for identifying effects of the deficiency state,

estimates of dietary requirements, and hence recommended allowances, must be based to a large extent on surveys of blood tocopherol levels and the average daily consumption in typical diets. The results of population and dietary surveys may be compared to experimental data on requirements in laboratory animals for the purpose of extrapolating to a requirement level in humans. Reliance on findings in animals, however, is risky and should not be used except in the context of a guide for defining human needs.

Because surveys of blood tocopherol concentrations in the North American population have been of great importance in arriving at a definition of the human being's requirement for vitamin E, it is pertinent to review the results of such investigations (see Sec. II.A for additional detail). Before doing so, however, the following caution mentioned previously must be interjected once again: since tocopherols in plasma are associated with lipids and distributed according to the fat content of each lipoprotein fraction, the capacity of the noncellular portion of blood to carry vitamin E is highly dependent upon its lipid content. Thus, it has been well documented [21, 202] that plasma tocopherol levels correlate with plasma cholesterol or total lipid concentrations, particularly the latter. In fact, the concentration of total tocopherols in plasma is sufficiently dependent upon circulating lipids that a given value for the former may be meaningless if not accompanied by an estimate of plasma lipids. Unfortunately, all large population surveys to date have measured plasma or serum tocopherols alone and have not recorded these as a function of lipid levels.

With these limitations in mind, the results of selected evaluations of healthy, control subjects are presented in Fig. 1 and Table 11. Data from the large surveys of Harris et al. [27] and Bieri et al. [28] indicate that the normal mean level of tocol tocopherols in adult serum or plasma equals 1.05 mg/dl but that the range is wide. As discussed previously relative to Fig. 1, the values essentially follow a normal distribution for adults with the two standard deviation range being 0.50-1.6 mg/dl. Since the total lipid concentration in adult serum averages 0.6 g/dl, a normal mean ratio of 1.8 mg tocopherol per gram of total lipid can be readily calculated. This represents more than twice the level which Horwitt et al. [21] consider minimal in accordance with their estimates of blood lipids in the Elgin Project.

From the results listed for adults in Table 11, it is evident that the mean level of total tocopherols found in serum or plasma ranges from 0.7 to 1.2 mg/dl in the surveys conducted to date. Analyzing the data collectively, it may be concluded that the weighted average concentration in the 1001 North American adults evaluated was 1.0 mg/dl. If greater than 0.5 mg/dl is accepted as the definition of vitamin E adequacy, it appears upon reviewing available figures that approximately 7% of the adult

TABLE 11 Blood Tocopherol Concentrations in Random Populations of Control Subjects: Results of Selected Surveys

Investigator(s)	N[a]	Serum or plasma tocopherol (mg/dl)[b]	Population evaluated
Total tocopherols			
Binder et al. [115]	8	0.71 ± 0.16	Adults
Baker et al. [281]	630	0.90 ± 0.30	Children (10–13 years old)
Bieri et al. [28]	132	1.05 ± 0.26	Adults (17–55 years old)
Bennent and Medwadowski [282]	19	0.81 ± 0.17	Children (2–10 years old)
Bunnell et al. [202]	30	1.01 ± 0.20	Adults (20–40 years old)
Chieffi and Kirk [283]	188	0.98 ± 0.30	Adults (16–101 years old)
Darby et al. [163]	10	1.06 ± 0.06	Adults
Ferguson et al. [39]	74	0.89 ± 0.20	Adults
Goldbloom [114]	36	$0.77 \ (0.53–1.32)^{c}$	Adults
Goldbloom [114]	58	$0.62 \ (0.28–1.06)^{c}$	Children (2–12 years old)
Gordon et al. [112]	46	0.73 ± 0.19	Children (2–12 years old)
Harris et al. [27]	197	1.05 ± 0.32	Adults (17–64 years old)
Harris et al. [284]	70	1.04 ± 0.30	Young adults
Hillman and Rosner [285]	14	0.83 ± 0.39	Adults (22–40 years old)
Klatskin and Krehl [000]	23	1.23 ± 0.31	Adults (20–40 years old)
Lemley et al. [287]	21	1.09 ± 0.17	Adults (15–88 years old)
Leonard et al. [162]	17	0.74 ± 0.21	Adults
Levine et al. [30]	17	0.53 ± 0.13	Children (2–10 years old)

Levine et al. [30]	21	0.79 ± 0.20	Young adults
McWhirter [29]	13	0.75 ± 0.24	Children (4–6 years old)
McWhirter [29]	14	0.92 ± 0.28	Children (8–10 years old)
Muller et al. [120]	21	0.80 ± 0.18	Children
Nitowsky et al. [50]	15	0.75 ± 0.15	Adults
Postel [288]	30	1.20 ± 0.22	Adults (19–68 years old)
Quaife and Harris [289]	17	1.20 ± 0.22	Young adults
Scrimshaw et al. [290]	17	1.05 ± 0.27	Young adults
Urbach et al. [291]	30	1.08 ± 0.29	Adults
Wechsler et al. [292]	12	0.96 ± 0.33	Young adults (23–30 years old)
Witting and Lee [293]	24	1.09 ± 0.25	Young adults (20–23 years old)
α –Tocopherol			
Bieri and Prival [25]	40	0.92 ± 0.30	Adults
Farrell and Bieri [202]	18	0.65 ± 0.14	Young adults
Farrell et al. [144]	11	0.73 ± 0.25	Young adults
Herting and Drury [294]	37	0.36 ± 0.02	Adults
Underwood and Denning [117]	41	0.76 ± 0.17	Young adults
Wo and Draper [295]	62	0.81 ± 0.26	Children (6–17 years old)
Wo and Draper [295]	54	1.21 ± 0.57	Adults

a Number of subjects evaluated.
b Mean ± SD.
c Range is shown since SD was not reported.

population falls below this level [27]. Although concentrations less than
0.5 mg/dl correlate with a tendency for erythrocyte hemolysis to occur in
the presence of hydrogen peroxide, it must be kept in mind that subjects
with relatively low blood lipid levels are not necessarily deficient in
vitamin E and do not always show in vitro hemolysis [30].

The investigations presented in Fig. 1 and Table 11 have dealt primarily with young and middle-aged adults and there is a need to assess the
pediatric and geriatric populations in more detail. Surveys on infants and
children discussed previously (see Sec. II.A) have disclosed lower plasma
total tocopherol concentrations in agreement with, but not entirely attributable to, the lower blood lipid content [29,30]. In addition, some evidence
suggests that plasma tocopherol levels increase with age, probably because
of elevated blood lipids [283].

Dietary surveys of tocopherol levels have been limited in number but
have yielded fairly consistent results. Because the recently revised
Recommended Dietary Allowance for vitamin E has been established
according to the amounts present in balanced diets, the importance of
accurately measuring the tocopherol content of the "average" diet cannot
be overemphasized. The results of five such studies designed to determine the daily consumption of vitamin E are listed in Table 12 which also
provides a description of the diet. Harris and Embree [296] first recorded
data on the tocopherol content and PUFA level of isolated foodstuffs available for consumption, although they did not actually measure these
substances in representative diets. They calculated that foods marketed
in 1960 would provide 14.9 mg or 22.4 IU α-tocopherol daily. Bunnell
et al. [297] followed this report in 1965 with an analysis of a variety of
foods from eight typical breakfasts, lunches, and dinners. These investigators reported an average daily α-tocopherol content of 7.4 mg and a
range from 2.6 to 15.4 mg. More recently, Slover [299] published values
for three categories of foods (natural, processed, and prepared for
immediate consumption) and provided data on the distribution of the tocopherol isomers. He also pointed out, as supported by additional studies
[300], that techniques used for processing various dietary elements lead to
a significant reduction in tocopherol content.

In a key study dealing with the tocopherol consumption of working
adults, Bieri and Evarts [24] focused attention on the amount of vitamin E
ingested daily by analyzing composite samples of foods from a hospital
cafeteria in Maryland. These investigators selected meals representative
of a variety of eating habits, ranging from low to high caloric content and
varying in the amount of fat supplied. They also measured the PUFA con-
tent of the diets and evaluated the α-, γ-, and δ-isomers of tocopherol.
From this survey, it was determined that the average α-tocopherol intake
per day was 9.0 mg with a range of 4.4-12.7 mg. This may be extrapolated
to an average intake of 13.5 IU vitamin E with corresponding range figures

TABLE 12 Estimated Average Daily Intakes of Vitamin E and PUFA in North America

Type of diet or foods evaluated	α-Tocopherol (mg)		Other tocopherols average (mg)	PUFA average (g)	Reference number
	Average	Range			
1. Major classes of foods available to the average U.S. consumer in 1960	14.9[a]	–[b]	–[b]	24.2	296
2. Prepared foods corresponding to a "typical" U.S. diet of 1965	7.4	2.6-15.4	–[b]	–[b]	297
3. Representative breakfasts and lunches of 1972 from a U.S. hospital cafeteria	9.0	4.4-12.7	29.2[c]	21.2	24
4. Convenience dinners and composite Canadian diets of 1973 (processed foods)	6.4	–[b]	–[b]	12.4	298
5. Representative prepared meals from a U.S. college dormitory cafeteria (1975)	7.5	2.9-15.3	21.2[d]	19.5	293

[a] Calculated for a "representative" diet from published values on the tocopherol content of major food classes; no allowance made for losses in processing and cooking.
[b] Data not reported.
[c] 77% γ-tocopherol and 23% δ-tocopherol.
[d] 83% γ-tocopherol and 17% δ-tocopherol.

figures of 6.6 IU and 19.1 IU. It is of considerable interest to note that
γ-tocopherol rather than the α-isomer was the predominant vitamer in
these diets leading to a 20% contribution by γ-tocopherol to the total
vitamin E activity of the diet (see Table 12). In addition, Bieri and Evarts
[123] also reported that the relative content of γ-tocopherol in human
tissues was considerably higher in 1973 as compared with previous assess-
ments in 1949 [301] and 1958 [302]. This finding emphasizes the importance of making appropriate allowance for γ-tocopherol in calculating the
dietary intake and requirement of humans.

Witting and Lee [293] recently utilized an approach similar to that of
Bieri and Evarts [24] and analyzed the tocopherol content of 17 representative diets fed to female students in a college dining hall in Texas. It
was found that the total tocopherol consumption averaged 28.7 mg/day and
was comprised of 60% γ-, 25% α-, and 12% δ-tocopherols. The intakes
of α-tocopherol ranged from 2.9-15.3 mg/day and averaged 7.5 mg/day.
This corresponds to an average consumption of 14 IU vitamin E per day,
allowing for the activity of isomers other than α-isomers.

The dietary survey results of Bieri and Evarts [24] and Witting and
Lee [293] challenge the calculated values of Harris and Embree [296] and
suggest that considerably less vitamin E is actually being consumed in the
United States than was suspected when the original recommended allowances were established. In fact, the determined average daily consumption of vitamin E in adults from the Maryland and Texas surveys is less
than half the 30 IU recommended for male adults by the Food and Nutrition
Board in 1965. Still lower dietary intakes have been found elsewhere. In
assessing a composite Canadian diet providing 2780 calories/day,
Thompson et al. [298] found an α-tocopherol concentration of 6.4 mg.
This level approximates the value of 5 mg/day found by Smith et al. [303]
in their appraisal of meals ingested by patients in a British hospital. It
must be mentioned, however, that the diets evaluated by Smith and associates were of marginal quality with respect to various nutrients and were
not representative of the average American diet in terms of caloric content
and PUFA level.

B. Recommended Dietary Allowances

The Recommended Dietary Allowances or RDA are determined for each
essential nutrient and published by the Committee on Dietary Allowances
of the Food and Nutrition Board (National Academy of Sciences, National
Research Council). These figures are greatly emphasized by educators
and are extensively cited in the literature; however, they have been frequently misinterpreted. For this reason, a brief description of the nature
of the RDA is appropriate before discussing requirements for vitamin E in
selected population groups in the United States.

Recommended Dietary Allowances are defined as "levels of intake of essential nutrients considered . . . on the basis of available scientific knowledge to be adequate to meet the known nutritional needs of almost every healthy person" [218,304,305]. The recommendation therefore refers to the amount of a given nutrient that should be consumed without considering losses during food processing. Moreover, the RDA for vitamins pertain specifically to maintenance of health and not to additional needs associated with illness. Further, the levels recommended by the Food and Nutrition Board are not meant to be "optimal" nor "ideal" intakes; rather, they represent the average requirements for almost every healthy person. Thus, the RDA are estimates of amounts of essential nutrients that an average individual in the American population must consume in order to provide reasonable assurance that physiological needs will be met. They only apply to individuals already healthy and make no allowance for repletion of exhausted stores. Relative to premature infants, previously untreated patients with intestinal malabsorption, and those with protein-calorie malnutrition, the RDA figures for vitamin E are clearly not applicable. Low birthweight infants have in fact been excluded from consideration by the most recent Committee on Dietary Allowances.

Scientists serving on the Food and Nutrition Board must exercise judgment in defining adequacy of intake, particularly when information available on a nutrient is imprecise and of questionable reliability. Because judgment plays an important role in the decision, RDA figures can readily become a source of contention. Indeed, the lowering of the RDA for vitamin E by 50% in 1974 has already promoted a lively controversy.

Although RDA were first published in 1943, it was not until 1968 that vitamin E was included on the roster [306]. It must be understood that satisfactory data on average dietary consumption were unavailable to the committee responsible for issuing the first recommendations relative to vitamin E intake. Thus, the first specifications for α tocopherol were based to a large extent on extrapolation from animal studies and on information concerning the vitamin E intake of subjects studied in the Elgin Project [307] (see Sec. II.C.f). Specifically, the extrapolation of Harris [308] on vitamin E requirements by 11 different animals was utilized in establishing the first RDA. Taking the observation that a good relationship existed between the average tocopherol requirement and the 0.75 power of body weight, the following formula was derived:

$$\text{IU required} = (1.25)(\text{kg body wt})^{0.75}$$

The 1.25 correction factor is derived from Harris's observations [308]. Calculations with the above formula revealed an estimate of 5 IU

for infants and 30 IU for a 64-kg man. These figures were included as the
first RDA for vitamin E. Soon after the publication of these recommendations, however, it became recognized that the average composition of
American diets is such that 30 IU/day could only be provided if the diet was
highly enriched in PUFA. Data from the Elgin Project may have been misleading in retrospect because subjects during the later stages of the study
were consuming diets now recognized as unusual in their high content of
polyunsaturated fat. Thus, the RDA figures issued for tocopherol in 1968
were unrealistically high. In fact, few diets adequate in all other nutrients
meet the allowance originally recommended for vitamin E.

In order to correct the unattainable allowances and to reflect the
present level of PUFA consumption, as well as the known distribution of
tocopherol isomers in current diets, the most recent Committee on Dietary
Allowances significantly lowered the RDA for vitamin E. The present
values are listed in Table 13. In deriving these levels of recommended
average daily intake, allowance was made for the contribution of isomers
other than α-tocopherol, principally the γ-vitamer. The Committee
stressed the view that a fixed recommendation for any age and sex group is
not realistic but that a range of 10-20 IU total vitamin E activity should be
present in adult diets supplying 1800-3000 calories. It was further acknowledged that a high intake of PUFA can increase vitamin E requirements.
Fortunately, most oils that contain large amounts of polyunsaturates are
also relatively high in vitamin E [181].

In addition, the 1975 Food and Nutrition Board report [218] has specifically pointed out that since the fatty acid composition of tissues can be
influenced by the type of dietary fat, it is not possible to establish a fixed
allowance for a desirable ratio of vitamin E:PUFA. Such a posture represents somewhat of a departure from the view maintained by many nutritional scientists during the 1960s when considerable emphasis was placed
on vitamin E:PUFA relationships. Relying on the data of Harris and
Embree [296] suggesting that a figure of 0.6 mg α-tocopherol per gram of
dietary PUFA might enable one to set a fixed ratio, earlier authors paid
considerable attention to this guideline in attempting to define dietary vitamin E adequacy [308,309]. Subsequently, from evaluations of many
species, it has become apparent that a constant E:PUFA ratio cannot be
reliably specified [12,181]. In this connection, it is noteworthy that
according to the recent dietary surveys [24,293] described in Table 12, the
ratio in the average American diet approximates 0.4 mg α-tocopherol per
gram of PUFA. This is of course less than the 0.6 level which was prematurely accepted before adequate experimental confirmation [309].
Because of the limitations in the E:PUFA ratio, it would appear that until
more information becomes available on dietary factors that influence vitamin E needs other than polyunsaturates, this relationship should not be
employed in the formulation of RDA for vitamin E.

TABLE 13   Recommended Dietary Allowances of the Food and Nutrition
Board - 1974

Group	Age (years)	Maximum weight (kg)	Vitamin E activity (IU/day) [a, b]
Infants	0–0.5	6	4
	0.5–1.0	9	5
Children	1–3	13	7
	4–6	20	9
	7–10	30	10
	11–14	44	12
Adolescent and adult males	>15	70	15
Adolescent and adult females	>15	58	12
Pregnant and lactating females	−[c]	−[c]	15

[a] Recommended level of daily intake for healthy Americans consuming an average diet; see text for further explanation of RDA.
[b] Total vitamin E activity, estimated to be comprised of 80% α-tocopherol and 20% other tocopherols.
[c] Not specified.

With further reference to the revised RDA figures, the data of Table 12 make it abundantly clear that the average American diet can now conform to the official recommendations. It is worthwhile noting once again, however, that the levels specified are for maintenance of good nutrition of almost every healthy person in the United States. In concluding this discussion of Recommended Dietary Allowances, the author also wishes to emphasize that it would be short-sighted to accept the 1975 figures as immutable. Just as the allowances required modification after 1968, the present recommendations may also need revision. Additional research is particularly needed in regard to the tocopherol content of diets consumed by the pediatric population, as well as data on plasma tocopherol levels in large groups of normal infants and children.

E.   Recent Developments

1.   Survey status.   Although there is still a pressing need for more data
on the vitamin E status of infants and children, results from recent surveys
have clearly shown that lower levels of tocopherol are normally present in
the pediatric population as compared to adults.   In addition, these observations support the concept of expressing serum or plasma tocopherol values
on the basis of total lipid concentrations.   Farrell et al. [310] found in a
study of 1 to 12 year old children, as contrasted with young adults evaluated
concurrently, that 36% of the pediatric population had tocopherol values less
than 0.5 mg/dl, the previously recognized "lower limit of normal;" however,
none of these subjects showed excessive erythrocyte hemolysis in vitro when
RBC suspensions were incubated in the presence of peroxide.   Almost all of
the children had tocopherol/total lipid ratios above 0.8 mg/g, the "minimal"
level proposed by Horwitt [21] for normal vitamin E status.   Thus, Farrell
et al. [310] concluded that the range of normality established for adults with
respect to tocopherol concentrations and tocopherol/lipid ratios cannot be
applied to children, and that new norms need to be used in assessing pediatric patients.   To establish a reliable range of normal for infants and children,
more survey data are required from larger pediatric populations.   Such studies will be facilitated by the recent development by Bieri et al. [311] of a
rapid, accurate micro-assay method for α-tocopherol using high pressure
lipid chromatography.

2.   Tocopherol supplementation in hemolytic anemia.   Recent clinical investigations have supported the potential importance of tocopherol's antioxidant
function in stabilizing the erythrocyte membrane.   Patients with inborn errors
of metabolism leading to inadequate glutathione reducing capacity offer a unique
opportunity to examine red cells in relation to vitamin E, and have been studied
by Dr. Joseph Schulman and associates at the NIH [312].   Patients with glu-
cose-6-phosphate dehydrogenase deficiency have been found to show significantly increased red cell half-life values and decreased reticulocyte counts
after tocopherol treatment.   In addition, a patient with glutathione synthetase
deficiency (5-oxoprolinuria) showed similar improvement after taking 30 IU/kg
of α-tocopheryl acetate for three months [312].

3.   Vitamin E and the lung.   Clinical evidence that vitamin E may have a protective influence on the human repiratory system has been obtained in a controlled trial of parenteral tocopherol, the results of which suggest that premature infants with severe respiratory distress syndrome (hyaline membrane
disease) may benefit from this treatment [313].   Specifically, none of the nine
infants receiving daily injections of α-tocopherol (20 mg/kg) developed bronchopulmonary dysplasia ("pulmonary oxygen toxicity"), whereas 6 of 13 controls
showed clinical and radiographic evidence of the disease.   These impressive
results are prelimiary, but agree with data obtained in studies with various
animal species and should encourage further investigation of the clinical role
of vitamin E with respect to the developing respiratory system.   Such research
should be stimulated by the fact that two major chronic pediatric pulmonary
diseases (cystic fibrosis and bronchopulmonary dysplasia) occur in children
who are susceptible to severe tocopherol deficiency.

ACKNOWLEDGEMENTS

The author is grateful to Dr. John G. Bieri for many stimulating discussions and helpful suggestions during the preparation of this article. In addition, the expert secretarial and editorial assistance of Mrs. Penny Colbert is acknowledged and appreciated.

REFERENCES

1. E. V. McCollum, A History of Nutrition. Cambridge, Mass., Riverside, 1957.
2. J. Green, Ann. N.Y. Acad. Sci. 203:29 (1972).
3. M. L. Scott, in The Fat Soluble Vitamins. Edited by H. F. DeLuca and J. W. Suttie. Madison, Univ. Wisconsin, 1969, p. 355.
4. K. E. Mason and M. K. Horwitt, in The Vitamins. Edited by W. H. Sebrell and R. S. Harris. New York, Academic, 1972, p. 272.
5. L. L. Tureen, P. M. Farrell, and R. R. Cova, Proc. Soc. Exp. Biol. Med. 119:28 (1965).
6. P. A. Young and L. L. Tureen, Acta. Neuropathol. 6:279 (1966).
7. V. H. Cohn, in Pharmacological Basis of Therapeutics. Edited by L. Goodman and A. Gilman. London, Macmillan, 1970, p. 1960.
8. Vitamin E, Med. Lett. 17:69 (1975).
9. K. E. Mason and M. K. Horwitt, in The Vitamins. Edited by W. H. Schrell and R. S. Harris. New York, Academic, 1972, p. 293.
10. M. K. Horwitt, Vit. and Horm. 20:541 (1962).
11. M. K. Horwitt, in Modern Nutrition in Health and Disease, 5th ed. Edited by R. S. Goodhart and M. E. Shils. Philadelphia, Lea and Febiger, 1973, p. 175.
12. J. G. Bieri, Nutr. Rev. 33:161 (1975).
13. H. H. Gordon and H. M. Nitowsky, in Modern Nutrition in Health and Disease. Edited by M. G. Wohl and R. S. Goodhart. Philadelphia, Lea and Febiger, 1968, p. 238.
14. M. K. Horwitt, C. C. Harvey, G. D. Duncan, and W. C. Wilson, Amer. J. Clin. Nutr. 4:408 (1956).
15. M. K. Horwitt, Amer. J. Clin. Nutr. 8:451 (1960).
16. M. K. Horwitt, C. C. Harvey, B. Century, and L. A. Witting, J. Amer. Diet. Assn. 38:231 (1961).
17. H. H. Gordon and H. McNamara, Amer. J. Dis. Child. 62:328 (1940).
18. H. J. Kayden, Ann. Rev. Med. 23:285 (1972).
19. T. Fujii, H. Shimizu, and I. Eda, J. Vitaminol. 18:84 (1972).
20. H. S. Jacob, S. H. Ingebar, and J. H. Jandl, J. Clin. Invest. 44:1187 (1965).

21. M. K. Horwitt, C. C. Harvey, C. H. Dahm, and M. T. Searcy, Ann. N.Y. Acad. Sci. 203:223 (1972).

22. J. De La Huerga, C. Yesinick, and H. Popper, Amer. J. Clin. Pathol. 23:1163 (1953).

23. M. L. Quaife, N. S. Scrimshaw, and O. H. Lowry, J. Biol. Chem. 180:1229 (1949).

24. J. G. Bieri and R. P. Evarts, J. Amer. Diet. Assn. 62:147 (1973).

25. J. G. Bieri and E. L. Prival, Proc. Soc. Exp. Biol. Med. 120:554 (1965).

26. G. Brubacher and H. Weiser, Wiss. Veroeff. Deut. Ges. Ernaehrung 16:50 (1967).

27. P. L. Harris, E. G. Hardenbrook F. P. Dean, E. R. Cusack, and J. L. Jensen, Proc. Soc. Exp. Biol. Med. 107:381 (1961).

28. J. G. Bieri, L. Teets, B. Belavady, and E. L. Andrews, Proc. Soc. Exp. Biol. Med. 117:131.

29. W. R. McWhirter, Acta Pediatr. Scand. 64:446 (1975).

30. S. L. Levine, A. J. Adams, M. D. Murphey, and P. M. Farrell, Pediatr. Res. 10:356 (1976).

31. D. S. Frederickson and R. I. Levy, in The Metabolic Basis of Inherited Disease. Edited by J. B. Stanbury, J. B. Wyngaarden, and D. S. Frederickson. New York, McGraw-Hill, 1972, p. 531.

32. L. A. Cibils and F. P. Zuspan, Clin. Obstet. Gynecol. 16:199 (1973).

33. A. Norman, B. Strandvik, and O. Ojamae, Acta Pediatr. Scand. 61:71 (1972).

34. P. M. Farrell and M. E. Avery, Amer. Rev. Resp. Dis. 111:657 (1975).

35. L. J. Filer, Amer. J. Clin. Nutr. 21:3 (1968).

36. K. C. Davis, Amer. J. Clin. Nutr. 25:933 (1972).

37. D. K. Melhorn and S. Gross, J. Pediatr. 79:569 (1971).

38. J. V. Straumfjord and M. L. Quaife, Proc. Soc. Exp. Biol. Med. 61:369 (1946).

39. M. E. Ferguson, E. Bridgforth, M. L. Quaife, P. M. Martin, R. O. Cannon, W. J. McGanity, J. Newhill, and W. J. Darby, J. Nutr. 55:305 (1955).

40. J. S. Vobecky, J. Vobecky, D. Shapcott, R. Blanchard, R. Lafond, D. Cloutier, and L. Munan, Can. J. Physiol. Pharmacol. 52:384 (1974).

41. M. Tateno, Acta Obstetr. Gynaecol. Jap. 20:19 (1973).

42. M. Mino and H. Nishimo, J. Nutr. Sci. Vitaminol. 19:475 (1973).

43. P. J. Leonard, E. Doyle, and W. Harrington, Amer. J. Clin. Nutr. 25:480 (1972).

44. W. C. Owens and E. U. Owens, Amer. J. Ophthalmol. 32:1 (1949).

45. W. T. Moyer, Pediatrics 6:893 (1950).

46. S. W. Wright, L. J. Filer, and K. F. Mason, Pediatrics 7:386 (1951).
47. P. Gyorgy, G. Cogan, and C. S. Rose, Proc. Soc. Exp. Biol. Med. 81:537 (1952).
48. H. H. Gordon and J. P. de Metry, Proc. Soc. Exp. Biol. Med. 79:446 (1952).
49. J. B. Mackenzie, Pediatrics 13:346 (1954).
50. H. M. Nitowsky, M. Cornblath, and H. H. Gordon, AMA J. Dis. Child. 92:164 (1956).
51. H. Hassan, S. A. Hashim, T. B. Van Itallie, and W. H. Sebrell, Amer. J. Clin. Nutr. 19:147 (1966).
52. F. A. Oski and L. A. Barness, J. Pediatr. 70:211 (1967).
53. F. A. Oski and L. A. Barness, Amer. J. Clin. Nutr. 21:45 (1967).
54. S. Gross and D. K. Melhorn, Ann. N.Y. Acad. Sci. 203:141 (1972).
55. D. K. Melhorn, S. Gross, G. A. Lake, and J. A. Leu, Blood 37:438 (1971).
56. R. T. Gross, R. Bracci, N. Rudolph, E. Schroeder, and J. A. Koche, Blood 29:481 (1967).
57. S. Younkin, F. A. Oski, and L. A. Barness, Amer. J. Clin. Nutr. 24:7 (1971).
58. M. K. Horwitt and P. Bailey, Arch. Neurol. Psychiatr. 1:312 (1959).
59. A. Minkowski, Sang 22:701 (1951).
60. H. M. Nitowsky, K. S. Jus, and H. H. Gordon, Vit. and Horm. 20:559 (1962).
61. A. B. Reese, M. J. King, and W. E. Owens, Amer. J. Ophthalmol. 36:1333 (1953).
62. R. A. Dilley and D. G. McConnell, J. Membrane Biol. 2:317 (1970).
63. V. E. Kinsey, Arch. Ophthalmol. 56:481 (1956).
64. V. E. Kinsey and J. F. Chisholm, Amer. J. Ophthalmol. 34:1259 (1951).
65. R. D. Zachman and S. N. Graven, Amer. J. Dis. Child. 128:165 (1974).
66. P. M. Farrell and R. V. Kotas, Adv. Pediatr. (1976). In press.
67. A. Llewellyn and P. Swyer, in Care of the High Risk Neonate. Edited by M. H. Klaus and A. A. Fanaroff. Philadelphia, Saunders, 1973, p. 152.
68. A. S. DeLeon, J. H. Elliott, and D. B. Jones, Pediatr. Clin. N. Amer. 17:309 (1970).
69. A. S. Muskin, Trans. Ophthalmol. Soc. U.K. 94:251 (1974).
70. A. Patz, Trans. Amer. Ophthalmol. Soc. 66:940 (1968).
71. J. T. Flynn, Devel. Med. Child. Neurol. 17:525 (1975).
72. J. S. Curran, S. J. Cantolino, W. C. Edwards, and T. C. Van Cader, Pediatr. Res. 9:364 (1975).
73. L. Johnson, D. Schaffer, and T. R. Boggs, Amer. J. Clin. Nutr. 27:1158 (1974).

74. H. L. Newmark, W. Pool, J. C. Bauernfeind, and E. DeRitter, J. Pharmacol. Sci. 64:655 (1975).

75. F. A. Oski and J. L. Naiman, Hematologic Problems in the Newborn, 2nd ed. Philadelphia, Saunders, 1972, p. 1.

76. J. A. Stockman, Sem. Hematol. 12:163 (1975).

77. L. A. Barness, F. A. Oski, M. L. Williams, G. Morrow, and S. B. Annand, Amer. J. Clin. Nutr. 21:40 (1968).

78. J. H. Ritchie, M. B. Fish, V. McMasters, and M. Grossman, N. Engl. J. Med. 279:1185 (1968).

79. M. A. Chadd and A. J. Fraser, Int. J. Vit. Res. 40:610 (1970).

80. S. S. Lo, D. Frank, and W. H. Hitzig, Arch. Dis. Child. 48:360 (1973).

81. D. K. Melhorn and S. Gross, J. Pediatr. 79:581 (1971).

82. D. K. Melhorn, S. Gross, and R. J. Izant, J. Pediatr. 81:753 (1974).

83. S. Gross and D. K. Melhorn, J. Pediatr. 85:753 (1974).

84. D. K. Melhorn, Ohio State Med. J. 69:751 (1973).

85. M. L. Williams, R. J. Shott, P. L. O'Neal, and F. A. Oski, N. Engl. J. Med. 292:887 (1975).

86. T. C. Panos, B. Stinnett, G. Zapata, J. Eminians, B. V. Marasigan, and A. G. Beard, Amer. J. Clin. Nutr. 21:15 (1968).

87. R. B. Goldbloom and D. Cameron, Pediatrics 32:36 (1963).

88. P. Sartain, J. L. Kay, and P. M. Dorn, So. Med. J. 60:1371 (1967).

89. S. A. Hashim and R. H. Asfour, Amer. J. Clin. Nutr. 21:7 (1968).

90. J. E. Richards, R. B. Goldbloom, and R. L. Denton, Pediatrics 20:92 (1957).

91. B. A. Abrams, J. M. C. Gutteridge, J. Stocks, M. Friedman, and T. L. Dormandy, Arch. Dis. Child. 48:721 (1973).

92. Panel on the Diagnostic Applications of Radioisotopes in Hematology, International Committee for Standardization in Hematology, Recommended methods for radioisotope red cell survival studies, Blood 38:378 (1971).

93. J. W. Hollingsworth, J. Lab. Clin. Med. 45:469 (1955).

94. S. Foconi and S. Sjolin, Acta Pediatr. Scand. 48:18 (1959).

95. E. Kaplan and K. S. Hsu, Pediatrics 27:364 (1961).

96. A. V. Gilardi and P. Miescher, Kindern. Schweiz. Med. Wschr. 87:1456 (1957).

97. H. J. Suderman, F. D. White, and L. G. Israels, Science 126:650 (1957).

98. H. A. Pearson and K. M. Vertrees, Nature 189:1019 (1961).

99. G. R. Buchanan and A. D. Schwartz, Blood 44:347 (1974).

100. M. Davidson, Pediatr. Clin. N. Amer. 17:913 (1970).

101. R. E. Wood, T. F. Boat, and C. F. Doershuk, Amer. Rev. Resp. Dis. 113:833 (1976).

102. P. A. di Sant'Agnese and R. C. Talamo, N. Engl. J. Med. 277:1399 (1967).

103. A. Lapey, J. Kattwinkel, P. A. di Sant'Agnese, and L. Laster, J. Pediatr. 84:328 (1974).

104. L. W. Matthews and S. Spector, Pediatrics 27:351 (1961).

105. P. M. Farrell, J. C. Fratantoni, J. G. Bieri, and P. A. di Sant'Agnese, Acta Pediatr. Scand. 64:150 (1975).

106. C. C. Lobeck, in The Metabolic Basis of Inherited Disease, 2nd ed. Edited by J. B. Stanbury, J. B. Wyngaarden, and D. S. Frederickson. New York, McGraw-Hill, 1960, p. 1300.

107. F. Mullins, R. Talamo, and P. A. di Sant'Agnese, JAMA, 192:741 (1965).

108. P. A. di Sant'Agnese and P. M. Farrell, in Clinical Biochemistry of the Neonate. Edited by D. S. Young and J. M. Hicks. New York, Wiley, 1976, in press.

109. J. Kattwinkel, L. M. Taussig, B. E. Statland, and J. I. Verter, J. Pediatr. 82:234 (1973).

110. W. J. Darby, M. E. Ferguson, R. H. Furman, J. M. Lemley, C. T. Ball, and G. R. Meneely, Ann. N.Y. Acad. Sci. 52:328 (1949).

111. L. J. Filer, S. W. Wright, M. P. Manning, and K. E. Mason, Pediatrics 8:388 (1951).

112. H. H. Gordon, H. M. Nitowsky, J. T. Tildon, and S. Levin, Pediatrics 21:673 (1958).

113. H. M. Nitowsky, J. T. Tildon, S. Levin, and H. H. Gordon, Amer. J. Clin. Nutr. 10:368 (1962).

114. R. B. Goldbloom, Can. Med. Assn. J. 82:28 (1970).

115. H. J. Binder, D. C. Herting, V. Hurst, S. C. Finch, and H. M. Spiro, N. Engl. J. Med. 273:1289 (1965).

116. J. T. Harries and D. P. R. Muller, Arch. Dis. Child. 46:341 (1971).

117. B. A. Underwood and C. R. Denning, Pediatr. Res. 6:26 (1972).

118. C. W. Darby, A. G. F. Davidson, and I. D. Desai, Arch. Dis. Child. 48:72 (1973).

119. B. W. Taylor, J. L. Watts, and A. S. Fosbrooke, Arch. Dis. Child. 48:657 (1973).

120. D. P. R. Muller, J. T. Harries, and J. K. Lloyd, Gut 15:966 (1974).

121. P. M. Farrell, J. G. Bieri, J. C. Fratantoni, R. E. Wood, and P. A. di Sant'Agnese, J. Clin. Invest., 60:233 (1977).

122. B. A. Underwood, C. R. Denning, and M. Navab, Ann. N.Y. Acad. Sci. 203:237 (1972).

123. J. G. Bieri and R. P. Evarts, Amer. J. Clin. Nutr. 28:717 (1975).

124. J. G. Bieri and R. K. H. Poukka, Int. J. Vit. Res. 40:344 (1970).

125. E. H. Oppenheimer, Bull. Johns Hopkins Hosp. 98:353 (1956).

126. J. G. Bieri, in The Fat Soluble Vitamins. Edited by H. F. De Luca and J. W. Suttie. Madison, Univ. Wisconsin Press, 1969, p. 307.

127. R. E. Olson and P. C. Carpenter, Adv. Enz. Reg. 5:325 (1967).
128. A. Cantarow and M. Trumper, Clinical Biochemistry, 6th ed. Philadelphia, Saunders, 1962, p. 180.
129. T. L. Munsat, R. Baloh, C. M. Pearson, and W. Fowler, JAMA 226:1536 (1973).
130. M. W. Thompson, E. Murphey, and P. J. McAlpine, J. Pediatr. 71:82 (1967).
131. P. M. Farrell, E. E. Eyerman, and L. L. Tureen, Ann. N.Y. Acad. Sci. 138:102 (1966).
132. J. W. C. Bird and F. Carabello, Nature (Lond.) 210:95 (1966).
133. P. M. Farrell and L. L. Tureen, Proc. Soc. Exp. Biol. Med. 127:678 (1968).
134. P. M. Farrell and L. G. Tomasi, unpublished observations.
135. K. E. Mason, in The Structure and Function of Muscle, Vol. 30. Edited by G. H. Bourne. New York, Academic, 1960, p. 171.
136. K. E. Mason, in The Vitamins, Vol. 5. Edited by W. H. Sebrell and R. S. Harris. New York, Academic, 1954, p. 514.
137. P. M. Farrell and W. K. Engel, unpublished observations.
138. S. Levin, M. H. Gordon, H. M. Nitowsky, C. Goldman, P. A. di Sant'Agnese, and H. H. Gordon, Pediatrics 27:578 (1961).
139. A. R. McGiven, Arch. Dis. Child. 37:656 (1962).
140. W. Kintzen, Int. Z. Vitamin-forsch 22:273 (1950).
141. E. H. Oppenheimer and J. R. Easterly, Hopkins Med. J. 133:252 (1973).
142. C. Nezelof and P. Lancret, Arch. Franc. Pediatr. 16:1035 (1959).
143. H. H. Gordon, H. M. Nitowsky, and M. Cornblath, Amer. J. Dis. Child. 90:669 (1955).
144. P. M. Farrell, J. C. Fratantoni, R. E. Wood, V. W. Fischer, and J. G. Bieri, Fed. Proc. 33:672 (1974).
145. J. G. Bieri and R. K. H. Poukka, J. Nutr. 100:557 (1970).
146. P. T. Kuo and N. N. Huang, J. Clin. Invest. 44:1924 (1965).
147. R. Caren and L. Corbo, J. Clin. Endocr. Metab. 26:470 (1966).
148. M. L. Rosenlund, H. K. Lim, and D. Kritchevsky, Nature (Lond.) 251:719 (1974).
149. J. P. W. Rivers and A. G. Hassan, Lancet 2:642 (1975).
150. L. A. Witting and M. K. Horwitt, J. Nutr. 82:19 (1964).
151. J. G. Bieri and R. K. H. Poukka, J. Nutr. 100:557 (1970).
152. B. L. Shapiro, Q. T. Smith, and W. J. Warwick, Proc. Soc. Exp. Biol. Med. 144:181 (1973).
153. W. A. Blanc, J. D. Reid, and D. H. Anderson, Pediatrics 22:494 (1958).
154. I. Kerner and R. B. Goldbloom, AMA J. Dis. Child 99:597 (1960).
155. D. M. Borel and J. K. Reddy, Arch. Pathol. 96:269 (1973).
156. W. Volwiler, Amer. J. Med. 23:250 (1957).

157. C. Morin and M. Davidson, Gastroenterol. 52:565 (1967).
158. J. G. Bieri, Ann. N.Y. Acad. Sci. 203:181 (1972).
159. C. W. Woodruff, Amer. J. Clin. Nutr. 4:597 (1956).
160. D. P. R. Muller and J. T. Harries, Biochem. J. 122:28P (1969).
161. A. S. Minot, J. Lab. Clin. Med. 29:772 (1944).
162. P. J. Leonard, M. S. Losowsky, and C. N. Pulvertaft, Gut 7:578 (1966).
163. W. J. Darby, M. E. Cherrington, and J. M. Ruffin, Proc. Soc. Exp. Exp. Biol. Med. 63:310 (1946).
164. I. Ramirez, R. Santini, J. Corino, and P. J. Santiago, Amer. J. Clin. Nutr. 26:1045 (1973).
165. J. Pomeranze and R. J. Lucarello, J. Lab. Clin. Med. 42:700 (1953).
166. C. J. Glueck, R. C. Tsang, R. W. Fallat, and B. A. Scheel, Pediatrics 54:51 (1974).
167. M. T. MacMahon and G. Neale, Clin. Sci. 38:197 (1970).
168. B. Bramwell and R. Muir, Quart. J. Med. 1:1 (1908).
169. T. Weinberg, H. H. Gordon, E. H. Oppenheimer, and H. M. Nitowsky, Amer. J. Pathol. 34:565 (1958).
170. H. M. Nitowsky, H. H. Gordon, and J. T. Tildon, Bull. Johns Hopkins Hosp. 98:361 (1956).
171. H. J. Binder and H. M. Spiro, Amer. J. Clin. Nutr. 20:594 (1967).
172. P. J. Leonard and M. S. Losowsky, Amer. J. Clin. Nutr. 24:388 (1971).
173. A. M. Pappenheimer and F. Victor, Amer. J. Pathol. 22:395 (1946).
174. H. Braunstein, Gastroenterology 40:224 (1961).
175. F. A. Bassan and A. L. Kornzweig, Blood 5:381 (1959).
176. I. S. Friedman, H. Cohn, M. Zymaris, and M. S. Goldner, Arch. Intern. Med. 105:112 (1960).
177. E. R. Simon and P. Ways, J. Clin. Invest. 43:1311 (1964).
178. H. J. Kayden and R. Silber, Trans. Amer. Assn. Physicians 78:344 (1965).
179. I. Molenaar, F. A. Hommes, W. G. Braams, and H. A. Polman, Proc. Nat. Acad. Sci. 61:982 (1968).
180. J. T. Dodge, G. Cohen, H. J. Kayden, and G. B. Phillips, J. Clin. Invest. 46:357 (1967).
181. J. G. Bieri and P. M. Farrell, Vit. and Horm., in press (1976).
182. K. Wallis, M. Gross, J. L. Zaidman, and A. Julsary, Pediatrics 48:669 (1971).
183. J. D. L. Hansen, in Calorie Deficiencies and Protein Deficiencies. Edited by R. A. McNance and E. M. Widdowson. London, Churchill, 1967, p. 33.
184. R. E. Olson, Protein-Calorie Malnutrition. New York, Academic, 1975.

185. R. W. Vilter, in Protein-Calorie Malnutrition. Edited by R. E. Olson. New York, Academic, 1975.

186. N. S. Scrimshaw, M. Behar, G. Arroyave, C. Tejada, and F. Viteri, JAMA 164:555 (1957).

187. D. S. McLaren, E. Shirajian, H. Loshkajian, and S. Shadarevian, Amer. J. Clin. Nutr. 22:863 (1969).

188. A. S. Majaj, J. S. Dinning, S. A. Azzam, and W. J. Darby, Amer. J. Clin. Nutr. 12:374 (1963).

189. H. H. Sandstead, M. K. Gabr, S. A. Azzam, A. S. Shuky, R. J. Weiler, O. M. E. Din, N. Mokhtar, A. S. Prasad, A. E. Hifney, and W. J. Darby, Amer. J. Clin. Nutr. 17:27 (1965).

190. O. Thanangkul, J. A. Whitaker, and E. G. Fort, Amer. J. Clin. Nutr. 18:379 (1966).

191. S. J. Baker, S. M. Pereira, and A. Begum, Blood 32:717 (1968).

192. C. H. Halstead, N. Sourial, S. Guindi, K. A. H. Mourad, A. K. Kattab, J. P. Carter, and V. N. Patwardhan, Amer. J. Clin. Nutr. 22:1371 (0000).

193. P. Kulapongs, in Protein-Calorie Malnutrition. Edited by R. E. Olson. New York, Academic, 1975, p. 263.

194. J. S. Dinning and P. L. Day, J. Exp. Med. 105:395 (1957).

195. J. A. Whitaker, E. G. Fort, S. Vimokesant, and J. S. Dinning, Amer. J. Clin. Nutr. 20:783 (1967).

196. R. Y. Asfour and S. Firzli, Amer. J. Clin. Nutr. 17:158 (1965).

197. A. Stekel and N. J. Smith, Amer. J. Clin. Nutr. 23:896 (1970).

198. C. A. Finch, in Protein-Calorie Malnutrition. Edited by R. E. Olson. New York, Academic, 1975, p. 247.

199. M. K. Horwitt, B. Century, and A. A. Zeman,,Amer. J. Clin. Nutr. 12:99 (1963).

200. R. H. Bunnell, E. De Ritter, and S. H. Rubin, Amer. J. Clin. Nutr. 28:706 (1975).

201. J. C. Bauernfeind, H. Newmark, and M. Brin, Amer. J. Clin. Nutr. 27:234 (1974).

202. P. M. Farrell and J. G. Bieri, Amer. J. Clin. Nutr. 28:1381 (1975).

203. M. Briggs and M. Briggs, Med. J. Aust. 1:434 (1974).

204. L. E. Rosenberg, N. Engl. J. Med. 281:146 (1969).

205. L. Pauling, Proc. Natl. Acad. Sci. 68:2678 (1971).

206. P. S. Hench, E. C. Kendall, C. H. Slocumb, and H. E. Polley, Arch. Intern. Med. 85:545 (1950).

207. C. R. Scriver, Pediatrics 46:493 (1970).

208. J. Marks, Vit. and Horm. 20:573 (1962).

209. Tocopherex, Squibb and Sons, Princeton, N.J.

210. Aquasol E, USV Pharmaceutical Corp., Tuckahoe, N.Y.

211. A. L. Tappel, Ann. N.Y. Acad. Sci. 203:12 (1972).

212. M. K. Horwitt, Amer. J. Clin. Nutr. 27:1182 (1974).
213. A. L. Tappel, Vit. and Horm. 20:483 (1962).
214. M. K. Horwitt and K. E. Mason, in The Vitamins. Edited by W. H. Sebrell and R. E. Harris. New York, Academic, 1972, p. 309.
215. H. Larsson and K. Haeger, Pharmacol. Clin. 1:72 (1968).
216. E. V. Shute and H. Bailey, Vitamin E, Your Key to a Healthy Heart. New York, Arc Books, 1968.
217. W. E. Shute, Ann. N.Y. Acad. Sci. 52:63 (1949).
218. Food and Nutrition Board, Recommended Dietary Allowances. Washington, D.C., National Academy of Sciences, National Research Council, 1974).
219. R. W. Hillman, Amer. J. Clin. Nutr. 4:603 (1956).
220. O. A. Roels, Nutr. Rev. 24:129 (1966).
221. J. Winberg and R. Zetterstrom, Acta Pediatr. 45:96 (1956).
222. B. E. March, E. Wong, L. Seier, J. Sim, and J. Biely, J. Nutr. 103:371 (1973).
223. A. Vogelsang and E. V. Shute, Nature (Lond.) 157:772 (1946).
224. W. E. Shute, E. V. Shute, and A. Vogelsang, Med. Record 160:91 (1947).
225. W. E. Shute and H. J. Taub, Vitamin E for Ailing and Healthy Hearts. New York, Pyramid, 1969.
226. I. S. Ravin and K. A. Katz, N. Engl. J. Med. 240:331 (1949).
227. S. H. Rinzler, H. Bakst, Z. H. Benjamin, A. L. Bobb, and J. Travell, Circulation 1:228 (1950).
228. T. W. Anderson, Can. Med. Assn. J. 110:401 (1974).
229. R. E. Hodges, J. Amer. Diet. Assn. 62:638 (1973).
230. R. E. Olson, Circulation 48:179 (1973).
231. R. W. Anderson and D. B. Reid, Amer. J. Clin. Nutr. 27:1174 (1974).
232. K. Haeger, Vasa 2:280 (1973).
233. K. Haeger, Amer. J. Clin. Nutr. 27:1179 (1974).
234. A. M. Boyd, A. H. Ratcliffe, R. P. Jepson, and G. W. H. James, J. Bone Joint Surg. 31B:325 (1949).
235. A. H. Ratcliffe, Lancet 2:1128 (1949).
236. P. D. Livingstone and C. Jones, Lancet 2:602 (1958).
237. H. T. G. Williams, D. Fenna, and R. A. Macbeth, Surg. Gynecol. Obstet. 132:662 (1971).
238. R. F. Cathcart, JAMA 219:216 (1972).
239. S. Baer and W. I. Heine, JAMA 139:733 (1949).
240. M. Hamilton, G. M. Wilson, P. Armitage, and J. T. Boyd, Lancet 1:367 (1953).
241. A. Fajgelj, K. Haeger, S. E. Lindell, and N. M. Olsson, Vasc. Dis. 4:280 (1967).

242. C. K. Donegan, A. L. Messer, E. S. Orgain, and J. M. Ruffin, Amer. J. Med. Sci. $\underline{217}$:294 (1949).

243. H. Levy and E. P. Boas, Ann. Intern. Med. $\underline{28}$:1117 (1948).

244. A. Vogelsang, Angiology $\underline{21}$:275 (1970).

245. H. P. Helwing, H. Hochrein, and B. Helwing, Arzneimittel-forsch. $\underline{21}$:335 (1971).

246. A. Ochsner, N. Engl. J. Med. $\underline{271}$:211 (1964).

247. A. Ochsner, M. D. De Bakey, and P. T. De Camp, JAMA $\underline{144}$:831 (1950).

248. H. Hammerl and O. Pichler, Wein. Klin. Wschr. $\underline{72}$:468 (1960).

249. D. E. Gray and J. M. Loh, Can. J. Biochem. $\underline{36}$:269 (1958).

250. T. Davies, J. Kelleher, and M. S. Loskowsky, Clin. Chim. Acta $\underline{24}$:431 (1969).

251. D. W. Woolley, J. Biol. Chem. $\underline{159}$:59 (1945).

252. K. L. Zierler, D. Grob, and J. L. Lilienthal, Amer. J. Physiol. $\underline{153}$:127 (1948).

253. J. J. Corrigan and F. I. Marcus, JAMA $\underline{230}$:1300 (1974).

254. L. J. Machlin, R. Filipski, A. L. Willis, D. C. Kuhn, and M. Brin, Proc. Soc. Exp. Biol. Med. $\underline{149}$:275 (1975).

255. L. J. Machlin, R. Filipski, C. Dalton, W. Hope, A. L. Willis, D. Kuhn, and M. Brin, Fed. Proc. $\underline{34}$:912 (1975).

256. K. Korsan-Bengtsen, D. Elmfeldt, and T. Holm, Thrombos. Diathes. Haemorrh. $\underline{31}$:505 (1974).

257. M. Steiner and J. Anastasi, J. Clin. Invest. $\underline{57}$:732 (1976).

257a. M. Steiner and J. Anastasi, Clinical Res. $\underline{24}$:498a (1976).

258. M. Okuma, M. Steiner, and M. Baldini, J. Lab. Clin. Med. $\underline{75}$:283 (1970).

259. A. Nordoy and E. Strom, J. Lipid. Res. $\underline{16}$:386 (1975).

260. A. L. Bacharach, Br. Med. J. $\underline{1}$:890 (1940).

261. W. J. Darby, R. O. Cannon, and M. M. Kaser, Obstet. Gynecol. Survey $\underline{3}$:704 (1948).

262. D. Solomon, D. Strummer, and P. Nair, Ann. N.Y. Acad. Sci. $\underline{203}$:103 (1972).

263. A. A. Abrams, N. Engl. J. Med. $\underline{272}$:1080 (1965).

264. L. Zannos-Mariolea, F. Tzortzaton, K. Dendaki-Svolaki, C. Katerellos, M. Kavallari, and N. Matsaniotis, Br. J. Hematol. $\underline{26}$:193 (1974).

265. C. B. Hyman, B. Fanding, R. Alfin-Slater, L. Kozak, J. Weitzman, and J. A. Ortega, Ann. N.Y. Acad. Sci. $\underline{232}$:211 (1974).

266. J. Stocks, E. L. Offerman, C. D. Modell, and T. L. Dormandy, Br. J. Hematol. $\underline{23}$:713 (1972).

267. C. Choremis, V. Kyriakides, and E. Papadakis, J. Clin. Pathol. $\underline{14}$:361 (1961).

268. C. B. Modell, J. Stocks, and T. L. Dormandy, Br. Med. J. 3:259 (1974).
269. H. P. Ehrlich, H. Tarver, and T. K. Hunt, Ann. Surg. 175:235 (1972).
270. V. W. Stuyvesant and W. B. Jolley, Nature (Lond.) 216:585 (1967).
271. L. L. Pennock, Ann. N.Y. Acad. Sci. 52:413 (1949).
272. J. M. Goodson, in Diet, Nutrition and Periodontal Disease. In press.
273. T. K. Cureton, Amer. J. Physiol. 179:628 (1954).
274. L. Prokap, Sportarztl. Prax. 1:19 (1960).
275. I. M. Sharman, M. G. Down, and R. N. Sen, Br. J. Nutr. 26:265 (1971).
276. P. P. Nair, E. Mezey, H. S. Murty, J. Quartner, and A. I. Mendeloff, Arch. Intern. Med. 128:411 (1971).
277. C. J. Watson, I. Bossenmaier, and R. Cardinal, Arch. Intern. Med. 131:698 (1973).
278. P. Mustajoki, JAMA 221:714 (1972).
279. J. N. Roehm, J. G. Hadley, and D. B. Menzel, Arch. Environ. Health 24:237 (1972).
280. D. Harman, J. Gerontol. 26:451 (1971).
281. H. Baker, O. Frank, S. Feingold, G. Christakis, and H. Ziffer, Amer. J. Clin. Nutr. 20:850 (1967).
282. M. J. Bennent and B. F. Medwadowski, Amer. J. Clin. Nutr. 20:415 (1967).
283. M. Chieffi and J. E. Kirk, J. Gerontol. 6:17 (1951).
284. P. L. Harris, K. C. D. Hickman, J. L. Jensen, and T. D. Spies, Amer. J. Public Health 36:155 (1946).
285. R. W. Hillman and M. C. Rosner, J. Nutr. 64:605 (1958).
286. G. Klatskin and W. A. Krehl, J. Clin. Invest. 29:1528 (1950).
287. J. M. Lemley, R. G. Gale, R. H. Furman, M. E. Cherrington, W. R. Darby, and G. R. Meneely, Amer. Heart J. 37:1029 (1949).
288. S. Postel, J. Clin. Invest. 35:1345 (1956).
289. M. L. Quaife and P. L. Harris, J. Biol. Chem. 156:499 (1944).
290. N. S. Scrimshaw, R. B. Greer, and R. L. Goodland, Ann. N.Y. Acad. Sci. 52:312 (1949).
291. C. Urbach, K. C. D. Hickman, and P. L. Harris, Exp. Med. Surg. 10:7 (1952).
292. I. S. Wechsler, G. G. Mayer, and H. Sobotka, Proc. Soc. Exp. Biol. Med. 47:152 (1941).
293. L. A. Witting and L. Lee, Amer. J. Clin. Nutr. 28:571 (1975).
294. D. C. Herting and E. E. Drury, Amer. J. Clin. Nutr. 17:351 (1965).
295. C. K. W. Wo and H. H. Draper, Amer. J. Clin. Nutr. 28:808 (1975).
296. P. L. Harris and N. D. Embree, Amer. J. Clin. Nutr. 13:385 (1963).

297. R. H. Bunnell, J. Keating, A. Quaresimo, and G. K. Parman, Amer. J. Clin. Nutr. 17:1 (1965).

298. J. N. Thompson, J. L. Beare-Rogers, P. Erdody, and D. C. Smith, Amer. J. Clin. Nutr. 26:1349 (1973).

299. H. T. Slover, Lipids 6:291 (1971).

300. A. C. Frazer and J. G. Lines, J. Sci. Food Agr. 18:203 (1967).

301. M. L. Quaife and M. Y. Dju, J. Biol. Chem. 180:263 (1949).

302. M. Y. Dju, K. E. Mason, and L. J. Filer, Amer. J. Clin. Nutr. 6:50 (1958).

303. C. L. Smith, J. Kelleher, M. S. Losowsky, and N. Morrish, Br. J. Nutr. 26:89 (1971).

304. A. E. Harper, Nutr. News 37:5 (1974).

305. A. E. Harper, Nutrition Today 9:15 (1974).

306. Food and Nutrition Board, Recommended Dietary Allowances. Washington, D.C., National Academy of Sciences, National Research Council, 1968.

307. M. K. Horwitt, Amer. J. Clin. Nutr. 27:1182 (1974).

308. P. L. Harris, Ann. N.Y. Acad. Sci. 52:240 (1949).

309. L. A. Witting, Amer. J. Clin. Nutr. 25:257 (1972).

310. P. M. Farrell, S. L. Levine, M. D. Murphey, and A. J. Adams, Am. J. Clin. Nutr. 31:1720 (1978).

311. J. G. Bieri, T. J. Tolliver, and G. L. Catignani, Am. J. Clin. Nutr. 32:2143 (1979).

312. S. Spielberg, L. A. Boxer, L. M. Corash, and J. D. Schulman, Ann. Intern. Med., 90:53, 1979.

313. R. A. Ehrenkranz, B. W. Bonta, R. C. Ablow, and J. B. Warshaw, New Eng. J. Med. 299:564, (1978).

Part 11B/ Interpretation of Human Requirements for Vitamin E

MAX K. HORWITT
St. Louis University School of Medicine
St. Louis, Missouri

I.	Introduction	621
II.	Frank Deficiencies	621
III.	Requirements to Prevent Hidden Deficiencies	622
	A. Erythrocyte Survival	623
	B. Significance of Peroxide Hemolysis Test	625
	C. Problems Affecting Choice of Daily Requirements	626
IV.	Pharmacological Effects of Large Doses of Vitamin E	630
	A. Air Pollutants	631
	B. Effects of α-Tocopherylquinone	632
	C. Prolongation of Blood Clotting	633
	References	634

I. INTRODUCTION

A discussion of the use of vitamin E by humans might properly be divided into three sections. In the first section, one can include information relating to deficiencies that are associated with demonstrable pathology. The second section will deal with the important, but relatively small and difficult to measure, changes which may take place as a consequence of undesirable oxidations of cellular material at borderline levels of dietary intake. The third section will discuss the possible pharmacological effects of ingesting vitamin E at levels many times the apparent nutritional requirements.

II. FRANK DEFICIENCIES

Usually such cases are limited to infants who have not yet achieved any stores of vitamin E and who have deficiencies of lipid absorption. One should also include in this group some infants receiving intravenous feeding and those whose intake may be grossly inadequate for other reasons.

Deficiencies in children have been discussed in detail in previous chapters, but information on one case that was published in a journal not usually read by nutritionists should be added.

Dr. Percival Bailey, the eminent neurosurgeon whose histopathological work is impeccable, was collaborating in a study of the effects of different dietary fats and oils on the development of encephalomalacia in chicks [1]. He was particularly interested in the loss of Purkinje cells in the cerebellum after hemorrhages developed. Serendipitously, an infant's brain brought to him for pathological evaluation showed alterations in the cerebellum that were remarkably similar to changes in the brains of chicks with vitamin E deficiency [2]. After further evaluation, it was learned that the child had been a severe nutritional problem for 8 weeks, requiring feeding through a Levine tube. During her last 3 weeks, she had received intravenous feedings, with most of the calories provided by a commercial emulsion containing 15% cottonseed oil that had approximately 50% linoleic acid. The vitamin preparations administered did not include any vitamin E. It is noteworthy that it takes about 3 weeks to produce encephalomalacia in a chick on a vitamin E-deficient diet. In evaluating the observation made by Dr. Bailey, it should be emphasized that he had previously studied hundreds of brains, including those from alcoholics and others with nutritional deficiencies, and had never before seen the same histopathology in humans. The changes were quite different from the encephalopathy observed in Wernick's disease. His paper on chick pathology [1] and the report on the child [2] were published separately. Generally, one can state that, in humans, a deficiency of the tocopherols to a degree sufficient to produce the spectrum of severe pathology demonstrable in young animals will rarely be observed. Such pathology is so debilitating and so often irreversible that human beings might not have evolved to their present state if they did not have the capacity to store some vitamin E in all of their lipids. To prevent such extreme deficiencies of vitamin E, it is apparent that relatively small amounts of α-tocopherol are required. However, such minimal levels must be provided, and more importantly, they must be absorbed. When the mechanisms of absorption are deficient, it may be necessary to provide much larger amounts to overwhelm the deficiency in the absorptive processes.

III. REQUIREMENTS TO PREVENT HIDDEN DEFICIENCIES

Perhaps of greater concern than frank deficiencies of vitamin E is the determination of how much is needed to maintain optimum health in the sense used by those who evaluate nutritional requirements.

A. Erythrocyte Survival

Relatively small alterations in the level of hemoglobin in patients are so
common that physicians are perhaps less concerned about hemoglobin
levels that are slightly low than they might be. The level of hemoglobin
may be considered to be controlled by two opposing forces: the rate of
production and the rate of destruction. Accordingly, where erythropoietic
mechanisms are not accelerated when the erythrocytes are destroyed at a
faster rate one may have a decrease in the hemoglobin level. A decrease
in the number of erythrocytes triggers an increase in erythropoiesis, in
order that the erythrocyte count may be maintained at its original level.
In such a case, in the absence of information about the rate of erythrocyte
turnover, no information that more erythrocytes were destroyed is
obtained. Reticulocyte counts, when at low levels, may have a 50%
increase as from 0.4 to 0.6%, without one being able to attach any significance to the count.

Nevertheless, it is important to know that more tissue cells may be
destroyed when there is too little antioxidant present and that the theoretical implications of the in vitro peroxide hemolysis test may have practical
significance. The animal studies which first called attention to the possibility that erythrocytes may be destroyed during vitamin E deficiency
were first reported by Dinning, Day, and their collaborators [3-6] during
the time period when the Elgin Project on vitamin E requirements was in
progress. This alerted us to look for similar effects in the much milder
deficiencies being studied in the adult males [7].

Many of the details of the Elgin Project are described in Chap. 11A
and will not be repeated here. The hemoglobin levels of the subjects
on the diet which provided about 5 IU were routinely tested, and they
continued for several years at a slightly low, but so-called normal range.
A slightly elevated reticulocyte level in some of the subjects had given
some clues in the early years of the study, but it was not studied carefully
since all other blood sampling would have had to be interrupted to make a
careful examination of erythrocyte turnovers. It was not until the 72nd
experimental month that all other tests were stopped and a well-controlled
study of erythrocyte survival was initiated [7]. Because half-life time
data were not fully trusted, the evaluations were continued for the full
4 months of erythrocyte life. The results obtained showed that the erythrocytes of the subjects fed the diet low in vitamin E were being destroyed
at a rate 8-10% faster than in the subjects in the control group. The subjects with the lowest hemoglobin level (12.7 g%) had the shortest erythrocyte survival time (102 days). The 4-month test of erythrocyte life span
was repeated on three of the depleted subjects, each of whom was paired
with a subject from the "hospital diet" group on the day of analysis in order
to minimize technical errors. The replication was excellent. Soon after,

the depleted subjects were supplemented with α-tocopherol. It should be understood that the experimental diet was only marginally deficient. The objective was not so much to produce deficiency but to determine adult requirements. It is logical to predict that if the diet had been more deficient in vitamin E, more severe pathology would have developed.

One must emphasize that we do not know how soon in the study the decrease in erythrocyte survival time began. It could not possibly have been observed at all by normal clinical procedures, since a 10% increase in erythrocyte turnover, although not desirable, is well within the hematopoietic repair potential of the body. However, one must ask the question whether some of the other cells of the body, not so easily removable for study as the erythrocytes, might also have their life cycle similarly affected when there is an inadequate concentration of antioxidant in the cellular membrane phospholipids.

Confirmation of a decrease in erythrocyte survival in humans when serum tocopherol levels are decreased has been published by several laboratories. Oski and Barness [8] reported moderately shortened red cell survival in premature infants deficient in vitamin E. Binder et al. [9] reported a "significant decrease in survival" of red cells in three or six patients with markedly reduced serum tocopherol levels. None of these latter patients had anemia or any other evidence of hemolysis or bleeding which led to their doubt whether the [51Cr]labeling technique was adequate. Subsequently, Richie et al. [10] reported that the erythrocyte survival times were "strikingly short" in premature infants who had low levels of serum tocopherol. They resolved the question raised by Binder et al. [9], about the adequacy of the [51Cr]labeling technique by showing that the [51Cr] elution time was not a detrimental factor and that labeling with [32P]di-isopropyl-fluorophosphate gave the same results. They further stated that "the prompt lengthening of erythrocyte survival coincident with the rise in tocopherol is direct in vivo evidence of the role of tocopherol in preventing red-cell hemolysis."

Confirmation of the effect of α-tocopherol in prolonging red cell survival in vitamin E-deficient adults was provided by Leonard and Losowsky [11]. Using [51Cr]tagged cells they reported a marked increase in the erythrocyte half-life time after administration of α-tocopheryl acetate in five of eight subjects who had low plasma tocopherol levels.

There is less agreement about whether the reticulocyte count is increased when α-tocopherol is administered to a subject who is deficient in vitamin E. Logically, when the destruction of erythrocytes is prevented by adding α-tocopherol, one would expect the reticulocyte level to decrease. A slight increase in reticulocyte count was obtained after supplementation with vitamin E in adults in the Elgin Study [7]. Majaj et al. [12], Marvin and Audu [13] and Whitaker et al. [14] claimed there was a stimulation of erythropoiesis by vitamin E given to malnourished infants. These reticulocyte increases after supplementation with α-tocopheryl acetate are difficult to understand and may have been a secondary reaction to the general improvement in nutritional state. A more logical result was obtained by Ritchie et al. [10] who reported an increase in hemoglobin and a decrease in reticulocytes when α-tocopheryl acetate was given to vitamin E-deficient infants. After some years of evaluation of the conflicting data, this writer has concluded that one should not anticipate α-tocopherol to have an erythropoietic effect except as it may be simultaneously related to a general improvement in physiological state. Furthermore, most reports have shown that when no demonstrable anemia was present before tocopherol was administered, no reticulocyte increase was obtained—nor should it have been expected.

B. Significance of Peroxide Hemolysis Test

The confirmation of an increased erythrocyte turnover with low serum tocopherol levels lends credence to the significance of data obtained from the in vitro peroxide hemolysis tests in controlled dietary studies of vitamin E requirements. It has been shown [15] that the concentration of the hydrogen peroxide, the rate at which it is added to the erythrocyte suspension, the temperature, and the elapsed time of incubation all can have large effects on the amount of hemolysis obtained. All of these variables can be controlled to give reproducible results from a chosen set of them applied to a given sample of erythrocytes. The problem was to cerify that one had chosen the proper set of variables to distinguish between blood samples that have different levels of vitamin E so that one could separate depleted subjects from those consuming adequate amounts of the tocopherols. One can easily choose conditions at which all normal blood would hemolyze or, conversely, where no deficient blood would hemolyze [15].

There has been general agreement that serum levels of less than 0.5 mg/100 ml are suspect since at levels below 0.5 mg/100 mg one begins to obtain evidence of an increase in the data obtained from the peroxide hemolysis test as it is now being used in most laboratories. This choice is fortuitous since one does not obtain signs of a more rapid erythrocyte turnover in subjects that have as much as 0.5 mg/100 ml of tocopherol in their blood. Most reports in the literature of the more rapid erythrocyte turnover have been at serum tocopherol levels of less than 0.3 mg/100 ml. These are the same levels at which the peroxide hemolysis test results become strongly positive. From such information one should conclude the dietary intake of tocopherols should not be less than the amount needed to keep the serum levels above the critical level of 0.5 mg/100 ml. If a safety factor to cover individual variations is included in such a recommendation, the amount fed should be increased considerably.

In the Elgin Project [16], at the time when the linoleic acid content of the erythrocyte lipids had approximately doubled, the erythrocytes were more sensitive to the effects of peroxide in producing hemolysis. The erythrocytes of patients on the experimental diet, who had been supplemented with tocopherol for many months, showed a much more rapid increase in sensitivity to peroxide after tocopherol supplementation was stopped than other subjects whose erythrocyte lipids had been less unsaturated.

The level of tocopherol in the serum is not just a function of the amount of tocopherol consumed. The effects of malabsorption in decreasing the levels of vitamin E in all the tissues and circulatory fluids is well recognized. Less well publicized in the scientific literature is the fact that the level of lipoprotein in the serum may, in some circumstances, have a greater effect than the diet in determining the amount of tocopherol in the serum [17-19]. Just about every physiological event that decreases the cholesterol of every other serum component of the serum total lipids also decreases the level of serum tocopherol [19]. Thus, when triiodothyronine was given to eight patients who continued to be supplemented with 15 mg α-tocopheryl acetate·a day, there was a rapid drop in serum tocopherols from an average of 1.07 to 0.58 mg/100 ml [20]. This decrease was accompanied by a similar decrease in serum cholesterol. In this writer's experience all subjects with pathologically high levels of lipoprotein have, to date, all shown either elevated or high normal levels of serum tocopherols. Conversely, infants with low lipoprotein levels, for any cause, have all shown low levels of serum tocopherol. Thus, infants with protein-calorie malnutrition have low serum cholesterol and tocopherol in most cases. As soon as they are fed a better diet, albeit low in vitamin E, their serum lipoproteins return to normal and the serum levels of α-tocopherol are increased [19]. Apparently, there was a reserve of α-tocopherol in the tissues but it could not be transported to and by the blood. This means that it is possible for the erythrocyte to be in a deficient environment and subject to possible oxidative trauma while other tissues are less deficient in vitamin E.

C. Problems Affecting Choice of Daily Requirements

Assuming normal lipoprotein levels, what level of dietary tocopherols is required to keep the serum total tocopherols level at a respectable 1.0 mg/100 ml serum? The latter figure is chosen because it is the average level of total tocopherols found in adults with cholesterol levels of about 180 mg/100 ml [19]. Fortunately, by going back to unpublished data from the Elgin Project an answer to the question is available. Ten adult males were housed in the same metabolic unit as the experimental subjects on controlled diets but were fed separately, in an adjoining space, the same meals consumed by all the other patients who were housed in the other hospital buildings. This diet, called the "hospital diet," which was planned to be adequate in all respects, varied with the season in the same manner as other diets of noninstitutionalized subjects in the midwestern section of the United States. Frequent analysis showed that the daily allotment provided 8-12 mg α-tocopherol per day, an average of 10 mg. The polyunsaturated fatty acid content (PUFA) varied from 5 to 11% of the dietary fat or from 4 to 7 g per day. This is probably less PUFA than the amount consumed by the average American adult. To confirm the latter statement, it should be noted that the linoleate content of the depot fat of the subjects in the hospital diet group ranged from 5 to 11% [21]. The consumption of 10 mg α-tocopherol or approximately 15 International Units (IU) was not sufficient to prevent the peroxide hemolysis data from being greater than 10% on many occasions over a 6-year period. Despite dozens of replications of the results, some subjects consistently had erythrocytes that were more susceptible to peroxide hemolysis than anticipated at the level of intake. It is perhaps this observation more than any other that has influenced the author of this chapter to believe that an allowance of 15 IU per day of vitamin E is inadequate to cover the needs of all adults on average diets.

One of the problems that confronts the investigator making judgments on requirements for vitamin E lies with the sparsity of easily recognized pathological symptoms when the consumption of tocopherols is less than adequate. Most other vitamins have specific functions in either biochemical equations or hormonal activities which, when interrupted, produce more easily identifiable pathological symptoms. Most of the functions of vitamin E appear to be related to its activity as an antioxidant, and unless the deficiency is extreme, the replacement of damaged tissue cells can be accomplished without any readily apparent symptoms of a physiological disorder. As has been noted above [19], while other tissues may have an apparent sufficiency, it is possible for the blood to have tocopherol levels that are inadequate to protect the erythrocytes, as a result of either low concentrations of serum lipoproteins to transport the tocopherols or because of recent inadequate consumption. One must ask whether it is worth the effort to increase the consumption of vitamin E to prevent changes that can only be determined by specialized laboratory techniques.

Does it make any difference over the course of a lifetime if the rate of cellular turnover is accelerated by 5%? Given a choice, it would seem desirable to have an amount of vitamin E sufficient to prevent the destructive action of oxidative agents on the PUFA in the cellular phospholipids, or of other compounds susceptible to undesirable oxidation. When the diet is relatively low in PUFA, the evidence at hand indicates [21] that 10 mg α-tocopherol per day for the average adult male is the minimal amount that can prevent measurable undesirable sequelae. This amount is approximately equivalent to the 15 IU that is currently being recommended as the daily allowance by the Food and Nutrition Board [22] and allows for little or no safety for deviation from normalcy. It is half the previously recommended allowance [23] for adult males and is an amount that has been shown to be inadequate when corn oil was the major dietary fat [21].

An important fact that must be emphasized is the destructive effect of ferric ion on the tocopherols. In the early days of vitamin E research ferric salts were used to destroy the tocopherols in experimental diets. More recently it has been observed that when medicinal iron is administered to otherwise normal premature infants [24], a vitamin E-dependent anemia is produced.

Premature infants are particularly susceptible to vitamin E deficiency probably because the placenta does not transfer α-tocopherol to the fetus in adequate amounts. It should be noted that the anemia of prematurity and its relationship to a deficiency of the tocopherols has now been demonstrated by at least six different groups of investigators [8, 11, 24-27]. Apparently, additional α-tocopherol should be provided to premature infants not only to prevent the onslaught of retrolental fibroplasia [28] but also to minimize the destruction of erythrocytes. An amount of vitamin E equivalent to 15 IU per day, orally, has been recommended for all premature infants [26] within a few weeks after birth to minimize decreases in hemoglobin concentration.

One of the factors considered to be important by those who made the decision to decrease the allowance of vitamin E to the amount recommended in 1974 [23] was the development of chromatographic methods that could more easily distinguish between α- and γ-tocopherols. This development led to a change in the method of calculating the average American consumption of vitamin E. Older estimates of the average consumption of total tocopherols and tocotrienols in the daily adult American diet, give figures of about 15 mg per day [29]. Since then, the consumption of γ-tocopherol has greatly increased due to the greater use of soybean oil which contains about 6 times more γ- than α-tocopherol [30]. In addition, analyses of cereal grains have been shown to contain 0.9-1.7 mg α-tocotrienol and β-tocotrienol per 100 g [31]. The α-tocopherol in the average diet of 2500 kcal has been estimated in three studies to be between 6.4 and 9.0 mg (9.5-13.4 IU) [32-34]. From such data, after allowance of 20% activity for the γ-tocopherols in the diet (apparently without considering the other tocopherols and tocotrienols) a daily allowance of 15 IU of vitamins was considered proper for adults [30]. Apparently, the reasoning was that if no frank deficiency were noted in the population at this level of intake, 15 IU was adequate.

There are several inadequacies in the use of data which led to the above conclusion. First, it was not sound to use the figure of 6.4 mg α-tocopherol per day in calculating the averages from which a desirable consumption was to be estimated. This level was considered to be inadequate by those [32] who reported this figure. Furthermore the only long-term study of vitamin E [21] on the effects of voluntary consumption of balanced diets on blood levels and peroxide hemolysis gave contrary data. The α-tocopherol level of these diets ranged from 8 to 12 mg per day and at these levels of intake, blood plasma levels of less than 0.5 mg/ 100 g per day and peroxide hemolysis results of more than 10% were obtained at least 10% of the time. Such data were absorbed in the averages obtained when monthly results over a 6-year period are computed, but they are worth noting as effects on individual subjects. Another point not previously emphasized but recognized by those who have done repetitive determinations of the peroxide hemolysis test, is that some subjects consistently require a higher level of serum tocopherols than other subjects to minimize the amount of hemolysis obtained in the test. Two out of the ten subjects in the hospital diet group consistently presented high peroxide hemolysis results that were out of line with their serum tocopherol levels. Although the food consumption of the patients on the hospital diet was not recorded, frequent weight checks showed that they were consuming their food. Month after month, nearly all the subjects in this group had peroxide hemolysis test results which were appreciably higher than those obtained simultaneously from the subjects who were in the group on the controlled diet who were supplemented with α-tocopheryl acetate [16]. These higher data were obtained despite the fact that the depot fat of the hospital diet group subjects contained only 10-30% as much linoleate as subjects on the controlled diets. It was this observation, more than any other, that confirmed the impression that 15 IU per day was an inadequate level of intake of vitamin E at current levels of consumption of polyunsaturated fats.

Two items should be considered important. First, no investigator should publish a report on levels of α-tocopherol in the blood without simultaneous information on the amount of total tocopherols and tocotrienols present. The latter is easily determined by any one of the classical reduction techniques. Secondly, all records of the amount of vitamin E in the serum should be accomplished by some estimate of the level of the lipids in the blood. "Total lipids" may be preferred, but where not easily obtained, a record of the level of serum cholesterol or triglycerides is almost as useful. It does not yet seem to be fully recognized that at low or high levels of serum lipids, the dietary intake of vitamin E is of secondary importance in evaluating the significance of serum tocopherol data [19]. When the serum lipid levels are lower than normal the erythrocytes may be at risk, despite adequate consumption of vitamin E.

In order to determine how many International Units of vitamin E are being consumed, it is necessary to improve our knowledge of the activity of all the tocopherols and tocotrienols relative to α-tocopherol. This has become more important in recent years as the consumption of compounds with vitamin E activity other than α-tocopherol has increased in the American diet. Of these compounds, γ-tocopherol has received the most attention. It is now present in human tissues in surprisingly large amounts. The ratio of γ- to α-tocopherol in the tissues of patients who died in 1973 has been shown [35] to be from 28 to 80% in the liver, from 29 to 95% in the lipids, and about 50% in the heart. These figures appear to be higher than those normally found in the serum probably because the γ-tocopherol turns over more rapidly in the serum [36]. The relative activity of γ-tocopherol based on in vivo assays [37] is about 11% that of α-tocopherol. These workers also observed a synergistic effect of γ-tocopherol on a α-tocopherol activity. Bieri et al. [38] have reported the relative activity of γ-tocopherol to α-tocopherol to be 38% in the dialuric hemolysis test on rat blood in vitro. Significantly, Scott and Desai [39] have observed that nutritional muscular dystrophy in chicks is prevented by similar plasma concentration of α-, β-, and γ-tocopherol. An important conclusion of the latter study was that the prevention of pathology correlated best with total plasma tocopherol levels, although when fed separately there were large differences in relative activity. Accordingly, while it is important to know how much α-tocopherol is being consumed, one should not neglect the simple, and more easily reproducible, determination of the total tocopherols and tocotrienols. If "total tocopherols" in the diet are given the credence they once had, and still deserve, there would be less justification for a daily dietary allowance of 15 IU for adults.

The most important question to be asked is should frank deficiency, a state of pathology obtained only in young animals with essentially zero levels of tocopherols in their blood, be considered the criterion of tocopherol inadequacy, or should one strive for levels in the blood which protect at least 99% of the population from the type of erythrocyte fragility that can be measured by currently accepted techniques? Admittedly, the healthy hematopoietic system has no apparent difficulty in repairing the damage caused when a few more erythrocytes are destroyed. However, until we know that other cells in the body are not similarly affected, there is little choice but to make a decision on the side of safety.

IV. PHARMACOLOGICAL EFFECTS OF LARGE DOSES OF VITAMIN E

Any discussion of the biological usefulness of vitamin E should distinguish between the amount required as an essential nutrient and amounts provided to produce possible pharmacological activity. The levels of the latter may be many times the amounts recommended by nutritional scientists.

Excluding those who have done surveys on dietary intake, few have conducted experiments on the use of vitamin E by adults and the remainder seem to be divided into two categories: those strongly against supplementation with vitamin E and those strongly in favor of such supplementation. Most of those who have performed controlled research on the effects of supplementation with larger amounts of α-tocopherol have made judgments that are somewhere between the two extremes.

It may be that vitamin E suffers from what may be termed "the boy who cried wolf" syndrome. Many noninfectious diseases that have recurrent exacerbations and remissions have been treated with vitamin E. Understandingly, there has been a reaction by many biological scientists against such treatment when there was neither a good rationale known for the therapy nor controls established to prove that the patients would not have done as well without the treatment. Nevertheless, through the years reports of beneficial effects, often by individuals who had set out to disprove a therapeutic effect, have served to keep the possible usefulness of α-tocopherol an active subject. The question that remains to be answered is whether or not tocopherol in large amounts, or some metabolite of α-tocopherol, has physiological functions that can be observed and measured. As for the antioxidant function of the tocopherols, one must admit that larger amounts of an antioxidant should protect tissues susceptible to oxidative stress more efficiently than would smaller amounts. In this respect vitamin E differs from vitamins involved in enzymatic reactions, for example, thiamin and riboflavin where increases in the consumption of thiamin- and riboflavin-containing coenzymes beyond the amounts needed for normal rates of reaction do not cause the in vivo rate of the reaction to change. As for a function for a metabolite of α-tocopherol, only one such compound, α-tocopherylquinone, the first oxidation product of α-tocopherol, is a candidate for a possible physiological function.

A. Air Pollutants

One activity of α-tocopherol that has received attention in recent years is the possible salutory effect on lungs exposed to oxidative compounds in the atmosphere. A number of investigators, stimulated by increased attention to environmental and pollution problems, have claimed that α-tocopherol protects the lungs from damage caused by ozone and nitrogen dioxide [40-42]. Menzel et al. have also studied the phenomenon [43] to show that Heinz bodies are produced in normal human erythrocytes in the presence of ozone and unsaturated lipids. When mice fed the usual laboratory chow were exposed to ozone (0.85 ppm) for 4 hr, Heinz bodies occurred in approximately one-half the erythrocytes. Large doses of vitamin E were needed to prevent the formation of Heinz bodies in cells exposed to ozone.

In one study [42], an amount of vitamin E comparable to "average American consumption" was fed to rats. These animals had marked lung damage when exposed to 0.1 ppm ozone for 7 days. When another group of rats were fed 6 times as much vitamin E (6.6 mg/100 g rat diet) the undesirable effects were essentially absent.

The kinds of pollutants now found in our atmosphere represent a relatively new phenomenon in human experience. Perhaps it will be necessary to take what most nutritionists would consider unorthodox action to protect ourselves from this threat to our health—much more work in this field is indicated.

B. Effects of α-Tocopherylquinone

The biological activity of any drug is a function not only of its intact molecule, but also of its metabolite products. While the amounts of such metabolite products may not be significant when the tocopherols are ingested in amounts normally considered to be in the dietary range, their biological concentrations may be increased to levels that produce physiological effects when large amounts of vitamin E are ingested.

When α-tocopherol is in contact with ferric iron, α-tocopherylquinone is formed. It is not yet clear how much remains in animal tissues after it is formed, but when large amounts of α-tocopherol are ingested an appreciable amount of the quinone must be formed in the intestinal tract.

Both d-α-tocopheryl and d-α-tocopherylquinone can be reduced to form d-α-tocopheryl hydroquinone. Both the quinone and the hydroquinone can cure nutritional muscular dystrophy in animals [45,46]. The hydroquinone will also protect vitamin E-deficient rats during gestation [47]. Mauer and Mason [48] have shown that d-α-tocopheryl hydroquinone can prevent injury to the testes of vitamin E-deficient rats and rabbits. In addition, Rao and Mason [49] have demonstrated that d-α-tocopheryl hydroquinone has antivitamin K activity. Woolley [50] found that α-tocopherylquinone could function as an antimetabolite of vitamin K. This latter effect, when interpreted with other data, makes it possible to give some logical impetus to the theory that vitamin E may have something to do with vascular physiology. As Woolley has shown, there is a striking resemblance between parts of the molecules of phylloquinone (vitamin K_1) and α-tocopherylquinone. The latter could be a competitive inhibitor of vitamin K. In evaluating this possibility, it should be recalled that a large proportion of vitamin K is formed in the intestinal tract where much of the α-tocopherylquinone is also expected to be formed.

C. Prolongation of Blood Clotting

Korsan-Bengstan et al. [51] have reported that patients who had recovered from myocardial infarctions had a shorter plasma clotting time than a general population sample of the same age and sex. This stimulated these investigators to study the effects of long-term treatment with α-tocopherol on the plasma clotting time and rate of fibrinolysis [52]. After a 5-week period of study to establish basal levels, nine male subjects who had had myocardial infarctions within 5 years were given 300 mg α-tocopherol a day and observed for 64 weeks. The subjects were not decompensated and did not receive any drugs that could influence serum lipids or hemostasis. There was a prolongation of plasma clotting time, with and without the presence of Russell viper venom which started after 6 weeks of treatment. Some support for this work has been published by Corrigan and Marcus [53]. They observed clinical evidence of vitamin K deficiency during the course of treating a patient with warfarin and clofibrate. Upon learning that the patient had been taking 1200 IU vitamin E per day, they studied the combined effects of the therapy the patient was receiving. They were able to show that by adding or subtracting dl-α-tocopheryl acetate to the therapeutic regimen of warfarin and clofibrate that the vitamin E had an additional effect in depressing the vitamin K-dependent coagulation factors. After the vitamin E ingestion had been discontinued for 2 months, the patient was given 0.25 mg warfarin per day, 500 mg clofibrate 4 times/day and 800 mg dl-α-tocopheryl acetate daily. The baseline was double the normal level because of the effect of the known vitamin K inhibitors. The additional effect of the vitamin E was apparent by the 28th day. There was a drop in prothrombin time when the vitamin E ingestion was stopped for 7 days.

Schrogie [54] confirmed the potentiation of warfarin activity by vitamin E in rats given warfarin. Subsequently, three human volunteers were given 42 IU vitamin E for 30 days and no potentiation by vitamin E of the effect of 150 mg dicumarol was obtained. Apparently larger amounts of vitamin E for longer periods are needed to obtain a measurable effect.

Whether or not α-tocopherylquinone is responsible, at least in part, for the prolongation of blood clotting which has been reported is yet to be proven by additional research. At present, one may say that the evidence is rather convincing. An earlier controversy as to whether the quinone can be found in animal labeled d-α-tocopherol to prove the occurrence of small quantities of tocopherylquinone in the livers and muscle extracts of rats and pigs. Plack and Bieri [56] repeated the work of Draper and co-workers [57] to confirm the presence of tocopherylquinone in the tissues using different analytical techniques. It is noteworthy that Weber and Wiss [58] reported that relatively large amounts of α-tocopherylquinone were present in the depot fat of rats. More was present in animals fed a diet with coconut oil. More recently the kinetics of the accumulation of α-tocopherylquinone in the liver after intraperitoneal administration of large amounts of α-tocopheryl acetate to mice has been reported [59].

Although in vitro production of the quinone by $FeCl_3$, or other oxidative agents is a simple procedure, we do not know whether the amounts of quinone in the blood are sufficiently large to have an effect on blood-clotting mechanisms. There should be less question about the amounts of tocopherylquinone in the intestine, where much of the vitamin K is produced, since much of a large dose of α-tocopherol is excreted by way of the intestinal tract.

Attempts to explain claims for the use of vitamin E in the treatment of peripheral vascular and thromboembolic disease has led to research on the inhibition of plasmin-mediated fibrinolysis by vitamin E. Moroz and Gilmore [60] have recently reported a direct effect of vitamin E on the fibrinolytic system, namely, "in vitro inhibition of plasmin-mediated fibrinolysis at physiological concentrations of the vitamin and the enzyme."

Another aspect of blood-clotting relationships to vitamin E therapy has been studied by Machlin et al. [61]. If the peroxidation of arachidonate in platelets is inhibited by vitamin E, platelet aggregation may also be inhibited. To support this hypothesis it is shown that collagen-induced platelet aggregation was increased in vitamin E-deficient rats. In a later report, these workers [62] studied the influence of dietary vitamin E on prostoglandin biosynthesis in rat blood, since the endoperoxide of some of the prostoglandins biosynthesized by aggregating human platelets may cause extensive platelet aggregation. Their experiments with rats suggested that in vivo α-tocopherol may inhibit the generation of platelet-stimulating endoperoxides.

Do physicians who have presceibed vitamin E for its possible beneficial effects for vascular disorders have a better rationale now than they had before? It is hoped that there will be a resurgence of research on vitamin E to answer this question.

REFERENCES

1. B. Century, M. K. Horwitt, and P. Bailey, Arch. Gen. Psychiat. 1:420 (1959).
2. M. K. Horwitt and P. Bailey, Arch. Neurol. 1:312 (1959).
3. J. S. Dinning and P. L. Day, J. Exp. Med. 105:395 (1957).
4. H. N. Marvin, J. S. Dinning, and P. L. Day, Proc. Soc. Exp. Biol. Med. 105:473 (1960).
5. H. N. Marvin, Amer. J. Clin. Nutr. 12:88 (1963).
6. C. D. Fitch and F. S. Porter, J. Nutr. 89:251 (1966).

7. M. K. Horwitt, B. Century, and A. A. Zeman, Amer. J. Clin. Nutr. 12:99 (1963).
8. F. A. Oski and L. A. Barness, J. Pediatr. 70:211 (1967).
9. H. J. Binder, D. C. Herting, V. Hurst, S. C. Finch, and H. M. Spiro, N. Engl. J. Med. 273:1289 (1965).
10. J. H. Ritchie, M. B. Fish, V. McMasters, and M. Grossman, N. Engl. J. Med. 279:1185 (1968).
11. P. J. Leonard and M. S. Losowsky, Amer. J. Clin. Nutr. 24:388 (1971).
12. A. S. Majaj, J. S. Dinning, S. A. Azzam, and W. J. Darby, Amer. J. Clin. Nutr. 12:374 (1963).
13. H. N. Marvin and I. S. Audu, W. African Med. J. 13:3 (1964).
14. J. A. Whitaker, E. G. Fort, S. Vimokesant, and J. S. Dinning, Amer. J. Clin. Nutr. 20:783 (1967).
15. M. K. Horwitt, C. C. Harvey, G. D. Duncan, and W. C. Wilson, Amer. J. Clin. Nutr. 4:408 (1956).
16. M. K. Horwitt, Amer. J. Clin. Nutr. 8:451 (1960).
17. H. M. Rubenstein, A. A. Dietz, and R. Srinivasan, Clin. Chim. Acta 23:1 (1969).
18. T. Davies, J. Kelleher, and M. S. Losowsky, Clin. Chim. Acta 24:431 (1969).
19. M. K. Horwitt, C. C. Harvey, C. H. Dahm, and M. T. Searcy, Ann. N.Y. Acad. Sci. 203:223 (1972).
20. B. J. Meyer, B. Century, A. C. Meyer, and M. K. Horwitt, Arch. Gen. Psychiatr. 2:528 (1960).
21. M. K. Horwitt, Amer. J. Clin. Nutr. 27:1182 (1974).
22. Food and Nutrition Board, N.R.C. Recommended Dietary Allowance, 7th ed. National Academy of Science, Washington, D.C., 1968.
23. Food and Nutrition Board, N.R.C. Recommended Dietary Allowance, 8th ed. National Academy of Science, Washington, D.C., 1974.
24. D. K. Melhorn and S. Gross, J. Pediatr. 79:569 (1971).
25. M. A. Chadd and A. J. Frazer, Int. J. Vet. Res. 40:610 (1970).
26. S. S. Lo, D. Frank, and W. H. Hitzig, Arch. Dis. Child. 48:000 (19).
27. H. Hassan, S. A. Hashim, T. B. Van Itallie, and W. H. Sebrell, Amer. J. Clin. Nutr. 19:147 (1966).
28. L. Johnson, D. Schaffer, and T. R. Boggs, Jr., Amer. J. Clin. Nutr. 27:1158 (1974).
29. P. L. Harris and N. D. Embree, Amer. J. Clin. Nutr. 13:385 (1963).
30. J. G. Bieri, Nutr. Rev. 33:161 (1975).
31. H. T. Slover, Lipids 6:291 (1971).
32. R. H. Bunnell, J. Keating, A. Quaresimo, and G. K. Parman, Amer. J. Clin. Nutr. 17:1 (1965).
33. J. G. Bieri and R. Poukka Evarts, J. Amer. Diet. Assn. 62:147 (1973).

34. P. L. Harris, E. G. Hardenbrook, F. P. Dean, E. R. Cusack, and J. L. Jensen, Proc. Soc. Exp. Biol. Med. 107:381 (1961).
35. J. G. Bieri and R. Poukka Evarts, Amer. J. Clin. Nutr. 28:717 (1975).
36. M. K. Horwitt, C. C. Harvey, and E. T. Harmon, Vit. Horm. 26:487 (1968).
37. J. G. Bieri and R. Poukka Evarts, J. Nutr. 104:850 (1974).
38. J. G. Bieri, R. Poukka Evarts, and J. J. Garts, J. Nutr. 106:124 (1976).
39. M. L. Scott and I. D. Desai, J. Nutr. 83:39 (1964).
40. C. K. Chow and A. L. Tappel, Lipids 7:518 (1972).
41. D. B. Menzel, J. N. Roehm, and S. O. Lee, Agr. Food Chem. 20:481 (1972).
42. M. G. Mustapha, Nutr. Rep. Interm. 11:473 (1975).
43. D. B. Menzel, R. J. Slaughter, A. M. Bryant, and H. O. Jauregui, Arch. Environ. Health 30:296 (1975).
44. M. K. Horwitt, Amer. J. Clin. Nutr. 29:00 (1976).
45. J. B. MacKensie, H. Rosenkrantz, S. Ulick, and A. T. Milhorat, J. Biol. Chem. 183:655 (1950).
46. J. B. MacKensie and C. G. MacKensie, J. Nutr. 67:223 (1959).
47. J. B. MacKensie and C. G. MacKensie, J. Nutr. 72:322 (1960).
48. S. I. Mauer and K. E. Mason, J. Nutr. 105:491 (1975).
49. G. H. Rao and K. E. Mason, J. Nutr. 105:495 (1975).
50. D. W. Woolley, J. Biol. Chem. 159:59 (1945).
51. K. Korsan-Bengsten, L. Wilhelmsen, D. Elmfeldt, and G. Tibblin, Atherosclerosis 16:83 (1972).
52. K. Korsan-Bengsten, D. Elmfeldt, and T. Holm, Thromb. Diath. Haemorrhag. 31:505 (1974).
53. J. J. Corrigan and F. I. Marcus, JAMA 230:1300 (1974).
54. J. J. Schrogie, JAMA 232:19 (1975).
55. A. S. Csallany, H. H. Draper, and S. N. Shah, Arch. Biochem. Biophys. 98:142 (1962).
56. P. A. Plack and J. G. Bieri, Biochem. Biophys. Acta 84:729 (1964).
57. H. H. Draper, A. S. Csallany, and S. H. Shah, Biochem. Biophys. Acta 59:527 (1962).
58. F. Weber and O. Wiss, Helv. Physiol. Pharmacol. Acta 21:131 (1963).
59. S. A. Aristarkhova, Y. B. Barlokova, and N. G. Khrapova, Biofizika 19:703 (English trans.) (1973).
60. L. A. Moroz and N. J. Gilmore, Nature (Lond.) 259:235 (1976).
61. L. J. Machlin, R. Filipski, A. L. Willis, D. C. Kuhn, and M. Brin, Proc. Soc. Exp. Biol. Med. 149:275 (1975).
62. W. C. Hope, C. Dalton, L. J. Machlin, R. J. Filipski, and F. M. Vane, Prostglandins 10:557 (1975).

12 EPILOGUE

LAWRENCE J. MACHLIN
Hoffmann-La Roche Inc.
Nutley, New Jersey

In this chapter, I wish to briefly discuss some highlights of this book and my view of several aspects of vitamin E research. These comments are presented with the hope of stimulating further discussion and experimental research on vitamin E.

I. FOOD SOURCES

Plant foods vary considerably in vitamin E content depending on genetics, growing conditions, harvesting, storage, processing and cooking factors (see Chapter 4). As a result, there is poor agreement between estimates of vitamin E intake based on tabular data and those obtained by direct analysis. However, more information is now becoming available on the content of tocopherol and tocotrienol isomers in food. As this information accumulates, nutritionists will be able to estimate the vitamin E contribution not only from α-tocopherol, but from the other isomers as well.

The feeding of vitamin E to cattle, pigs, and poultry results in increased levels of the vitamin in meat, milk, and eggs, and if given in sufficient quantity is effective in preventing oxidative rancidity and resultant off-flavors in these foods (see Chapter 9).

II. ABSORPTION, TRANSPORT, AND TISSUE STORAGE

Intestinal absorption via the lymphatic system of tocopherol is dependent on simultaneous absorption of dietary lipids and the presence of bile acids (see Chapter 5A). The rate of absorption can be enhanced by simultaneous administration of medium-chain triglycerides. Tocopherol is transported

in the lipoprotein fractions of the blood. There is currently no evidence
for a specific transport protein. There is a high correlation between total
plasma lipid and plasma tocopherol. The uptake of tocopherol into tissues
varies directly with the logarithm of the tocopherol intake. This represents a departure from most vitamins, which usually have distinct thresh-
olds in tissues other than the liver, and may provide the explanation for
pharmacological effects of vitamin E. Adipose tissue, liver, and muscle
represent major storage depots of the vitamin. Adrenal and pituitary
glands and platelets have the highest concentration of the vitamin. The
rate of depletion of tocopherol after feeding a vitamin E-deficient diet
varies considerably from tissue to tissue, being relatively rapid in plasma
and liver, slower in skeletal and heart muscle, and very slow in adipose
tissue.

III. BIOCHEMICAL FUNCTION

The most reasonable single explanation of vitamin E function is that the
vitamin protects the integrity of cellular membranes against free radical
attack. α-Tocopherol is probably located within the membrane as a complex with the polyunsaturated fatty acids (PUFA) of the phospholipids. The
tocopherol may be specifically located near membrane-bound enzyme
complexes that can generate free radicals, such as the mixed-function
oxidases, prostaglandin synthetase, and reduced nicotinamide adenine
dinucleotide phosphate (NADPH) oxidase systems. The positioning of
tocopherol near these membrane-bound enzymes would facilitate the
trapping of free radicals and thus protect the membrane from damage.

   These concepts are elegantly presented by McCay and King (Chapter 5E.1); Molenaar and his co-workers (Chapter 5G); and Walton and
Packer (Chapter 10B). Thus, the many biochemical and pathological
effects of vitamin E inadequacy may be explained on the basis of alteration
in membrane structure and function without involving tocopherol in a specific role as a coenzyme or regulator of the synthesis of specific proteins.

   Vitamin E could also protect cells against damage by free radicals
from exogeneous sources (Chapter 10A). For example, inhalation of ozone
might lead to free radical damage in lung tissue. Consumption of carbon
tetrachloride and a variety of drugs might increase free radical production
in the liver.

   The ability of selenium to alleviate some of the consequences of
vitamin E inadequacy can be explained by its role as a component of glutathione peroxidase. This enzyme can also prevent free radical formation
by reducing H_2O_2 and other peroxides.

   It is interesting to note that almost all of the enzymes affected by
vitamin E status (Chapter 5E.2) are either membrane-bound or are

concerned with the glutathione peroxidase system. Thus, the concept that
vitamin E is primarily concerned with the protection of cellular membranes
from damage resulting from both endogeneous and exogenous sources of
free radicals is supported.

This concept does not necessarily exclude the possibility that vitamin E
may have some more specific role in metabolism and the recent findings of
binding protein for tocopherol in the liver nucleus (Chapter 5E.2) keep
alive such speculation.

IV. PATHOLOGY OF VITAMIN E DEFICIENCY

Recent histopathological studies using electron microscopic techniques
reinforce the concept that initial damage to tissues of vitamin E deficient
animals involves membranes, and in particular, microsomal and mito-
chrondrial membranes (see Chapters 5G and 7). The exact mechanism
involved in pathogenesis of cellular injury is still not known.

Blood vessels, particularly the capillaries, are often an early site of
tissue injury and in these cases, pathology is secondary to vascular injury
(Chapter 5G). An example of this occurs in development of nutritional
encephalomalacia in chickens. The earliest detectable changes in the
endothelial cells indicate lysosomal activation. This is followed by the
onset of neurological signs or the development of parenchymal necrosis.
The lesions developed are similar to infarcts caused by occulsive vascular
disease. In other E deficiency syndromes such as embryopathology,
exudative diathesis, and cardiomyopathy, there is also evidence that
vascular injury may be an early event.

In addition to injury to the endothelial cells, there is increased
tendency for platelet aggregation in plasma of vitamin E-deficient animals.
Thrombi are observed in cerebellum capillaries of chickens with encephalomalacia and also in the hearts of pigs with cardiomyopathy resulting from
vitamin E deficiency. The relevance of these observations to the etiology
of stroke, myocardial infarction, and other vascular diseases in humans
remains to be defined.

V. DISEASE RESISTANCE: IMMUNE RESPONSE

Tengerdy and his co-workers (see Chapter 8) have demonstrated enhanced
humoral immunity in animals and increased phagocytosis with vitamin E
supplements. Their studies are very provocative. Can cellular immunity
also be stimulated by vitamin E? Since cellular immunity is suppressed
by prostaglandins [1] and vitamin E reduces prostaglandin synthesis
(Chapter 5F), there is some theoretical basis for predicting such an

effect. It would be of considerable interest to determine whether vitamin E
can enhance the immune response in humans, particularly in immuno-
deficient populations such as the aged and those with cancer.

VI. AGING

The free radical hypothesis of aging provides a reasonable basis for proposing that vitamin E will extend the life span (Chapter 10B). The best
evidence for an extension of life span with vitamin E comes from studies
using <u>Drosophila melanogaster</u> or nematodes. The total number of population doublings observed in diploid human cell cultures increases with vitamin E treatment. This effect may only be related to the protection of the
cells against toxic effects of oxygen.

   The reports of increased life span of rodents treated with vitamin E
have not been convincing to many gerontologists. The reduction of the
"age" pigment (lipofuscin) in tissues of vitamin E animals supports but
does not prove the value of vitamin E in inhibiting the aging process.
Thus, unequivocal evidence for a role of vitamin E in the extension of life
span is not available. It is of some interest that the vitamin E requirement of rats increases with age [2] and it would be desirable to determine
whether this applies to humans. From a practical view, any effect of
vitamin E on improving the immune response or in preventing vascular
disease would have a profound effect on life span, even if the free radical
hypothesis was not an important mechanism. However, such effects also
remain to be proven.

VII. HUMAN DEFICIENCY STATES

In humans, the best studied examples of vitamin E deficiency are premature
infants and patients with cystic fibrosis (see Chapter 11A). Both conditions
are characterized by low blood tocopherol (less than 0.5 mg %), and in vitro
and in vivo hemolysis of erythrocytes.

   The typical syndromes appear at 4-6 weeks of age in infants of birth-
weights less than 1500 g and are characterized by reticulocytosis, thrombocytosis, and low hemoglobin values in the range of 7-10 g/dl. Some
infants have edema of the lower extremeties and scrotal area. This type
of anemia cannot be prevented by iron or vitamin B_{12} and it rarely responds
to folic acid therapy. The deficiency is usually associated with consumption
of infant formulas which are high in linoleic acid and low in vitamin E. The
administration of vitamin E intramuscularly during the first week of life
followed by daily oral administration of 25 mg vitamin E reverses all
symptoms. In addition, administration of vitamin E to premature infants

exposed to high oxygen environments reduces the incidence and severity of retrolental fibroplasia and bronchopulmonary dysplasia [3].

Cystic fibrosis patients are the best-studied "experiment of nature" involving prolonged vitamin deficiency in the young growing human. Many of the signs observed in vitamin E-deficient animals are found in these patients. There is some in vivo hemolysis as evidenced by decreased red blood cell (RBC) survival times. Some subjects with cystic fibrosis have elevated urinary creatine excretion and elevated plasma creatine phosphokinase (CPK), both indices of myopathy, although there is no clinical evidence of muscular weakness. As many as 10%, however, may display evidence of cardiomyopathy. Some sexually mature males have testicular dysfunction as evidenced by low semen volume, low sperm counts, and a high incidence of sperm abnormalities. In patients greater than 2 years old, lipofuscin accumulates in the smooth mouth muscle and other tissues.

The experience with premature infants and cystic fibrosis patients as well as with experimental nutritional deprivation in humans (the Elgin Project) (Chapter 11B) and with experimental animals indicates that blood levels of less than 0.5 mg% are usually associated with both in vitro and in vivo hemolysis. Although this rarely results in anemia, it might be considered a stress on the erythropoietic system, since RBC life is decreased. From studies of cystic fibrosis patients it is suggested that prolonged vitamin E deficiency, at least in children, can result in skeletal myopathy and cardiomyopathy and accumulation of lipofuscin in tissues. Thus, there is some justification for the proposal that blood levels of less than 0.5 mg% tocopherol should be considered indicative of vitamin E deficiency, and should be corrected. The major difficulty with this criterion is that plasma tocopherol levels are highly correlated with plasma cholesterol or total plasma lipids. As a result, subjects with hyperlipemia or hypolipemia might have plasma tocopherol levels that do not truly reflect the tissue tocopherol. In these cases, plasma tocopherol values would have little meaning. It has been suggested that a ratio of 0.8 mg total tocopherol per gram of total plasma lipids be used as a more meaningful index of vitamin E status in adults. In children 0.6 mg/g lipid may be the "lower limit" of normal [4].

Based on plasma tocopherol levels, another vitamin E-deficient population has been identified, β-thalassemia patients. These subjects have low blood tocopherols accompanied by deposits of lipofuscin in their tissues [5,6]. Although vitamin E therapy has not significantly reduced the transfusion requirements, the RBC half-life has been prolonged in about half the subjects with β-thalassemia [7]. Thalassemia intermedia subjects also have extremely low blood tocopherol values and should be studied more thoroughly as another "natural" human model of a vitamin E deficiency.

Patients with another genetic hemolytic anemia, sickle-cell anemia, have also been found to have low blood tocopherol levels [8]. Administration

of vitamin E to these patients results in a considerable reduction in the
percent of circulating irreversibly sickled cells [9]. Whether vitamin E
will ameliorate the anemia and other clinical manifestations of the disease
remains to be determined.

VIII. FACTORS INFLUENCING NUTRITIONAL REQUIREMENTS

As indicated by the several authors in this book (see Chapters 5D and 11A),
establishment of nutritional requirements is replete with difficulties. In
animals, selenium and sulfur amino acids will prevent certain vitamin E
deficiency symptoms. In the United States, a deficiency of either of these
latter nutrients is rare. However, we are aware of no controlled studies
in humans that have been concerned with such interrelationships. Although
polyunsaturated fatty acids (PUFA) increases the vitamin E requirement in
animals, a similar quantitative relationship in humans has been more difficult to establish.

Vitamin E ameliorates the effects of a large number of insults to
experimental animals. These include high oxygen tension, ozone, nitrogen
dioxide, mercury, lead, alcohol, carbon tetrachloride, nitrosamine
[10,11], and drugs (acetaminophen, digitalis, and adriamycin) (see Chapter 10A) [12,13].

α-Tocopherol prevents nitrosamine formation in vitro by destroying
nitrite anion and in vivo by preventing the nitrosative cleavage of the amine
to a nitrosamine [10,11]. Since 80% of nitrosamines are carcinogenic, the
prevention of nitrosamine formation is of considerable potential significance
for the prevention of cancer. A recent report [14] has shown that administration of vitamin E to humans results in over a 90% reduction in mutagenic
activity in feces. This is presumptive evidence that vitamin E might
reduce nitrosamine-induced carcinogenesis in humans. Verification and
extension of such studies in humans would be most welcome.

The effect of vitamin E therapy in protecting against the consequences
of high oxygen atmosphere in premature infants (retrolental fibroplasia,
pulmonary dysplasia) has recently been reported [3]. The role of
vitamin E in protecting humans against the harmful effects of many other
toxicants deserves investigation. Ethical considerations preclude experimentation with heavy metals and most drugs. However, a study of the
interrelationship of alcohol intake and E status could be undertaken. The
effect of tocopherol on adriamycin toxicity could also be investigated,
since the drug is being used in cancer treatment in spite of the risks of
cardiomyopathy. Oral contraceptive users have reduced plasma tocopherol
levels. The significance of this observation could be explored. Finally,
the role of vitamin E in the human immune response demands further consideration. This should be investigated in both normal and immune deficient subjects.

IX. TREATMENT OR PREVENTION OF DISEASE

As Farrell has pointed out (Chapter 11A), proving the efficacy or the lack
of efficacy of a treatment for many diseases is fraught with experimental
difficulties. Although the literature on vitamin E therapy is enormous, the
number of well-controlled studies with adequate numbers of subjects is
still quite small.

The efficacy of vitamin E in the treatment of intermittent claudication
appears reasonably established. Beyond that, good objective evidence for
therapeutic effects from vitamin E appears meagre. However, a number
of recent findings provide a theoretical basis for reinvestigation of the role
of vitamin E in treatment of vascular and inflammatory diseases. For
one, it is now clear that platelet physiology can be altered by vitamin E
status. Platelets normally have an extremely high tocopherol concentration compared to other tissues of the body and this content can be varied,
depending on tocopherol intake. There is some evidence that platelet
aggregation [15, 16] and platelet factor-3 release can be inhibited by
vitamin E [17]. Thus, vitamin E status may affect thrombosis both by a
direct effect on aggregation and indirectly by influencing blood coagulation
as mediated by platelet factor-3. Further confirmation of the influence of
vitamin E on platelet physiology in humans is definitely needed. The
observations in animals of early pathological changes in small blood
vessels also suggest that vitamin E might influence peripheral blood flow.

Another recent observation in animals which should be confirmed and
extended is the inhibitory effect of vitamin E on prostaglandin synthesis
(see Chapter 5F) [18]. Some, but not all trials have indicated that vitamin E has an antiinflammatory effect in animals [19, 20]. Preliminary
information in humans with inflammatory skin lesions [21] and periodontal
disease [22] suggests that vitamin E can alleviate these diseases. Examination of the concept that vitamin E can influence the inflammatory process should also be encouraged.

In summary, vitamin E deficiency (defined as less than 0.5 mg%
plasma tocopherol) resulting from low intakes or malabsorption or both,
generally results in a reduced RBC half-life, but no anemia. Anemia is
observed in premature infants and children with protein-calorie deficiency,
but RBC synthesis may be limited in these cases by factors other than vitamin E. In thalassemia and sickle-cell anemia, plasma tocopherol levels are
low but the clinical consequences of these low levels have not been clearly
established. With a very prolonged deficiency in children such as occurs in
cystic fibrosis, a mild myopathy may occur in some patients, but muscle
dysfunction has not been reported. Cardiomyopathy and testis degeneration
have also been observed in some of the cystic fibrosis patients, although a
relationship of these symptoms to vitamin E status has yet to be proven.

In adults, a deficiency of vitamin E would be expected to put some
strain on the haemopoietic system, but would have no other obvious conse-

quence. The major question facing us is: What are the less obvious consequences? Can marginal vitamin E deficiency over a long time span cause serious consequences? Is the immune system and/or inflammatory process compromised? Is the body less able to cope with environmental insults (i.e., air pollutants, alcohol, nitrosamines, other xenobiotics)? Is peripheral blood flow altered? Is there a greater susceptibility to peripheral blood flow altered? Is there a greater susceptibility to peripheral vascular disease? Can vitamin E ameliorate the clinical manifestations of sickle-cell anemia? Only when we have answers to these questions will the role of vitamin E in animal and human health be adequately defined.

REFERENCES

1. O. J. Plescia, A. H. Smith, and K. Grinwich, Proc. Natl. Acad. Sci. USA 72:1848 (1975).

2. S. R. Ames, Amer. J. Clin. Nutr. 27:1017 (1974).

3. R. A. Ehrenkranz, B. W. Bonta, R. C. Ablow, and J. B. Warshaw, N. Engl. J. Med. 299:564 (1978).

4. P. M. Farrell, S. L. Levine, M. D. Murphy, and A. J. Adams, Amer. J. Clin. Nutr. 31:1720 (1978).

5. C. B. Hyman, B. Landing, R. Alfin-Slater, L. Kozak, J. Weitzman, and J. A. Ortega, Ann. N.Y. Acad. Sci. 232:211 (1974).

6. E. A. Rachmilewitz, B. H. Lubin, and S. B. Shohet, Blood 47:495 (1976).

7. E. A. Rachmilewitz, A. Shifter, and I. Kahane, Amer. J. Clin. Nutr. 32:1850 (1979).

8. C. Natta and L. J. Machlin, Amer. J. Clin. Nutr. 32:1359 (1979).

9. L. J. Machlin, C. Natta, and M. Brin, Fed. Proc. 38:609 (1979).

10. J. J. Kamm, T. Dashman, H. Newmark, and W. J. Mergens, Toxicol. Appl. Pharmacol. 41:575 (1977).

11. W. J. Mergens, J. J. Kamm, H. L. Newmark, W. Fiddler, and J. Pensabene, in Environmental Aspects of N-Nitroso Compounds. Edited by E. A. Walker, M. Castegnaro, L. Griciute, and R. E. Lyle. Lyon, IARC Scientific Pub. No. 19, 1978, p. 199.

12. J. Kelleher, M. P. Keaney, B. E. Walker, M. S. Nosowsky, and M. F. Dixon, J. Int. Med. Res. 4:138 Suppl. 4 (1976).

13. C. E. Myers, W. McGuire, and R. Young, Can. Treat. Rep. 60:961 (1976).

14. W. R. Bruce, A. J. Varghese, S. Wang, and P. Dion, in Naturally-Occurring Carcinogens: Mutagens and Modulation of Carcinogenesis. Proc. of the 9th Princess Takamatso Symposium, Tokyo 1979, Univ. Park, Baltimore. In press.

15. L. J. Machlin, R. Filipski, A. L. Willis, D. C. Kuhn, and M. Brin, Proc. Soc. Exp. Biol. Med. 149:275 (1975).

16. J. Anastasi and M. Steiner, Clin. Res. $\underline{24}$:498A (1976).

17. K. Korsan-Bengsten, D. Elmfeldt, and T. Holm, Thromb. Diath. Haemorrhag. $\underline{31}$:505 (1974).

18. W. C. Hope, $\overline{C}$. Dalton, L. J. Machlin, R. J. Filipski, and F. M. Vane, Prostaglandins $\underline{10}$:557 (1975).

19. V. W. Stuyvesant and $\overline{W}$. J. Jolley, Nature (Lond.) $\underline{216}$:587 (1967).

20. M. Kamimura, J. Vitaminol. $\underline{18}$:204 (1972).

21. M. Jaratt, South. Med. J. $\underline{69}$:113 (1976).

22. J. M. Goodson, in Diet, Nutrition and Peridontal Disease. Edited by S. P. Hazen. Chicago, Ill., American Society for Preventative Dentistry, 1975, p. 53.

INDEX

Abetalipoproteinemia, 523, 563-566, 575, 577
  peroxidative hemolysis test, 578
Abortion, 594-595
Absorption, 170-189, 637
  effect of bile and pancreatic juice, 180-181, 185-186, 189
  effect of dietary lipid, 181-183, 189
  efficiency of, 179, 189
  inhibitors of, 103-104
  lymphatic, 175-177, 180-182, 187-188
  intestinal, 171-183
  methods, 171-175
  sites of, 176-179
Acanthocytes, 418
Accessory sex glands, 349-351
Acetaminophen toxicity, 642
Acid phosphatase, 322
ACTH (adrenocorticotropic hormone), 284, 357-364
Adducts, 244-246
Adenylate cyclase, 370
Adherent cells, 433
Adipose tissue, 83
  analysis, 83

[Adipose tissue]
  depletion of tocopherol, 266-229
  peroxidation of, 386
Adrenal, 206-208, 217, 248, 353-364
Adrenal function, 353-364
Adriamycin toxicity, 642
Age, influence on tissue content, 201-203
Aging, 640
  free radical hypothesis, 495-512, 640
  immune response, 442
  neuropathology, 415
Air pollutants, 474, 480, 630-631
Alanine amino transferase, 322
Alcohol toxicity, 484-485, 642
Aldolase, 322
Algae, 84-87, 392
Alfalfa, 102-103, 106, 446
Aminopyrine demethylase, 322
Amaurotic family idiocy, 422
Amyotrophic lateral sclerosis, 415
Analysis, 65-97
  automated, 91
  colorimetry, 70-71, 91
  column chromatography, 73

[Analysis]
  electrochemical (polarographic),
    79, 91
  of foods and feeds, 84-85
  gas-liquid chromatography, 78-79
  high performance liquid
    chromatography, 73-74, 91
  paper chromatography, 74
  of pharmaceuticals, 85-86
  sample preparation, 68
  molecular distillation, 69-70
  saponification, 68-69
  spectrofluorometry, 72-73, 91
  spectrophotometry, 71-72
  thin layer chromatography, 75-78
  of tissues, 81-84
Androgen, 350-352, 382
Anemia, 418, 574
    (see also Hemolytic anemia)
  of protein-calorie malnutrition,
    568
  of premature infant, 418-419,
    523-540
Angina pectoris, 586-587
Antibody production, 431-434
Anti-coagulant activity, 593-594
Anti-inflammatory, 248, 597, 643
Antioxidant, function of vitamin E,
    23, 50   292-296
Antioxidant theory, 281-282,
    289-309, 334-335, 342, 465
Antioxidants, 280-282, 335
  and aging, 506-512
  and anti-body production, 431-433
  and cancer, 510-512
  and encephalomalacia, 407
  and lipopigments, 422
Anti-vitamin K activity, 593, 631
Arachidonic acid, 300, 343,
    378-379, 381, 482-483, 504
  in lungs, 482
  ratio to tocopherol, 382, 385
Arachidonic acid metabolism, 479
Arterial blood flow, 590-591

Arteritis, 407
Arteriolocapillary fibrosis, 500,
    502
Arteriosclerosis, 284, 582
Ascorbic acid, 284, 357, 500, 508,
    509
Aspartate amino transferase, 89,
    322
Ataxia, 407, 413
Atherosclerotic plaque, 278
ATPase, 290, 332, 335-336, 341
    383, 420
Autofluorescence, 420
Autofluorescent granules, in brain
    capillaries, 410-411
Axon, degeneration of, 409,
    413-417

Bacteria, 268
Baking of foods, 113-115, 122
Batten's disease, 422
Benzylyl radical, 232
BHA (butylated hydroxy anisole),
    280, 284, 445, 510
BHT (butylated hydroxy toluene),
    280, 284, 445, 453, 508-510
Bile, 180, 185-186, 250-252, 559
Biliary atresia, 557-559, 575, 577
  neuropathology, 415
Biliary cirrhosis, 557-558
Biliary obstruction, 557, 560-561
Bilirubinemia, 538
Binding protein for tocopherol, 329
Bioassay, 86-90
Biochemical function, 638
Biogensis (see biosynthesis)
Biological activity, relation to
    structure, 49-51
Biosynthesis, 48-49, 101, 268-271
Bleaching, 112
Blood,
  analysis, 81, 87
  clotting, 632-633

[Blood]
coagulation, 593
flow, 590-591
Blood tocopherol (see also Plasma
and Serum tocopherol)
in adult humans, 525, 599-602
in children, 600-602
in cystic fibrosis patients, 543-544
relationship to lipid, 599, 625, 628
Bone marrow abnormalities, 418
Brain,
glutathathione peroxidase content,
227
pathology, 407-413
Bread, 138-139
Breakfast cereals, 133-135

Calves,
myopathy, 406
Cancer, 436, 441-442, 496,
505-512, 642
Canning, 115-116
Capillaries,
degeneration in brain, 407-408,
410-411, 503
lysosomal changes, 407-413
Capillary fragility, 530
Capillary leakage, 417
Carbamyl phosphate synthetase,
322
Carbon tetrachloride,
source of free radicals, 303-306,
484-485
toxicity, 303-306, 484, 489
Carcinogenesis, 305
Carcinogens, 496, 505-506,
510-511, 642
Cardiomyopathy, 549-550
Cardiovascular disease, 580-581,
586-594
Cardiovascular system, pathology,
417-418
Catalase, 298-299, 500, 511

Cathepsins, 322
Celiac disease, 541, 557, 560-561
Cell culture, 343-344, 506-507
Cell structure, 373
Cellular immunity, 434-435
Central nervous system lesions,
399, 407-417
Cereal grains
effect of expanding, puffing,
rolling, shredding, 110
losses in refining, 118
Cereal grain baked products,
138-142
Cereal grain products, 135-138
Cerebrospinal fluid, analysis, 82,
87
Ceroid, 291, 398-399, 420-422,
496, 500, 502, 565, 575
(see also lipofuscin)
accumulation in nerves, 413
Chelators, 295, 339
Chemistry, 7-65
chromatography, 28-29
esterification, 24-25
hydrogenation of tocotrienols, 40
nomenclature, 14-18
oxidation, 15, 20-23, 231-237
physicochemical properties,
infra red spectra, 28
mass spectra, 28
melting point, 26
optical activity, 26-27
ultra violet spectra, 26
x-ray diffraction, 28
stereoisomers, 10-14
stereochemistry, 10-14
synthesis, 29-47
thermolysis, 16, 24
structure, 9-14
tocopherols, 10-14
tocotrienols, 10-14
Chickens,
antibody production, 431
disease protection, 435

[Chickens]
encephalomalacia, 407-413
exudative diathesis, 417
Children, blood tocopherol levels,
    525
Chloroplasts, 270-271, 391-192
Cholesterol, 382, 507, 510
    in membranes, 376, 378, 380,
    382, 386
Cholesterol hydroperoxide, 381,
    507
Cholesterol-lowering effect, 592
Choline, 284-285
Choline deficiency, 417
Chromanol ring, in membranes,
    380, 384
Chromanoxyl radical, 231
Chromatography, 28, 29
    column, 70, 73
    gas-liquid, 78-80
    high-performance liquid, 73-74
    paper, 74
    thin-layer, 75-78
Chromium-51 RBC half-life (see
    red blood cell survival)
Chylomicrons, 186, 194
Cirrhosis, 541
Clotting time, 632-633
Codeine demethylase, 323
Cod liver oil,
    effect on flavor, 449
Coenzyme Q (see ubiquinone)
Cold, common, 580
Colitis, 557, 559
Collagen, 500-501
Cooking of foods, 113-115
Conjugated dienes, 304
Congestive heart failure, 592
Copper, 446, 501-502
Corn, 107-110
Corticosterone, 353-354, 358, 382
Creatine phosphokinase, 321-324,
    547-549
Creatinuria, 546-547, 574, 641

Cross-linking of DNA and protein,
    497, 501
Cyclic AMP, 434
Cyclic AMP phosphophodiesterase,
    322
Cyclic peroxides, 487-492
Cystic fibrosis, 541-556, 575,
    578, 640-641
    neuropathology, 415
Cystic mastitis, 595
Cytochrome, 306-309, 450
Cytochrome oxidase, 323
Cytochrome c reductase, 333, 336
Cytosol, 338

Dairy products, 147-148
Deficiency,
    in animals, 521
    in humans, 520-579, 620-621,
    640
    subclinical, 523
Dehydration of food, 115-116
Delayed-type hypersensitivity, 434
Diastereomers, 14, 31
Dibutyrl cyclic AMP, 357, 363
Dietary intake, 126-127, 273
Dietary requirements,
    influence of other nutrients,
    272-284
    of animals, 273, 465
    of humans, 598-608, 620-633
Dietary surveys, 273, 602-604
Digitalis toxicity, 592, 642
Dimer, 53, 232, 236, 244-246,
    337
Disease protection, 435-439, 639
DNA, 319-320, 497, 501, 503,
    510-511
DNA-protein adducts, 497
DNA polymerase, 508
DNA repair, 501
DNase, 323
Diplock-Lucy hypothesis, 343-385

Dog,
  testicular atrophy, 399
DPPD (N, N'diphenyl-p-phenylene
  diamine), 280-281, 303, 431,
  445, 485
Drosophila melanogaster, 502, 508
Drug metabolism, 309-311
Drug metabolism system, 306-307
Drug toxicity, 642
Ducks, oxidation of meat, 463
Dystrophic axons, 415

Edema, 417, 535
Eggs and egg products, 147-148
Electron spin resonance (ESR)
  spectroscopy, 302, 305,
  505-506
Electron transport system, 342, 380,
  384-385
Elgin project, 522-523, 525,
  569-574, 622-623, 625
Embryopathy, 398-399
Emmerie-Engel reaction, 70-71
Encephalomalacia, 90, 277,
  279-280, 503, 621
  (see also Necrotizing
  encephalopathy)
  in man, 530
  pathology, 407-413
Endoperoxide, 294, 479, 487-491
Endoplasmic reticulum, 304-305,
  376, 378, 387
Endothelial cell injury, 407,
  410-414
Enteropathies, 556-566
Enzymes,
  membrane bound, 382-384, 386
Enzyme function, 321-324, 383
Epimers, 13-14, 31
Epoxide, 23, 50, 235, 505, 510
Erythrocyte (see Red blood cell)
Erythrocyte-hemolysis test,
  88-89

Erythropoiesis, 319, 418, 568,
  574, 623-624
Ethane, 282, 489
Ethoxyquin, 280-281, 290, 445,
  453, 509-510
Exercise, 597-598
Experimental deprivation, 569-574
  (see also Elgin project)
Excretion, 250-252, 257
Extraction, 68
Exudative diathesis, 276, 417

Fats, 120-122
  (see also Vegetable oils)
Fat (see also adipose tissue)
  analysis, 87
  tocopherol content, effect of
  intake, 464
Fat cells, glucose oxidation,
  352-353
Fatty acid composition of liver,
  378-379, 382
Feeds,
  analysis, 84
  effect of drying, 105-106
  effect of organic acids, 107
Fetal blood, tocopherol concentra-
  tion, 527-529
Fetal resorption, 398
Fetal-resorption test, 87-88
  (see also Resorption-gestation)
Fetus,
  tocopherol content, 202-205, 526
Fibrinolysis, 633
Fibroblasts, 503, 506-507
Fish, 146-147, 394
Fishy flavor, 449, 452, 463
Fish oils, effect on flavor, 449,
  463
Flavin sensitized reactions, 507
Flavor preservation, 445-465
Flour, 108-109, 118-119
Fluorescence, 72-73, 91

Food processing, 104
Foods, 156-157, 637
  analysis, 84
  influence of storage, 116, 117
Free radicals, 231-233, 290-307,
    480, 487-490, 495-512, 638
  in membranes, 383, 385
  damage to membrane phospho-
    lipids, 499
  endogenous sources, 296-303,
    384, 494
  formed from exogeneous sources,
    303-306
  hypothesis of aging, 497-512
  of tocopherol, 496
  in mitochondria, 381
Freezing of food, 115-116, 126
Fruit, 124-143
Fruit products, 142-143
Frying, 113-114, 116
Fumigation, 110
Function, 638

Galactosidase, 323
Gamma tocopherol (see γ Tocopheral)
Gastrectomy, 557, 559
Gene transcription, 329
Germinal epithelium, degeneration
    of, 399-401
Germination, 101
Glucose-6-phosphatase, 383
Glucose-6-phosphate dehydrogenase,
    323
Glucuronidase, 323
Glutathione, 279, 299, 521
Glutathione, in red blood cells,
    478, 535, 555
Glutathione peroxidase, 277-279,
    298-301, 323, 385, 417,
    490-491, 499, 509, 511
Glutathione reductase, 278, 299,
    322
Glycoproteins, 376, 384, 475-476

Golgi complex, 376, 378, 381
Gonadal function, 349-352
Grains, effect of milling, 107-108
Grasses, effect of maturity and
    weather, 102
Growth, 90
  of plants, 101
Guinea pigs,
  fetal death, 398
  myopathy, 402
  testicular atrophy, 399

Haber-Weiss reaction, 297
Hallervorden-Spatz disease, 415
Hamster,
  testicular atrophy, 399
Heating of foods, 113-115
Heart,
  depletion of tocopherol, 226-229
  tocopherol content
    of subcellular fractions, 377
    in cystic fibrosis, 546
Heart disease, 417-418, 586-588,
    592
  ischemic, 586-588
Heart lipopigment, 421, 503
Hematopoietic disorders, 418-419
Heinz bodies, 478, 486
Heme synthesis, 307-309, 568
Hemolysis, 88-89, 381
  peroxidative, 523, 528-530
Hemolytic anemia, 282, 500
  in premature infants, 533-540
  genetic, 641-642
Hepatic necrosis (see Liver
    necrosis)
History, 1-6, 8-9
  antioxidant function, 2-3
  fertility, 1-2
  isolation, 3
  muscular dystrophy, 2-4
  synthesis, 4
Homogentisic acid, 263-269

Hormonal function, 348-370
Horse,
  cardiomyopathy, 418
  myopathy, 406
Humoral immunity, 430-434
Hyaline membrane disease, 531-532
Hyaluronidase, 322
Hydrogen peroxide, 297-303, 498,
  504-505, 529
Hydroperoxide, 294, 299, 487-492,
  498-499
  of fatty acids, 277-278
Hydroxyacyl Co A dehydrogenase,
  322
Hydroxy fatty acids, 278
Hydroxyl radical, 297-303, 498-499
6-Hydroxy-2,5,7,8-tetramethyl-2-
  chroman-carboxylic acid
  (Trolox-C), 23-24, 298
Hyperlipidemia, 524
Hypertension, 592
Hypoxia, 431, 502

Immune response, 384, 430-442,
  639
Immunoglobulins, 431-434
Induction period, 454, 463-464
Infant foods, 125-126, 143-146
Infantile neuroaxonal dystrophy, 415
Infants,
  content of tissues, 202-205
  premature anemia, 418, 640
  (see also Premature infants)
Injectable preparations, 578, 582
Insects, 393-394
Integral proteins, 375-376, 384-385
Interceroids, 420
Intermittent claudication, 502, 583,
  588-592, 643
Interstitial cells (Leydig), 399-400
Intestinal lymphangectasia, 557,
  559, 561
Intestinal resection, 557

Intestinal transport, 183-185, 189
  passive diffusion, 189
Intestinal ultrastructure, 556
Intestinal ultrastructure in
  abetalipoproteinemia, 566
Intestine, ceroid in, 555, 565
Invertebrates, 393-394
Ionophore function, 290
Iron, 282-283, 297, 302, 308-309
  effect on hemolytic anemia, 537,
  627
  in infant formulae, 527
Irradiation, 110-111
Irreversibly sickled cells, 642
Isocitric dehydrogenase, 322
Isomers, contribution to dietary
  biological activity, 275
Isoprenoid side chain, relationship
  to biological activity, 50
Isoprenyl-containing compounds,
  248-249

α Ketoglutarate, oxidation, 335-341
Krebs cycle, 336, 340

Lactic dehydrogenase, 89, 322
Latex, 392
Lead toxicity, 309, 480, 485-486
Leaves, 84, 87
Light damage, 507
Linoleic acid
  causative agent of enceopolo-
  malacia, 407
  effect on absorption, 182, 211
  in adipose tissue, 626
  in erythrocytes, 625
Lipid peroxidation, 290-296,
  498-499, 501-502, 509-511
  in adrenal, 353-362
  in tissues, 355, 421
Lipofuscin, 282, 420-423, 502-503
  (see also Ceroid)

[Lipofuscin]
  in smooth muscle of malabsorption
    patients, 555-556, 563
Lipopigments, 420-422, 502
  (see also Ceroid, lipofuscin)
Lipoic acid, 339
Lipolysis, 352-353
Lipoproteins, 187, 194-200
Lipoproteins in serum, effect on
    tocopherol level, 625
Lipoxygenase, 322, 479
Liver,
  analysis, 82, 87
  depletion of tocopherol, 226-229
  tocopherol content
    in cystic fibrosis patients, 544,
      546
    in chicken and turkeys, 455
    of subcellular fractions,
      relation to intake, 458-461
Liver necrosis, 90, 276, 279, 303,
    335, 337, 419-420, 484-485
Liver parenchymal cells, 378, 383
Liver-storage tests, 89-90
Lucy hypothesis, 311, 343, 380, 381
  (see also Diplock Lucy theory)
Lung, tocopherol content,
  of subcellular fractions, 377
  relationship to intake, 214
Lymph, very low-density lipo-
    proteins (VLDL), 187, 194-197
Lymphocyte, 433, 434
Lysosomal enzymes, 89, 381
Lysosomal membrane, 374, 376,
    381
Lysosomes, in capilliary
    endothelium, 410-412

Macrophase, 223-224, 433
Macrophages, ceroid pigment in,
    398-399, 421
Malabsorption, 523, 540-569, 575

Malaria, 436
Malate dehydrogenase, 322
Malondialdehyde, 292, 306, 342,
    478, 496, 500, 507
Malondialdehyde, in poultry meat,
    450-453, 457-462
Malondialdehyde cross-linking,
    478
Margarine, 121-122
Maternal blood tocopherol
    concentration, 527-528
Maternal-fetal ratio of blood
    tocopherol, 527-528
Meat, 146-147
Mechanically deboned turkey (MDT)
    meat, 455, 457
Medium chain triglycerides, effect
    on absorption and tissue
    distribution, 182-185, 189,
    212
Megavitamin Therapy (see
    Pharmacologic effects)
Membrane, 222, 290, 296, 301,
    344, 372-387, 475-480,
    498-499, 504, 511, 638
  antioxidant structure, 475
  of fat globule, 448
  plasma, 372, 376, 385, 388, 419
  proposed localization of
    tocopherol, 385
Membrane fluidity, 343
Membrane fragility, 380, 383
Membrane models, 374-375
Membrane permeability, 381-382,
    386
Membrane phospholipids, 376-380
Membrane proteins, 376, 382-383
Membrane recognition, 384
Membranous subcellular fractions,
    tocopherol content, 376-377
Menaquinone, 248-249
2-Mercaptoethanol, 433
Mercury, 642

Metabolites of tocopherol, 20,
51-53, 246-248, 250-252,
255-256
unidentified in bile, 250-252
Metabolism of tocopherol, 193-257,
380
Mice
fetal death, 398
myocardial disease, 417
testicular atrophy, 399
Micelle, 183
Microbes, 392
Microcirculation,
in myopathy, 403
in central nervous system, 407
Microsomes, 221, 290, 304,
338-339, 379, 382
Milk, 123-124
seasonal effect, 104-105
oxidized flavor, 446, 448
Milling, 107
Mitochondria, 221-223, 290, 332,
498, 504, 507
Mitochondrial membranes, 378-380,
382-383, 385, 504
Mitochondrial metabolism, 332-345
Mixed function oxidase, 309-311,
384-386, 450, 505, 509
(see also Drug metabolism,
cytochrome)
Mobilization from tissues, 226-230
Molecular distillation, 69-70
Molenaar hypothesis, 384-387
Monkey,
anemia, 418
testicular atrophy, 398
Mulberry heart disease, 418
Muscle,
depletion of tocopherol, 226-229
excessive respiration, 335
oxygen consumption, 335, 406
tocopherol content
correlation with therapy, 590

[Muscle]
[tocopherol content]
in cystic fibrosis, 544, 546,
458
of chickens and turkeys, 455,
458-461
relationship to intake, 215,
458-461, 463, 582-583
Muscular dystrophy (see also
Myopathy)
activity of lysosomal enzymes,
381, 403
bioassay, 89
Duchenne (genetic), 521
effect of antioxidants, 280
effect of ubiquinone, 285
effect of selenium, 276, 278-279
effect of tocopheryl quinone, 285
Muscular strength, 549
Muscle necrosis, 402-406
Mutagenesis, 511
Mutagens, 642
Mutation, 496-497, 505
Myelin sheath, 413
Myocardial disease, 417-418, 639
Myopathy, 276, 402-406, 548
(see also Muscular dystrophy)
Myopathy,
human, 406, 576
in cystic fibrosis, 546-549
in malabsorption disease, 561-562
pathogenesis, 403-404
ultrastructural changes, 403

NAD-cytochrome c reductase,
333-334
NADH, 341
NADPH-dependent enzymes, 378,
380, 384
NADPH oxidation, 297-303
Necrotic liver degeneration
(see Liver neccosis)

Necrotizing arteritis, 417
Necrotizing encephalopathy (see
    also Encephalomalacia), 503
Necrotizing myopathy (see Myopathy)
Nematode, lifespan, 508
Neonate, 528-529
Neuraminadase, 322
Neurological symptoms, 407, 410
  in abetalipoproteinemia, 565-566
Neuroaxonal dystrophy, 415
Neuropathology in vitamin E
    deficiency, 407-417
Nerves (see Neuropathology)
Nitrates, 104
Nitroanisole-O-demethylase, 322
Nitrogen dioxide toxicity, 474,
    480-483, 498, 630
Nitrosamine, 510, 642
Nomenclature, 14-15, 18-19, 66-67
None-heme iron, 385
Nordihydroguaiaretic acid, 509
Nucleic acid metabolism, 318-320
5' Nucleotidase, 322, 383
Nutritional encephalomalacia
    (see Encephalomalacia)
Nutritional muscular dystrophy,
    402, 406
Nutritional requirements, 598-608
Nutritional status, 524-526
Nuts, 122, 148-149

Oral contraceptives, 642
Ornithine-keto acid aminotrans-
    ferase, 323
Oxaloacetic acid, 340
Oxidative phosphorylation, 341-342,
    386, 406
Oxygen consumption, of muscle,
    335, 406
Oxygen toxicity, 502, 507, 531-532,
    598, 642
Ozone toxicity, 474, 478, 480-484,
    498, 598, 630-631
Ozonides, 478, 481

Palm oil, 120
Pancreatic carcinoma, 541, 559
Pancreatic fibrosis, 277-279
Pancreatic insufficiency, 542
Pancreatic lesions, 394
Pancreatitis, 541, 559-561
Paralysis, 402, 413
Parenteral administration, 221,
    532, 558, 565, 577, 578, 582
Pasture, 447
Pathology, 398
Pentane, 489
Periodontal disease, 597, 643
Peripheral vascular disease,
    587-592
Peroxidase deficiency, 422
Peroxidative hemolysis, 528-530,
    571
  correlation with blood tocopherol,
    543, 550, 571
  during tocopherol depletion of
    normal adults, 571, 572
  in abetalipoproteinemia, 565
  in cystic fibrosis, 550-551
Peroxidation
  in tumors, 511
  in vivo, 281-284, 342-343, 386,
    475-482
  of brain lipids, 407
  of membranes, 386
Peroxide hemolysis test, 524, 571,
    624-625
Peroxides, 498, 500
  in adipose tissue in vivo, 417
  in poultry meat, 452
  lipid, in tissues, 281-283
  reduction of, 298
Phagocytosis, 436, 438-349
  of muscle fibers, 403-405
Pharmacologic effects, 579-598,
    629-633, 638
Photosensitizers, 505
Photosynthetic electron transport,
    504
Phospholipase, 322, 381

Photosynthesis, 391, 392
Phylloquinone, 248-249
Phytol, synthesis of, 44
Phytyl chain, complex with
    arachidonate, 380, 384
Pigs, 283
  anemia, 418
  fetal death, 398
  myocardial pathology, 417-418
  testicular atrophy, 399
Pituitary, 367
Placental abnormalities, 398-399
Placental barrier, 199
Placental transport, 527
Plants, 101, 391-392
  biosynthesis in, 268-271
  influence of genetics on content,
    103
Plasma lipid, relationship to
    tocopherol level, 524-526, 641
Plasma tocopherol,
  analysis, 81, 87, 197
  correlation with malabsorption,
    545
  distribution in lipids, 198-200
  in adults consuming supplementary
    vitamin E, 582-583
  influence of lipids, 199-200,
    524-526, 584
  in children, 525
  in normal adults, 525, 574
  transport in, 197-200
Platelet aggregation, 418, 491, 593,
    633, 643
Platelet count, 419, 593
Platelets, 643
  analysis, 82, 87
  tocopherol content, 593
  relationship to plasma
    concentration, 216
Polycyclic hydrocarbons, 505
Pork, rancidity and off-flavors,
    462-465
Porphyria, 598
Polyunsaturated fatty acids, 504
  effect on absorption, 181-182

[Polyunsaturated fatty acids]
  effect on fatty acids in tissues, 297
  effect on requirements, 273-276,
    606, 626
  effects on tocopherol depletion,
    510-571
  in infant formulas, 534
  ratio to vitamin E, 274-276, 606
  ratio to tocopherol in plasma and
    erythrocytes, 554
Poultry meat, 449-462
Posterior column degeneration,
    413-417
Premature infant, blood tocopherol,
    527, 577
Premature infants (see also Infants),
    523, 526-540, 575, 627
Prostacyclin, 479
Prostaglandins, 364-368, 434, 479,
    482, 484-491, 504, 594
Preceroids, 420
Propyl gallate, 509
Protein-calorie deficiency, 523,
    566-569, 575, 643
Protein metabolism, 318, 320-321
Prothrombin time, 632
Pyruvate kinase, 322

Quinol, 233-235
Quinone, 235-236, 285
0-Quinone methide, 233

Rabbits,
  myocardial disease, 413
  myopathy, 402
  testicular atrophy, 399
Radiation, 496, 498, 510
Rancidity, 450, 452, 457-462
Rat,
  anemia, 418
  fetal death, 398
  myopathy, 402
  testicular atrophy, 399
  myocardial disease, 417

Receptor proteins, 476-477
Recommended Dietary Allowances
    (RDA), 272-273, 602, 604-607
Red blood cell,
    analysis, 81, 87
    deformation and budding 507
    exchange of tocopherol with plasma,
        200-201
    filterability, 486, 496
    lifespan, 622
    membrane, 201, 380-381, 383,
        385, 530
    peroxidative hemolysis, 418,
        528-530, 550-551, 565, 578
    ratio of tocopherol to
        arachidonate, 385
    ratio of tocopherol to PUFA, 199,
        554, 565
    survival, 534-540, 576
        in cystic fibrosis, 552-554
        in pancreatitis and idiopathic
            steatorrhea, 562-563
        in tocopherol-deprived adults,
            572-573, 622-624
    stability, 550-555
    tocopherol content,
        in abetalipoproteinemia, 565
        in cystic fibrosis, 546
    tocopherol quinone in, 242
Refining of foods, 107-109, 112-113,
    118
Regional enteritis, 541, 557-559
Repair of DNA, 501
Repressor of enzyme synthesis,
    321
Reproductive system, 398-402
Requirements, 598-608, 620-633
Resorption-gestation, effect of
    antioxidants, 281
Respiratory decline, 90, 377-341
Reticulocytosis, 289, 535-538,
    574, 622-623
Reticuloendothelial system,
    223-226
Retina, tocopherol in, 531
Retinal vasculopathy, 531-533
Retinopathy of prematurity, 532
Retrolental fibroplasia, 527,
    530-533, 627, 641-642

Reverse electron transport, 341
Riboflavin, 507
RNA, 319-320
RNA polymerase, 323
RNase, 323
Rotifer, 290, 369, 393
Rubber, 120, 392
Ruminants, myocardial disease,
    417

Safety of high doses, 584-586
Seeds, 101
Selenium, 228, 276-279, 298, 311,
    337, 385-386, 500, 507-510
    effect on cancer, 441, 510
    exudative diathesis, 417
    immune response, 440-441
    in plasma of cystic fibrosis
        patients, 555
    in myopathy, 403
Selenoproteins, 279
Seminiferous tubules, 399-400
Serine dehydratase, 323
Sertoli cells, 399-400
Serum, analysis, 81, 87
Sheep,
    cardiomyopathy, 418
    myopathy, 406
Shikimic acid pathway, 268
Simon's metabolites, 243, 246-248
Singer-Nicolson model, 375, 384
Sickle cell anemia, 641-642
Singlet oxygen, 23, 50, 295
Skin, 220
    tocopherol content of chicken and
        turkey, 454
Smooth endoplasmic reticulum,
    372-373, 387
Smooth muscle, 398, 555
Snail, 393
Spermatogenesis, 349-351, 399
Spielmeyer-Vogt-Batten disease,
    422
Spleen, 436
Spleen weight, 432-433
Spinal cord pathology, 413,
    415-416, 421

Spontaneous abortion, 594-595
Sprue, 541, 557
Stability in foods, 116-117
Spectrophotometry, 71-72
Spectrofluorometry, 72-73
Steatorrhea, 541, 559-561, 564
Stereoisomers of tocopherol, 11-13
Sterility, 350
Steroidogenesis, 357-352, 382, 386
Storage, 220, 575
Stroke, 639
Structure—biological activity, 49-51
Subcellular particles, 221
Subcellular fractions, tocopherol
    content, 377
Succinate-cytochrome C reductase,
    333
Succinate oxidation, 335-341, 382-383
Succinoxidase, 336
Sulfhydryl groups, 338-341
Sulfhydryl group, in xanthine
    oxidase, 325
Sulfhydryl inhibitors, 338
Sulfur amino acids, 279-280, 419
Superoxide anion, 23, 292, 295,
    297-298, 301
Superoxide dismutase, 23, 300, 500
Surveys, 598, 608

Testicular atrophy, 399-402
Testicular disfunction, 641
Testis, 382, 387
Testicular degeneration, 90, 349-352
Testosterone, 351-352
Thallasemia intermedia, 641
Thalassemia major, 283, 502,
    595-596, 641
Therapy, 576-579
Thiobarbituric acid test (TBA),
    353, 387-491
  in poultry meat, 450-453,
    457-462
Thrombocytosis, 418, 535
Thrombocytothemia, 82
Thrombosis, 82, 419, 592, 643
  of small blood vessels, 407-408,
    413-414, 639

Thromboxane, 479, 483, 484
Thymus, 436
Thyroid, 367-368
  lipofuscin in, 556
Tissue depletion of tocopherol,
    556, 570-571
Tissue uptake, relationship to oral
    dose, 214
Tissues,
  tocopherol content,
    effect of age, 201-203
    in chickens and turkeys, 450,
      452-456, 458-462
  tocopherol distribution, 201-230
Tocol structure, 10-14, 100
α-Tocopheramine, 49
  absorption, 173, 179
α-Tocopherol, structure, 2
β-Tocopherol, structure, 11
γ-Tocopherol,
  biological activity, 525
  content of tissues, 629
  control of diet, 604, 627
  in plasma, 524, 525
  structure, 11
  tissue turnover, 229, 256
δ-Tocopherol, structure, 11
Tocopherol isomers in plasma, 524
α-Tocopheronic acid, 51, 243, 247,
    254-255
α-Tocopheronolactone, 247-248,
    254-255
  anti-inflammatory activity, 28
α-Tocopheroxide, 19
α-Tocopherlylacetate, absorption,
    173, 175-179
α-Tocopheryl acetate, 253
  analysis, 85
  use in fortification, 130-131
  stability, 113-115, 130
  water miscible, 530, 534, 536,
    541, 577-578, 581
α-Tocopheryl cinnamate, 253
α-Tocopheryl esters
  hydrolysis of, 184-186, 189,
    252-253
  absorption of, 189, 253

α-Tocopheryl hydroquinone,
    243-244, 391, 631
  biological activity, 285, 631
α-Tocopheryl nicotinate
  absorption, 173, 179
  excretion, 250-252
  tissue distribution, 209-211, 218,
    223-226, 253
α-Tocopheryl p-aminobenzoate,
    253
α-Tocopherylquinone, 15-17,
    233-235, 295, 630-632
  anti-vitamin K activity, 631
  biological activity, 49, 241, 285
  conversions of, 25
  effect on nematode lifespan, 508
  in photosynthetic electron
    transport, 391
  occurrence in plants, 237, 241,
    392
  occurrence in animal tissue, 52,
    237-244, 254-256, 632
α-Tocopheryl semiquinone radical,
    294-296
α-Tocopheryl succinate, 578
  absorption of, 179
Tocotrienols, 10-11, 13, 18-19,
    100, 628
  biosynthesis, 268-271
α-Tocotrienol, structure, 11
β-Tocotrienol, structure, 11
γ-Tocotrienol, structure, 11
δ-Tocotrienol, structure, 11
Tortillas, 117
Transport, 193-257, 638
  from lymph to blood, 194-197
  in plasma, 198-200
Transport protein, 638
Trolox C (see 6-hydroxy-2,5,7,8-
    tetramethyl-2-chroman-
    carboxylic acid)
Tropical sprue, 541
Tryptophan, 280
Trienol structure, 10-14, 100
Tumor, 510-511
Turkey meat, 449-462
Turkeys, disease protection, 435

Ubiquinone, 285, 391, 436, 439
Ulcers, 597
Uncoupled oxidative phosphoryes-
    tion, 335
Urine, 247, 250
Uterus, ceroid pigment in, 38

Vascular fragility, 530
Vascular integrity, 489-491
Vascular pathology, 417-419, 633,
    639
  of fetus, 399
  of brain, 407-413
  in retina, 530-533
Vascular permeability, 410,
    417
Vegetables, 124-125, 153-155
Vegetable oils, 84, 112, 120-122,
    149-153, 156
  effect of processing,
    112-113
Vitamin A, 280, 283-284, 402,
    439-440
Vitamin A toxicity, 284
Vitamin C
  (see ascorbic acid)
Vitamin K, 593, 631
Vitamin K inhibitors, 632

Warafarin, 632
Water-miscible tocopherol, 530,
    534, 536, 541, 565
Wheat, 107-111, 118
  germ, 118
  germ oil, 120-121
Whipple's disease, 557
White muscle disease, 276
Wound healing, 597

Xanthine dehydrogenase, 323-324
Xanthine oxidase, 323-329
Xanthine-xanthine oxidase system,
    297